Life Choices

Hastings Center Studies in Ethics

A SERIES EDITED BY

Mark J. Hanson and Daniel Callahan

This series of books, published by The Hastings Center and Georgetown University Press, examines ethical issues in medicine and the life sciences. Established in 1969, The Hastings Center, located in Garrison, New York, is an independent, nonprofit, and nonpartisan research organization. The work of the Center is mainly carried out through research projects, the publication of the *Hastings Center Report* and *IRB: A Review of Human Subjects Research,* and numerous workshops, conferences, lectures, and consultations. **The Hastings Center Studies in Ethics** series brings the ongoing research of The Hastings Center to a wider audience.

Life Choices:

A Hastings Center
Introduction to Bioethics
Second Edition

EDITED BY
Joseph H. Howell and William F. Sale

FOREWORD BY
Daniel Callahan

GEORGETOWN UNIVERSITY PRESS / WASHINGTON, D.C.

2 64262

JAN 3 0 2002

Georgetown University Press, Washington, D.C. 20007
© 2000 by Georgetown University Press. All rights reserved.
Printed in the United States of America
10 9 8 7 6 5 4 3 2 1   2000
THIS VOLUME IS PRINTED ON ACID-FREE ∞ OFFSET BOOK PAPER

Library of Congress Cataloging-in-Publication Data
Life choices : a Hastings Center introduction to bioethics / edited by
  Joseph H. Howell and William F. Sale ; foreword by Daniel Callahan.
  —2nd ed.
      p.   cm. — (Hastings Center studies in ethics)
    Includes bibliographical references.
    ISBN 0-87840-757-X (pbk.)
    1. Medical ethics.   I. Howell, Joseph H.   II. Sale, William F.
  (William Frederick)   III. Series.
  R724.L496.2000
  174'.2—dc21   99-29971
                                                        CIP

Contents

Preface to the Second Edition

This book represents what we believe are some of the very best articles published in the *Hastings Center Report* over the past twenty-eight years. While most of the articles were published in the last fifteen years, a number of "classic" articles were included. We selected articles that addressed the major bioethical issues of our time. In the foreword to the first edition, Daniel Callahan stated the two-fold purpose of this collection: to provide a challenging text for classrooms and study groups and to serve as a testimony to the achievements of the Hastings Center in the study of bioethics.

The changes in the second edition include a new section on The Goals and Allocation of Medicine. Articles from an international study of the goals of medicine introduce this section by focusing on the purposes of medicine and its limitations. A new section on the cloning of human beings provides a positive and negative response to the National Bioethics Advisory Commission's report. Additional articles on ethical theory, the duty to die, and genetics are included.

In addition to the acknowledgments from the first edition, we would again like to thank Mark Hanson and Bette Crigger for their advice and considerable help on the second edition. We would also like to thank Deborah Weiner, editorial and production manager of Georgetown University Press.

Joseph H. Howell
William Frederick Sale

DANIEL CALLAHAN

Foreword to the First Edition

I write this during the twenty-fifth-anniversary year of The Hastings Center. When the work of the Center began in 1969, there was then no idea that it could be valuable and useful to have a publication. On the contrary, we all had a sense that there were too many magazines and journals about and that another would be one too many.

We soon changed our minds about that. The field of bioethics was developing even more rapidly than we had guessed, and it soon became clear that there was a place for a journal devoted to the topic. Unlike the present situation, the medical journals at that time rarely published anything to do with ethics, and the ethics journals rarely published anything to do with medicine or biology. That meant there were few outlets for those who wanted to write about bioethics, and few outlets as well for the emerging work of The Hastings Center. Those rare people then teaching courses in the field had no texts, relying instead on their personal collection of articles drawn from scattered sources.

The *Hastings Center Report* was born in 1971. At first it was little more than a large newsletter, with short articles and bits of news. We soon came to feel the need for a more scholarly journal and created the *Hastings Center Studies* to complement the *Report*. That proved to be a cumbersome solution, and the publication of two journals was just a little too much for our small staff. We then decided to combine the *Report* and *Studies* into a much-expanded, new version of the *Report*. The idea was to combine news and short features about the field with more scholarly articles, much as the magazine *Science* has so successfully done over the years. That was a happy solution for us, and the *Hastings Center Report* as it now appears was born.

No doubt a historian will someday study the contents of the *Report* to trace the trends and developments in bioethics. Over the years it has tracked the innumerable debates, arguments, and intellectual developments that have marked a lively, never-still field. It is a pleasure to see how many of the articles from its pages have stood the test of time, as useful and timely as ever to both scholars and lay people, to veterans in the field and to students just coming to it.

We have been proud to publish the *Hastings Center Report*. Its editors over the years have been a smart and critical group: Bruce Hilton, Margaret and Peter Steinfels, Courtney Campbell, Carol Levine, and Bette Crigger. They have been joined by an able group of associate editors—Mark Hanson, Hilde Nelson, Joyce Bermel, and Nancy deKoven, among others—and helped as well by staff members of the Center. This collection of articles bears the imprint of their hard work. We believe it will be of great use in classrooms and study groups. We also believe it will stand as a nice testimony indeed to the first quarter century of the life of The Hastings Center.

DANIEL CALLAHAN

President

Acknowledgments

We would like to acknowledge the contributions of several groups and individuals who made this collection possible. First, we thank The Hastings Center for providing the articles gathered here from the pages of the *Hastings Center Report*. Special thanks to Daniel Callahan, President; Mark Hanson, Associate for Religious Ethics; Bette Crigger, Editor of the *Hastings Center Report*; and other readers at The Hastings Center for their advice and critical comments. Second, we thank the Florida Humanities Council, and especially Joan Bragginton, Project Director, for their assistance in the initial research that eventually led to the current collection. Third, the following libraries were most helpful in preparing this collection of readings: the Law Library and Strozier Library at Florida State University and the Gulf Coast Community College Library. Fourth, we thank our colleagues at Gulf Coast Community College who provided advice and assistance in the editing process. Finally, we thank our beloved secretary, Marie Z. Fuller (1942–1994); it is in her memory that we dedicate this collection of articles.

JOSEPH H. HOWELL
Professor of History and Humanities

WILLIAM FREDERICK SALE
Associate Professor of Philosophy
and Chair of the Social Sciences
Gulf Coast Community College

PART I: Introduction: Can Ethics Provide Answers?

JAMES RACHELS
Can Ethics Provide Answers?

SIDNEY CALLAHAN
The Role of Emotion in Ethical Decisionmaking

CARL ELLIOTT
Where Ethics Comes From and What to Do About It

"Bioethics" refers to the application of moral reasoning to issues raised by medical treatments, technologies, and the life sciences. Bioethical decisions are quite simply "life choices"—choices regarding the meaning of life, its beginning, the quality of its continuation, and its end. Bioethical issues include the allocation of health care resources, life-prolonging treatments, organ transplantation, euthanasia, physician-assisted suicide, abortion, new reproductive technologies, and recent advances in genetic diagnosis and therapy. Such issues often prove controversial and divisive. Occasionally, bioethical questions leave us puzzled and confused: new medical treatments and technologies often do not come with sufficient precedents to guide our moral reasoning.

The challenges of bioethics to private moral choice and public policy formulation raise numerous difficult questions. What resources offer the best guiding principles for forming personal values? How are these values, once formed, best applied to specific bioethical concerns? What happens when a circumstance is so difficult or complex that strongly held values are brought into sudden and sharp conflict? How do personal values shape public policy? Is a consensus of values possible in these challenging areas? And if it is, what methods can be implemented to raise the consciousness of individuals and groups to forge such a consensus?

Many will turn to a religious or ethical tradition to provide a framework of values for approaching these difficult choices. Some will appeal to deeply-held religious values which spring from a commitment to a higher being or a higher set of laws. These values act as an umbrella—a "sacred canopy" in the words of sociologist Peter L. Berger—over all other values in the lives of the religiously committed. Creedal statements and sacred scriptures affirm these values over time and give structure to enduring religious institutions. Others will appeal to historic ethical traditions which emphasize one of the following: character (virtues or traits that constitute the highest good in human life), moral law (principles, generally based upon reason, that provide justification for moral choice), maximizing happiness (moral judgments based upon creating the greatest good for the greatest number of persons), or social justice (the fair distribution of the benefits and burdens of society). The various religious and ethical traditions are not mutually exclusive of one another but may provide a rich deposit of resources from which the individual may choose.

But there are many for whom these traditional moral "voices" offer little, or at best incomplete, direction. For some, "emotions energize the ethical quest," providing motivation for clear ethical thinking and action. Others turn to social custom for moral direction—that is, to values which have so long endured in the life of a community that they appear self-evident and in no need of rational justification. For others, scientific discovery and technological innovation have created a new "voice of authority": the voice of scientific expertise which may define and restrict the ways non-experts approach ethical choices.

Three articles will introduce the larger collection of readings. These articles focus on the "hard choices" of ethical questions, the limits of rationalistic answers and ethical theory, and the need for a multifaceted approach to bioethical decisionmaking. The introductory articles are:

- James Rachels' **Can Ethics Provide Answers?** responds to the challenges of cultural relativism (moral values determined by custom) and emotivism (moral values based on expressions of strong feelings). While admitting the limits of rationality, Rachels nevertheless argues for the worth of rational methods in moral inquiry.
- Sidney Callahan's **The Role of Emotion in Ethical Decisionmaking** attempts to balance the rationalist critique of emotion's role in decisionmaking by portraying reason and emotion as "mutually corrective."
- Carl Elliott's **Where Ethics Comes From and What to Do About It** argues that ordinary people rarely consider ethical theory when making decisions about particular problems. These decisions are based upon cultural influences that are often beyond the individual's control. Elliott acknowledges that ethical theories may influence moral decisions but do so indirectly.

James Rachels

Can Ethics Provide Answers?

No great powers of observation are needed to see that American people are not as optimistic or confident as they once were. Even as the Vietnam war and the Watergate scandals recede into memory, other concerns take their place. The energy crisis and a growing rate of inflation are the visible signs of an uncertain economy—an economy which, in addition to creating a general sense of insecurity, makes it harder than ever to satisfy demands for social justice. Technology, which was supposed to save us, now presents as many problems as solutions—witness the controversy over nuclear energy, for example. Pessimism seems not only understandable, but rational.

Ethics and Ethical Theory

In this bleak situation the study of ethics flourishes. Perhaps moral guidance is most needed when times are hardest, because then temptation is greatest. But there is a curious pessimism even about ethics itself. Recently I saw a proposal, written by a distinguished professor of business, to add a course in ethics to his department's curriculum. It was an enthusiastic statement, detailing the benefits of such an offering. But it concluded with the remark that "Since there are no definite answers in ethics, the course should be offered on a pass-fail basis." I don't know why he thought that, lacking definite answers, it would be any easier to distinguish passing from failing work than "B" work form "C" work, but what struck me most was the casual, offhand manner in which the remark was made—as though it were *obvious* that, no matter how important ethical questions might be, no "definite answers" are possible.

Philosophers have given a great deal of attention to this issue, but the result, unfortunately, has been a great deal of disagreement. There are generally two schools of thought. On one side there are those who believe that ethics is a subject, like history or physics or mathematics, with its own distinctive problems and it own methods of solving them. The fundamental questions of ethics are questions of conduct—what, in particular cases, should we do?—

and the study of ethics provides the answers. On the other side are those who, like the professor of business, deny that ethics is a proper subject at all. There are ethical questions, to be sure, and they are important; but since those questions do not have definite answers, there cannot be a subject whose business it is to discover them.

In this essay I shall discuss whether in fact ethics can provide answers. As a preliminary to that discussion, however, I need to say something about the relation between ethics and ethical theory. Ethics is the subject that attempts to provide directions for conduct: should a manufacturer advertise a product as being better than it is? Should a lawyer suppress evidence that tends to show that his client is guilty? Should a physician help a dying patients who, because of constant misery, wishes to end his life sooner? And so on, endlessly.

Ethical theory, on the other hand, concerns itself with questions *about* ethics. These questions divide naturally into two categories. First, ethical theorists want to know about the relations between the various principles that are used in justifying particular moral judgments. Can they be fitted together into a unified theory? Can these diverse principles be reduced to one ultimate principle, which underlies and explains all the rest? Much of modern moral philosophy has consisted in the elaboration of such theories: egoism, Kantianism, and utilitarianism, each purporting to have discovered *the* ultimate principle of ethics, are the most familiar. Second, there are questions about the status of ethics. Are there any objective truths in ethics, which our moral judgments may correctly or incorrectly represent? Or, are our moral judgments nothing more than the expression of personal feelings, or perhaps the codes of the societies in which we live? Often it is helpful to analyze the meaning of moral concepts—to examine what is meant by such words as "good," "right," and "ought."[1]

Twenty years ago the prevailing orthodoxy among English-speaking philosophers was that ethical theory, but not ethics itself, is the proper concern of philosophy. Philosophers, it was said, are theoreticians, not ministers or guidance counselors. The more radical philosophers even excluded what I have called the first part of ethical theory from their purview; they restricted their attention entirely to the analysis of moral language. The result was a body of literature that seemed, to those outside academic circles, curiously empty and sterile.

Today this attitude has been almost completely abandoned; the best writing by moral philosophers combines ethical theory with a concern for concrete ethical issues. Part of the reason for this change is that the traumas of the past two decades—especially the protest movements against racism, sexism, and the Vietnam war—forced philosophers to rethink their role in society. But there is a deeper reason, internal to philosophy itself. The rejection of ethics was the result of a preoccupation among philosophers during the first half of this century with understanding the different kinds of inquiry. Science, mathematics, religion, and ethics are very different from one another; and as philosophers tried to sort out the differences, the idea took hold that philosophy's distinctive contribution is to analyze and clarify the concepts used in each area. It was an appealing idea, with ample historical precedent. After all, the patron saint of philosophy, Socrates, had conceived of his work mainly as an investigation of definitions; and Aristotle and Kant had appealed, at key points in their work to linguistic considerations for support. Philosophers, then, were not to study ethics but only the language of ethics. That philosophers are not ethicists seemed as natural a conclusion that philosophers are no scientists or mathematicians.

By the mid-1960s, however, it was becoming clear that the recognition of differences between kinds of inquiry does not require that they be pursued in isolation from one another. Indeed, separation may not be desirable or even possible—one cannot do physics without mathematics. Today philosophers generally do not recognize sharp boundaries between their own work and work in other areas. Thus W.V. Quine, whom many consider the most eminent living American philosopher, regards his work as continuous with that of theoretical science. While Quine's writing can be read with only a layman's knowledge of science, much contemporary philosophy of science cannot. The reuniting of ethical theory with ethics, then, is merely a part of a larger movement within philosophy, bringing back into proper relation the disparate inquiries.

The Case Against Ethics

The professor of business whose statement I quoted is not unusual; a great many people, including many philosophers, believe that there are no "answers" in ethics. It is a remarkable situation: people make judgments every day about what should or should not be done; they feel strongly about those views, and sometimes they become angry and indignant with those who disagree. Yet, when they reflect on what they are doing, they profess that their judgments are no more "true" than the contrary ones they reject so vehemently. The explanation of this puzzling situation goes deep into our history, and into our understanding of the world and our place in it.

Throughout most of western history there was thought to be close connection between ethics and religion. In Plato's *Euthyphro* Socrates offered powerful arguments for separating the two, but this point of view did not prevail. (Socrates, it will be remembered, was tried and convicted of impiety.) Right and wrong continued to be defined by reference to God's will, and human life came to be regarded as meaningful only because of its place in God's plan. The church, therefore, was the guardian of the moral community and its main authority.

By the eighteenth century these ideas had begun to lose their grip on people's minds, largely because of changes that had taken place in the conception of the physical world. The physical sciences had successfully challenged the ancient belief that the earth is the center of the cosmos; instead, it was recognized to be a relatively insignificant speck. The next step would be the realization that, from a cosmic point of view, human beings are themselves insignificant. In his famous essay on suicide, published posthumously in 1783, Hume took that step, declaring that "The life of a man is of no greater importance to the universe than that of an oyster."[2] The aim of this essay was to defend the permissibility of suicide; in doing that, Hume was particularly eager to separate religious from moral notions, and to dispel the idea that human life is a gift from God that can rightly be taken only by God. This belief he considered to be a compound of "superstition and false religion," and he held that the purpose of our thinking should be to replace superstition and false religion with reason and understanding. The truth, in his view, is that *we* care about human life, because we are human, and that is all there is to it. Our lives have no more, and no less, importance than that. If he had lived to see it, Hume would no doubt have felt vindicated by the second great modern change in our conception of the world and our place in it that came from the biological sciences. The thought that we are the products of an evolutionary history much like that of all the other animals has further eroded confidence about any special place for humanity in the scheme of things.

In our own time, however, it has been the social sciences that have presented the greatest challenge to traditional ideas about human beings. In particular, the understanding of human nature derived from contemporary sociology and psychology has seemed to many people incompatible with a belief in the objectivity of ethics—that is, with a belief in objective standards of right and wrong.

The sociologists have impressed upon us that moral standards differ from culture to culture; what the "natural light of reason" reveals to one people may be radically different from what seems obvious to another. This, of course, has been known for a long time. Herodotus made the point very clearly in the fifth century B.C.:

> Darius, after he had got the Kingdom, called into his presence certain Greeks who were at hand, and asked—"What he should pay them to eat the bodies of their fathers when they died?" To which they answered, that there was no sum that would tempt them to do such a thing. He then sent for certain Indians, of the race called Callatians, men who eat their fathers, and asked them, while the Greeks stood by, and knew by the help of an interpreter all that was said—"What he should give them to burn the bodies of their fathers at their decease?" The Indians exclaimed aloud, and bade him forbear such language. Such is men's wont herein; and Pindar was right, in my judgment, when he said, "Custom is the king o'er all."[3]

Today any educated person could list countless other examples: the Eskimos allow first-born daughters to die of exposure; the Moslems practice polygamy; the Jains will not eat meat. With communications media providing constant contact with other parts of the world, it may now seem simply naive to think that our moral views are anything more than one particular cultural product.

Psychological studies tend to undermine confidence in the objectivity of ethics in a different way, by making us aware of the nonrational ways in which moral beliefs are formed in the individual. The general picture remains remarkably constant even when we consider radically different psychological theories. Freud and Skinner, for example, tell much the same story. The key idea in Freud's account is that of the "pleasure principle." The child learns from an early age that certain types of behavior will be followed by pleasure, often in the form of parental approval, and that other actions produce unpleasant consequences. Thus he learns to behave in some ways and to avoid others, and when his vocabulary has become sufficiently rich he calls the former acts "right" and the latter "wrong." Skinnerian psychology could hardly be more different from Freudian thought; nevertheless their fundamental ideas concerning moral development are almost identical. Where Freud speaks of pleasure, Skinner speaks of "positive reinforcement": the individual is positively reinforced (rewarded) when he performs certain acts, and so tends to repeat that behavior; he is negatively reinforced (punished) for other acts, which he subsequently tends not to repeat. The concepts of good and evil become attached to the two kinds of behavior. Skinner goes so far as to suggest that "good" may be *defined* as "positively reinforcing." On both theories, a person who had been raised differently would have different values. The suggested conclusion is that the belief that one's values are anything more than the result of this conditioning is simply naive.

Thus, in many people's minds, sociology and psychology swallow up ethics. They do not simply explain ethics; they explain it *away*. Ethics can no longer exist as a subject having as its aim the discovery of what is right and what is wrong; for this supposes, naively, that there *is* a right and wrong independent of what people already happen to believe. And that is precisely what has been brought into doubt. Ethics as a subject must disappear, to replaced, perhaps, by something like "values clarification." We can try to become clearer about what our values are, and about the possible alternatives. But we can no longer ask questions about the truth of our convictions.

With such impressive intellectual forces behind it, it is not surprising that this way of thinking about ethics has been tremendously influential. However, most contemporary philosophers have, with good reason, taken a dim view of these arguments. In the first place, the fact that different societies have different moral codes proves nothing. There is also disagreement from society to society about scientific matters: in some cultures it is believed that the earth is flat, and that disease is caused by evil spirits. We do not on that account conclude that there is no truth in geography or in medicine. Instead, we conclude that in some cultures people are better informed than in others. Similarly, disagreement in ethics might signal nothing more than that some people are less enlightened than others. At the very least, the fact of disagreement does not, by itself, *entail* that truth does not exist. Why should we assume that, if ethical truth exists, everyone must know it?

Moreover, it may be that some values are merely relative to culture, while others are not. Herodotus was probably right in thinking that the treatment of the dead—whether to eat or to burn them—is not a matter governed by objectively true standards. It may be simply a matter of convention that respect is shown in one way rather than another. If so, the Callatians and the Greeks were equally naive to be horrified at each other's customs. Alternative sexual customs—another favorite example of relativists—might also by equally acceptable. But this does not mean that there are *no* practices that are objectively wrong: torture, slavery, and lying, for example, could still be wrong, independently of cultural standards, even if those other types of behavior are not. It is a mistake to think that because some standards are relative to culture, all must be.

The psychological facts are equally irrelevant to the status of ethics as an autonomous subject. Psychology may tell us that beliefs are acquired in a certain way—perhaps as the result of positive and negative reinforcements—

but nothing follows from this about the nature of those beliefs. After all, *every* belief is acquired through the operation of some psychological mechanism or other, including the simplest factual beliefs. A child may learn to respond "George Washington" when asked the name of the first president, because she fears the disapproval of the teacher should she say anything else. And, we might add, if she were reinforced differently she might grow up believing that some one else first held that office. Yet it remains a matter of objective fact that Washington was the first president. The same goes for one's moral beliefs: the manner of their acquisition is logically independent of their status as objectively true or false.

Thus the outcome of the psychological account of ethics is reminiscent of the fate of nineteenth-century attempts to reduce mathematics to psychology. In the late 1800s there was considerable interest in explaining mathematics by reference to psychological theories of human thought—but that interest waned when it was realized that little light was being shed on mathematics itself. Regardless of how it might be related to our thought processes, mathematics remained a subject with its own integrity—its own internal rules, procedures, problems, and solutions—in short, its own standards of truth and falsity. The reason ethics resists explanation by sociology or psychology, or, for the matter, the most recent pretender, sociobiology, is that, like mathematics, it is also a subject with its own integrity.

While contemporary philosophers have not been impressed by the social scientific arguments concerning ethics, they have nevertheless found certain other arguments against ethics to be plausible. Those arguments go back to Hume, who maintained that belief in the very possibility of an objectively correct ethical system is part of the old "superstition and false religion." Stripped of false theology, Hume said, we should come to see our morality as nothing more than the expression of our feelings.

But Hume did not merely assert this; he attempted to prove it by giving arguments. His most influential argument was based on the idea that there is a necessary connection between moral belief and conduct. The test of whether we sincerely believe that we ought to do something is whether in fact we are motivated to do it; if I say that I believe I ought to do such-and-such, but have not the slightest inclination to do it, my statement is not to be believed. Thus having a moral belief is at least in part a matter of being motivated to act, or, as Hume put it, of having a sentiment. On the other hand, a person's capacity to discern truth and falsehood—in Hume's terms, his reason—has no necessary connection with his conduct at all: "Morals move men to act; reason alone is utterly impotent in this particular." The point is that, if moral belief is conceived as the perception of truth or falsity, its connection with conduct remains mysterious; whereas if it is regarded as an expression of sentiment, this connection is made clear.

In our own time Hume's thoughts have been adapted to support a theory according to which moral judgments are not really judgments at all, but disguised imperatives. According to this theory, known as emotivism, when one makes a moral judgment such as,

It is wrong to make someone the subject of an experiment without his permission,

One is actually saying no more than,

Don't make someone the subject of an experiment without his permission.

Alternately, as it was sometimes said, one is doing nothing more in making these judgments than expressing one's attitude, and urging others to adopt that attitude. Even though they may be sincere or insincere, imperatives and expressions of attitude are neither true nor false—and so, moral judgments are neither true nor false.[4]

If *this* is what moral judgments are, then once again ethics has lost its status as a subject. There are no truths for it to investigate. It cannot even be a branch of psychology, for although psychology is concerned with attitudes, it is only concerned with nonmoral truths *about* attitudes, which, unlike expressions *of* attitude, are true or false.

Among English-speaking philosophers, emotivism has been the most influential theory of ethics in the twentieth century. Earlier I remarked on some of the reasons that led philosophers to reject normative ethics as part of their subject. Clearly, the influence of emotivism was another important element in this rejection, and little was written by philosophers on concrete moral issues until fairly recently—the mid-1960s—when emotivist ideas had begun to lose their influence. Until then, the literature on moral issues was mainly the work of the theologians, who, standing firmly against the trends of thought I have been describing, never lost confidence in the integrity of ethics as a subject.

There is now an extensive philosophical literature cataloguing the deficiencies of emotivism. One of the main problems with the theory was its failure to account for the place of reason in ethics. It is a point of logic that moral judgments, if they are to be acceptable, must be founded on good reasons: if I tell you that such-and-such action is wrong, you are entitled to ask *why* it is wrong; and if I have no adequate reply, you may reject the advice as unwarranted. The emotivists were able to give only the most anemic account of the relation between moral judgments and the reasons that support them. Moral reasoning, on this theory, turned out to be indistinguishable from propaganda. If moral judgments are merely expressions of attitude, then reasons are merely considerations that influence attitudes. It was a natural outcome of the theory that *any* fact that influences attitudes counts as a reason for the attitude produced; thus, if the thought that Jones is black causes you to think badly of him, then "Jones is black" becomes a reason in support of your judgment that he is a bad man.

Obviously, something had gone wrong. Not just any fact can count as a reason in support of just any judgment. For one thing, the fact must be relevant to the judgment, and psychological influence does not necessarily bring relevance with it. But this is only the tip of an iceberg. Arguments in support of moral judgments can be criticized, and found adequate or inadequate, on any number of other grounds. Once this is realized, however, we have taken a big step away from emotivism, and all the other trends of thought I have been describing, toward the recognition of ethics as an autonomous subject.

Ethics and Rationality

Ultimately the case against ethics can be answered only by demonstrating how moral problems are amenable to solution by rational methods. In any particular case the right course of action is the one that is backed by the best reasons. Consider, for example, euthanasia. We may determine whether mercy-killing is right or wrong by formulating and assessing the arguments that can be given for and against it.[5] This is at bottom what is wrong with psychological and cultural relativism: if we can produce good reasons for thinking that this practice is wrong, and show that the arguments in its support are unsound, then we have proven it wrong regardless of what belief one has been conditioned to have, or what one's cultural code might say. And emotivism runs afoul of the same fact: if a stronger case can be made for euthanasia than against it, then mercy-killing *is* permissible, no matter what one's attitude might be.

The first and most obvious way that a moral argument can go wrong is by misrepresenting the facts. A rational case for or against a course of conduct must rest on some understanding of the facts of the case—minimally, facts about the nature of the action, the circumstances in which it would be done, and its likely consequences. Even the most skeptical thinkers agree that reason has this role to play in moral judgment: reason establishes the facts. Unfortunately, however, attaining a rational view of the facts is not always a simple matter. In the first place, we often need to know what the consequences of a course of action will be, and this may be impossible to determine with any precision or certainty. Opponents of euthanasia sometimes claim that, if mercy-killing were legalized, it would lead to a diminished respect for life throughout the society, and we would end up caring less about the elderly, the mentally retarded, and so forth. Defenders of euthanasia, on the other hand, heatedly deny this. What separates the two camps is a disagreement about "the facts," but we cannot settle the issue in the same easy way we could settle an argument about what would happen if Coca-Cola were boiled. We seem to be stuck with different estimates of what would happen if euthanasia were legalized, which may be more or less reasonable, but which we cannot definitively adjudicate.

Moreover, it is often difficult to determine the facts because the facts are distressingly complex. Take, for example, the question of whether the government of South Vietnam, which the United States supported during the late war was democratic. This question figured prominently in some of the debates of the time. I take it to be primarily a matter of fact, but it was not a *simple* matter of fact. In order to decide the matter, one had to fit together into a pattern all sorts of other facts about the operation of that government and its relation to its citizens. That the government was, or was not, democratic was a kind of conclusion resting on those other facts; it was a matter of what the simpler facts added up to.

Suppose, though, that we have a clear view of the relevant facts, so that our arguments cannot be faulted on that ground. Is there any other test of rationality that the arguments must pass? Hume's official view was that, at this point, reason has done all it can do, and the rest is up to our "sentiments." Reason sets out the facts; then sentiment takes over and the choice is made. This is a tempting idea, but it only illustrates a common trap that people fall into. Philosophical theses may seduce with their beautiful simplicity; an idea may be accepted because of its appeal at a high level of generality, even though it does not conform to what we know to be the case at a lower level. In fact, when Hume was considering concrete ethical issues, and not busy overemphasizing the role of sentiment, he knew very well that appeals to reason are often decisive in other ways. In the essay on suicide to which I have already referred, he produced a number of powerful arguments in support of his view that a person has the right to take his own life, for example, when he is suffering without hope from a painful illness. Hume specifically opposed the traditional religious view that, since life is a gift from God, only God has the right to decide when it shall end. About this he made the simple but devastating observation that we "play God" as much when we save life as when we take it. Each time a doctor treats an illness, and thereby prolongs a life, he has decreed that the patient's life shall not end *now*. Thus if we take seriously that only God may determine the length of a life, we would have to renounce not only killing but saving life as well.

This point has force because of the general requirement that our arguments be consistent, and consistency, of course, is the prime requirement of rationality. Hume did *not* argue that the religious opponent of suicide has got his facts wrong—he did not insist that there is no God, or that God's will had been misunderstood. If Hume's objection were no more than that, then no religious person need be bothered by it. Hume's objection was much stronger; for he was pointing out that we may appeal to a general principle (such as "Only God has the right to decide when a life shall end") only if we are willing to accept *all* its consequences. If we accept some of them (the prohibition of suicide and euthanasia), but not others (the abandonment of medicine), then we are inconsistent. This point, which has fundamental importance, will be missed if we are blinded by overly simple doctrines like "Reason establishes the facts; sentiment makes the choice."

There are other ways in which an ethical view may fail to pass the test of consistency. A person may base his ethical position on his "intuitions"— his prereflective hunches about what is right or wrong in particular cases— and, on examination, these may turn out to be incompatible with one another. Consider the difference between killing someone and "merely" allowing someone to die. Many people feel intuitively that there is a big moral difference between these two. The thought of actively killing someone has a kind of visceral repulsiveness about it that is missing from the more passive (but still unpleasant) act of standing by and doing nothing while someone dies. Thus it may be held that, although euthanasia is wrong, since it involves direct killing, nevertheless it is sometimes permissible to allow death by refraining from life-prolonging treatment.

To be sure, if we do nothing more than consult our "intuitions," there seems to be an important difference here. However, it is easy to describe other cases of killing and letting die in which there does *not* not seem to be such a difference. Suppose a patient is brought into an emergency room and turned over to a doctor who recognizes him as a man against who he has a grudge. A quick diagnosis reveals that the patient is about to die, but can be saved by a simple procedure—say, an appendectomy. The doctor, seeing his chance, deliberately stalls until it is too late to perform the life-saving procedure, and the patient dies. Most of us would think, intuitively, that the doctor is not better than a murderer, and the fact that he did not directly kill that patient, but merely let him die, makes no difference.

In the euthanasia case, the difference between killing and letting die seems important. In the grudge case, the difference seems unimportant. Is the difference important, or isn't it? Such cases show that unexamined intuitions cannot be relied upon. Our intuitions may be nothing more than the product of prejudice, selfishness, or cultural conditioning; we have no guarantee that they are perceptions of the truth. And when they are not compatible with one another, we can be sure that one or the other of them is mistaken. In the case of killing and letting die, we need to ask *why* the distinction does, or does not, make a moral difference. It certainly does not matter, from the patient's point of view, whether he is killed or allowed to die: either way, he ends up dead. (In the euthanasia case, it may matter to the patient that he die sooner rather than later, because he is suffering—therefore, it may be preferable that he be killed, because it is quicker. But what governs choice here is an argument about suffering, not the importance of killing vs. letting die *as such*.) Perhaps the reason why there *seems* to be a difference is that killings are so often accompanied by bad motives, while acts of letting die are usually done from acceptable motives. Thus it is the difference between the motives, and not the difference between the acts themselves, that is morally significant.

Recently there has been a lot of discussion of this distinction in the philosophical literature, and at first it was largely a matter of the different writers citing their intuitions, with each one producing cases in which the favored intuition "seemed" correct. Now, however, the debate has reached a more profitable stage in which the emphasis is on investigating whatever reasons can be produced to support one view over the other.[6]

Let me mention one other way in which the requirement of consistency can force a change in one's moral views. I have been emphasizing that a moral judgment, if it is to be acceptable, must be backed by reasons. Consistency requires, then, that if there are exactly the *same* reasons in support of one course of conduct as there are supporting another, those actions are equally right, or equally wrong. We cannot say that X is right, but that Y is wrong, unless there is a *relevant difference* between X and Y. This is a familiar principle in many contexts: it cannot be right for a teacher to give students different grades unless there is a relevant difference in the work that they have done; it cannot be right to pay workers different wages unless there is some relevant difference between the jobs they do; and so on. This principle underlies the social ideal of equality.

It has recently been noticed that this principle has even more radical implications than egalitarians have realized, for if applied consistently it would require that we rethink our treatment of animals. We routinely perform experiments on chimpanzees that we would never perform on humans—but what is the difference between chimps and humans that justifies this difference in treatment? One answer might be that humans are far more intelligent and sensitive than chimpanzees; but this only invites a further query: suppose the humans are mentally retarded, so that they are *less* intelligent than chimps? Would we then be willing to experiment on retarded humans in the same way? And if not, why not? What is the difference between the individuals in question, which makes it all right to experiment on one but not the other? At this point the defender of the status quo may be reduced to asserting that, after all, the humans are *human*, and that's what makes the difference. This, however, is uncomfortably like asserting that, after all, women are *women*, or blacks are *black*, and that's why *they* may be treated differently. It is the announcement of a prejudice, and nothing more.[7]

I have left until last a matter that many moral philosophers believe is at the heart of their subject. In many instances we cannot make progress in moral deliberation until we become clearer about the meaning of the concepts that are employed in our arguments—and the analysis of concepts has always been the philosopher's special concern. The most important concepts for ethics in general are the concepts of rightness, goodness, and obligation. We want first to be clear about what *they* mean, and this is not merely a matter of idle curiosity, but a necessity for making progress in our thinking. In this essay I have, without announcing the fact, made a number of points that depend on the analysis of these concepts: that the right thing to do is the course of action supported by the best reasons, and that in the absence of relevant differences it cannot be right to treat individuals differently, are, in my opinion, propositions that follow directly from the meaning of the moral concepts.

The importance of conceptual analysis may not be obvious, however, if we concentrate only on such general concepts. Where particular moral issues are concerned, the analysis of more specific concepts may be crucial. By now it obvious that the argument over whether fetuses are persons, and so fall under the protection of the moral rules governing the treatment of persons, is not an argument over "the facts." We all know what sort of biological and psychological entity a fetus is, or we think we do, and yet disagreement persists about whether fetuses are persons. What divides the parties on this point is their differing understandings of what it means to be a person—the analysis of the concept.

Opponents of abortion like to show photographs of fetuses, to underscore the point that it is not merely a blob of tissue that is destroyed in an abortion.

What makes the photographs effective is that they seem to show *people*, albeit very tiny and helpless ones, just like you and me: yet, the pro-choice advocate might point out, what the pictures show is only that the fetus has the *physical* characteristics normally associated with persons. In addition, persons have psychological characteristics—consciousness, beliefs, desires, hopes, and so forth—which define their lives as individuals. Since the fetus does not have this complex of psychological characteristics, the pro-choice advocate can argue plausibly that they are not persons in any morally important sense. The whole argument hinges on what in meant by "person."

In one respect I believe that the pro-choice advocates are right. It is a person's psychological characteristics, and not the fact that he or she has a certain kind of body, that is important from a moral point of view. That is why, when some one has become irreversibly comatose, it seems pointless to maintain him or her alive by artificial means. Without consciousness, with all that it involves, being alive does one no good. Indeed many are tempted to say that such unfortunate people are already dead, in recognition of the fact that their biographical lives are over, even though biologically they are still alive. The case of the fetus is, however, different, because although the fetus may lack the psychological characteristics of a person, it nevertheless *will* have them if it is allowed a normal development. The major unresolved question about the morality of abortion is how much, if at all, this potentiality counts. People have differing intuitions on the matter, but I am not aware that anyone has produced a convincing argument either way.

The Limits of Rationality

The preceding discussion will not have dispelled all the nagging doubts about ethics. Rational methods can be used to expose factual error and inconsistency, in the ways I have described, but is that enough to save ethics from the charge that, at bottom, there is no "truth" in its domain? Couldn't two people who are equally rational—who have all the relevant facts, whose principles are consistent, and so on—still disagree? And if "reason" were inadequate to resolve the disagreement, wouldn't this show that, in the end, ethics really is only a matter of opinion? These questions will not go away.

There is a limit to what rational methods can achieve, which Hume described perfectly in the first appendix to his *Inquiry Concerning the Principles of Morals* (1752):

> Ask a man *why he uses exercise*; he will answer, *because he desires to keep his health*. If you then inquire *why he desires health*, he will readily reply,

because sickness is painful. If you push your inquiries further and desire a reason *why he hates pain*, it is impossible he can ever give any. This an ultimate end, and is never referred to any other subject.

Perhaps to your second question, *why he desires health*, he may also reply that *it is necessary for the exercise of his calling.* If you ask *why he is anxious on that head,* he will answer, *because he desires to get money.* If you demand, *Why? It is the instrument of pleasure,* says he. And beyond this, it is an absurdity to ask for a reason. It is impossible there can be a progress *in infinitum*, and that one thing can always be a reason why another is desired. Something must be desirable on its own account, and because of its immediate accord or agreement with human sentiment and affection.[8]

The impossibility of an infinite regress of reasons is not peculiar to ethics; it applies in all areas. Mathematical reasoning eventually ends with axioms that are not themselves justified, and reasoning in science ultimately depends on assumptions that are not proven. At some point reasoning must always come to an end, no matter what the subject.

The *difference* between ethics and other subjects is in the involvement of the emotions. In order for anything to count as an ultimate reason for or against a course of conduct, one must *care* about that thing in some way. In the absence of any emotional involvement, there are no reasons for action. The fact that the building is on fire is a reason for me to leave only if I care about not being burned; the fact that children are starving is a reason for me to do something only if I care about their plight. (On this point the emotivists were right, whatever defects their overall theory might have had.) It is the possibility that people might care about different things, and so accept different ultimate principles between which "reason" cannot adjudicate, which continues to undermine confidence in the subject itself.

However, one other point needs to be considered before we reach any conclusions. What people care about is itself sensitive to pressure from the deliberative process, and can change as a result of thought. A person might not care very much about something prior to thinking it through, but come to feel differently once he has thought it over. This fact has been considered extremely important by some of the major philosophers. Aristotle, Butler, and others emphasized that responsible moral judgment must be based on a full understanding of the facts; but, they added, after the facts are established a separate cognitive process is required for the agent to fully understand the import of what he or she knows. It is necessary not merely to know the facts, but to rehearse them carefully in one's mind, in an impartial, nonevasive way. *Then* one will have the kind of knowledge on which moral judgment may be based.

Aristotle even suggested that there are two distinct species of knowledge: first, the sort of knowledge possessed by one who is able to recite facts, "like the drunkard reciting the verses of Empedocles," but without understanding their meaning; and second, the sort of knowledge possessed when one has thought carefully through what one knows. An example might make this clearer. We all know, in an abstract sort of way, that many children in the world are starving; yet for most of us this makes little difference to our conduct. We will spend money on trivial things for ourselves, rather than spending it on food for them. How are we to explain this? The Aristotelian explanation is that we "know" the children are starving only in the sense in which the drunkard knows Empedocles' verses—we simply recite the fact.[9] Suppose, though, that we thought carefully about what it must be *like* to be a starving orphan. Our attitudes, our conduct, and the moral judgments we are willing to make, might be substantially altered.

A few years ago a wire-service photograph of two Vietnamese orphans appeared in American newspapers. They were sleeping on a Saigon street; the younger boy, who seemed to be about four, was inside a tattered cardboard box, while his slightly older brother was curled up around the box. The explanation beneath the photograph said that while they begged for food during the day, the older boy would drag the box with them, because he didn't want his little brother to have to sleep on the sidewalk at night. After this photograph appeared, a large number of people contacted relief agencies offering to help. What difference did the picture make? I don't believe it was a matter of people being presented with new information—it wasn't as though people did not know that starving orphans have miserable lives. Rather, it brought home to people in a vivid way things that they already knew.

In ordinary moral discussion we recognize that thinking through what one knows is a separate matter from merely knowing. Those who favor voluntary euthanasia ask us to consider what it is like, from the point of view of the dying patient, to suffer horribly. Albert Camus, in his essay on capital punishment, "Reflections on the Guillotine," argued that people tolerate the death penalty only because they think of it in euphemistic terms ("Pierre paid his debt to society") rather than attending the sound of the head falling into the basket.[10] And as I have already mentioned, opponents of abortion show us pictures of fetuses, to force you to pay attention to what it is that is killed. Often this method of argument is dismissed as involving nothing more than a demagogic appeal to emotion, which ought to have no place in rational discussion. Sometimes the charge is true. However, this type of argument may also serve as an antidote for the self-deception that Bishop Butler saw as corrupting moral thought. When we do not *want* to reach a certain conclusion about what is to be done, for whatever reason—perhaps we would rather spend money on ourselves than give it for famine relief—we may refuse to face up to what we know in a clear-minded way. Facts that would have the power to move us are put out of mind, or are thought of only bloodlessly and abstractly. Rehearsing the facts in an imaginative way is needed.[11]

Now let us return to the question of ethical disagreement. When disagreement occurs, two explanations are possible. There could be some failure of rationality on the part of one or the other person, or they could simply be different, in that they care about different things. In practice, when important matters are at issue, we always proceed on the first hypothesis. We present arguments on the assumption that those who disagree have missed something: they are ignorant of relevant facts, they have not thought through what they know, they are not consistent, and so on. We do not credit the idea that they are "different."

Is this procedure reasonable? Are there any real-life examples of ethical disagreement where the explanation is that the people who disagree, while being rational enough, simply care about different things? If there are, they are notoriously hard to find. The familiar examples of the cultural anthropologists turn out upon analysis to have other explanations. The eskimos who allow their first-born daughters to die of exposure, and who abandon feeble old people to a similar fate, do not have less respect for life than other peoples who reject such practices. They live in different circumstances, under threat of starvation in a hostile environment, and the survival of the community requires policies which otherwise they would happily renounce. The Ik, an apparently crude and callous people indifferent even to the welfare of their own children, took on those characteristics only after a prolonged period of near-starvation, which virtually destroyed their tribal culture. There may be some disagreements which reflect cultural variables—I have already mentioned Herodotus' Greeks and Callatians, for example—but beyond that, and barring the kind of disaster that reduced the Iks, it is plausible to think that people are enough alike to make ethical agreement possible, if only full rationality were possible.

The fact that rationality has limits does not subvert the objectivity of ethics, but it does suggest a certain modesty in what can be claimed for it. Ethics provides answers about what we ought to do, given that we are the kinds of creatures we are, caring about the things we will care about when we are as reasonable as we can be, living in the sort of circumstances in which we live. This is not as much as we might want, but it is a lot. It is as much as we can hope for in a subject that must incorporate not only our beliefs but our ideals as well.

Who Provides the Answers?

In one of Charles Schulz's "Peanuts" cartoons, Lucy wonders aloud: "Are there more bad people in the world or are there more good people?" With an expansive gesture, Charlie Brown responds: "Who is to say? Who is to say who is bad or who is good?" "I will," says Lucy.

Lucy has the right idea. Of course there is no central authority who decrees what is good and what is bad; each person must make his or her own judgments. This should come as no surprise, for exactly the same is true of ordinary factual matters. "Who is to say how many books are on the shelf?" The answer is, obviously, anyone who cares to count. Similarly, where moral matters are concerned, anyone who cares to think things through can "say" what is good or bad.

This parallel between factual and moral issues can be pushed one step further. We are not tempted to ask for the help of an "authority" when the question at issue is as simple as the number of books on a shelf. We can easily figure this out for ourselves. However, other factual issues may be so difficult or complicated that laypersons cannot figure things out for themselves; technical competence is required. In these cases we do look for help from authorities. Similarly, we are all competent to judge relatively simple moral matters: we need no expert consultants to tell us that murder, rape, or pointless lying is wrong. But some moral matters are more complicated, and here we may wish the guidance of "experts," if there are any.

As one might expect, remembering our discussion of rational choice, there are two kinds of expertise required for dealing with complicated moral issues. The first is expertise concerning relevant facts. Suppose the issue is nuclear energy: we need to know about the costs of this source of energy; the likelihood of accidents at power plants; the probable consequences of such accidents; the disposal of radioactive wastes; and so on. We also need to know about the possibilities of alternate sources of energy. There are difficult matters even for those who devote their professional lives to them, and quite beyond the comprehension of laypersons who have not bothered to do a lot of studying. It would be easy to give other examples of the same kind; to mention a different area, competent judgment in many matters of public policy requires a distressingly broad knowledge of economics. Clearly, laypersons need the guidance of the experts here; and when the experts disagree, the rest of us may not know what to think.

The other area of expertise concerns more abstract matters: the critical assessment of arguments, the formulation and testing of principles, the analysis of concepts, and so forth. These are the traditional skills of philosophers and theologians, and that is why it has seemed natural to look to these thinkers as moral guides—*not* because they are better people, or because they are blessed with some kind of occult insight. I say "philosophers and theologians" although I have a certain reservation about theology. The theologian is most helpful when he is least theological. Morality concerns everyone, religious and nonreligious alike. Arguments that appeal only to the faithful will have limited value. Theologians themselves realize this, and often present their arguments entirely in secular terms. It may be emphasized that certain values are espoused within a religious tradition, but at the same time it is assumed that those values can be discussed and defended independently.

There are, then, "experts" on ethical matters—people who have informed themselves as to the relevant facts and who have studied the arguments and concepts involved. We have already begun to make use of such people in special contexts. For example, institutions conducting research with human subjects have special review boards to consider, from an ethical point of view, the permissibility of particular projects. It would be foolish to think that every decision made by such boards is wise; even leaving aside political considerations, infallibility is not to be expected. Nevertheless, the very existence of such panels acknowledges that there are ethical matters that cannot be dealt with responsibly apart form special knowledge and study. Egalitarian sentiments notwithstanding, one person's opinion is not always as good as another's.

This conclusion may easily be misinterpreted. Sometimes it is wise and even necessary for the rest of use to leave certain ethical decisions to experts, especially those concerning matters with which we have little experience. This does not mean that moral life is a game of follow-the-leader. Lucy was right. People who are not able to spend a lot of time studying ethical questions ought to pay attention to the results of those who have. But that is a matter of where we find guidance, not where we find bosses. A slavish follower is not a moral agent. In the end, moral agents must answer the question "Who is to say?" as Lucy did. If, in the hard cases, different agents come up with different answers, that is why we need politics as well as ethics.

QUESTIONS FOR CONSIDERATION

1. How does Rachels characterize the relationship between ethics and ethical theory?
2. According to Rachels, the social sciences (psychology and sociology) explain away ethics in the minds of some people. How does he answer the charges of psychological and cultural relativism?

3.   What are the deficiencies of emotivism that Rachels identifies?
4.   How does Rachels characterize the rational methods for solving moral problems? What is the role of accurately determining the facts of a case in solving moral problems? What is the test of consistency relative to moral problems? Why does Rachels believe that motives are morally significant in making decisions? What is the significance of the analysis of moral concepts?
5.   What are the "limits of rationality" that Rachels identifies? How does emotional involvement or care provide motivations for moral choices?
6.   What role does Rachels see for the "experts" on ethical issues?

NOTES

1. William Frankena's book *Ethics* (Englewood Cliffs, N.J.: Prentice-Hall, second edition, 1973) is a helpful introduction to ethical theory. For information about particular topics and theories, various articles in the eight-volume *Encyclopedia of Philosophy*, edited by Paul Edwards (New York: Macmillan & Free Press, 1967) are useful. The reader should not be put off by the fact that it is "merely" an encyclopedia; it is a splendid work with which everyone should be familiar.

2. The essay on suicide, together with other relevant works, is conveniently reprinted in *Hume's Ethical Writings*, edited by Alasdair MacIntyre (New York: Collier, 1965). Of the many commentaries on Hume, Rachel Kydd's *Reason and Conduct in Hume's Treatise* (New York: Russell & Russell, 1964) is especially recommended.

3. *The History of Herodotus*, translated by George Rawlinson, adapted by John Ladd in *Ethical Relativism* (Belmont, Cal.: Wadsworth, 1973), p.12. *Ethical Relativism* is a good collection of articles on the relation of ethics to culture.

4. The classic defense of emotivism is Charles L. Stevenson, *Ethics and Language* (New Haven: Yale University Press, 1944). J.O. Urmson, *The Emotive Theory of Ethics* (London: Hutchinson, 1968), provides a critical assessment.

5. A survey of the relevant arguments may be found in James Rachels, "Euthanasia," in *Matters of Life and Death*, edited by Tom Regan (New York: Random House, 1980), pp. 28–66.

6. James Rachels, "Active and Passive Euthanasia," *The New England Journal of Medicine*, 292 (1975), 78–80, argues that there is no morally important difference between killing and letting die. This article is reprinted, together with a response by Tom L. Beauchamp, "A Reply to Rachels on Active and Passive Euthanasia," in Tom L. Beauchamp and Seymour Perlin, eds., *Ethical Issues in Death and Dying* (Englewood Cliffs, N.J.: Prentice-Hall, 1978). Richard L. Trammell, "Saving Life and Taking Life," *Journal of Philosophy* 72 (1975), 131–37, is an excellent defense of the distinction. James Rachels, "Killing and Starving to Death," *Philosophy* 54 (1979), 159–71, continues the attack and criticizes some of Trammell's arguments.

7. These arguments are advanced with great vigor by Peter Singer in his book *Animal Liberation* (New York: New York Review/Random House, 1975).

8. *Hume's Ethical Writings*, p. 131.

9. Aristotle, *Nicomachean Ethics*, 1147b.

10. Albert Camus, *Resistance, Rebellion, and Death* (New York: Knopf, 1961), 175–234.

11. Among contemporary philosophers, this point has been made most forcefully by W. D. Falk. See his "Action-Guiding Reasons," *Journal of Philosophy* 60 (1963), 702–18.

SIDNEY CALLAHAN

The Role of Emotion
in Ethical Decisionmaking

What is the moral significance of my feelings when I hear that newly dead human bodies are used in car crashes for research on automobile safety? What should I make of the emotions aroused by the news that dying old persons will have their food and water withdrawn, or in other instances, be straitjacketed and forcibly fed? And does my emotional response to the dilemmas presented by AIDS and surrogate motherhood count? Everyone agrees that bioethical decisions, involving as they often do matters of life, death, sex, reproduction, and familial and professional loyalties, can arouse emotional responses. What is not agreed upon is whether, or how, one should weigh emotions when trying to resolve an ethical dilemma.

A completely rationalist view dismisses the role of emotions with the assertion that "arguments are one thing, sentiments another, and nothing fogs the mind so thoroughly as emotion."[1] Adherents of this negative estimate of emotion would advise a person confronting an ethical dilemma to arrive at a decision using rational considerations alone. As Tristram Engelhardt, Jr. says in his widely hailed book on bioethics, we should see the affirmations of one's feelings as "irrational, *surd*," and seek to become impartial reasoners "whose only interests are in the consistency and force of rational argument."[2]

Other philosophers may begrudgingly admit the inevitability of emotive intuitions, or gut feelings in moral argumentation but vigorously resist employing them. As James Rachels puts it, "The idea cannot be to avoid reliance on unsupported 'sentiments' (to use Hume's word) altogether—that is impossible. The idea is always to be suspicious of them, and to rely, on as few as possible, only after examining them critically, and only after pushing the arguments and explanations as far as they will go without them."[3]

Joel Feinberg contends that emotions always should be subordinated to reason in the process of decisionmaking. Feinberg is not unappreciative of moral emotions, but they can never serve as an ethical criterion. A sentimental attachment to fetuses, corpses, or body parts should not be allowed to thwart the interests of actual living persons who need abortions, organ transplants, or automobile safety research. For emotions to count in any applied ethical decisions, they must be justified on independent grounds.[4]

I propose a model for the mutual interaction of thinking and feeling in ethical decisionmaking. Certainly, reason should monitor reason as in traditional philosophical critiques, and reason should tutor the emotions as in Feinberg's model. But I would also claim that emotion should tutor reason and that emotion should monitor emotion. The ideal goal is to come to an ethical decision through a personal equilibrium in which emotion and reason are both activated and in accord.

Human Emotions in Psychology

What do we now think we know about the functioning of human beings that should make us take emotions more seriously in ethical enterprises?

The human emotional system is a universal component of human functioning, the primary motivating system of all activity, including of course, thinking about ethical dilemmas. Following Darwin's lead, psychological theorists now see human emotions, like human cognitive capacities, to have been selected through evolution to ensure the survival of individuals and the group.[5] Emotions are energizing and adaptive, and serve communicating, bonding, and motivating functions. They seem to be distinct from either physiological drives or cognitive processes, although complex interactions and learned associations occur. Without emotions or affects to amplify physiological drives and infuse cognitive processing with subjective meaning, human beings would not care enough to stay alive, much less mate, nurture offspring, create kinship bonds, or pursue art, science, literature, or moral philosophy.

Emotions can be loosely defined as distinctly patterned human experiences that, when consciously felt, produce qualitatively distinct subjective feelings and predispositions: "I am angry and want to attack"; "I am afraid and want to flee"; "I love and wish to approach."[6] Theorists argue over the correct boundaries of definition: How long does an emotion last? How intense must it be? Must it always involve awareness? Others focus upon how cognition, learning, and the social environment influence emotional experiences. I take an inclusive approach that sees feelings, sentiments, and moods as forms of emotional experience.

The different emotions appear to be constituted of distinctly patterned responses of the neurobiochemical, facial, and motor systems.[7] Evidence from cross-cultural and infant research points to panhuman constancies in emotional response and expression—from New York to New Guinea, the same facial expressions communicate the same emotions.[8] A limited set of basic emotions have been described which, like the primary colors, can be blended, differentiated, and elaborated. These primary emotions are usually differentiated as interest-excitement, enjoyment-joy, surprise-startle, distress-anguish, anger-rage, disgust-revulsion, contempt-scorn, fear-terror, shame-humiliation, and for many, guilt-remorse, and love.

As human beings we come equipped with evolved emotional and cognitive capacities that operate interactively. While emotions and cognitions are often combined, emotions differ from cognitions in their subjective intensity, specificity, and nonverbal richness.[9] The emotional system also seems to respond to and encode in memory nonverbal, qualitative dimensions of experience. Reason as verbal, symbolic, cognitive processing, is a faculty more detached, mobile, and quick in operation than emotion. But the existence of such complex subsystems in the human organism seems an overall advantage: one system can always serve as a corrective to the others. Emotion and thinking are, in sum, complementary, synergistic, parallel processes, constantly blending and interacting as a person functions.

Thinking and deciding take place in self-conscious, aware, motivated human beings who are constantly experiencing what William James called the stream of consciousness. Thinking will interact with a person's emotive, perceptual, physiological, and motor systems. Emotions also interact in the stream of consciousness in complex ways, especially through memory.

As we think through a problem we call upon our memory. Memory networks may be activated by either a feeling or an idea; calling up one part of a scenario may activate the feelings or ideas stored with it.[10] Thinking about death may activate sad feelings; feeling sad may activate thoughts of death. Emotional states have been shown to affect all sorts of cognitive processes: selective content and efficiency of memory, problem-solving or learning ability, predictions of the future, social evaluations of persons, self-estimates, altruistic decisions, aggressive assessments, and even perception of physical stimuli in the environment.

Researchers on the development of emotion in children present a helpful image of the continual dynamic of thinking and feeling in consciousness. Finding inadequate linear models that posited that cognition causes emotion, or that emotion causes cognition, these researchers "developed a third model based on the metaphor of a musical fugue . . . in this model, the cognitive-emotional relationship is depicted as a complex interplay of processes, similar to the themes of a fugue, which are often lost and reappear."[11] The interweaving process goes on in human beings throughout life: emotions induce thoughts that may induce emotion.[12] This interplay between thinking and feeling in personal consciousness can become open to introspection, and long before experimental psychologists began their studies these inner processes were depicted in poetry, drama, fiction, philosophy, and religious writing.

Emotions and Moral Reasoning

Indeed, the emotions are particularly important in moral and ethical functioning. In every culture children develop emotional reactions of guilt and shame at the same age. They seem to have an innately programmed predisposition to be morally socialized and to enter into moral discourse, for which full development of emotional response is necessary.[13] Studies of psychopaths indicate that they are below average or deficient in emotional responsiveness. A lack of anxiety, guilt, empathy, or love devastates moral functioning. Persons may have a high I.Q and be able to articulate verbally the culture's moral rules, but if they cannot feel the emotional force of inner obligation, they can disregard all moral rules or arguments without a qualm.

Emotions energize the ethical quest. A person must be emotionally interested enough and care enough about discerning the truth to persevere despite distractions. Even more, a person who wrestles with moral questions is usually emotionally committed to doing good and avoiding evil. A good case can be made that what is specifically moral about moral thinking, what gives it its imperative "oughtness," is personal emotional investment. When emotion infuses an evaluative judgment, it is transformed into a prescriptive moral judgment of what ought to be done.

Moreover, it appears that the building blocks of moral thinking are imbued with emotion. The human mind gives evidence of actively creating units consisting of fused thoughts and emotions and then storing these constructions in long-term memory. These cognitive-affective constructs, the thing and the feeling-about-the-thing, appear to be encoded in complex networks of memory, some of which may be complex or extensive enough to be called narratives, "scripts," "scenes," or "scenarios."[14] Moral sentiments consist of such fusions of things joined with feelings about the thing, as for instance, "torture wrong, disgusting," or "truthtelling good." As we think through a moral conflict or question we call up memory stores and inevitably have our thinking shaped by the linked associations.

Personally invested emotional commitments shape selective attention. A person always enters the ethical decisionmaking process in midstream, influenced by his or her past experiences and the operation of long-term memory. Evidence is accruing that the emotions or thoughts that seem to "pop" spontaneously into our heads are not at all random. Extensive preconscious selection and filtering interact with long-term memory to determine what reaches conscious awareness.[15] The selective filtering activity that brings a thought or feeling to consciousness will have personal significance and may serve adaptive or defensive purposes.[16] High level thinking, much less a creative intellectual solution ("Aha, I've got it!"), can happen only when a person has been prepared through past effort. So too, emotional responses, especially moral sentiments, indicate the achievement of self-development and those "habits of the heart" known as moral character.

As the philosopher Iris Murdoch has expressed this:

> If we consider what the work of attention is like, how continuously it goes on, and how imperceptibly it builds up structures of value round about us, we shall not be surprised that at crucial moments of choice most of the business of choosing is already over. This does not imply that we are not free, certainly not. But it implies that the exercise of our freedom is a small piecemeal business which goes on all the time and not a grandiose leaping about unimpeded at important moments. The moral life, in this view, is something that goes on continually.[17]

Moral lapses, "sudden" betrayals, or acts of heroism are influenced by past choices.

The Tutoring Role of Reason

Methods for the rational assessment of thinking and the rational tutoring of emotions in ethical decisionmaking have been highly developed and elaborated. There have also been many attempts to broaden and deepen the concept of reason—and thereby implicitly recognize and recapture the role of emotion in thinking. Human reasoning is no longer identified solely with the calculating and analytic capacities displayed by computers; human intelligence is more imaginative, holistic, and playful (more emotive?) than narrowly focused logical or critical analysis.

By certain traditional criteria, such as consistency, logic, rules of evidence, appropriateness, coherence, clarity, completeness, and congruence with reality, human thinking can be assessed as ranging from the highly rational to the seriously inadequate. Moral thinking, as a form of structured thought, can be assessed by the traditional canons of rationality, and moral philosophers are adept in this analysis.

We can almost always assess rationally (at least in others) the appearance of childish, immature, emotional responses, fused with childish thinking, that endanger ethical decisions. Humans wish to avoid pain and seek pleasure. Initiated and abetted by psychoanalysis, the psychology of self-deception has made us acutely aware of the emotional and cognitive maneuvers that produce self-protective feats of selective attention, sometimes called "vital lies."[18] All of the "defenses" enumerated in psychoanalytic thinking are activations of cognitive-affective structures to deploy attention away from painful reality, or if that fails, to distort what is perceived and felt. Persons who constantly and rigidly use these strategies to avoid pain finally so cripple their emotional capacities that their cognitive and emotional functioning becomes maladaptive by any standards, whether one talks about neurosis, regression, or moral immaturity.

Psychology now sees the person as constantly acting. The "id" is no longer reified as a force, but is characterized as the regressed, childish way a person feels and thinks:

> It is a way of acting erotically or aggressively that is more or less infantile in its being irrational, unmodulated, unrestrained, heedless of consequences and contradiction, thoroughly egocentric, and more than likely associated with those vivid and diffuse physiological processes that fall under the common heading of excitement or arousal.[19]

The emotions and moral thinking displayed are those of a child, whether the person is a bright young physician under stress, an old person facing death, an adolescent facing life, or even a middle-aged philosopher undergoing a second adolescence. Regression can occur at any time in the life cycle, and can produce irrational emotions entwined with irrational thinking. Other emotional disorders have the same effect, so that "reasoning with a person suffering from mania is like reasoning with a five-year-old."[20] Depressed persons are equally resistant to the rational tutoring of their emotions. When people are in such an excessively stressed or regressed state, they cannot make mature moral or ethical decisions.

Such disturbed states are fairly dramatic and have given rise to the equating of all emotion with those particular infantile passions that are dangerous to moral functioning. Excessive conditions of disordered emotion and thinking result in qualitatively different states of addiction and obsession; feelings and thoughts are flooding, intrusive, inappropriately repeated and recycled, with the felt loss of flexible control of attention.

While the circular interaction of thinking and feeling ensures that they both deteriorate together, it is easier to notice the more dramatic disorders of the emotions. Thus traditional rationalist philosophers and Freudian theorists, and those proposing models of decisionmaking, have stressed the bias involved in emotions.

Regression and Moral Conflict

The working model of moral conflict has been that of emotion warring against reason, with only reason's mastery offering trustworthy guidance. A more careful analysis of the regressed state would see that the moral conflict is usually a case of one immature thinking-emotive moral scenario in conflict with another more wholly owned and appropriately mature moral scenario. Rational tutoring of self or others assesses the inappropriate responses and substitutes others. Reasoning can affect mood and emotions as stoic strategies, psychotherapy, and ordinary self-control regularly prove.

Rational persons may have a more difficult time noticing and assessing those less dramatic but equally disabling disorders consisting of deficits of emotion. In philosophical arguments the problem of such deficits is regularly ignored and that of excessive emotion emphasized. Yet in our technological culture perhaps the greatest moral danger arises not from sentimentality, but from devaluing feeling and not attending to or nurturing moral emotions. Numbness, apathy, isolated disassociations between thinking and feeling are also moral warning signals. Psychopaths, persons under stress, persons who have coped by ignoring or denying their emotions, suffer from deficit problems in moral emotions.

Some persons are too "burned out" from stress to see or care about moral dilemmas. Others are so accustomed to isolating and not attending to their emotions that when they inadvertently must confront feeling, they are overwhelmed by what seems to them an alien external force. They are all the more susceptible to moral collapse and making poor ethical decisions.

Habits of numbing or suppressing emotion spread to other domains in a personality and impair moral thinking as surely as excessive, infantile emotions do. The human mind for brief periods can go into detached, depersonalized overdrive and function automatically like a computer. We have seen detached analysis destructively employed by the best and the brightest. The maintenance of moral emotions and the care and cultivation of moral sentiment should be seen as all-important; after all, the rational tutoring of emotion depends upon people who already possess a highly developed emotional repertoire. Those concerned with educating health care workers know that the absence of emotional responses of empathy and sympathy become critical bioethical issues.[21]

The Tutoring Role of Emotion

But the more controversial claim being made here is that just as reason tutors and monitors emotion, so too can our emotions tutor reason. Why so? And how? There are positive and negative ways this can happen as the dynamic interactive stream of human consciousness proceeds. We are sometimes morally restrained, and on the other hand, sometimes activated by our emotions to go beyond our habitual moral framework. Given the knowledge of the preconscious filtering process needed for consciousness, and knowing the innate capacity of the emotional system to respond to reality, even momentary emotions can be seen as a message to myself, from myself and all that has shaped me. We should pay attention, for our emotions constitute reflexive personal signals, or "vital signs" informing us of inner processes or of interactions with the environment.[22]

As we think through moral options or pursue arguments there can arise negative emotional responses ranging from mild feelings of aversion to intense feelings of repugnance. A rational argument without any apparent logical flaws may be presented—in, for instance, proposals for using torture, or harvesting neomorts, or refusing to treat AIDS—but our moral emotions prevent us from giving assent. When we feel strongly and persistently that this is wrong, wrong, wrong, but we can't articulate why, we withhold assent. Our discomfort induces us to continue looking beyond the proposed arguments, to keep searching and broaden the review. Later we may be able to understand the emotional reaction and feel profoundly grateful that we were not carried away by abstractions.

Emotions also tutor moral reasoning in positive ways. Much of our creativity in moral thinking emerges as ideas and emotions are activated in memory and produce new reverberations. Many moral revolutions have been initiated by empathy felt for previously excluded groups: slaves, women, workers, children, the handicapped, experimental subjects, patients in institutions. As I emotionally respond to another person or group, I may be forced to confront a conflicting moral attitude concerning the group. Novel emotional responses of sympathy clash with previously accepted moral principles, an inconsistency and unsettling discrepancy that can then prompt a creative moral readjustment.

The emotion of love, defined minimally as joyful interest with a predisposition to approach and attachment, most aptly tutors reason. Love engenders attention and concern, and minimizes fear and indifference. It motivates the resistance necessary to withstand automatic dismissals. At the other end of the emotional spectrum, anger, especially vicarious anger, can also tutor moral reasoning. Since the time of the Old Testament prophets, the experience of indignation or anger has moved persons to call for a drastic revision of their moral ideas. Present experiences of anger at what happens to an AIDS patient, a dying old person, or the mentally retarded in institutions, may cause a drastic reappraisal of moral thinking.

In a more subtle process, even more difficult to elucidate or articulate, one emotion can monitor and tutor another. Love and sympathy neutralize many negative emotions, as for instance when in the treatment of the diseased or handicapped, sympathy overcomes disgust. Love can quell anger or mitigate contempt for a person's moral lapse or betrayal. On the other hand, anger can transform sadness, depression, and apathy into active assertion or aspiration. Much of both psychotherapy and moral socialization can be seen not only as teaching rational control, but also as trying to substitute and transform one emotion by inducing the feeling of another.

As Iris Murdoch has expressed it:

> It is also a psychological fact, and one of importance in moral philosophy, that we can all receive moral help by focusing our attention upon things which are valuable: virtuous people, great art, perhaps the idea of goodness itself. Human beings are naturally "attached" and when an attachment seems painful or bad it is most readily displaced by another attachment. . . .[23]

An attachment or emotion can be experienced as painful or bad, both by its intrinsic experience of awfulness, as in envy or jealousy, and/or because our reason has judged it to be bad in this situation.

Loving attachments to virtuous persons influence and tutor my own emotions and moral sentiments. In ethical decisionmaking, I can assess an emotional response by comparing it to the response of those I admire and love. Their moral authority and persuasiveness arise from my emotional response to their goodness. In the same way, my emotional aversion to a person's life and moral being can make me distrust their reactions to a moral dilemma.

Our trust in the moral sentiments of those we hold to be good is not irrational, but neither is it infallible, since they too can be mistaken. Nonetheless, we are drawn even more persuasively to those we think to be rationally acute as well as good. If emotion and reason are inevitably intertwined, then the traditionally acclaimed guidance of persons communally held to be wise and good is most to be trusted. A good person's lifelong cultivation of appropriate emotions will help protect him or her from those deformations of moral reasoning that afflict the immature, regressed, or selfishly willful person undergoing stress or conflict. While a diseased physician can cure a sick patient, it is unlikely that an amoral or evil person can make wise and good ethical judgments solely through logical analysis.

The Art of Ethical Decisionmaking

If one would decide wisely and well, the best strategy would include both trusting and skeptical awareness of all of one's capacities and reactions. An individual is far too complex and personal consciousness (and preconsciousness) operates too instantaneously, for simple linear processing. It is essential to engage in fully extended, fully inclusive, circular, parallel processing of the dynamic interplays of consciousness.

While I am assessing my reasoning and arguments by rational criteria, I should pay attention to emotions, even those fleeting negative feelings that may be most in danger of defensive suppression. In the same process my emotional responses are in turn being rationally and emotionally assessed for appropriateness, or for their infantile or qualitative characteristics. Deficits and numbness should also be considered. As rational argument proceeds I can seek to enrich the process with emotional intuitions and associations, imagined moral scenarios, and the testimony of the wise and good. Can these emotions become universal, can they produce good consequences, are these feelings consistent with my other best emotions? Communication about my feelings with others would be a further test: Certainly, I should also continually compare my rational arguments to the critical reasoning of reflective experts, as found, say, in analytic articles or ethical guidelines. New ideas, arguments, or emotions should be continually checked and mutually adjusted.

The philosopher Jonathan Bennett recommends "checking of one's principles in the light of one's sympathies. . . It can happen that a certain moral principle becomes untenable—meaning one cannot hold it any longer— because it conflicts intolerably with the pity or revulsion or whatever that one feels when one sees what the principle leads to." Even more interestingly, Bennett sees principles themselves "as embodiments of one's best feelings, one's broadest and keenest sympathies. On that view principles can help one across intervals when one's feelings are at less than their best, that is through periods of misanthropy or meanness or self-centeredness or depression or anger."[24]

Philosophers rehabilitating emotions and emotional commitments are recognizing what Mary Midgley has called "the unity of the moral enterprise."

In her view, solving moral problems involves "three inseparable aspects—(1) a changing view of 'the facts,' (2) a change of feeling, and (3) a change in action, arising out of a changing sense of what action can decently be contemplated and what cannot." She thinks it has been a "real misfortune" that many philosophers "have tended to concentrate entirely on separating these factors and putting them in competition as if they were alternatives, rather than on investigating the highly complex relation between them and pointing out where it goes wrong."[25] Heart and mind should no longer be seen as antagonistic adversaries in the moral enterprise.

As one wrestles with an ethical decision the goal is an emotively grounded reflective equilibrium in which all systems are integrated, all tests are satisfied, and a wholehearted decision can be made. The person as knower or whole self, has done the best he or she can after a fully personal engagement. But one may still have to deal with further conflict arising from disagreements with others, either as personal individuals or collective professional groups or institutions. What about other persons and their differing moral sentiments? Their lack of emotion, or different emotions combined with different reasoning may lead to very different resolutions in direct conflict with my own. What then? Must I resign, resist, persuade, sue, or politically organize? Since such social conflicts and challenges present new ethical dilemmas, I may have to repeat my whole decision-making process again to deal with the consequences of an ethical decision.

One conclusion I would have to draw, however, is that I must respect the differing moral sentiments of others. Just as in my reasoning I would be open to correction from better arguments, so I should be open to the possibility that the moral emotions of others may be more valid and morally sound than my own. Unlike Feinberg, I would be especially slow to label the moral sentiments or responses of others as squeamishness, or sentimentality, or irrationality. I would be especially aware that graver moral danger arises from a deficit of moral emotion than from emotional excess.

Even if a person cannot articulate or defend his or her emotions philosophically, that would not necessarily prove them wrong. The requirement that everyone must be able to articulate and defend rationally their moral sentiments seems excessive. This requirement may be hard even for moral philosophers, and might be beyond many people's resources. Since emotions and moral sentiments arise partially from nonverbally encoded interpersonal experiences that a person may not quickly retrieve from memory, persons with developed intuitive emotional responses may still lack the vocabulary or skill to compete in philosophical or political debate. They may need intellectual advocates to articulate and defend their moral sentiments. The newest developments in psychology and philosophy indicate that in the future of bioethics, there will be more analysis and defense of the role of emotions in ethical decisionmaking.

QUESTIONS FOR CONSIDERATION

1. What are the primary emotions identified by Callahan? What is the role of these emotions in energizing, communicating, bonding, motivating, thinking, and forming memory?
2. What does Callahan see as the role of emotions in moral reasoning?
3. How does Callahan characterize the tutoring role of reason?
4. How does Callahan characterize the tutoring role of emotion? Do you agree that strong feelings should sometimes overrule reason?

NOTES

1. Quoted in Joel Feinberg, "Sentiment and Sentimentality in Practical Ethics," Presidential Address delivered before American Philosophical Association in Sacramento, California, March 26, 1982; see also "The Mistreatment of Dead Bodies: The Moral Trap of Sentimentality," *Hastings Center Report* 15:1 (February 1985), 31–37.

2. H. Tristram Engelhardt, Jr., *The Foundations of Bioethics* (New York: Oxford University Press), 10.

3. James Rachels, *The End of Life: Euthanasia and Morality* (Oxford: Oxford University Press, 1986), 149.

4. Feinberg, "Sentiments and Sentimentality in Practical Ethics."

5. Robert Plutchik, *Emotion: A Psychoevolutionary Synthesis* (New York: Harper and Row, 1980).

6. See Carroll E. Izard, "Emotion-Cognition Relationships and Human Development," in *Emotions, Cognition & Behavior,* Carroll E. Izard, Jerome Kagan, and Robert B. Zajonic, eds. (Cambridge: Cambridge University Press, 1984), 17–37. A counter view holding that most emotions are cognitive systems or rules of behavior can be found in James R. Averill, "Emotion and Anxiety: Sociocultural, Biological, and Psychological Determinants," In *Explaining Emotion,* Amelie O. Rorty, ed. (Berkeley: University of California Press, 1980), 37–72.

7. Ross Buck, *The Communication of Emotion* (New York: The Guilford Press, 1984).

8. Paul Ekman, "Expression and the Nature of Emotion," in *Approaches to Emotion*, Klaus R. Scherer and Paul Ekman, eds. (Hillsdale, NJ: Lawrence Erlbaum, 1984), 319–43.

9. Douglas Derryberry and Mary Klevjord Rothbart, "Emotion, Attention and Temperament," in *Emotions, Cognition & Behavior,* 132–66; for a philosophical treatment of "magnetizing dispositions" and the "tenacity" of emotions, see Amelie O. Rorty, "Explaining Emotions," in *Explaining Emotions,* 103–26.

10. Stephen G. Gilligan and Gordon Bower, "Cognitive Consequences of Emotional Arousal," in *Emotions, Cognition & Behavior,* 547–88.

11. Michael Lewis and Linda Michalson, *Children's Emotions and Moods* (New York: Plenum Press, 1983), 88.

12. Joseph DeRivera, "Development and the Full Range of Emotional Experience," in *Emotion in Adult Development,* Carol Zander Malatesta and Carroll E. Izard, eds. (Beverly Hills, CA: Sage Publications, 1984), 45–63.

13. Richard A. Dienstbier, "The Role of Emotion in Moral Socialization," in *Emotions, Cognition & Behavior,* 484–514; Drew Westen, *Self & Society: Narcissism, Collectivism, and the Development of Morals* (Cambridge: University Press, 1985), especially Chapter 2, "Emotion: A Missing Link Between Psychodynamic and Cognitive-Behavioral Psychology?", 22–96; for a philosophical reappraisal see Roberto Mangabeira Unger, *Passion: An Essay on Personality* (New York: The Free Press, 1984).

14. Silvan S. Tomkins, *Affect, Imagery and Consciousness,* Cognition and Affect, 3 (New York: Springer, 1982).

15. Daniel Goleman, "Part Two, The Machinery of Mind," in *Vital Lies, Simple Truths: The Psychology of Self-Deception* (New York: Simon and Schuster, 1985).

16. Roy Schafer, "The Psychoanalytic Vision of Reality," in *A New Language for Psychoanalysis* (New Haven: Yale University Press, 1976) 22–56.

17. Iris Murdoch, *The Sovereignty of Good* (London: Ark Paperbacks, 1985), 37.

18. Goleman, *"Part Two, The Machinery of Mind,"* 22.

19. Schafer, "The Psychoanalytic Vision of Reality," 195.

20. Silvano Arieti and Jules Bemporad, *Severe and Mild Depression: The Psychotherapeutic Approach* (New York: Basic Books, 1978), 17.

21. Mary Howell, "Caretakers' Views on Responsibilities for the Care of the Demented Elderly," *Journal of the American Geriatrics Society* 32:9 (September 1984), 657–60; Christine K. Cassel, "Ethical Dilemmas in Dementia," *Seminars in Neurology* 4:1 (March 1984), 92–97; Kathleen Nolan, "In Death's Shadow: The Meanings of Withholding Resuscitation," *Hastings Center Report* 17:5 (October/November 1987), 9–14.

22. Willard Gaylin, *Feelings: Our Vital Signs* (New York: Harper & Row, 1979).

23. Iris Murdoch, *The Sovereignty of Good,* 56.

24. Jonathan Bennett, "The Conscience of Huckleberry Finn," *Philosophy* 49 (1974), 123–34.

25. Mary Midgley, "The Flight from Blame," *Philosophy* 62 (1987), 271–91.

CARL ELLIOTT

Where Ethics Comes From and
What to Do About It

One of the most alarming aspects of describing an ethical problem, and of hearing it described by others, is discovering just how many ways it can be done. How a moral problem is described will turn on an array of variables: the role and degree of involvement in the case of the person who is describing it, the person's particular profession or discipline, her religious and cultural heritage—indeed, all of the intangibles that have contributed to her character. What is more, the description any person offers will also vary—notoriously— according to whether an ethical decision has been made or is still to come, whether that decision is now judged to be a sound one or a poor one, whether the consequences were unintended or foreseen.

Consider a relatively common case: a middle-aged man with multisystem organ failure, poor but not hopeless prognosis, now incompetent, experiencing what seems to be considerable pain, whose family is faced with the decision about whether to continue his medical treatment. Think of the possible alternatives to the brief and inadequate description I have offered here. A clinician will describe the patient's medical problems, his hospital course, his treatment, his laboratory work, and so on. A moral philosopher will be less interested in the medical details of the case than she will the moral ones, and her description will be constructed from a vocabulary of terms such as autonomy, justice, and beneficence, and the patient's goals, values, and wishes. The patient's wife will not describe a "case," but a continuing chapter in her life. A chaplain, social worker, nurse, or hospital administrator will offer still another description, as will the patient's daughter, his minister, his friends, his colleagues, and his enemies. The perceptions of each of these will change as the patient's story unfolds: what seemed to be minor decisions at one time now appear disastrous; incidents that might have been overlooked now seem to be portents. And any description offered will reflect whether the patient is in a Tel Aviv teaching hospital, a Heidelberg *Krankenhaus*, or a Chicago V.A. facility.

Perhaps the most frustrating feature of describing a moral problem is the gulf between moral description and moral experience. No description, it seems, can do justice to the realities of our moral problems.[1] It is extraordinarily difficult, if not impossible, to capture the countless subtleties that go into the perceptions and judgments of each person involved: the hopes, fears, prayers, guilt, pride, and remorse; the conflicting emotions which accompany irrevocable decisions; the self-imposed pressure to carry through with an action once a decision has been made. Much of what goes into actual moral choices remains unarticulated. To express these things, even to perceive them consciously, requires a talent possessed by few of us other than novelists or poets.

A second problem comes from the realization that in describing a given case, one has done much of the ethical work already. A person's moral judgment is reflected in what he chooses to include in a description: whether he mentions that the patient's wife has visited her critically ill husband only twice over the past three weeks, whether he reports a bed shortage in the ICU, whether he notes that the patient's children stand to inherit the dying man's estate, how he describes the patient's prognosis, whether he brings up the option of palliative care, whether he notes that the nursing staff feels strongly that treatment should be stopped, whether he mentions that the patient was an IV drug abuser. One of the most interesting and disturbing discoveries to be made in a medical ethics case conference is how one's moral institutions change as each player in the drama says his piece, as another perspective is added to one's own. One begins to suspect that it is self-deception to think any description free of ideology, to believe that any viewpoint can approximate an impartial spectator.

A third problem is that to make sense of a particular case, one has to have some sort of conceptual framework in which to place it. This conceptual framework structures one's perception of the case. Medical students know this as well as ethicists: it is only with time, as more patients are encountered and filed within certain conceptual categories, that one begins to understand how to think about specific cases—what to ask, what to examine, what is relevant and what is not. But concepts of necessity involve generalities, not particulars, types of cases, not individual ones. We swap precision for simplicity. As Nigel Barley says, "Generalizations always tell a little lie in the service of greater truth."[2] But if general conceptual frameworks are psychologically essential in ethics, they also make it easy to overlook those aspects of our moral experience that are not easily generalized. Let me mention only a few examples. In theory, it is often said that moral concerns override other concerns, but in practice, one can often readily understand their being overridden themselves, perhaps by practical considerations. In theory, it seems that moral dilemmas can be solved, but in practice they often cannot. In theory, we speak of beings who rationally choose what they believe to be the best action, but in practice we find ourselves making irrational decisions under the sway of seemingly inscrutable desires. In theory, guilt is an emotion that we feel (or rationally should feel) when we have acted wrongly, but in practice we sometimes feel guilty when we have done nothing at all. Indeed, a caricature history of ethics could be written merely by cataloguing various attempts to make our moral experience more intelligible by describing it in terms of something else: moral goodness can be defined in terms of happiness; our moral sense is like of physical senses; moral expressions are like expressions of approval or disapproval. All of this is not to imply, I hasten to say, that all theories are caricatures. Such an implication would itself be a caricature. I only point out that moral theories trade in generalities and simplifications, which make it easy to forget how particular and complicated our moral experience is.

Implicit in these problems is a tension between the ethics of description (and consequently of theory), and the experience of making ethical judgments in concrete cases. The ethics of description and theory seems necessary to make sense of such a wide range of cases, but as with narrative fiction and reality, moral description differs from our actual moral experience. To make sense of ethical problems, we must impose some sort of artificial order on the story we tell, whether we do it in terms of a narrative, or ethical principles, or a medical case history. The order imposed on it affects how we respond to it; thus, we treat differently the cases we have heard described and those we have actually experienced. In fact, not even those cases we experience first hand are innocent of theory. Our moral judgments change how we describe those cases to ourselves. Joan Didion puts this well:

> We look for the sermon in the suicide, for the social or moral lesson in the murder of five. We interpret what we see, select the most workable of the multiple choices. We live entirely, especially if we are writers, by the imposition of a narrative line upon disparate images, by the "ideas" with which we have learned to freeze the shifting phantasmagoria which is our actual experience.[3]

For those who make a living by talking and writing about ethics, it is often easy to forget that ethics never came in flavors of deontology and consequentialism. The principles of justice and autonomy and utility are not intrinsic properties of ethical principles—or more fashionably, of a communitarian or a narrative ethics. Yet we find these useful ways of thinking about ethics because they are self-standing conceptual systems by which we can impose some sort of order upon ethical problems. But in reality, ethics does not stand apart. It is one thread in the fabric of a society, and it is intertwined with others. Ethical concepts are tied to a society's customs, manners, traditions, and institutions—all of the concepts that structure and inform the ways in which a member of that society deals with the world. When we forget this we are in danger of leaving the world of genuine moral experience for the world of moral fiction—a simplified, hypothetical creation suited less for practical difficulties than for intellectual convenience.

Theory and Practice

It is sometimes thought that the job of applied ethics is to apply normative ethical theories to particular practical problems. Recent years have shown growing dissatisfaction with such an approach, and the reason is simple: it does not work. The problems are becoming increasingly well rehearsed.[4] In the first place, as there is no shortage of ethical theories, one must be able to adjudicate among rival theories to decide which to apply to any given ethical problem. This can be difficult, especially when intuition does not incline us in a particular direction. When we do have strong moral intuitions, they are usually concerned with a particular case, and not with a theory.

Moreover, theories are tested not only against moral intuitions: they are also tested against other theories. As moral theories present problems arising out of their own internal tensions—how to mediate between conflicting moral principles, how to account for exceptions to principles—adjudicating between rival theories is usually done by appeal to tests such as clarity, economy, comprehensiveness, and coherence. But while it is obviously easier to understand and apply theories that are clear, economical, comprehensive, and coherent, it is not at all plain why we should expect a moral theory to measure up to such test, when our own moral beliefs are often genuinely unclear, uneconomical, noncomprehensive, and incoherent. To put it rather bluntly, the conflict here is one between tidiness and truth: we want our theories to be simple and elegant, but also true, and the only measure of the "moral truth" of a theory seems to be our own inconsistent, untidy moral intuitions.

But the most trying problems for ethical theorists is how we should understand the equilibrium in a particular case between our moral intuitions and the mandate of an ethical system. On the one hand, ethical theories are supposed to corroborate and justify our moral judgments, but on the other, particular judgments are also supposed to count against theories. That is, theorists expect particular moral judgments to be backed by principles and theories, but it may also be considered a failing for a theory if that theory yields an especially counterintuitive judgment. Most of us would consider it sufficient to dismiss a given ethical theory, for example, if it told us that betraying one's friends and torturing the innocent were morally obligatory. Yet why do ethical theories justify some moral judgments and not others? How are we to decide if the theory counts against the judgment, or the judgment against the theory? Our problem is understanding this practical check on ethical theory. For clearly, if a given problem does in fact yield moral disagreement, then any theory that does its job will be counterintuitive for someone, in generating a judgment that runs squarely against that person's sincerely held moral beliefs.

The practical difficulty with applying ethical theories is that ordinary people pay little attention to theories when they make their moral decisions. Moral decisions are, of course, often influenced by theories of one sort or another, but this influence is usually indirect rather than explicit. (I myself refer to no specific moral theories or doctrines in making moral judgments, but I have no illusions that these judgments are independent of the fact that I grew up as a Presbyterian in South Carolina.) What is more, the rules for moral argument in the ethics of theory seem to differ from the rules that carry weight in the ethics of ordinary life. In theory, one is likely to be criticized for making illogical jumps and deriving illegitimate conclusions. In ordinary life one persuades, cajoles, jokes, threatens, coerces, reminds, harasses, begs, and forgives. One tells stories, makes analogies, sermonizes, moralizes, holds grudges, and gets righteously indignant. This is not to say that one never behaves this way in academic ethics, of course—or that all forms of moral argument are equally valid. But one need only compare the discussion of an ethical issue in a medical journal, a theological journal, and a philosophy journal to see that even in the circumscribed world of American academe, and even in the subculture thereof that has devoted itself to discussing ethics, there are strikingly different methods of ethical argument. And the differences between the conduct of moral argumentation in ordinary experience and in academic ethics presents certain barriers to the academic who is concerned with influencing practical decisions. It is difficult to say how a theory can be applied, or even whether it should be applied, if it is alien not only in content but in structure to the way that people are accustomed to making their moral choices.

What, then, accounts for the attractiveness of moral theories? For clearly, a notion so deeply entrenched in moral philosophy cannot be entirely useless. One obvious answer is the theories' psychological appeal. This is not just to say that most of us seem to have some sort of ground-level preference for simple explanations, though there is probably some truth to that. It is also that we need to impose some degree of order on our moral judgments, and theory gives us that order. We do not need order to the degree conventionally required of a moral theory, but it would be psychologically impossible to have a completely random, unrelated, orderless set of moral judgments. We speak and think in terms of concepts, and concepts impose at least a minimal degree of order on our moral experience.[5]

But another reason for the appeal of moral theories, one that moral antifoundationalists tend to overlook, is the extent to which moral theories are genuinely helpful. Simplifying a complicated case to "autonomy versus beneficence" does tell a little lie (many little lies, in fact), but we should not ignore the truth in that simplification—or its usefulness. I can still recall the startling clarity that emerged out of the seeming chaos of numberless cases when I learned to classify them in certain ways: autonomy and beneficence, beneficence and truthtelling, acting and refraining. The simplifications eventually crumble, but it is only because the cases have first been simplified that a critique of simplification is possible. What is more, the truths carried by these simplified ways of seeing often help to sort out the problems in these cases: they capture and summarize the kinds of intuitions that we (at least we in the West) often come to when we think about such problems. It may not help a doctor "solve" an ethical problem to know that it exemplifies a conflict between beneficence and autonomy, but it does often help her clarify her own thoughts about the matter—not least because it orders and focuses a wide range of disparate intuitions.

And finally, we should not forget theory's rhetorical power. Even if a moral theory is not the sort of thing that can be rigidly "applied," it is one of the tools of rational persuasion, and thus powerful fuel for moral argument. The consistency of a moral theory may point out the inconsistencies in conventional moral thinking, which may in turn result in real changes in moral values. (Think of natural rights theory and the French and American Revolutions, or, to take a more recent example, Peter Singer's application of utilitarianism to animals.) Where we go wrong, on the other hand, is in beginning to expect more from a moral theory than it can provide.

Choosing Ethics

When we analyze ethical problems, we are able to choose the ethical principles, values, and beliefs that we think should apply to that problem and govern its resolution. Thus we tend to see ethics not as an intrinsic part of society, but as some sort of abstract system to be imposed upon, chosen by, or rejected by a society. The temptation to think of ethics in this way can be especially strong in the United States, where one is likely to encounter individuals with moral beliefs varying over a wide range. Ethics becomes a microcosm of politics, and the question, What shall I do? becomes instead, What is the best moral system for us to have?

In some cases this approach is fine—if, for instance, the question to be addressed is what sort of policy we want in general for our society, and if this is a question about which we are genuinely undecided. And it would be foolish to think that the ethical decisions of individuals in particular cases do not influence the moral values of other individuals, and thus of society in general. The question of how a particular moral judgment will affect the course of moral thinking in a society is always a legitimate one to consider. This is why, in the previously mentioned case, it is appropriate not only to consider what would be the morally best course of action, but also whether that course of action reflects the sort of policy one would like to see influencing similar decisions elsewhere. The objections of some writers to active euthanasia reflect these sorts of concerns: they recognize that euthanasia may well be the best course of action in some few, individual cases, but fear that disastrous consequences would result if active euthanasia were a widely endorsed policy.

But in other situations the notion that ethics can be chosen might be quite misleading. We do not—we cannot—choose our moral beliefs at will, and consequently a society has only very limited and indirect control over the moral values it embraces. Here the contrast between morality and politics is helpful, because some political structures, when they are not tyrannical, are to some extent the product of willful control. In a democratic society we change our laws, policies, and (less easily) our political institutions. Our moral values, on the other hand, are primarily the result of cultural factors beyond our reach. They are subject to rational scrutiny, to be sure, and are also subject to change, but, like the broader aspects of character of which moral values are a part, they are largely out of our control.

The point here is that although they are often concerned with the same problems, questions about personal moral values differ fundamentally from questions about political and institutional policy. And while ethical theories are often genuinely helpful in addressing political and institutional questions, they are much less helpful in particular cases. The reason, of course, is that while we make policy, we do not make our values. We can quite easily choose the sort of principles we think should guide general policy about, say, the allocation of scarce medical resources, or about abortion, but we cannot choose, at least not in the same way, to change people's values, nor can we simply choose the values upon which our decisions about policy are made. Values are rooted much deeper than that.

Thus it is at least in some sense misguided, even futile, to call for a "new ethics," as seems to be increasingly common nowadays—be it a communitarian ethics, a return to premodern virtue, a narrative ethics, a family or citizen ethics—if what is intended by such calls is an actual change in our society's moral values.[6] To be sure, sometimes this is not what is intended: what is meant by a new ethics is sometimes a new ethical *theory*, a call for writers and consultants in ethics to pay attention to forgotten or overlooked values. But often, it seems, the point of a call for a new ethics is to promote in moral agents some new value or new way of thinking about values—to effect real change in the values of a society. And while one small step toward changing moral values is to criticize them and call attention to new ones, we cannot simply return to an Aristotelian world view, or adopt a communitarian ethics. Such sweeping changes in a society's moral values come about only with broader changes in a society's way of life—its traditions, political institutions, family structures, and so on—changes that occur, to a disturbing degree, as a consequence of events that are rarely planned and often undesired.

Calling for a society to adopt new moral values is one way of responding to moral pluralism, as a diversity of values might be the barrier to agreement. A similar and more common way of responding is to construct moral theories that treat individuals as abstractly as possible, appealing to the broadest and most general values that they share, and then constructing a theory on the foundations of these shared values. People are replaced by rational deliberators, bundles of pure will. The solution to moral disagreement is to construct a theory based on principles to which all rational persons can agree, and which will in turn yield conclusions to which they must also agree, if they are rational and consistent.

However, while this may be an adequate approach to political (policy, institutional, legal) differences, where the aim is a minimal degree of cooperation necessary for peaceful coexistence, contemporary moral debate often seems to overlook the fact that ethics can be a very intimate affair. It involves not only respecting rights, but also such things as gratitude, hurt feelings, embarrassment, and love. These things are deeply intertwined with culture and individual character. Policy and law set boundaries for human behavior, but because morality is bound up so tightly with family ties and cultural inheritance, with character, communication, and self-perception, moral agreement requires shared values above a basic minimum. It also requires shared institutions, cultures, and traditions. Moral differences are usually settled not by simply blunting individual differences, but by becoming individuals more like each other. (For all of the hostility United States nationalism understandably arouses abroad, it at least serves this effect: it provides shared ideals that individuals of widely divergent cultural backgrounds can embrace.)

Concepts and Disagreement

It is often taken for granted that the moral concepts of a society should reflect some underlying standard of order. If they do not, it is up to those who work in ethics to point out the disorder (incoherence, inconsistency) and perhaps work at correcting it, for this lack of order is at the root of moral disagreement. For instance, when in *After Virtue* Alasdair MacIntyre argues that moral language is in a "state of grave disorder" (p.2), he cites the existence of widespread, apparently irresolvable moral disagreement as evidence. "The most striking feature of contemporary moral utterance is that so much of it is used to express disagreements: and the most striking feature of debates in which these disagreements are expressed is their interminable character" (p.6). MacIntyre goes on to suggest that the reason for the disordered state of moral discourse is that we have inherited the conceptual fragments of a multitude of moral traditions, concepts which have been severed from those traditions which ground them.[7]

Part of the appeal of Macintyre's account of moral language stems from the extent to which it is obviously true: moral disagreement grows as traditions change and as individuals of divergent cultural traditions come to live together. But part of its appeal also comes from the way it plays upon the tacit assumption, widely shared among writers in ethics, that moral beliefs and values in society should reflect standards of order of the sort we expect in a moral theory—consistency, coherence, simplicity, and so on—with the result being that disorder becomes a phenomenon that needs explanation.

But what sort of order should we expect in our moral language? Or perhaps even more importantly, what is it for a moral language to be in a state of disorder? Surely it does not mean that individuals in a society have moral beliefs that are inconsistent with each other, or that conflict with the moral beliefs of others: in the West, anyway, this seems historically to have been a fairly constant feature of moral discourse. MacIntyre compares the state of contemporary moral discourse to that of a society which, through some catastrophe, has lost all knowledge of the content and methods of science, and whose scientific discourse must therefore struggle along with remnants of scientific knowledge and methods left from the old society. The image of a disordered language of morality called up by Macintyre's scenario resembles that described by Paul Auster in his novella, *The City of Glass*, where the world, once in the state of Eden, has collapsed into confusion, leaving in disarray the language that describes it:

> Nature became detached from things: words devolved into an arbitrary collection of signs: language became severed from God . . . .
>
> For our words no longer correspond to the world. When things were whole, we felt confident that our words could express them. But little by little things have broken apart, shattered, collapsed into chaos. And yet our words have remained the same. They have not adapted themselves to the new reality. Hence, every time we try to speak of what we see, we speak falsely, distorting the very thing we are trying to represent.[8]

But surely this state of affairs, in which language has somehow remained static while the world has changed and in which human beings can barely understand each other, is not the state of contemporary moral language. Whatever moral disagreement we find in society, contemporary moral discourse allows for communication among individuals with minimal confusion as to what is *meant* when a moral judgment is expressed. When I say that active euthanasia is wrong, you may disagree, but you understand what I mean. In fact, disagreement of this sort, far from being evidence of a disordered language of morality, *presupposes* understanding between speaker and hearer about what is meant when a moral judgment is expressed. Before you can disagree with my judgment that active euthanasia is wrong, you must know what I mean when I say it.

Yet the point at which Macintyre's account goes awry contains an important clue to the extent to which we should expect order in our moral language. We should not expect our moral language to reflect the underlying standards of order we might expect of a moral theory—the standard that insists that all our moral beliefs be consistent with each other and with those of others, formulable in principles for behavior upon which all rational persons would agree. Rather, we should expect our language to meet the minimal standards of order that would allow communication and understanding among those who use it.

How much order will this be? Quite a lot, as it turns out—and this will place limits on the extent of our moral disagreement. For moral terms such as *humane*, *cruel*, *wrong*, or *perverse* to gain currency in our language, speakers must understand what the terms mean. That is, they must understand that using these words to describe actions or persons reflects a certain *attitude* on the part of the speaker. Not "just" an attitude, of course, but an attitude of a certain sort, carrying all the baggage we normally attach to moral terms, such as extreme importance, certain characteristics related to universalizability and objectivity, and so on.

Agreement as to what moral words *mean* places constraints on the things to which they can be *applied*. My understanding of what is meant by *kind* or *cruel* is determined by the sorts of things to which these words are applied by the broader community of speakers. If there were not at least some minimal overlap as to the sorts of things to which this community of speakers applies the words *cruel* and *kind*, I would be unable to learn what these words meant. Mutual understanding of the word *cruel* would be impossible if one person applied it to the practice of causing needless pain, another used it to designate the practice of punishing and rewarding only people who deserve it, and a third used it to describe self-sacrifice in the service of one's fellows. Of course, because moral words do reflect attitudes that differ from one person to the next, we will not always have *complete* agreement about what actions or persons the words should be applied to. But we must have some minimal amount of agreement about certain paradigm examples of cruelty and kindness or perversity, or else moral words would cease to be tools of communication.[9]

It is not always easy, however, to see just how moral concepts are tied to a way of life, especially when that way of life is one's own. Clifford Geertz offers an instructive example from Balinese life with the concept of *lek*, which is occasionally translated as "shame," but which Geertz says is probably closer to "stage fright." However, to understand what the Balinese mean by *lek*, one must also have some understanding of the Balinese concept of self. The western notion of the self (or at least what is sometimes called, somewhat disparagingly these days, the Enlightenment concept of the self) is roughly circumscribed, independent, free, self-governing, and (more or less) rational. The Balinese notion of the self, says Geertz, is quite different: in contrast to the independent individualism of the Western self, in Bali "anything idiosyncratic, anything characteristic of the individual merely because he is who he is physically, psychologically, or biographically, is muted in favor of his assigned place in the continuing, and, so it is thought, never-changing pattern that is Balinese life." A person is identified by various labels: birth order, caste titles, kinship markers, sex indicators. These identify him as "a determinate point in a fixed pattern, as the temporary occupant of a particular, untemporary, cultural locus." In Bali, says Geertz, life is theater. As such, "it is dramatis personae, not actors, that endure: indeed, it is dramatis personae, not actors, that in a proper sense, really exist."[10]

Lek, then, is not just shame: it is fear of exposure, that fear that "the public performance to which one's cultural location commits one will be botched and that the personality—as we would call it but the Balinese, of course, not believing in such a thing, would not—of the individual will break through to dissolve his standardized public identity." Geertz says: "When this occurs, as it sometimes does, the immediacy of the moment is felt with excruciating intensity and men become suddenly and unwillingly creatural, locked into mutual embarrassment, as though they had happened upon each other's nakedness."[11]

The point her, of course, is that a moral concept such as *lek* cannot be understood apart from the Balinese concept of selfhood, which cannot be understood apart from Balinese ritual life, which cannot be understood apart from the Hindu, Buddhist, and Polynesian religions of Bali, and so on. Moral concepts are interwoven into the moral tapestry of a life. Oddly enough, this is easier to see by looking at another culture than by looking at one's own. We look at Bali through American eyes, with American values: but to look at American life requires that we do it with equipment made from the very stuff we are trying to judge.

I once heard it said (I cannot recall where) that if you want to understand America, first understand baseball. There is some truth to that remark—some truth about baseball, to be sure, but also some truth about how American concepts and American problems are inseparable from their broader cultural context. For instance, I have found that non-Americans occasionally find it difficult to understand all the fuss over the "right to die" debate in America, and the vehemence with which it is sometimes argued. Why would anyone want to continue treating a patient in a persistent vegetative state with virtually no chance for recovery? Ah, well, I usually explain, you must also understand how the right to die is related to the right to life, and to the debate over abortion, and to American churches, and to the role of the church in small-town life: you must also understand something about American hospitals and feminism and libertarianism and fundamentalism and natural rights and John Locke and Thomas Jefferson and so on and so on, ad infinitum. To understand America, I explain, you must first understand baseball.

Pluralism and Practical Action

The difficulty with moral concepts, of course, is that when we look at them in this way, as a part of a society's form of life, they start to seem "merely" one sort of concept among many, as "only" relative to the way in which a people live. Hence relativism, hence the subjectivity of morals, and hence all the myriad debates in which moral philosophy has mired itself over the years. I believe that the constraints placed on morality by language and concepts prevent such a slide into relativism, but this is not the place to rehearse that debate. More important for our purposes is the relationship of moral pluralism to practical action. It is all very well to say that morality is embedded in a form of life, but how should we respond?

For one thing, it is important to realize that the bare fact of moral pluralism does not minimize the importance of moral conviction. Whatever else a moral judgment is, it is something we take seriously: it is no accident that we speak of moral *values*, with all the weight that word carries. And moral convictions need not be diminished by the recognition that others have moral convictions that they take equally seriously. My recognition that others have differing moral beliefs about a given problem does not require me to sit back in respectful silence. One important mechanism for dealing with moral pluralism in the West is argument and rational persuasion. After all, communal living does require a certain amount of moral agreement.

Another more obvious but less often discussed consequence of recognizing pluralism is a redirection of one's intellectual energy. If moral concepts, and thus moral problems, are dependent on a culture's institutions, then clearly one important way to deal with those problems is to deal with the institutions. Cultural institutions are highly resistant to change, and it is not always clear what changes will solve problems and what changes will create them. But can anyone doubt that a great number of the problems in medical ethics are the result, for instance, of the way American doctors and medical students are trained? Or that many of these problems are fueled by the threat of malpractice lawsuits? Or that the abortion debate could ever be resolved without some broader changes in the circumstances that make abortion seem a necessary choice to so many women?

Yet if moral concepts are bound up in a society's way of life, then unless we expect all of the institutions, customs, and traditions of that society to be ordered and systematic, we should not expect moral concepts to meet the standards that we would require of a systematic theory. Like other institutions, morality evolves in haphazard fashion, and moral disagreement inevitably emerges in response to broader societal changes. In fact, disagreement is so much a part of our notion of morality that we should reflect for a moment on what else we would lose if moral disagreement were to disappear. The results would bear little resemblance to what, at least in the West, we call morality. The concept of conscientious objection would vanish: we would have no moral reformers and no civil disobedience. We would lose the notion of one's moral ideals being self-chosen, of making up one's own mind about a matter of moral discretion. Also gone would be the idea of moral maturity, which would be replaced by conformity to moral consensus. Moral reasoning would become like mathematical reasoning: all competent adults would agree which actions are right and wrong, and moral maturity would simply be a matter of acquiring the mental skills to reason correctly.

Moral disagreement will be with us as long as there is disagreement about what way of life is best for human beings. It is not at all obvious that there is a question that is answerable, even in principle.[12] There may be no best life, only better and worse lives. And if morality is tied to a form of life, then it is a mistake to think that we can eliminate moral differences without eliminating the differences in culture, and in individuals, to which morality is tied. Though the biological characteristics humans share will mean that some lives, and some features of lives, are necessarily good or bad for human beings, there is no compelling reason, universally applicable, for adopting any one particular sort of life over all others—even if we had the choice, which we do not. For this reason, we should expect diversity in the sort of lives that people live, as well as the moral differences that inevitably follow.

QUESTIONS FOR CONSIDERATION

1. How does Elliott characterize the description of a moral problem from different individuals' points of view?
2. Why does Elliott indicate that a person's moral judgment is expressed in his or her moral description?
3. What does Elliott mean by a general, conceptual framework for particular cases? What are some problems he identifies with such a framework?
4. Elliott comments that applying normative ethical theories to practical problems simply does not work. Do you agree "that ordinary people pay little attention to theories when they make their moral decisions"?
5. How does Elliott distinguish between applying ethical principles to public policy and to particular cases? Do you agree that moral values are "the result of cultural factors beyond our reach . . . out of our control"?
6. According to Elliott, what is the value of moral language?
7. How does Elliott argue that moral pluralism does not slide into relativism?

NOTES

1. See Grant Gillett, "Women and Children First," forthcoming in *Medicine and Moral Reasoning*, B. Fullford, G. Gillett, and J. Soskice, eds. (Cambridge: Cambridge University Press, 1988); also his "Euthanasia, Letting Die and the Pause," *Journal of Medical Ethics* 14, no. 2: 61–67.

2. Nigel Barley, *Not a Hazardous Sport* (New York: Henry Holt, 1988), p. 205.

3. Joan Didion, "The White Album," in *The White Album* (New York: Penguin, 1981), p. 11.

4. See, for example, Annette Baier, "Theory and Reflective Practices," in *Postures of the Mind* (Minneapolis: University of Minnesota Press, 1984), pp. 207–27; Robert L. Holmes, "The Limited Relevance of Analytic Ethics to the Problems of Bioethics," *Journal of Medicine and Philosophy* 15, no. 2 (1990): 143–59; and especially Stuart Hampshire, *Morality and Conflict* (London: Basil Blackwell, 1983).

5. Carl Elliott, "Everything is What It Is," *Inquiry* 34 (1992): 525–38; Grant Gillett, *Reasonable Care* (Bristol: Bristol Press, 1989).

6. For instance, see Alasdair Macintyre, *After Virtue* (Notre Dame, Ind.: University of Notre Dame Press, 1981); John Hardwig, "What About the Family?" *Hastings Center Report* 20, no. 2 (1990): 5–10; Marion Danis and Larry Churchill, "Autonomy and the Commonweal," *Hastings Center Report* 21, no. 1 (1991): 25–31; Steven H. Miles and Kathryn Montgomery Hunter, "The Case: A Story Lost and Found," Commentary and Overview, *Second Opinion* 15 (November 1990): 55–57.

7. See also the excellent criticism of MacIntyre's account of moral language in Paul Johnston, *Wittgenstein and Moral Philosophy* (London: Routledge, 1989), pp. 87–89.

8. Paul Auster, *New York Trilogy: City of Glass, Ghosts, The Locked Room* (New York: Viking Penguin, 1990).

9. For a more extended discussion of this broadly Wittgensteinian account of moral language, see in Paul Johnston, *Wittgenstein and Moral Philosophy*; Grant Gillett, *Representation, Meaning, and Thought* (New York: Oxford University Press, 1992).

10. Clifford Geertz, *Local Knowledge* (New York: Basic Books, 1983), pp. 62, 63.

11. Geertz, *Local Knowledge*, p. 64.

12. The best essay that I have read on this subject, and one I have drawn on here, is Stuart Hampshire's superb "Morality and Conflict" in *Morality and Conflict* (London: Basil Blackwell, 1983).

OVERVIEW OF READINGS

Both Rachels and Callahan agree that ethics can provide answers if we maintain a "certain modesty" in our approach to difficult moral questions. Rational methods do provide a logical process for our ethical problem solving, while emotions motivate us to deeply care about moral issues. This collection of articles, taken from the pages of the *Hastings Center Report,* focus on the following ethical topics that challenge both our reasoning and our caring:

The Goals and Allocation of Medicine—includes an international study of the goals of medicine. Four goals are identified and defended. Other articles focus upon the distribution and limits of health care.

Biomedicine, Rights, and Responsibilities—examines patient autonomy in contrast to the interests of family members, health care providers, and society as a whole.

Reproductive Freedom and Responsibility—reflects the ongoing debates on the issues involving abortion.

Termination of Treatment—analyzes the effects of biomedical technologies upon the distribution, limitations, and termination of health care.

Family, Parenthood, and New Reproductive Technologies—explores the moral conflicts that arise from new reproductive technologies such as in vitro fertilization, artificial insemination, embryo transfer, surrogacy, embryodiagnosis, and frozen embryos.

Organ Procurement and Transplantation—investigates the issues surrounding the removal of human organs and tissue, including property rights and the role of consent.

Genetics, Human Nature, Human Destiny—focuses upon the accumulation and use of genetic information and upon the application of gene therapy.

Cloning Human Beings: Responding to the National Bioethics Advisory Commision's Report—provides a summary of the recommendations of the NBAC's report on human cloning and reactions to the issues raised by the report.

PART II: The Goals and Allocation of Medicine

PART II:1: The Goals of Medicine: Setting New Priorities

A HASTINGS CENTER PROJECT REPORT
Executive Summary
Setting New Priorities
Specifying the Goals of Medicine

JONATHAN M. MANN
Medicine and Public Health, Ethics and Human Rights

PART II:2: The Allocation of Medicine

NORMAN DANIELS AND JAMES E. SABIN
Last-Chance Therapies and Managed Care: Pluralism,
Fair Procedures, and Legitimacy

PAUL T. MENZEL
Rescuing Lives: Can't We Count?

BARUCH BRODY
Public Goods and Fair Prices: Balancing Technological Innovations
with Social Well-Being

Extraordinary increases in health care cost in the United States have led to attempts to contain those cost in various ways. Health maintenance organizations (HMOs) and preferred-provider insurance (PPI) limit costs by means of managed care. Managed care limits what health care providers can charge for specific treatments and may prohibit certain medical procedures. In 1990 the state of Oregon developed a health care plan that focused upon allocation and rationing. This plan provided health care to a larger number of citizens, while setting priorities regarding the treatments to be funded. Such attempts to contain costs raise questions about the overall goals of medicine and fairness in allocating health care.

Part II:1: The Goals of Medicine: Setting New Priorities

• *Executive Summary* is an introduction to an international report on the goals of medicine. Two extended excerpts from that report are included in this section. The international group leaders that participated in this study include the following: Gebhard Allert of Germany, Bela Blasszauer of Hungary, Kenneth Boyd of Scotland, Daniel Callahan of the United States, Raanan Gillon of England, Joseph Glasa of the Slovak Republic, Diego Gracia of Spain, Fernando Lolas of Chile, Maurizio Mori of Italy, Lennart Nordenfelt of Sweden, Jan Payne of the Czech Republic, Peter Rossel of Denmark, Agus Suwandono of Indonesia, Henk ten Have of The Netherlands, and Lu Weibo of China.

• *Setting New Priorities* identifies the significant changes that have been brought about by the biomedical sciences and by the practice of medicine. Problems with these changes are acknowledged in both developed and developing nations. A fresh examination of the goals of medicine is advocated.

• *Specifying the Goals of Medicine* opens by defining the key terms of health, malady, disease, illness, and sickness. Four goals of medicine are identified and defended: the prevention of disease and injury and the promotion and maintenance of health, the relief of pain and suffering caused by maladies, the care and cure of those with a malady and the care of those who cannot be cured, and the avoidance of premature death and the pursuit of a peaceful death.

• Jonathan M. Mann's *Medicine and Public Health, Ethics and Human Rights* identifies new relationships in medicine: public health and human rights, the need for an ethics of public health, and human rights and the responsibilities of medicine and the medical professional. These new relationships have emerged in response to world events such as the AIDS epidemic and humanitarian emergencies throughout the world.

Part II:2: The Allocation of Medicine

• Norman Daniels and James E. Sabin's *Last-Chance Therapies and Managed Care* examines the issues of fairness and legitimacy in health plans that determine whether patients with life-threatening diseases will receive insurance coverage for unproven treatments. Using high-dose chemotherapy with autologous bone marrow transplantation for advanced breast cancer as their primary example, Daniels and Sabin trace the history of the response of various managed care organizations to the request for coverage of the treatment. They conclude by identifying some exemplary practices in managing last-chance therapy.

• Paul T. Menzel's *Rescuing Lives: Can't We Count?* describes the conflict between multiple organ recipients and those on the waiting lists seeking a single organ. He argues that one person receiving multiple organs will result in the denial of organs for several other people.

• Baruch Brody's *Public Goods and Fair Prices: Balancing Technological Innovation with Social Well-Being* raises the questions of how government can encourage private organizations to develop new technologies (such as drugs) and how the cost of those technologies may be contained? He notes that social well-being is enhanced by providing incentives for private organizations to develop new technologies. He also argues that reasonable prices must be maintained in order for those in need to be able to afford them.

PART II:1: The Goals of Medicine: Setting New Priorities

A Hastings Center Project Report

The Goals of Medicine: Setting New Priorities

Executive Summary

Economic, social, and scientific pressures on medicine in the late twentieth century are forcing policymakers throughout the world to attempt medical and health care reform. But these efforts will fail, or not reach their full potential, unless a new light is turned on the values at the core of medicine. That is the purpose of this report.

Our premise is that the *ends* of medicine and not only its means are at stake. The biomedical revolution, and the technological innovations it has spawned, are unsurpassed in human history for their positive impact on the health of people worldwide. Yet the advances of modern medicine present a double-edged sword—longer lives have often come at the price of greater suffering, illness, and higher costs. Balancing the advantages against the disadvantages of advanced medical technology is an increasingly important priority for policymakers in both the industrialized and developing world. And in the struggle to balance their budgets, governments of countries, rich and poor, must place medicine in competition with a range of other demands for scarce resources.

The Goals of Medicine

This reality led representatives of fourteen countries—industrialized and developing, rich and less so—to question afresh the traditional goals of medicine. The goals of medicine, this group has argued, should be four. Representing the core values of medicine, they will help medicine maintain

_____ 57 _____

its integrity in the face of political and social pressures to serve anachronistic or alien purposes.

The prevention of disease and injury and promotion and maintenance of health.
The relief of pain and suffering caused by maladies.
The care and cure of those with a malady, and the care of those who cannot be cured.
The avoidance of premature death and the pursuit of a peaceful death.

Practical Aims and Implications

A fresh look at the goals of medicine makes possible a practical approach to important questions about the future priorities of biomedical research, the design of health care systems, and how physicians should be trained. A model of research should be developed that would incorporate expertise in epidemiology and public health to provide a broader understanding of various diseases in society. Efforts to develop health care systems should begin with a solid core of primary and emergency care, and consider the needs of society's most frail humans. Medical students should be taught that death is inevitable, and that they will not always be able to cure. They must learn to address the problems of chronic illness. The new physicians must also be schooled in economics, the humanities, and the organization of health care to meet the economic realities of contemporary health care systems.

Mistaken Medical Goals and the Misuse of Medical Knowledge and Skills

The uses of medical knowledge and skills are many. Most are good, but some are evil. Unacceptable uses of medical knowledge include the use of public health information to justify undemocratically coercing large groups of people into changing their "unhealthy" behaviors. At the other extreme, medicine cannot have as a goal the ultimate well-being, beyond the aim of good health, of the individual. Medicine is also incapable of determining the overall good for society.

Looking Forward

Modern interpretations of the goals of medicine leave it open to abuse or misuse. Our purpose is to examine these premises and interpret them in a new light. Regardless of the political or geographic barriers, medicine should aspire:

to be honorable and to direct its own professional life;
to be temperate and prudent;
to be affordable and economically sustainable;
to be just and equitable; and
to respect human choice and dignity.

Only the common efforts of doctors and patients, medicine and society, can shape medicine's future well and satisfyingly. The place where that effort must always begin is with the goals of medicine itself.

Setting New Priorities

Few changes in human life have been so great as those wrought by the biomedical sciences and the practice of medicine. Life expectancy has been dramatically extended. An entire range of infectious diseases has been virtually eliminated. Genetic anomalies can be detected in utero, organs transplanted, reproduction controlled, pain relieved, and bodies rehabilitated in ways unimaginable a century ago. If to the advances in biomedicine are added those broader changes occasioned by better food, water, housing, and safety conditions in many parts of the world, nothing less than a profound transformation of human life has taken place. It has changed the way human beings think about the ancient threats of disease, illness, and death. It has no less changed the way in which societies organize the provision of health care.

Yet all is by no means well with these great changes. Optimism about the imminent conquest of disease has proven deficient. Infectious disease has not in fact been eliminated, especially in the developing nations. Even in the developed countries it is staging a comeback. The chronic and degenerative diseases of aging persist. Politically and economically, every nation is confronting a growing problem in financing health care. The developed nations are finding it more difficult to pay for all the medical needs and possibilities that present themselves. Everywhere there is a growing need to control costs and achieve greater efficiency. The idea of straight-line progress has run into both scientific and economic obstacles in the wealthy nations of the world. In the developing countries, where great strides have been made in reducing infant mortality and extending average life expectancy, basic questions are being faced about the extent to which they should try to emulate the models of the developed countries, with their expensive technologies and elaborate, costly health care systems. In almost every nation there are troubling anxieties about the future of medicine and health care in the face of aging populations, rapid technological change, and ever rising public demand. The emergence of a strong movement toward patient self-determination and an equitable medicine form an important moral backdrop to these developments.

The most common response to these problems has been essentially technical or mechanistic in nature. They are perceived and dealt with as a crisis of management and organization, calling for reformed methods of financing and delivery, for political and bureaucratic change, for more research and better means of assessing medical technologies. The language of reform is ordinarily dominated by discussions of the role of the market, privatization, incentives and disincentives, cost control and cost benefit analysis, deductibles and co-payments, various budgeting and organizational schemes, centralization versus decentralization. Those are important and understandable responses, but they are not enough. They focus primarily upon the means of medicine and health care, not upon their goals and ends. The intensity of the technical discussion has, ironically, obscured the poverty of discussion about the purpose and direction of medicine.

The premise of our study was different: the ends of medicine and not only its means are at stake. Too often it seems taken for granted that the goals of medicine are well understood and self-evident, needing only sensible implementation. Our conviction, however, is that a fresh examination of those goals is now necessary. Without such a reflection, the various reform efforts going on throughout the world may fail altogether or not achieve their full potential. The economic pressures on medicine provide one strong incentive for such an examination. The great expansion of medical knowledge and understanding and the social, moral, and political problems and possibilities attendant on that expansion provide a no less important motivation.

QUESTIONS FOR CONSIDERATION

1. What are some of the profound changes brought about by the biomedical sciences and the practice of medicine? What are some of the ongoing problems?
2. What are the limitations of the technical and mechanistic responses to these problems?
3. Why is the focus upon the goals of medicine important?

Specifying the Goals of Medicine

We want now to specify what we take to be appropriate contemporary goals for medicine and, at the same time, to justify those goals and to take account of the problems of meaning and interpretation that they pose. A preliminary step is necessary, that of defining some key terms. With that step behind us, the goals can be adequately addressed under four headings: the prevention of disease and the promotion of health, the relief of pain and suffering, the treatment of disease and the care of those who cannot be cured, and the avoidance of a premature death and the promotion of a peaceful death.

Defining "Health" and Other Key Concepts

It is hardly possible to talk about the goals of medicine without, at the same time, touching upon a cluster of ideas that fill out medicine's meaning and purpose. Medicine has an interest in health, but just what is health? If one reason we become unhealthy is disease, just what is that? And if unhealthiness manifests itself in illness and sickness, just what do those terms mean? A promising way into these questions is to begin where good medicine ordinarily begins, with a focus on the person, that human being who is ill and therefore seeks to be healthy. It has long been noted that good health has a paradoxical quality to it: it is a precious good, but when present in a person it is all but invisible. We do not notice our good health because our body functions without trouble or stress; it is simply there, our quiet and faithful servant.

This experience provides the foundation for a definition: by "health" we mean the experience of well-being and integrity of mind and body. It is characterized by an acceptable absence of significant malady, and consequently by a person's ability to pursue his or her vital goals and to function in ordinary social and work contexts. By this definition we aim to stress a traditional focus on bodily wholeness and general well-working, on the absence of malfunction, and on the resultant ability or capacity to act in the world.

Our definition differs from the influential 1947 definition of the World Health Organization, with its emphasis on health as "complete physical, mental, and social well-being." It is not possible now or ever for medicine to bring about "complete" well-being, even in the sphere of the physical, with which it is most familiar. Some degree of malady is part of the life of every person at some time or other, and all will succumb to it in the end. It is no less true, happily, that some degree of good health is part of the life of most people as well, and thus its maintenance takes a high place in the ends of medicine. Health and sickness are by no means a sharp dichotomy, just as disease can have a differential impact on people's lives.

If health is the central and most decisive concept for medicine—shaping the way much of its mission will be understood—there are other important concepts as well, notably malady, disease, illness, and sickness. The term "malady" is meant to cover a variety of conditions, in addition to disease, that threaten health. They include impairment, injury, and defect. With this range of conditions in mind it is possible to define "malady" as that circumstance in which a person is suffering, or at an increased risk of suffering an evil (untimely death, pain, disability, loss of freedom or opportunity, or loss of pleasure) in the absence of a distinct external cause. The phrase "in the absence of a distinct external cause" is meant to distinguish the internal sources of malady from a continuing dependence upon causes clearly distinct from oneself (e.g., the pain caused by torture or civil violence). The harm, in short, comes from within the person, not from the outside. By a "disease" we will mean a physiological or mental malfunction based on a deviation from statistically standard norms, that brings about illness or disability or increases the chance of a premature death. By "illness" we will mean a subjective feeling on the part of a person that bodily or mental well-being is absent or impaired and thus ordinary functioning in life is impaired. By "sickness" we will mean society's perception of the health status of a person, ordinarily encompassing an outside perception that the person is not functioning well, mentally or physically.

Four Goals of Medicine

With these definitions in hand we can turn to our effort to reinterpret the goals of medicine. It should be noted at the outset that there was considerable disagreement within our group on two questions. The first was whether it is helpful or reasonable to attempt to prioritize the goals of medicine. Are some goals comparatively more important than others or logically prior to others? After considerable debate a consensus developed that it is not helpful, nor really possible, to set fixed priorities. Different people will have different health needs, and the same person may have different needs at different times during the course of the same illness. There was, in this respect, also some debate on whether it would be better to speak of the "core values" of medicine rather than the goals of medicine, or to see the "goals" more as regulative ideals to be sought rather than formal goals. On the whole, it was agreed that the language of goals remains useful.

Part of the debate over prioritizing goals turned on a second question, that of the status to be assigned to health promotion and disease prevention as a goal of medicine. There was full agreement on the importance of health promotion and disease prevention. But since they require strategies that move well outside of the medical arena, and since too high a priority for primary prevention at least could seem to imply an abandonment of sick people, there was resistance to giving it even a logical priority. We want, then, only to stress its importance, which is true as well of the other goals we specify. We give none a fixed priority, and each will have a greater or lesser importance under different circumstances.

The Prevention of Disease and Injury and the Promotion and Maintenance of Health

Health promotion and disease prevention are core medical values for three reasons. First, common sense says that it is preferable to avoid disease and injury where that is possible. A primary duty of physicians and those who work with them will be to help patients stay well and to educate them in the best means to do so. Some would claim that physicians who help their patients remain healthy do them as great a service as those who care for them after injury, disease, and disability have occurred. The importance of health promotion in the case of children, who still die at a high rate in many parts of the world, can scarcely be exaggerated. An ancient aim of medicine has been to help people live more harmoniously with their environment, an aim that must be pursued from the beginning of life to its very end. Our group felt compelled to stress one instance of disease prevention in particular: the enormous danger to health posed by tobacco, and the need to educate the young so they will not start on its use, and older people to give up its use.

Second, there is accumulating, though not uncontroverted, evidence that some efforts to promote health and prevent disease will have beneficial economic consequences by reducing the extent and burden of morbidity and chronic disease later in life. At the same time, even if not inexpensive, such efforts are cost-effective ways of maintaining health. So too, a heavier emphasis on promotion and prevention can deflect interest away from dependence on high-technology, acute care rescue medicine and help reduce the sometimes excessive dominance and glamour of the latter.

Third, it is important to convey to the medical profession and the general public that medicine is more than a discipline that only rescues and works with those already sick, and that health care systems are more than simply "sick-care systems." To give a high place to health promotion and disease prevention would signal to everyone, within and outside of medicine, that considerable social and individual benefits would flow from a far stronger emphasis here.

In arguing for health promotion and disease prevention as a basic goal of medicine, we do not want to minimize two points: death can only be postponed, not conquered; and disease in general cannot be overcome, only some diseases, which in turn will be replaced by other diseases in the lives of people. The prevention of disease can, therefore, never be given an absolute priority over other medical goals. Everyone will eventually become ill, or be injured or disabled, and at that time the other goals of medicine will come to the fore.

Beyond those provisos, many obstacles stand in the way of health promotion and disease prevention. There is a dearth of good data on the full costs of health promotion programs and their cost-benefit ratios. It has sometimes also been argued that since the primary determinants of health status are income, class, education, and general social opportunities, there is little that medicine as such can do to make a significant difference to population health. It can at best only provide relief after people are sick. In the same vein, it has been contended that too intent a focus on influencing and changing individual behavior can amount to "blaming the victim," as if that behavior were the ultimate cause of bad health. Does not a public health perspective show that social factors are far more important than individual behavior in causing disease, and do not genetic and other forms of medical knowledge show that there are usually important genetic links in the expression of disease in individuals?

These are not irreconcilable viewpoints. While good data on cost-benefit ratios is important, there is no reason to single out health promotion for skepticism any more than any other part of medicine. As for the problem of "blaming the victim," even in the face of strong social pressures, individuals can and do change their health behaviors, whether to stop smoking, control drinking, lose weight, or begin to exercise. Individual behavior is the variable through which, in any case, much social influence is filtered. Even if total individual change is not possible or at least likely in many cases, from an economic and personal angle even relatively small changes can make a real difference. It should also be obvious that cultural differences, of a kind that can be changed for better or worse, significantly influence individual behavior.

Perhaps most important, by treating disease prevention and health promotion as core values in medicine no less than in public health, it might be possible in the years ahead to bring into closer working relationship two critical fields of health care medicine and public health—that too long have worked separately, often in competition with each other. Greater cooperation between them is badly needed. Public health is well positioned (when adequately supported financially) through its epidemiological capacities to track patterns of disease, accident, and disability and to make that knowledge available to physicians. Medicine, because of its access to and focus upon individual patients, is in a unique position to counsel them, and through family histories, testing, and other techniques, to identify those most at risk for disease. The more that public health and clinical medicine can coordinate their skills, the better off both will be. A sensitive approach to health promotion will be sharply aware of the importance of background living conditions—economic, occupational, and social—on health status. Medicine can and should therefore better integrate its efforts with other welfare-oriented social and government institutions.

The Relief of Pain and Suffering Caused by Maladies

While there are diseases, such as high blood pressure, that produce no immediate symptoms, most people seek the ministrations of medicine for the relief of pain and suffering. Their bodies hurt in some way and they want help, or they are psychologically burdened and seek relief; and often both pain and suffering are experienced together. Pain and suffering, however, while often joined in a patient, are not necessarily the same. Pain refers to extreme physical distress and comes in many varieties: throbbing, piercing, burning. Suffering, by contrast, refers to a state of psychological burden or oppression, typically marked by fear, dread, or anxiety. Severe and unrelenting pain can be a source of suffering, but pain does not always lead to suffering (particularly if the patient knows it is temporary or part of an eventual cure). Nor does suffering always entail pain: much of the suffering of mental illness, or simply the ordinary fears of life, does not necessarily include physical pain.

The relief of pain and suffering is among the most ancient duties of the physician and a traditional goal of medicine. For a number of reasons, however, contemporary medicine throughout the world often does not adequately meet that goal. For many years, studies have shown that physicians vary in how well they understand and practice the palliation of pain. Inadequate or inappropriate palliation is still all too common. That failure is often exacerbated by laws or customs concerning narcotics that intimidate physicians from making the best use of modern methods of palliation. In many parts of the world, the necessary narcotics are not even available; and ironically, this may be the case in countries that manage to find some money for expensive technological treatments, as in the case of cancer chemotherapy. In both the developed and developing countries, there are great inadequacies in education on pain relief, in the application of available knowledge, and in the medical and cultural support needed to make decent relief routinely available. Palliative care medicine is an emerging field of great importance, dealing with a complex and not yet fully understood subject. It should be well supported and vigorously advanced.

The relief of suffering is in no better a state. Even if there is a good knowledge of effective pharmacological approaches to pain relief, the mental and emotional suffering that can accompany illness is often not recognized or treated properly. Drugs are too often depended upon to do the work that more properly requires counseling and empathy. The failure of some physicians to take their point of departure from the patient as a whole person, not merely as a collection of organs, means that psychological suffering may be overlooked altogether or considered unimportant if noticed.

At a minimum, the failure here is to understand that the fear of bad health, of disease and illness, can often cause as much suffering as their reality. The threat that possible pain, disease, or injury represents to the self can be profound, equaling their actual effects on the body; and physicians are appropriately called upon to help allay such anxieties. It is perfectly plausible to speak of illness without disease, to capture a range of conditions and experience not reducible to organic failings. A holistic perspective on health will help to lay a new foundation for the care of that 50 percent or so of patients who need help but manifest none of the clinical symptoms of disease.

Of profound importance is the suffering occasioned by mental health problems, from severe conditions such as schizophrenia or depression to the milder, but still serious problems of the neuroses, phobias, and character disorders. Not all problems of mental health have disease as their cause, and it is important not to require a biological basis to justify taking mental health problems seriously. The full range of mental health conditions, well recognized medically, affects millions of people throughout the world. Even so, because their initial symptoms may be diffuse or undifferentiated expressions of suffering, mental health problems are too frequently ignored or minimized in primary health care settings, where the tendency is strong to look principally for conditions with clear disease pathologies.

The disparity between subsidized care for the physically ill, and the often more limited health care for the mentally ill signifies a lingering stereotype: that mental illness is less important than physical illness. Mental illness can, in fact, impose every bit as much suffering and disability as physical maladies. It is important, moreover, that there be a good medical understanding of the difference between disease conditions with an organic basis and those functional conditions that may express harmful social conditions. And medicine must recognize that many forms of human suffering—war, violence, the betrayal of trust—have nothing to do in their causes with poor health or disease.

How far should medicine go in the relief of suffering? Our group was divided, for instance, on the issue of euthanasia and physician-assisted suicide both historically forbidden by most medical ethics—as a medical response to the suffering of those who are terminally or incurably ill. It was agreed, nonetheless, that the issue will be important in the years ahead as medicine works to better understand its duties, and the limits of those duties, toward those who suffer. Some of the suffering that attends disease is readily understood to be a response to the disease itself. It can cause fear, despair, a profound sense of fatigue, anxiety about the future, and a sense of great futility and helplessness. To these the physician and other health care workers should respond with caring and empathy and, where possible, counseling. But some suffering, particularly when connected with a chronic or terminal condition, can raise for patients questions about the meaning of life itself, of good and evil, of personal fate and destiny—questions commonly thought of as spiritual or philosophical, not medical, in nature.

Why am I sick? Why must I die? What is the point of my suffering? Medicine, as such, can offer no answers to such questions; they are not in its domain. And yet, as human beings, physicians and nurses will be looked to for some kind of response. Here, we suggest, the caregiver will have to call upon his or her own experience and perception of the world, simply being one human being with another human being, looking not only to medical knowledge but also to compassion and fellow-feeling. At times, however, even the most empathetic caring and the most advanced palliative care will reach their limit. Here medicine will have to recognize its own boundaries; not all of life can be controlled or managed by a medicine as finite in its possibilities as those human beings it serves are finite in theirs.

The Care and Cure of Those with a Malady, and the Care of Those Who Cannot Be Cured

People typically turn to medicine because they feel ill, have been injured, or because they are impaired mentally or physically. Medicine, for its part, responds by looking for a cause of the malady, the characteristic presumption being that it may be found in an injured or diseased organ or limb. When that proves to be the case, medicine seeks to cure the malady and return a patient to a state of normal well-being and function. Yet people do not ordinarily present doctors with diseased organs, even if they know or suspect that is why they feel ill. Patients usually seek something more than cure only; they look for empathy and understanding. Patients as persons bring illness and injury to doctors; that is what they most directly experience subjectively and what most ordinarily motivates them to seek relief. They present themselves, and it is from those selves that cure and care should take their point of departure.

In its eagerness to cure patients, modern medicine has sometimes neglected its caring function—as if to say that, if cure might be found, who needs caring? That way of thinking is profoundly mistaken. In many cases, to be sure, utterly impersonal technique is acceptable enough, even a virtue, as in emergency tracheotomies, cardiopulmonary resuscitation, and many forms of high-technology surgery. But far more common is the need for caring. Caring is not simply the manifestation of concern, empathy, and a willingness to talk with patients. It is also a capacity to talk and listen in a way that is cognizant of those supportive social and welfare services needed to help people and their families cope with the wide range of nonmedical problems that can and usually will accompany their illness. Of necessity, good caring demands technical excellence as a crucial ingredient.

A sick parent unable to care properly for his children may suffer far more from that situation than directly from his disease, just as the spouse caring for someone with Alzheimer's may be as much in need of help as the patient herself. The healing function of medicine encompasses both curing and caring, and healing may in a broader sense be possible even in those cases where medicine cannot cure. It can heal by helping a person cope effectively with permanent maladies.

Rehabilitation is an important and growing part of modern medicine, stimulated by the development of many means of enabling injured or diseased patients to regain vital functions and be enabled to return to society. It is a form of medicine that falls somewhere between curing and caring: it may in some cases restore normal function, in other cases do so only partly, and in some cases help to slow down progressive degeneration. Either way, rehabilitation ordinarily requires a great deal of time and attention to be successful, and in that respect needs a strong and sustained spirit of caring and social support. Healing is a very real possibility even when the body cannot be restored to a well-functioning state.

In aging societies, where chronic disease is the most common cause of pain, suffering, and death where, in other words, the illness will continue over time regardless of what is done medically—caring becomes all the more important, coming back into its own after an era in which it always seemed a second-best choice. In cases of chronic illness patients must be helped to make personal sense of their condition, and helped to learn how to cope with it and live with it, perhaps permanently. By their sixties, most people will have at least one chronic condition, and by their eighties, three or more. For those over eighty-five, at least half will need some significant help in carrying out the ordinary activities of daily living. Because the chronically ill must learn to adapt to a new and altered self, much of the work of the medical professional must focus on the management, not the cure, of disease, and in this case "management" should mean the empathetic and continuing psychological care of a person who must, one way or another, come to terms with the reality of illness. It has indeed been noted that medicine may have to help the chronically ill person forge a new identity.

This is hardly a situation restricted to the elderly, even if they are likely to be the most numerous among the chronically ill. Those with AIDS, or disabled children, or injured young adults, will no less need care. Indeed, the very success of medicine in saving lives—whether low birthweight babies at the beginning of life, or nonagenarians at the end of life—has increased, not decreased, the overall burden of morbidity. People are now able to live with illnesses, sometimes well and sometimes not, that would have killed them a generation or two ago. They are, consequently, not only candidates for more curative medicine, but just as surely candidates for more caring medicine.

The Avoidance of Premature Death and the Pursuit of a Peaceful Death

The struggle against death in many of its manifestations is an important goal of medicine. Yet it should always remain in a healthy tension with medicine's duty to accept death as the destiny of all human beings. Medical treatment should be provided in ways that enhance, rather than threaten, the possibility of a peaceful death. Contemporary medicine, unfortunately, has too often treated death as the supreme enemy. This it has done by giving lethal disease too high a proportion of research money, by sometimes extending life beyond any point of human benefit, and by woefully neglecting the humane care of the dying—as if the dying patient had forfeited medicine's claim to attention, human presence, and effective palliation.

Avoiding premature death. In medicine's struggle against death, an appropriate aim first and foremost is to reduce premature death, in populations generally and individuals particularly. A secondary purpose is to care appropriately for those whose deaths would no longer be considered premature, but who could nonetheless benefit from medical treatment. It will, broadly speaking, be the primary duty of medicine and health care systems to help the young become old, and then, that accomplished, to help those who are old live out the remainder of their lives in dignity and comfort.

The notion of a "premature" death will be relative to history, culture, and the state of available medical knowledge, skills, and technology. A premature death may be said generally to take place when a person dies before having had an opportunity to experience the main possibilities of a characteristically human life cycle: the chance to pursue and gain knowledge, to enter into close and loving relationships with others, to see one's family or other dependents safely into their own adulthood or independence, to be able to work or otherwise develop one's individual talents and pursue one's life goals, and, most broadly, to have the chance and capacity for personal flourishing. Within an individual life cycle a death may be premature if, even at an advanced age, life could be preserved or extended with no great burden on the individual or society.

If avoiding premature death should be a high goal for medicine, it would be a mistake to act as if all death is premature, no less than to overemphasize eliminating death at the expense of other important health needs. The pursuit of increased life expectancy for its own sake does not seem an appropriate medical goal. The average life expectancy in the developed countries allows citizens a full life, even if many of them might like longer lives. This is surely not an unacceptable personal goal, but given the costs and difficulties of achieving significant additional gains through technological innovation, it is doubtful that this is a valid global or national goal, or a goal for medical research more generally.

Pursuing a peaceful death. Since death will come to all, and the patients of every doctor must eventually die as surely as the doctor herself, medicine must give a high place to creating those clinical circumstances in which a peaceful death is most likely. A peaceful death can be defined as one in which pain and suffering are minimized by adequate palliation, in which patients are never abandoned or neglected, and in which the care of those who will not survive is counted as important as the care of those who will survive. Medicine can of course never fully guarantee a peaceful death nor can it be responsible for what people bring to their own dying. But medicine can avoid treating death as if it is an avoidable biological accident, a medical failure. Death is, as it has always been, the inevitable outcome, sooner or later, of even the best medical treatment. At some point in every life, life-sustaining treatment will be futile; the final limit of medical skills will be reached. Thus the humane management of death is the final and perhaps most humanly demanding responsibility of the physician, who is forced to recognize in her patient both her own fate and the inherent limitations of the science and art of medicine, whose compass is mortal, not immortal, beings.

Terminating life-sustaining treatment. Modern medicine has made death a more, not less, complex problem. In the face of medical progress and constantly changing technology, every society will have to work out moral and medical standards for the appropriate cessation of life-sustaining medical treatment of the terminally ill. It is important that patients and families have a significant role in such decisions when possible. Criteria for the cessation of treatment will include the burden of the treatment upon the patient, the likely benefit of the treatment in sustaining a kind of life acceptable to the patient, and the availability of resources to carry out aggressive acute care procedures. The demands upon the physician, given his great power in this circumstance, can be considerable: to balance patient needs and medical integrity and to facilitate a peaceful death. The appropriate goal of medicine in such cases is to promote the welfare of the patient, to sustain life where possible and reasonable, but to recognize that because of its necessary place in the human life cycle, death as such is not to be understood as the enemy. It is death at the wrong time (too early in life), for the wrong reasons (medically avoidable or treatable at a reasonable cost), and coming to the patient in the wrong way (full of relievable pain and suffering and excessively prolonged) that are the appropriate enemies.

QUESTIONS FOR CONSIDERATION

1. How do the authors define the following terms: health, malady, disease, illness, and sickness?

2. What are the three justifications for the goal of the prevention of disease and the promotion of health? What are the limitations on the medical profession in achieving this goal?

3. How can public health and clinical medicine cooperate in achieving this goal?

4. In addressing the goal of the relief of pain and suffering caused by maladies, how is pain contrasted with suffering?

5. How do the authors criticize contemporary medicine regarding the relief of pain and suffering? What is needed to improve palliative care?

6. What is the role of care in the cure of those with a malady and those who cannot be cured? How is this care uniquely extended to the aging, those with AIDS, disabled children, and injured young adults?

7. What is the healthy tension between avoiding a premature death and the pursuit of a peaceful death?
8. How do the authors characterize a premature death?
9. How can medicine assist in achieving a peaceful death?
10. What are the implications for terminating life-sustaining treatments in achieving a peaceful death?

Jonathan M. Mann

Medicine and Public Health, Ethics and Human Rights

The relationships among medicine, public health, ethics, and human rights are now evolving rapidly, in response to a series of events, experiences, and struggles. These include the shock of the worldwide epidemic of human immunodeficiency virus and AIDS, continuing work on diverse aspects of women's health, and challenges exemplified by the complex humanitarian emergencies of Somalia, Iraq, Bosnia, Rwanda, and now, Zaire.

From among the many impacts of these experiences, three seem particularly salient. First, human rights thinking and action have become much more closely allied to, and even integrated with, public health work. Second, the long-standing absence of an ethics of public health has been highlighted. Third, the human rights-related roles and responsibilities of physicians and other medical workers are receiving increased attention.

Public Health and Medicine

To explore the first of these issues—the connections between human rights and public health—it is essential to review several central elements of modern public health.

Medicine and public health are two complementary and interacting approaches for promoting and protecting health—defined by the World Health Organization (WHO) as a state of physical, mental, and social well-being. Yet medicine and public health can, and also must be differentiated, because in several important ways they are not the same. The fundamental difference involves the population emphasis of public health, which contrasts with the essentially individual focus of medical care. Public health identifies and measures threats to the health of populations, develops governmental policies in response to these concerns, and seeks to assure certain health and related services. In contrast, medical care focuses upon individuals—diagnosis, treatment, relief of suffering, and rehabilitation.

Several specific points follow from this essential difference. For example, different instruments are called for: while public health measures population health status through epidemiological, survey, and other statistically based methods, medicine examines biophysical and psychological status using a combination of techniques, including dialogue, physical examination, and laboratory study of the individual. Public health generally values most highly (or at least is supposed to) primary prevention, that is, preventing the adverse health event in the first place, such as helping to prevent the automobile accident or the lead poisoning from happening at all. In contrast, medicine generally responds to existing health conditions, in the context of either secondary or tertiary prevention. Secondary prevention involves avoiding or delaying the adverse impact of a health condition like hypertension or diabetes. Thus, while the hypertension or insulin deficiency exists, its effects, such as heart disease, kidney failure, or blindness, can be avoided or delayed. So-called tertiary prevention involves those efforts to help sustain maximal functional and psychological capacity despite the presence of both the disease, such as hypertension, and its outcomes, heart disease, stroke, or kidney failure.

Accordingly, the skills and expertise needed in public health include epidemiology, biostatistics, policy analysis, economics, sociology, and other behavioral sciences. In contrast, medical skills and expertise center on the exploration, analysis, and response to the biophysical status of individuals, based principally on an understanding of biology, biochemistry, immunology, pharmacology, pathology, pathophysiology, anatomy, and psychology.

Naturally, the settings in which public health and medicine operate also differ: governmental organizations, large-scale public programs, and various fora associated with developing and implementing public policy are inherently part of public health, while private medical offices, clinics, and medical care facilities of varying complexity and sophistication are the settings in which medical care is generally provided. Finally, the relationship between the profession and the people with whom it deals differs: in a sense, public health comes to you, while you go to the doctor. And expectations associated with each domain differ: from medicine, individual care and treatment are sought; from public health, protection against broad health threats like epidemic disease, unsafe water, or chemical pollution is expected.

Therefore, public health and medicine are principally distinguished by their focus on collectivities or on individuals, respectively, with a series of subsidiary differences involving methods of work, systems of analysis and measurement, emphasis on primary versus secondary or tertiary prevention, types of expertise and relevant skill, settings in which work is conducted, and client/public relationships and expectations.

Yet obviously, there is substantial overlap. Public health requires a sound biomedical basis, and involves many medical practitioners, whose services are organized in settings such as maternal and child health clinics, or immunization programs. Also, medical practice operates within a context highly influenced and governed by law and public policy. The potentially fluid relationship between public health and medicine is further suggested by recent proposals in this country that certain traditional public health functions be delegated to the private medical sector.

Despite these many differences, people equate medical care with health. Certainly, this basic confusion has informed the recent discussions of health care in the United States; and coverage of health issues in the popular press around the world reflects this perspective, in which access to medical care and the quality of that care are seen as the principal health needs of individuals and populations.

Medicine and Health

Yet the contribution of medicine to health, while undeniably important (and vital in certain situations), is actually quite limited. For example, it is estimated that only about one-sixth of the years of life expectancy gained in this country during this century can be attributed to the beneficial impact of medicine, medical care, and medical research. And it has been estimated that only about 10 percent of preventable premature deaths are associated with a lack of medical care. Similarly, the World Bank has estimated that a lack of essential clinical services is responsible for between 11 and 24 percent of the global burden of disease. Of course, none of these data, including also the notable decline in diseases like tuberculosis well before antimycobacterial therapy became available, suggest that medical care is irrelevant; rather, they suggest its limits.

In 1988, the United States' Institute of Medicine defined the mission of public health as "ensuring the conditions in which people can be healthy." This profound definition begs the most vital question for public health, namely, what are these essential conditions in which people can best achieve the highest possible level of physical, mental, and social well-being? If not medical care— its availability and quality—then what?

The vast majority of research into the health of populations identifies so-called "societal factors" as the major determinants of health status. Most of the work in this area has focused on socioeconomic status as the key variable, for it is clear, throughout history and in all societies, that the rich live generally longer and healthier lives than the poor. Thus, in the United Kingdom in 1911, the age-adjusted standardized mortality rate among members of the lowest social class was 1.6 times higher than for the highest social class. Interestingly, following creation of the National Health Services to ensure full access to medical care, and despite a dramatic change in major causes of death (from mainly infectious to mainly chronic diseases), in 1981 this societal gradient not only persisted, but increased, to a 2.1-fold higher standardized mortality rate among the lowest compared with the highest social class.

A major question arising from the socioeconomic status-health gradient is why there is a gradient. For example, among over 10,000 British civil servants followed for many years, health status and longevity were better for each successive category of civil servants, from lowest to highest. This raises two issues: first, while we believe we can—at least intuitively explain poor health among the destitute when compared with the rich, associated with a lack of good food, housing, and with poor sanitary conditions, even the lowest class of British civil servants cannot be considered poor. Secondly, why should the civil servants in the next-to-highest group, living in quite comfortable circumstances, experience poorer health than the highest group?

Beyond these unanswered issues, many recent studies have pointed to the limited explanatory power of socioeconomic status, generally measured in terms of current income, years of education, and job classification. Other measures, such as the extent of socioeconomic inequality within a community, the nature, level, and temporal pattern of unemployment, societal connectedness and the extent of involvement in social networks, marital status, early childhood experiences, and exposure to dignity-denying situations have all been suggested as powerful potential components of a "black box" of societal factors whose dominant role in determining levels of preventable disease, disability, and premature death is beyond dispute.[1]

An Ethics for Public Health

Public health, although it began as a social movement, has—at least in recent years—responded relatively little to this most profound and vital knowledge about the dominant impact of society on health. To illustrate: we all know that certain behaviors have an enormous impact on health, such as cigarette smoking, excess alcohol intake, dietary choices, or levels of exercise and physical fitness. How these behaviors are conceptualized determines how they will be addressed by public health. The basic question is whether and to what extent these behaviors can be considered, and therefore responded to, as isolated individual choices.

The curve represented in Figure 1 (replicable among public health practitioners in at least three countries) [Figure 1 not shown] reflects a strong belief that important health-related behaviors are substantially influenced by societal factors and context. Yet examining public health programs designed to address the health problems associated with these same behaviors reveals that they generally consist of activities which assume that individuals have essentially complete control over their health-related behaviors. Traditional public health seeks to provide individuals with information and education about risks associated with diet or lack of exercise, along with various clinic-based services such as counseling, or distribution of condoms and other contraceptives. However, while public health may cite, or blame, or otherwise identify the societal-level or contextual issues—which it acknowledges to be of dominant importance, both in influencing individual behavior and for determining health status more broadly—it does not deal directly with these societal factors.

At least three reasons for this paradoxical inaction may be proposed. First, public health has lacked a conceptual framework for identifying and analyzing the essential societal factors that represent the "conditions in which people can be healthy." Second, a related problem: public health lacks a vocabulary with which to speak about and identify commonalities among health problems experienced by very different populations. Third, there is no consensus about the nature or direction of societal change that would be necessary to address the societal conditions involved. Lacking a coherent conceptual framework, a consistent vocabulary, and consensus about societal change, public health assembles and then tries valiantly to assimilate a wide variety of disciplinary perspectives, from economists, political scientists, social and behavioral scientists, health systems analysts, and a range of medical practitioners. Yet while each of these perspectives provides some useful insight, public health becomes thereby a little bit of everything and thus not enough of anything.

With this background in mind, it would be expected that in the domains of public health and medicine, different, yet complementary languages for describing and incorporating values would be developed. For even when values are shared at a higher level of abstraction, the forms in which they are expressed, the settings in which they are evoked, and their practical application may differ widely.

Not surprisingly, medicine has chosen the language of ethics, as ethics has been developed in a context of individual relationships, and is well adapted to the nature, practice, settings, and expectations of medical care. The language of medical ethics has also been applied when medicine seeks to deal with issues such as the organization of medical care or the allocation of societal resources. However, the contribution of medical ethics to these societal issues has been less powerful when compared, for example, with its engagement in the behavior of individual medical practitioners.

Public health, at least in its contemporary form, is struggling to define and articulate its core values. In this context, the usefulness of the language and structure of ethics as we know it today has been questioned. Given its population focus, and its interest in the underlying conditions upon which health is predicated (and that these major determinants of health status are societal in nature), it seems evident that a framework which expresses fundamental values in societal terms, and a vocabulary of values which links directly with societal structure and function, may be better adapted to the work of public health than a more individually oriented ethical framework.

For this reason, modern human rights, precisely because they were initially developed entirely outside the health domain and seek to articulate the societal preconditions for human well-being, seem a far more useful framework, vocabulary, and form of guidance for public health efforts to analyze and respond directly to the societal determinants of health than any inherited from the past biomedical or public health tradition.

Public Health and Human Rights

The linkage between public health and human rights can be explored further by considering three relationships. The first focuses on the potential burden on human rights created by public health policies, programs, and practices. As public health generally involves direct or indirect state action, public health officials represent the state power toward which classical human rights concerns are traditionally addressed. Thus, in the modern world, public health officials have, for the first time, two fundamental responsibilities to the public: to protect and promote public health, and to protect and promote human rights. While public health officials may be unlikely to seek deliberately to violate human rights, there is great unawareness of human rights concepts and norms among public health practitioners. In stark contrast to the large number of bioethics courses available in medical educational settings, a recent survey of all twenty-eight accredited schools of public health in the United States and schools of public health in thirty-four other countries identified only seven formal courses in human rights for the presumed future leaders of public health.

Public health practice is heavily burdened by the problem of inadvertent discrimination. For example, outreach activities may "assume" that all populations are reached equally by a single, dominant-language message on television; or analysis "forgets" to include health problems uniquely relevant to certain groups, like breast cancer or sickle cell disease; or a program "ignores" the actual response capability of different population groups, as when lead poisoning warnings are given without concern for financial ability to ensure lead abatement. Indeed, inadvertent discrimination is so prevalent that all public health policies and programs should be considered discriminatory until proven otherwise, placing the burden on public health to affirm and ensure its respect for human rights.

In addition, in public health circles there is often an unspoken sense that public health and human rights concerns are inherently confrontational. At times, this has been true. In the early years of the HIV epidemic, the knee-jerk response of various public health officials to invoke mandatory testing, quarantine, and isolation did create a major clash with protectors of human rights. Even quite recently, an opinion piece in the *British Medical Journal* purports that excessive respect for human rights crippled public health efforts and is therefore responsible for the intensifying and expanding AIDS epidemic.

However, while modern human rights explicitly acknowledges that public health is a legitimate reason for limiting rights, more recently the underlying complementarity rather than inherent confrontation between public health and human rights has been emphasized. Again in the context of AIDS, public health has learned that discrimination toward HIV-infected people and people with AIDS is counterproductive. Specifically, when people found to be infected were deprived of employment, education, or ability to marry and travel, participation in prevention programs diminished. Thus, recent attention has been directed to a negotiation process for optimizing both the achievement of complementary public health goals and respect for human rights norms.

A second relationship between public health and human rights derives from the observation that human rights violations have health impacts, that is, adverse effects on physical, mental, and social well-being. For some rights, such as the right not to be tortured or imprisoned under inhumane conditions, the health damage seems evident, indeed inherent in the rights violation. However, even for torture, only more recently has the extensive, life-long, family and communitywide, and transgenerational impact of torture been recognized.

For many other rights, such as the right to information, to assembly, or to association, health impacts resulting from violation may not be initially so apparent. The violation of any right has measurable impacts on physical, mental, and social well-being; yet these health effects still remain, in large part, to be discovered and documented. Yet gradually, the connection is being established.

The right to association provides a useful example of this relationship. Public health benefits substantially—even requires—involvement of people in addressing problems that affect them. Because the ability of people concerned about a health problem to get together, talk, and search for effective solutions is so essential to public health, wherever the right to association is restricted, public health suffers. Taking a positive example from the history of HIV/AIDS: needle exchange—the trading-in of needles used for drug injection for clean needles, so as to avoid needle-sharing with consequent risk of HIV transmission—was invented by a union of drug users in Amsterdam. Needle exchange was a classic example of an innovative, local response to a pressing local problem. Needle exchange was not and would have been highly unlikely to have been developed by academics, government officials, or hired consultants! Yet the creative solution of needle exchange and respect for the right of association are closely linked. Thus, in societies in which people generally, or specific population groups, cannot associate around health, or other issues, such as injection drug users in the United States, or sex workers, or gay and lesbian people in many countries, local solutions are less able to emerge or be applied and public health is correspondingly compromised.

A third relationship between health and human rights has already been suggested; namely, that promoting and protecting human rights is inextricably linked with promoting and protecting health. Once again, this is because human rights offers a societal-level framework for identifying and responding to the underlying—societal—determinants of health. It is important to emphasize that human rights are respected not only for their instrumental value in contributing to public health goals, but for themselves, as societal goods of preeminent importance.

For example, a cluster of rights, including the rights to health, bodily integrity, privacy, information, education, and equal rights in marriage and divorce, have been called "reproductive rights," insofar as their realization (or violation) is now understood to play a major role in determining reproductive health. From an early focus on demographic targets for population control, to an emphasis on ensuring "informed consent" of women to various contraceptive methods, a new paradigm for population policies and reproductive health has recently emerged. Articulated most forcefully at the United Nations Conference on Population and Development in 1994 in Cairo, the focus has shifted to ensuring that women can make and effectuate real and informed choices about reproduction. And in turn, this is widely acknowledged to depend on realization of human rights.

Similarly, in the context of HIV/AIDS, vulnerability to the epidemic has now been associated with the extent of realization of human rights. For as the HIV epidemic matures and evolves within each community and country, it focuses inexorably on those groups who, before HIV/AIDS arrived, were already discriminated against, marginalized, and stigmatized within each society. Thus, in the United States the brunt of the epidemic today is among racial and ethnic minority populations, inner city poor, injection drug users, and, especially, women in these communities. In Brazil, an epidemic that started among the jet set of Rio and Sao Paulo with time has become a major epidemic among the slum-dwellers in the favelas of Brazil's cities. The French, with characteristic linguistic precision, identify the major burden of HIV/ AIDS to exist among "les exclus," those living at the margins of society. Now that a lack of respect for human rights has been identified as a societal level risk factor for HIV/AIDS vulnerability, HIV prevention efforts—for example, for women—are starting to go beyond traditional educational and service-based efforts to address the rights issues that will be a precondition for greater progress against the epidemic.

Ultimately, ethics and human rights derive from a set of quite similar, if not identical, core values. As with medicine and public health, rather than seeing human rights and ethics as conflicting domains, it seems more appropriate to consider a continuum, in which human rights is a language most useful for guiding societal level analysis and work, while ethics is a language most useful for guiding individual behavior. From this perspective, and precisely because public health must be centrally concerned with the structure and function of society, the language of human rights is extremely useful for expressing, considering, and incorporating values into public health analysis and response.

Thus, public health work requires both ethics applicable to the individual public health practitioner and a human rights framework to guide public health in its societal analysis and response.

At the hypothetical extreme of individual medical care, ethics would be the most useful language. However, to the extent that the individual practitioner is cognizant of the societal forces acting upon the individual patient, societal level considerations may also be articulated in human rights terms. At the other extreme of public health, human rights is the most useful language, speaking as it does directly to the societal level determinants of well-being. Nevertheless, the ethical framework remains critical, for public health is carried out by individuals within specific professional roles and competencies.

In practice, of course, positions between the hypothetical extremes of medicine and public health are more common, calling for mixtures of human rights and ethical concepts and language.

Professional Roles and Responsibilities

The placement of both human rights and ethics and public health and medicine at ends of a continuum suggests also that the interest domains of individuals and organizations can be "mapped", and areas calling for additional attention can be highlighted.

According to this mapping approach, the "French Doctors" movement can be seen as primarily medical, primarily ethics-based, yet with growing involvement in the public health dimensions of health emergencies and in human rights issues raised by these complex humanitarian crises. Similarly, many traditional, medical ethics-based institutes and centers can be placed on this map. At the Harvard School of Public Health, the Francois-Xavier Bagnoud Center for Health and Human Rights, along with several others, is now focusing on the health-human rights territory This map also suggests two major gaps in current work: on the ethics of public health, and on the relationships between medicine and human rights.

Where are the ethics of public health? In contrast to the important declarations of medical ethics such as the International Code of Medical Ethics of the World Medical Association and the Nuremberg Principles, the world of public health does not have a reasonably explicit set of ethical guidelines. In part, this deficiency may stem from the broad diversity of professional identities within public health. Yet, curiously, many of the occupational groups central to public health (epidemiologists, policy analysts, social scientists, biostatisticians, nutritionists, health system managers) have not yet developed, or are only now developing, widely accepted ethical guidelines or statements of principle for their work in the public health context. Thus, while a public health physician may draw upon medical ethics for guidance, the ethics of a public health physician have yet to be clearly articulated.

The central problem is one of coherence and identity: public health cannot develop an ethics until it has achieved clarity about its own identity; technical expertise and methodology are not substitutes for conceptual coherence. Or, as one student remarked a few years ago, public health spends too much time on the "p" values of biostatistics and not enough time on values.

To have an ethic, a profession needs clarity about central issues, including its major role and responsibilities. Two steps will be essential for public health to reach toward this analytic and definitional clarity.

First, public health must divest itself of its biomedical conceptual foundation. The language of disease, disability, and death is not the language of well-being; the vocabulary of diseases may detract from analysis and response to underlying societal conditions, of which traditional morbidity and mortality are expressions. It is clear that we do not yet know all about the universe of human suffering. Just as in the microbial world, in which new discoveries have become the norm—Ebola virus, hantavirus, toxic shock syndrome, Legionnaires' disease, AIDS—we are explorers in the larger world of human suffering and well-being. And our current maps of this universe, like world maps from sixteenth century Europe, have some very well-defined, familiar coastlines and territories and also contain large blank spaces, which beckon the explorer.

The language of biomedicine is cumbersome and ultimately perhaps of little usefulness in exploring the impacts of violations of dignity on physical, mental, and social well-being. The definition of dignity itself is complex and thus far elusive and unsatisfying. While the Universal Declaration of Human Rights starts by placing dignity first, "all people are born equal in dignity and rights," we do not yet have a vocabulary, or taxonomy, let alone an epidemiology of dignity violations.

Yet it seems we all know when our dignity is violated or impugned. Perform the following experiment: recall, in detail, an incident from your own life in which your dignity was violated, for whatever reason. If you will immerse yourself in the memory, powerful feelings will likely arise—of anger, shame, powerlessness, despair. When you connect with the power of these feelings, it seems intuitively obvious that such feelings, particularly if evoked repetitively, could have deleterious impacts on health. Yet most of us are relatively privileged, we live in a generally dignity-affirming environment, and suffer only the occasional lapse of indignity. However, many people live constantly in a dignity-impugning environment, in which affirmations of dignity may be the exceptional occurrence. An exploration of the meanings of dignity and the forms of its violation—and the impact on physical, mental, and social well-being—may help uncover a new universe of human suffering, for which the biomedical language may be inapt and even inept. After all, the power of naming, describing, and then measuring truly enormous child abuse did not exist in meaningful societal terms until it was named and then measured; nor did domestic violence.

A second precondition for developing an ethics of public health is the adoption and application of a human rights framework for analyzing and responding to the societal determinants of health. The human rights framework can provide the coherence and clarity required for public health to identify and work with conscious attention to its roles and responsibilities. At that point, an ethics of public health, rather than the ethics of individual constituent disciplines within public health, can emerge.

Issues of respect for autonomy, beneficence, nonmaleficence, and justice can then be articulated from within the set of goals and responsibilities called for by seeking to improve public health through the combination of traditional approaches and those that strive concretely to promote realization of human rights. This is not to replace health education, information, and clinical service-based activities of public health with an exclusive focus on human rights and dignity. Both are necessary.

For example, the challenges for public health officials in balancing the goals of promoting and protecting public health and ensuring that human rights and dignity are not violated call urgently for ethical analysis. The official nature of much public health work·places public health practitioners in a complex environment, in which work to promote rights inevitably challenges the state system within which the official is employed. Ethical dimensions are highly relevant to collecting, disseminating, and acting on information about the health impacts of the entire range of human rights violations. And as public health seeks to "ensure the conditions in which people can be healthy," and as those conditions are societal, to be engaged in public health necessarily involves a commitment to societal transformation. The difficulties in assessing human rights status and in developing useful and appropriate ways to promote human rights and dignity necessarily engage ethical considerations. For example, beyond accurate diagnosis, beyond efforts to cure, and even beyond the ever-present responsibility for relief of pain, the physician agrees to accompany the patient, to stand by the patient through her suffering, even to the edge of life itself, even when the only thing the physician can offer is the fact of his or her presence. Is this not as relevant to public health? For public health must engage difficult issues even when no cure or effective instruments are yet available, and public health also must accompany, remain with, and not abandon vulnerable populations.

That this work—added to, not substituted for, the current approach of public health—will require major changes in public health reflection, analysis, action, and education, is clear. That it is urgently required, in order to confront the major health challenges of the modern world, is equally clear.

Physicians and Human Rights

Finally, turning to the third issue raised by new challenges to the domains of public health, medicine, ethics, and human rights: what about the human rights role and responsibilities of medicine and the medical professional? To what extent and in what ways are—or might, or should medicine generally and physicians in particular be involved in human rights issues? Physicians have developed important roles in the context of human rights work. This work generally started from a corporatist interest in the fate of fellow physicians suffering human rights abuses, and then expanded in four directions. First, physicians created the "French Doctors" movement, providing medical assistance to populations in need, across borders. This dramatic and catalyzing work, including the concept of the right to assistance and the duty to intervene, expressed—in medical terms—the same transnational, universalist impulse as the modern human rights movement. Then, groups such as Physicians for Human Rights applied medical methods and analysis to detect and document torture, executions, and other similar human rights violations. In this manner, credible documentation, necessary also for redress and prosecution, has increasingly been made available. Meanwhile, Amnesty International has been concerned with the participation of physicians in human rights violations, usually in the context of torture and imprisonment under inhumane conditions. Finally, at a global level, physicians have articulated a role in seeking to prevent health catastrophes, exemplified by the Nobel Peace Prize-winning organization, International Physicians for Prevention of Nuclear War.

These historic and often courageous engagements with human rights issues have carried physicians to the frontiers of new challenges, exemplified by complex humanitarian emergencies, efforts to identify the full range of health consequences from human rights violations, and further struggle with societal issues inextricably linked with the health dimensions of conflict, economic consumption, and the degradation of the global environment. Increased physician participation and concern with these issues will inevitably blur preexisting boundaries between public health and medicine and create new interactive configurations between human rights and ethics.

Yet for individual medical practitioners, how is a human rights perspective relevant? Human rights and dignity will be engaged to the extent that the physician seeks to go beyond the usual, limited boundaries of medical care. Take two examples: a child with asthma, or a woman seeking emergency room care for injuries inflicted by her spouse. In each case, the limited medical perspective is vital. For the precipitating factors for asthma, and the likelihood of seeking early care as asthmatic attacks begin, lead directly to environmental conditions, economic issues, and discrimination. Similarly, domestic violence invokes, necessarily, societal issues in which the human rights framework will be useful, if not essential. Whether considering cancer, heart disease, lead poisoning, asthma, injuries, or infectious diseases, while the medical professional may start from a context dominated by individual relationships, a larger, societal set of issues will inevitably exist. The question then becomes, To what extent is the physician responsible for what happens outside the immediate context and setting of medical care? To what extent is a physician responsible for assuring access to care of marginalized populations in the community or helping the community understand the medical implications of public policy measures, or identifying, responding to, and preventing discrimination occurring within medical institutions?

Where, that is, does the boundary of medicine end? This seems a uniquely rich context for ethical discussion, at the frontiers of human rights and public health.

Of course, for those interested in the human rights dimensions of medicine, many may accuse physicians of "meddling" in societal issues that "go far beyond" their scope or competence. Also, issues of human rights inherently and inevitably represent a challenge to power—and health professionals are often part of, or direct beneficiaries of, the societal or institutional status quo that is challenged by the claims of human rights and dignity.

In conclusion, there is more to modern health than new scientific discoveries, or development of new technologies, or emerging or reemerging diseases, or changes in patterns of morbidity and mortality around the world. For we are living at a time of paradigm shift in thinking about health, and therefore about medicine and public health. Health as well-being, despite the World Health Organizations definition, lacks more than rudimentary definition, especially regarding its mental and societal dimensions. The universe of human suffering and its alleviation is being more fully explored. Awareness of the limits of medicine and medical care, growing recognition of the health impacts of societal structure and function, globalization and consequent interdependence, and the sometimes active, sometimes ineffectual actions of nation-states, all intersect to lead toward a new vision of health.

In the ongoing work on values and their articulation, we must acknowledge the provisional, untidy, and necessarily incomplete character of our understanding of the universe of health. In this context, medicine need not compete with public health, nor ethics with human rights; the search for meaning deserves to draw on all, as new constellations emerge and new relationships evolve.

Yet at such times of profound change, another kind of value becomes all the more vital. To build bridges—between medicine and public health, and between ethics and human rights—the critical underlying question may be,

Do we believe that the world can change? Do we believe that the long chains of human suffering can be broken? Do we agree with Martin Luther King that "the arc of history is long, but it bends towards justice?" Bioethical pioneers at the frontier of human history, we affirm that the past does not inexorably determine the future—and that it is precisely through this historic effort to explore and promote values in the world for which we share responsibility, articulated in philosophy and in action—that we express confidence in our own lives, in our community, and in the future of our world.

QUESTIONS FOR CONSIDERATION

1. What are the significant differences between medicine and public health?
2. What are some of the societal factors that are the major determinants of health status?
3. What are the reasons why public health fails to deal directly with societal factors? What does public health need to do to address these issues?
4. How does Mann describe the confrontational relationship between public health and human rights concerns?
5. What is the value of the language of human rights to public health?
6. What conditions does Mann identify as needed to develop an ethic of public health?
7. What examples does Mann cite of physicians engaged in human rights work?

NOTE

1. N. E. Adler et al., "Socioeconomic Status and Health: The Challenges of the Gradient," *American Psychologist* 49, no. 1 (1994): 15–24.

NORMAN DANIELS AND JAMES E. SABIN

Last-Chance Therapies and Managed Care: Pluralism, Fair Procedures, and Legitimacy

The most difficult and explosive responsibility for any health care system is deciding whether patients with life-threatening illnesses will receive insurance coverage for unproven treatments that they believe may make the difference between life and death.

Potentially life-saving treatments with proven efficacy and safety (proven net benefit) and quack treatments for which there is no scientific rationale rarely pose major problems about insurance coverage. In a country as wealthy as the United States, effective last chance treatments without alternatives generally are and should be covered virtually all the time. When shared resources from cooperative schemes are involved, as in public or private insurance, quack treatments will and should virtually never be covered, even if the patient or doctor passionately believe in the purported cure.

The difficult practical and ethical challenges come from promising but unproven last-chance treatments, for which we use high dose chemotherapy with autologous bone marrow transplant (ABMT) for advanced breast cancer as our key example.[1] Not covering treatments that ultimately prove to be effective lets curable patients die prematurely, and even if a treatment ultimately proves to be ineffective, not covering it may create the impression that critically ill patients are being abandoned in their moment of need. Covering treatments that ultimately prove to be ineffective or harmful reduces the quantity and quality of the patient's remaining life, wastes substantial resources, and undermines clinical research. These are the moral stakes in the decision.

There are also other costs and risks in these decisions. Denials of coverage for seriously ill people are highly visible. Even health plans that use impeccable science and patient-centered deliberation while trying to hold the traditional, contractually specified line against unproven therapies risk horrendous publicity, expensive litigation, and legislative mandates requiring coverage.

We shall later see that there is room for reasonable people to disagree about how to weigh the conflicting values and principles in these cases. There is no convincing, principled argument or social consensus for determining the relative importance of giving some (how much?) priority to meeting the urgent claims of patients in last-chance situations, providing stewardship of collective resources, producing the public good of scientific knowledge about the effectiveness of unproven therapies, and respecting patient autonomy through collaborative decisionmaking about risks and benefits.

We should not gloss over the ethical uncertainties in these cases by pretending that terms like "investigational," "experimental," and "medically necessary" tell us what to do. These terms explain little and dodge the genuine ethical dilemmas.[2] Without extensive explanation of the reasoning process, they will not—and should not—satisfy the public or the courts. The ethical challenges posed by unproven but promising last-chance technologies are not helped at all by the language of current medical insurance benefit contracts. They are also made harder to solve by the climate of distrust that surrounds insurers, including managed care organizations of all types.

Like other limit-setting decisions, the management of last-chance therapies poses a basic question in political philosophy: Why should the public accept as *legitimate* decisions made by managed care organizations that limit access to "unproven" last-chance therapies, especially if some responsible clinicians and their patients believe them to be effective? Under what conditions should the public grant authority to private, often for-profit organizations to make morally controversial decisions that affect our well-being in such fundamental ways?

In a three-year research project involving collaboration with a number of leading managed care organizations, we have been investigating, through a series of policy case studies, how insurers and health plans make coverage decisions about the adoption and application of new technologies.[3] In this policy discussion, we report on some very promising "exemplary practices" we have observed for managing last-chance therapies. We believe it would be premature to try to choose among these "exemplary practices." Because of the deep moral disagreement about the underlying issues, it would be wise for society to experiment with several promising strategies in order to learn more over time about how well they work and how morally acceptable they seem in light of actual practice.

Before describing the moral disagreement further, we shall begin with some background about the scientific and societal context in which the practices we describe have been developed.

A Brief Social History

By 1990 patients with advanced breast cancer, with the support of some clinicians, began to seek coverage for admittedly experimental use of autologous bone marrow transplant from managed care organizations, including our collaborating sites. Analogues to this treatment had proven effective for some lymphatic cancers, and there was some scientific rationale for extending the treatment to solid tumors. Despite the enthusiasm of the clinicians, and the desperate belief of the breast cancer patients, many of whom were well organized and informed, there was at the time no hard clinical evidence, and especially no controlled trials, that showed an advantage to the risky treatment over standard treatments. During this period in the early 1990s, technology assessment of the therapy was undertaken at a number of our collaborating managed care organizations and by the Medical Advisory Panel of the Blue Cross/Blue Shield Technology Evaluation Center (TEC).[4] The National Cancer Institute authorized four randomized clinical trials for ABMT in advanced breast cancer in 1991 (with support from TEC), but these results would not be available for some time. Early evaluations of this technology had to be based on weaker forms of evidence. Based on this early evidence regarding safety and efficacy, several managed care organizations (as well as the Oregon Health Services Commission) decided that the technology was not ready for standard coverage. (As early as 1990, one of our collaborating sites, Health Partners of Minnesota, provided coverage under "alternative funding" for participation in clinical trials.) Similarly, early evaluations by the Medical Advisory Panel found that there was inadequate evidence of efficacy or net benefit for ABMT for advanced breast cancer.

It was not until February 1996 that the BC/BS Medical Advisory Panel finally decided that the therapy did meet its criteria for status as a noninvestigational technology. At its February 1996 meeting, the panel evaluated evidence from the only published study of a randomized clinical trial,[5] as well as evidence from ongoing studies. The discussion suggested that the published study could not support conclusions about the greater efficacy of the therapy over standard treatments used in the U.S.,[6] but the advisory panel voted that its criteria were met. Those criteria are as follows:

1. The technology must have final approval from the appropriate government regulatory body.
2. The scientific evidence must permit conclusions concerning the effect of the technology on health outcomes.
3. The technology must improve the net health outcome.
4. The technology must be as beneficial as any established alternative.
5. The improvement must be attainable outside the investigational setting.

A consideration of the identical evidence in June 1996 by California State Blue Shield led to the opposite decision that the criteria were not yet satisfied.[7] As of mid-1996, several managed care organizations that had undertaken similar technology assessments also continued to believe that there was insufficient evidence to show that the therapy met reasonable criteria of safety and efficacy for advanced breast cancer in comparison to standard treatments—even if it had by then become nearly "standard" therapy.

Like HIV patients desperate to try "promising" drugs prior to full Food and Drug Administration testing, however, breast cancer patients in the early 1990s demanded that they be allowed to decide whether the risks were worth taking.[8] Yet, the "gatekeeper" for ABMT was not the FDA, charged with keeping unsafe pharmaceuticals off the market, but insurers, who by contract had no obligation to provide coverage for "investigational" treatments. When some managed care organizations with adequate evidence-based reason on their side insisted the therapy was still "investigational" and "unproven," and might even prove worse than standard therapies, patients pursued both litigation and legislation, and the media "exposed" the denials. As early as 1991, *60 Minutes* featured a story about Aetna declining coverage for ABMT for breast cancer. In California in 1993, the estate of Neline Fox won an $89 million suit against Healthnet, which had originally denied coverage, then provided it. The suit charged the delay cost Fox her life. This suit cast a pall over traditional procedures for assessing the status of last-chance therapies.

Throughout the early 1990s, many insurers were providing coverage for patients participating in approved clinical trials. Unfortunately, this coverage seemed "arbitrary and capricious" according to an important study in the *New England Journal of Medicine*, which said coverage was not correlated with pretreatment clinical characteristics of the patients, the design or phase of the study, or the response to induction therapy.[9] That study showed that as many as three out of four patients seeking coverage for participation in a trial were granted it, and another half of those who threatened legal action when initially denied also received coverage. Activism clearly paid off for patients seeking treatment.

Responding to well-organized and highly visible advocates for these women, some state legislatures mandated coverage as early as 1994 and 1995, despite protests—for example, in Minnesota and Massachusetts—that the mandates would make it impossible to continue proper clinical trials aimed at assessing efficacy. In other states, though legislative mandates were not passed, lawsuits in effect compelled coverage, since large punitive damages were imposed where coverage was denied or delayed. The resulting legal climate made it too risky and costly to deny what was still an unproven therapy.

Some insurers responded earlier than others to the handwriting on the wall, reading the message that traditional efforts to manage last-chance therapies by "holding the line" against investigational treatments were not working. Following the *60 Minutes* expose in 1991, Aetna, under the initiative of William McGivney, introduced a procedure in which an independent panel would be invoked when patients wanted a last-chance treatment for which internal review denied coverage. The same approach was adopted by Kaiser of Northern California in 1993. Other approaches were introduced in the same period, including Oregon Blue Cross Blue Shield's (1994) use of a transplant coordinator to manage the coverage of clinical trials for unproven last-chance therapies. In 1996 Health Partners introduced a special process for evaluating "promising therapies" that fall in the space between clearly investigational and standard treatment. It is this "new wave" of approaches that is the focus of our discussion below.

Before turning to the details of these newer approaches, we want to make three points. First, the social climate—including well-organized women's groups, a crusading media, committed practitioners, suspicious courts, and opportunistic legislators clearly made the standard "technology assessment" approach to holding the line against coverage for last-chance "investigational" therapies untenable. Second, the legal and political interventions compelling coverage also had the effect of making it more difficult to find out if high dose chemotherapy with stem cell support actually worked for advanced breast cancer by slowing enrollment in NIH-sponsored clinical trials. This public intervention frustrated another publicly supported goal in health care, namely, to make the system more efficient by pushing it to adopt "outcomes-based" medicine.

Third, the challenge to limit setting by managed care organizations has its international analogues in publicly administered and financed health care systems that offer universal coverage. "Bureaucratic decisions"—even if made by "legitimate" public agencies driven by budget limitations—seem to ignore the fact of urgent need in these cases. It would take us too far afield to discuss the similarities and differences between these cases (for example, in England,[10]

Norway, and New Zealand) and those in the United States, but it is important to see that the moral dimension of these issues arises across differences in institutional design, financing, national culture, and even incentives.

Moral Disagreement and Access to Last-Chance Therapies

Reasonable people disagree about the best way to manage access to last-chance therapies because they disagree about the relative importance of several values or principles that come into conflict in these cases. In a pluralist society, where the underlying disagreement may involve conflicts among more comprehensive and systematic moral views, this means there is no one way of managing last-chance therapies that all agree is morally superior. In effect, we may have to learn to live with alternative best practices, not agreement on one approach, even if, as we shall see, this raises a challenge to one aspect of our traditional thinking about fairness and justice.

The general and difficult moral problem that all health plans must solve is how to meet the diverse needs of the insured population under reasonable resource constraints. This problem involves balancing population-centered concerns against patient-centered ones. The major population-centered concerns are the prudent use of shared resources ("stewardship") and the promotion of public goods, including knowledge about safety and efficacy. Emphasizing these concerns leads to coverage only for last-chance treatments that meet a threshold of established net benefit and payment for unproven therapies only in the context of controlled clinical trials, in which a patient might receive a placebo or the standard treatment.

The key patient-centered concerns include: giving proper attention to patient needs, especially urgent needs as in the last-chance situations; avoiding harm, including the psychological harm that can arise from adversarialism; and managing uncertainties and risks through collaborative treatment planning. Emphasizing these concerns leads to toleration of lower standards of evidence for treatment coverage, to reluctance to require enrollment in controlled trials, and to giving patients and their clinicians more leeway in judging the relative weight of risks and benefits.

Reasonable people will differ, however, in the degree to which they want to trade population-centered values in favor of patient-centered ones because of the urgency of the situation. There is no higher level agreement on how much weight to give to the competing values or principles. Careful deliberation may resolve some of the conflicts, for often our views are not systematically considered, but it is unlikely to eliminate all of them. In many cases, the disagreement about weights may reflect significant differences in comprehensive moral views that people hold. For example, some "communitarians" will give more weight to guardianship of collective resources and the maximization of health benefits for a community that is cooperating to share resources than to meeting individually defined needs. Classic liberals will give more weight to respect for individual autonomy than to obligations of stewardship. "Communitarians" and "liberals" will recognize the relevance of the reasons to which the other gives priority since in other contexts these factors also count as reasons for them in their thinking about how to solve the general problem of meeting needs under resource constraints. But the disagreement about weights or priorities will probably persist.

This disagreement about weights will then lead people to have different views about the acceptability of different ways of managing last-chance therapies.

Some Exemplary Practices in Managing Last-Chance Therapies

Begin with the earliest approach to managing last-chance therapies, the terminal illness program William McGivney started at Aetna in 1991.[11] This program, used first primarily in an indemnity insurance context, was later adapted for use in a managed care setting by Northern California Kaiser Permanente and eventually became the model for the 1996 Friedman-Knowles legislation in California.

In the Aetna program, when medical directors in the field received a request for an unproven but promising last-chance cancer treatment that was not covered under established company policy, they referred the request to the home office at Hartford, where a consulting oncologist reviewed the clinical situation. A key feature of the program was that the home office oncologist was only empowered to approve requests. If the consulting oncologist believed the request did not represent reasonable clinical practice for the particular patient, the case was automatically referred outside the company for independent review by the Medical Care Ombudsman Program in Bethesda, Maryland.

The ombudsman program, which was founded by Grace Monaco in 1991, provides independent expert opinion about appropriate treatment in serious but ambiguous clinical situations. On a timetable that can be as short as twenty-four hours, the ombudsman program will put together a panel of two to three experts with no affiliation to the insurer or the provider of the proposed treatment to assess whether the proposed treatment has any scientific rationale for the particular patient. This is not a technology assessment of the new technology but an expert clinical assessment of the potential value of the technology for a particular patient. Typically, at least one of the experts is prepared to testify in court if the case should come to litigation.

Aetna did not restrict its own consulting oncologist from rendering negative coverage decisions because the consultant lacked competence. Any time that specialized technical expertise was needed, Aetna could have hired additional consultants at less cost to itself than using the ombudsman program. The problem Aetna was trying to solve with its terminal illness program was one of trust, not lack of technical expertise. The fact and appearance of "conflict of interest" was removed: if Aetna would say no only if an independent consultant said no, then the "no" should not be construed as a cost-driven decision. In circumstances of life-threatening illness and ambiguous information, the patient's trust in the decisionmaking process can be the difference between peace and outrage, or acceptance versus litigation.

In 1993 the Northern California region of Kaiser Permanente took the program that Aetna had developed in a primarily indemnity insurance context and adapted it for its own 3,600-physician prepaid group practice health maintenance organization. Kaiser's experience helps us understand the mechanism through which Aetna's innovative way of addressing the patient's concern about the insurer's potential conflict of interest helps the decisionmaking process.[12]

Like Aetna, Northern California Kaiser Permanente decided to let patients in last-chance situations know that they could go outside of Kaiser for an independent opinion from the ombudsman program if they were not satisfied with the internal decisionmaking process. This was a controversial step for Kaiser to take. Some Kaiser doctors worried that allowing automatic appeal outside the HMO would diminish the group's ability to manage care rationally and feared that the program itself might be very costly.

What actually happened was exactly the opposite. From 1994 to 1996, only six of the 2.5 million northern California members asked for referral to the ombudsman program. When the patients' concerns about insurer trustworthiness and potential conflict of interest were addressed in advance by the option of going outside of Kaiser for independent consultation, patients and families were much readier to enter into a reflective dialogue with their Kaiser physicians about what treatment approach really made sense for them.

The Aetna-Kaiser "last-chance" policy might simply be dismissed as a cost-benefit calculation made by the managed care organization. Put cynically, it is better to pay for a few treatments than face lawsuits, any one of which would be more costly than a bunch of treatments. But it also can be defended— and is by some managed care organizations that adopt it—on more explicitly moral grounds that connect its adoption with our earlier discussion.

The policy can be defended morally in this way. It recognizes the fundamental importance in a medical system of "shared decisionmaking" between patients and clinicians about risk-taking. If an unproven last-chance therapy is viewed by some acknowledged experts as the most appropriate treatment for the patient, and if the patient understands the risks as presented by parties on all sides, then organizations have no better option than to rely on the informed decision of the patient and her clinician. This is not the same as saying that a patient can be granted just any last wish regarding treatment; there must be some basis in evidence and expert view that the therapy is not quackery. In the external review model, that expert view is provided by the independent panel. Under those conditions, simply refusing to provide coverage fails to acknowledge the obligation not to impose paternalistically a plan's own judgment about acceptable risks and benefits on the choices of desperately ill patients with few options. To be sure, the role of the managed care organization as a guardian of shared resources is reduced. But this is defensible in light of both the urgency of the patients' needs, and the special importance, in light of the uncertainty and the severity of need, of promoting a climate of shared decisionmaking. Indeed, a proponent of this view might even say that the decision to hold to a hard-line denial is so likely to lead to a waste of resources in the legal and political climate that actually surrounds managed care organizations that the more efficient way to respect resources is to adopt the more lenient strategy toward last-chance therapies.

The Aetna-Kaiser approach has been embodied in recent legislation and is being advocated in other states and in recent consumer protection efforts nationally. Under the Friedman Knowles Experimental Treatment Act passed by the California legislature in 1996, the kind of independent consultation process that Aetna and Kaiser Northern California have piloted became mandatory for all California insurers on 1 July 1998. The provisions of the bill are quite detailed, but the basic concept is simple: If a patient with a condition that has no effective therapy and is likely to cause death within two years is denied coverage for a new treatment that has some scientific promise, an independent expert review of the decision must be offered.

What is so important about the Friedman-Knowles bill is the effort to use legislation to influence the quality of the decisionmaking process without making any attempt to mandate what the decisions themselves should be. The bill does not mandate any specific treatments, as so many states have done and continue to do. Rather, it mandates an organizational decisionmaking process designed to reduce fears about conflict of interest and increase deliberative reflection and clarity about the reasons for coverage decisions. (We note that in August 1997 the California legislature considered legislation that takes a step backward—mandating coverage for ABMT for breast cancer. Some proponents of the legislation say it eliminates "inequities" in coverage, since state employee benefits mandate ABMT but other insurers do not, an issue to which we shall return; critics say the state should not be making these disease-specific sorts of coverage decisions.)

Oregon Blue Cross Blue Shield has developed an approach to unproven bone marrow transplant regimens that reflects a slightly different moral framework. In 1993 in the aftermath of *Fox v. Healthnet*, Oregon Blue Cross Blue Shield created a new, full-time role of transplant coordinator. The transplant coordinator is a clinically experienced nurse whose job is to work directly with patients and families, transplant programs, employers, and the Oregon Blue Cross Blue Shield benefit systems to create mutually satisfactory individualized treatment plans.

Whereas Aetna and Kaiser use the option for independent review outside of the organization to allay patient concerns about conflict of interest and promote collaboration, Oregon Blue Cross Blue Shield's distinctive approach is an unusually open and accountable process of deliberation and reason-giving and an especially strong emphasis on supporting scientific treatment evaluation. Instead of the infamous "gag rule," the Oregon program has developed what might be called a "let's talk it over openly and at great length rule"!

In ethics classes at medical, nursing, and business schools we try to teach students to identify the key facts and values in a situation and to develop options to advance the most important values that apply. This is what the Blue Cross transplant coordinator does every day, except she does it in circumstances of time pressure and high emotion, not in a classroom. When we interviewed her for our research project, we told her that her role seemed to be one-third nurse clinician, one-third nurse manager, and one-third ethics professor.

Here are the kinds of things the transplant coordinator says in dealing with the multiple stakeholders in the decisionmaking process:

> To a confused and frightened patient: "Do you have this article about the treatment? Have you read this other one? I'm going to be at the library this afternoon—why don't you come and meet me there and we can go over the information together?"

To explain the importance of consistency to a wealthy patient: "Just because you're a VIP who lives in the West Hills, you don't really want to make me treat you any differently from the person who comes to clean your house, do you?"

To an employer who wants Blue Cross to cover an employee for a treatment that has no scientific justification: "But it's not based on sound science. Do you want to do the same thing for all the other women in your employee group? And even if you do, what will you tell their sisters who can't have the treatment? We want to be able to support scientific research that's going to answer the question."

And to a provider who is asking the insurer to cover an unproven treatment: "Then build your case to us, make your proposal so that when we make this decision, we can have sound rationale for a similar case on the next patient that you or someone else may send to us."

These comments illustrate the kind of deliberative dialogue that will have to happen hundreds of thousands and perhaps millions of times for doctors, patients, health plans, and society to move along a learning curve toward a more patient-centered, cost-effective, and ethical health care system.

The Oregon Blue process, like the Aetna-Kaiser, places its ultimate emphasis on encouraging open deliberation among patient, clinician, and, in this case, coordinator. When we asked the coordinator how she was able to achieve trust with patients without the promise of an external, independent review, as in the Aetna-Kaiser approach, she said that she would view an instance of a patient going to external review as a failure on her part to have engaged the patient in the kind of deliberative give and take that her approach requires. The promise of external review, she feared, could lure patients away from the need to engage in deliberation with her.

Although deliberation and shared decisionmaking were the key goals, Oregon Blue Cross Blue Shield has another priority as well—supporting clinically important research. If a promising but unproven last-chance treatment is available in a scientifically valid clinical trial, the plan will cover it. The coordinator claimed that as of our visit in June 1996, no patients had resorted to litigation, and a significant number decided that the unproven treatments they initially requested were, after careful thinking, not really what they wanted.

In contrast to the Aetna-Kaiser approach, Oregon Blue Cross Blue Shield appears to put more emphasis on redirecting its stewardship responsibility toward supporting research. At the same time, since outright denial of un-proven therapies was much less likely than in a traditional "hold the line" approach, it became possible to involve the patient in shared decisionmaking.

In 1996 Health Partners, a prominent HMO in Minnesota, began to develop a special policy regarding "promising" but still unproven therapies. For selected "promising treatments," Health Partners will provide coverage even though the technology still falls into the category of "investigational" and would traditionally be excluded from coverage by contract language. The rationale for singling out the category of "promising treatments" is to introduce consistent policy about a particular technology, thereby avoiding case by case responses to individual requests.

Although this approach clearly relaxes the traditional hard line about stewardship, it keeps the health plan in control of what counts as "promising." Compared to the case by case decisionmaking by Aetna, Kaiser of Northern California, and Oregon Blue Cross Blue Shield, the Health Partners approach appears to place more emphasis on the organizations stewardship role. It remains to be seen whether the approach of offering greater consistency technology by technology at the cost of less flexibility in deciding individual cases leads to more or less conflict and litigation.

Legitimacy and Fairness

Managed care organizations operate in a social climate of distrust. The vigorous effort at cost-containment initiated by large purchasers—employers and the government—has largely been invisible to the public. Instead, managed care organizations have taken the heat for cost containment and system change. In this climate of distrust, the issue of legitimacy noted earlier arises in a sharp form: Why should patients or clinicians who think they are being denied medically appropriate treatments, even unproven last-chance therapies, accept as legitimate the decisions of managed care organizations? More to the point, under what conditions should the public come to view these morally controversial decisions as legitimate?

Some might object that there is no special problem of legitimacy posed when medical insurers set limits any more than when other producers make decisions about the design of their products. Limits are legitimized and fair when consumers "consent" to purchase products at a fair market price. This consensual model fails, however, to dispel the legitimacy problem in our system. Half of all Americans have no choice of insurer. Those who do have choice of plans encounter limits only at a point when they are ill and cannot exercise further market choices. Finally, there is no assurance that the insurance market will produce a fair set of alternatives.[13]

Nor can we simply dispel the legitimacy problem by appealing to principles of distributive justice that tell us how to set these limits fairly. General principles of distributive justice fail to address a family of "unsolved rationing" problems, just as they fail to resolve the disputes about how to weigh population- and patient-centered values.[14] Even national commission proclamations about priorities in health care or the goals of medicine are unlikely to provide adequate guidance to many rationing choices. Consequently, we need an account of fair process to supplement whatever agreement we have on general principles, or legitimacy will fail.[15]

Elsewhere, we have argued that if the following four conditions were met, managed care organizations would take a large step toward earning legitimacy, at least over time:

1. Decisions regarding coverage for new technologies (and other limit-setting decisions) and their rationales must be publicly accessible.
2. The rationales for coverage decisions should aim to provide a reasonable construal of how the organization should provide "value for money" in meeting the varied health needs of a defined population under reasonable resource constraints. Specifically, a construal will be "reasonable" if it appeals to reasons and principles that are accepted as relevant by people who are disposed to finding terms of cooperation that are mutually justifiable.
3. There is a mechanism for challenge and dispute resolution regarding limit-setting decisions, including the opportunity for revising decisions in light of further evidence or arguments.
4. There is either voluntary or public regulation of the process to ensure that conditions 1 through 3 are met.[16]

These four conditions capture at least the central necessary elements of a solution to the legitimacy and fairness problems for coverage decisions about new treatments. Condition 1 requires openness or publicity, that is, clarity about the reasons for decisions. Condition 2 involves some constraints on the kinds of reasons that can play a role in the rationale; it recognizes the fundamental interest all parties have to finding a justification all can accept as reasonable. Condition 3 adds an element of "due process," and condition 4 ensures public accountability for meeting the other conditions.[17]

The guiding idea behind the four conditions is to convert the solutions to problems of limit setting of private managed care organizations into part of a larger public deliberation about a major, unsolved public policy problem, namely, how to use limited resources to protect fairly the health of a population with varied needs, a problem made progressively more difficult by the successes of medical science and technology. If met, these conditions help these private institutions to enable a more focused public deliberation that involves broader democratic institutions. They may indeed be a model for how solutions to this problem should be approached in public systems as well, since there is a tendency for these systems to establish highly visible, publicly accountable commissions, while remaining secretive and nonaccountable at the level where decisions are really made. The broader public deliberation envisioned here is not necessarily an organized democratic procedure, though it could include the deliberation underlying public regulation of the health care system. Rather, it may take place in various forms in an array of institutions, spilling over into legislative politics only under some circumstances.

The constraints here imposed on reasons have a bearing on a philosophical debate about the legitimacy of democratic procedures.[18] An aggregative or proceduralist conception of democratic voting sees it as a way of aggregating preferences. Where, however, we are concerned with fundamental differences in values, not mere preferences, an aggregative view seems inadequate. It seems insensitive to how we ideally would like to resolve moral disputes, namely, through argument and deliberation. An alternative "deliberative" view imposes constraints on the kinds of reasons that can play a role in deliberation. Not just any preferences will do. Reasons must reflect the fact that all parties to a decision are viewed as seeking terms of fair cooperation that all can accept as reasonable. Even if we have to rely on a majority vote to settle a disagreement where there are serious moral issues involved, if the reasons are constrained to those all must view as relevant, then the minority can at least assure itself that the preference of the majority rests on the kind of reason that even the minority must acknowledge appropriately plays a role in deliberation. The majority does not exercise brute power of preference but is instead constrained by having to seek reasons for its view that are justifiable to all fair-minded people, that is, to all who seek mutually justifiable terms of cooperation.

The procedures for managing last-chance therapies discussed above can meet these conditions. The first point to note is that the rationale for a plans adopting one procedure rather than another should itself be made public, as condition 1 requires. In such a rationale, giving more weight to responsibility for stewardship (as perhaps in the "promising therapy" strategy) than another strategy does is the type of reason that meets condition 2; so does the opposite weighting. Our main point in the preceding discussion is that each of the exemplary strategies could be defended publicly with reasons that meet these legitimacy conditions. What varies among these procedures is not the appeal to inappropriate reasons but the different weights reasonable people might give to relevant reasons.

In their implementation, any of these procedures should meet the other conditions as well. For example, in the procedure followed by Oregon Blue Cross Blue Shield in managing patients who may be left out of available clinical trials, there is an effort to engage the patient in reason-giving of exactly the sort required by condition 2. Similarly, the results of previous deliberations about particular cases could be made publicly available (still respecting confidentiality), so that they were accessible to other patients seeking to develop claims about coverage in their cases. In effect, a kind of case law should emerge that governs the operation of the managed care organization and is accessible to patients and clinicians. Similarly, the kind of deliberation engaged in by the external ombudsman program used by Aetna and Kaiser, and now mandated by California law, could also meet the publicity conditions and the restrictions on types of reason-giving.

We noted earlier that the legitimacy problem in the United States has its analogue in publicly administered systems. In other countries, even where public commissions have been established to approve "principles" for priority setting and limit setting in those systems, the agencies that make actual decisions often keep their results quiet, perhaps implicit in quietly made budget decisions, and fail to meet the conditions we articulate. We believe compliance with these conditions would contribute to establishing greater legitimacy for hard choices made in those systems as well.[19]

Formal versus Procedural Justice

There may not be just one best or fairest way to manage last-chance therapies. At least, reasonable people may not agree on what the best procedure is, and in light of that disagreement we should experiment with a family of "best practices," or so we have argued. There is a troubling implication of this view that some may see as a fatal objection. We see it not as a flaw in our approach but as a manifestation of an unavoidable moral uncertainty, which we must learn to respect and to live with.

Here is the problem. Suppose we have two patients, Groucho and Harpo, who are indistinguishable with regard to the relevant features of their cases. Both make the same claim that they need a particular high dose chemotherapy with stem cell support for their advanced cancers. Let us suppose that this treatment has not yet been shown to provide a net benefit for the condition, which is in any case fatal on standard treatments. Groucho belongs to BestHealth and Harpo to GreatCare, two responsible managed care organizations that manage last-chance therapies in different ways. For the sake of specificity, suppose BestHealth uses a version of the external appeal procedure (like Aetna or Kaiser) and that GreatCare covers people in clinical trials if they meet the protocols or can make a reasonable case that they should be so covered (like Oregon Blue Cross Blue Shield). Suppose finally that Groucho is denied the transplant but that Harpo is given it. When Groucho hears about Harpo, should we agree if he complains that one of them has been treated unfairly?

Groucho claims that a fundamental principle of justice has been violated, the formal principle that like cases be treated similarly. If his case is just like Harpo's in all relevant ways, then either both should get the treatment or neither should. The formal principle does not tell us how both should be treated, only that they should be treated similarly. Specifically, if there are reasons why Harpo should get the treatment, Groucho insists, then they apply equally to him, and he should receive it as well.

Groucho's complaint that a formal principle of justice is violated actually turns on there being a substantive reason or principle that grounds the decision to treat Harpo. To see this point, consider this variation on the case: in both managed care organizations, a coin is flipped about whether to give the treatment. Groucho loses and Harpo wins. When Groucho complains that like cases are being treated dissimilarly, we can now say to him, "The cases are unlike: there was a coin toss, and you lost and he won." There is no violation of the formal principle if there is a non-reason based procedure used to distinguish the cases, as there is in the case of a coin toss. Alternatively, we can construe this as a case in which a principle is appealed to and uniformly applied, namely the principle that winners but not losers of coin-tosses (or other random processes) will get the treatment.

Neither BestHealth nor GreatCare flips coins, however. Within their different procedures, each encourages the giving of reasons and deliberation about cases in light of reasons. We presuppose that the difference in their procedures for managing these cases rests on a difference in the ways the two organizations weight certain values, that is, the values of urgency, stewardship, and shared decisionmaking with patients. Suppose further that we are right to claim there is no argument we all can accept that shows that one weighting (and thus one procedure) is clearly morally more justifiable than the other. That weighting, and thus the choice of fair procedure, is itself the focus of reasonable disagreement.

Generally, when there is a violation of the formal principle of justice we are challenged to evaluate the weight attributed to a reason or principle that was applied in one case but not the other. We are asked to find a difference in the cases, that is, to show that they were not really similar in all relevant ways, or to affirm the uniform application of that reason or principle or of some alternative principle. But in the condition of moral pluralism we face, we have no candidate principle that purports to enjoy "our" endorsement independently of the fair procedure we are employing. A reason that may seem compelling or decisive in one process may not have that force in another. To be sure, we are not flipping coins in either case. We are deliberating carefully in a reason-driven and reason-giving way. But the weight given reasons in each setting is a reasonable reflection of other moral disagreements and moral uncertainty—the very uncertainty about what counts as a just outcome that compels us to adopt a procedural approach to fair outcomes. Groucho can be told this: Harpo was given the treatment because his plan reasoned about his case differently from your plan, and both ways of reasoning are relevant and arguably fair.

How tolerable would a system be if it produced situations in which a Groucho and Harpo were treated differently? We might think it makes a difference how centralized or decentralized a system is. In a decentralized system such as ours, for example, it may be difficult to require that insurance schemes use one rather than the another procedurally fair way of deliberating about cases (though legislation such as the Friedman-Knowles Experimental Treatment Act imposes uniformity, at least at one stage of decisionmaking). On what basis should the choice between procedures and weightings be made? Can we show a superior outcome to insisting on one such process rather than another? Without such a compelling regulatory reason, we might have trouble justifying public regulation requiring just one form of managing last-chance cases.

Despite the decentralization in our health care system, however, our courts arguably can impose a kind of unifying framework. Groucho might sue BestHealth, saying that not only does he want the treatment, and not only does some clinician he prefers say it is appropriate, but GreatCare has given the treatment to someone just like him. In practice, the courts could make unworkable an effort to experiment with different fair procedures to see what their advantages and disadvantages really are. On the other hand, what has often carried the day in actual suits on these matters is a demonstration of a lack of fair process and a kind of arbitrariness within an organization. If each of the fair procedures constitutes a reasonable defense against that sort of claim, then the courts might welcome an effort to rely more directly on fair procedures applied within plans. An analogy here would be the way in which the courts have welcomed decisionmaking by ethics committees in hospitals as preferable to having these kinds of cases continuously adjudicated in the courts.

Would it be a compelling regulatory reason that we find differential treatment unacceptable and have to avoid it, if only by insisting on uniform process by convention? That might be true in a decentralized system, but it seems even more likely to be true in a national health care system. In the United Kingdom, for example, it might seem more troubling that Groucho did not get his transplant in London but Harpo got his in Manchester. Here too, however, there might be disagreements among meaningful political units, the districts, about what constituted the "best" procedure. If that is true, then there might be even more reason to tolerate variation than there is in the United States where people are grouped into insurance schemes, not meaningful political units that have ways of selecting their procedures in a democratic fashion.

How acceptable differential treatment would be seems to depend, then, on whether a persuasive political rationale for uniformity can be developed. In a decentralized system, the political rationale would have to be sufficient to override the presumption that "private" insurers have the authority to select from among a set of comparably fair procedures. Of course, the political rationale might simply be that the legal system would not allow differential treatment; but that too remains to be seen.

In a national health care system, the political rationale for uniformity would have to show that differential treatment among districts was less acceptable than giving them the autonomy to select their own procedures. If meaningful political units, like districts, felt strongly enough about their choices of procedures, the costs of uniformity might be too high. For the problem we are facing, then, it remains unclear how unacceptable it would be for Harpo to get a last chance when Groucho does not.

Making decisions and policies about payment for promising but unproven last-chance therapies presents the most difficult moral and clinical policy challenge a health care system can face. Important values, all of which command respect and attention, inevitably come into conflict in these difficult situations, especially giving some (how much?) priority to meeting the urgent claims of patients in last-chance situations, providing stewardship of collective resources, producing the public good of scientific knowledge about the effectiveness of unproven therapies, and respecting patient autonomy through collaborative decisionmaking about risks and benefits.

General principles of distributive justice do not tell us how to weigh the relative claims of these competing considerations. Nevertheless, the insurers and managed care organizations whose programs we describe have developed procedures for making decisions and policies that can be defended on the basis of justifiable—although different—weights they give to the different values. In our decentralized, competitive system—largely in response to political and legal pressures patients and clinicians have brought to bear on these plans—an important social experiment has emerged. Different procedural "solutions" to the problem of limit setting in the case of new technologies are being developed and honed in practice. What can we learn from the experiment?

If we as a society can tolerate the inevitable differences in decisions and policies that the different configurations of values will create, we will have an opportunity to learn from the dialectic between principles and practice. We will see more clearly through a legacy of specific decisions and their outcomes just what the moral and nonmoral benefits and costs of the different approaches are. What we learn will help us refine our notions of fair procedure and in turn help us produce better solutions to the general problem of limit setting in health care that all societies are struggling with. In the last twenty to thirty years we have learned much and seen important changes in how individual clinicians and patients negotiate the difficult issues of clinical planning in the context of threats to life itself. If we have enough societal fortitude, and a modicum of strong political leadership, close study of the experiences generated by the kinds of programs we have described can help us do the same at the level of social policy.

Acknowledgments

Research for this paper has been generously supported by the Greenwall Foundation, the National Science Foundation, the Retirement Research Foundation, the Robert Wood Johnson Foundation, and the Harvard Pilgrim Health Care Foundation. We wish to thank our collaborating sites (Harvard Pilgrim Health Care, Kaiser Permanente of Northern California, Group Health Cooperative of Puget Sound, Health Partners, Oregon Blue Cross/Blue Shield, the Oregon Health Resources Commission, Aetna Insurance Company, and the Technology Evaluation Center of Blue Cross/Blue Shield Association) and our research associate, Susann Wilkinson, for help in gathering material for this project, and our research assistant, Roxanne Fay, for help in preparing Figure 1

[Figure 1 not shown]. The section on legitimacy and fairness is based on a more extended discussion of legitimacy and democratic deliberation in Norman Daniels and James Sabin, "Limits to Health Care: Fair Procedures, Democratic Deliberation, and the Legitimacy Problem for Insurers," *Philosophy and Public Affairs* 26, no. 4 (1997): 303–50.

QUESTIONS FOR CONSIDERATION

1. What do Daniels and Sabin identify as the possible consequences of not covering life-threatening treatments such as ABMT? What are the possible consequences of covering such treatments?
2. What has been the effect of the social climate and the legal and political interventions upon last-chance therapies?
3. Contrast the population-centered concerns (stewardship) with patient-centered concerns.
4. What were the main features of the Aetna and the Kaiser programs in managing last-chance therapies?
5. What was significant about the Friedman Knowles bill?
6. What was the Oregon Blue Cross emphasis upon deliberation, reason giving, and scientific treatment evaluation?
7. Describe the "climate of distrust" that Daniels and Sabin say that managed care organizations operate within.
8. Identify the four conditions that Daniels and Sabin argue will earn legitimacy for managed care organizations.
9. How does the example of Groucho and Harpo exemplify the use of different approaches to last-chance therapies without violating the principle of justice?

NOTES

1. We distinguish the case of promising but unproven last chance therapies from the case of treatments that professionals decide are futile. This kind of case is marked by clear professional judgment rooted in considerable *certainty about the evidence*. In the last-chance cases we are concerned with, it is professional *uncertainty*, not certainty, that is key.

2. See Norman Daniels and James Sabin, "When Is Home Care Medically Necessary?" *Hastings Center Report* 21, no. 4 (1991): 37–38; also James Sabin and Norman Daniels, "Determining 'Medical Necessity' in Mental Health Practice: A Study of Clinical Reasoning and a Proposal for Insurance Policy," *Hastings Center Report* 24, no. 5 (1994): 5–13.

3. Case studies completed to date include, James Sabin and Norman Daniels, "How MCOs Deliberated about Coverage for Lung Volume Reduction Surgery: A Focal Case Study," unpublished manuscript, and Susann Wilkinson, James Sabin, and Norman Daniels, "How MCOs Decided to Cover Pallidotomy for Advanced Parkinson's Disease: A Focal Case Study," unpublished manuscript. See also Norman Daniels and James Sabin, "Limits to Health Care: Fair Procedures, Democratic Deliberation, and the Legitimacy Problem for Insurers," *Philosophy and Public Affairs* 26, no. 4 (1997): 303–50.

4. Other technology assessment centers not affiliated with managed care organizations, such as ECRI, also undertook influential evaluations.

5. W. R. Bezwoda, L. Seymour, and R. D. Dansey, "High Dose Chemotherapy with Hematopoietic Rescue as Primary Treatment for Metastatic Breast Cancer: A Randomized Trial," *Journal of Clinical Oncology* 13 (1995): 2483–89.

6. The South African study used as its control a regimen of standard chemotherapy that was inferior in outcomes to the conventional therapy that would standardly be available in the United States and elsewhere. Showing that high-dose chemotherapy was superior to a conventional regimen that itself was far inferior to conventional therapy commonly in use should not persuade us of the superior efficacy of the high-dose regimen.

7. The California Blue Shield evaluation took place in a public setting, the only such open technology assessment process that we know of aside from Oregon Health Resources Commission. At its discussion, the panel seemed comfortable supporting its conclusion only after it was assured that no one actually wanting the high dose chemotherapy was unable to get it, despite its investigational status.

8. See Norman Daniels, *Seeking Fair Treatment: From the AIDS Epidemic to National Health Care Reform* (New York: Oxford University Press, 1995), ch. 6.

9. William P. Peters and Mark C. Rogers, "Variation in Approval by Insurance Companies for Coverage of Autologous Bone Marrow Transplantion for Breast Cancer," *NEJM* 330 (1994): 473–77.

10. For a detailed discussion of a famous British case that arrives at views similar to ours, see Chris Ham and Susan Pickard, *Tragic Choices in Health Care: The Story of Child B* (London: London Kings Fund Institute, 1998).

11. This program served as Aetna's *modus operandi* until the end of 1996, after Aetna purchased and merged with US Healthcare.

12. D. Blair Beebe, Arthur B. Rosenfeld, and Nancy Collins, "An Approach to Decisions about Coverage of Investigational Treatments," *HMO Practice* 11, no. 2 (1997): 65–67.

13. For fuller discussion, see Daniels and Sabin, "Limits to Health Care," pp. 308–14. See also Marc Rodwin, "The Neglected Remedy: Strenghening Consumer Voice in Managed Care," *The American Prospect* 34 (1997): 45–50.

14. See Norman Daniels, "Rationing Fairly: Programmatic Considerations," *Bioethics* 7, nos. 2-3 (1993): 224–33, reprinted in Norman Daniels, *Justice and Justification: Reflective Equilibrium in Theory and Practice* (New York: Cambridge University Press, 1997), ch. 15. Others have also argued, but for different reasons, that liberal principles of distributive justice will not address rationing problems. See Daniel Callahan, *Setting Limits: Medical Goals in an Aging Society* (New York: Simon and Schuster, 1987); Daniel Callahan, *What Kind of Life: The Limits of Medical Progress* (New York: Simon and Schuster, 1990); Ezekiel J. Emanuel, *The Ends of Human Life: Medical Ethics in a Liberal Polity* (Cambridge, Mass.: Harvard University Press, 1991). Callahan argues for societal specification of the goals of medicine: "Goals of Medicine: Setting New Priorities," *Hastings Center Report* 26, no. 6 (1996): S1–S28; but see also Norman Daniels, "Justice, Fair Procedures, and the Goals of Medicine," *Hastings Center Report* 26, no. 6 (1996): 10–12.

15. See also Len Fleck, "Just Caring: Rational Democratic Deliberation, Health Care Rationing, and Managed Care." Paper presented at the American Association of Bioethics meeting, San Francisco, November 1996, and "Just Caring: Oregon, Health Care Rationing, and Informed Democratic Deliberation," *Journal of Medicine and Philosophy* 19 (1994): 367–88.

16. See Daniels and Sabin, "Limits to Health Care," pp. 32–43.

17. These conditions were developed independently but fit reasonably well with the principles of publicity, reciprocity, and accountability governing democratic deliberation cited by Amy Gutmann and Dennis Thompson, *Democracy and Disagreement* (Cambridge: Harvard University Press, 1996). For reservations about their account, see Norman Daniels, "Enabling Democratic Deliberation." Paper presented to Pacific Division of the American Philosophical Association, Berkeley, Calif., March 1997.

18. See Daniels and Sabin, "Limits to Health Care," pp. 33–40. Important discussions of legitimacy and democratic deliberation can be found in Joshua Cohen, "Deliberation and Democratic Legitimacy," *in The Good Polity*, ed. Alan Hamlin and Phillip Petit (Oxford: Blackwells, 1989), pp. 17–34; and more recently, "Procedure and Substance in Deliberative Democracy," in *Democracy and Difference: Changing Boundaries of the Political*, ed. Seyla Benhabib (Princeton: Princeton University Press, 1996), pp. 95–119; Cass Sunstein, *The Partial Constitution* (Cambridge, Mass.: Harvard University Press, 1993).

19. See Ham and Pickard, *Tragic Choices in Health Care.*

PAUL T. MENZEL

Rescuing Lives: Can't We Count?

On 16 September 1993, five-year old Laura Davies of Manchester, England, received small and large intestines, stomach, pancreas, liver, and two kidneys in a fifteen-hour transplant operation at Children's Hospital of Pittsburgh. The National Health Service paid for little of her care, but scores of private donors responded to newspaper publicity and her parents' appeals to provide the half-million pounds or more required for her various operations. In this case, where was medical technology taking us?

Laura died on 11 November. According to her Manchester physician at the time of the operation, however, Laura had a "better than 50-50 chance." After all, the three previous child recipients of multiple organs at Pittsburgh since the advent of a new antirejection drug in 1992 are still alive. It is thus difficult to dismiss the willingness of Laura's parents and the physicians to proceed as using her for their own emotional or scientific purposes. Though surely "experimental," the surgery was the only choice Laura had.

And if anyone, either then or now in light of her death, claims that the 50-50 odds were inflated, a straightforward reply is available: maybe you're right, but let us employ this procedure, now and at other times, to see. Plucky Laura herself seemed to put the "guinea pig" charge to rest. "I'm not worried," she told reporters at a press conference. Then she ended the session with a song.

A standard objection to high expense-to-benefit care also does not apply: funded privately by response to special appeal. Laura's care does not come at the expense of anyone else whom limited funds might have saved. With a child like this and the money pouring in from donations, why should we dispute her parents' and physicians' decision? On a medical mission? Sure. Carried away? In the circumstances, seemingly not.

Still, something has been missed that is very problematic about Laura's care: in the attempt to save her, a greater number of lives were sacrificed.

It is a straightforward function of the marked scarcity of organs. Nearly half of the children now on organ transplant waiting lists die before they get them. We all should be able to see the big picture: if one person at the head of the queue gets four scarce organs instead of one, four others somewhere down the queue, not one, never get any.

Both the British and U.S. publics seem reluctant to recognize this. Take Pennsylvania's Governor Casey last spring. At first his waiting only a few days before receiving a heart-liver transplant met with skepticism: had he been allowed to jump the queue because of his political status? The Pittsburgh transplant center quickly replied: absolutely not, he was treated as any other multiple organ failure patient would have been. Because of the multiple failure, his need was more urgent. With the political queue-jumping charge rebuffed, the critics backed off.

But if organs are scarce, and those used in multiple scarce organ transplants could virtually always have saved more lives if used on others, what can possibly justify any multiple organ transplant candidate's elevation to the top of the queue? Except in the event of an extremely rare match, only two readily understandable explanations seem available, and neither justifies what was done.

One is pushing outward the medical frontier: carry out Casey's and Davies's more challenging operations despite the current sacrifice of a greater number of others' lives, and we will eventually develop new, effective forms of lifesaving. But this sort of argument represents the most extreme kind of medical adventurism. With the scarcity of organs virtually certain to continue—especially for children and infants, where we are already getting close to maximum contribution—what is the likelihood that multiple organ transplants will *ever* cease to use up on one person what could have saved several? A foolishly optimistic view of future organ drives the "experimental development" argument. We should experiment with multiple scarce organ transplants only if we have good reason to believe that sometime in the future we will have ample supply. But there is every reason to think we will *never* have that!

The other readily understandable explanation is the odd view of "urgency." The Pittsburgh surgeons appear to regard the failure of both a heart and liver as constituting more urgent need. This too falls apart upon examination. Certainly I am as close to death's door if "just" my heart fails as I am if my heart and liver both fail. Where, in "only heart failure," is there any lack of real urgency?

To say that Governor Casey or Laura Davies have greater medical need because they require two or seven organs instead of one betrays, I suppose, a kind of "Dunkirk Syndrome": thinking that the more *difficult* the rescue was, the greater was the need at the time. Admittedly, nations and doctors understandably feel in such circumstances that they have pulled off something more *miraculous*—in fact they have! But where in that pride in greater effort or thankfulness for greater luck is hidden any more urgent *need*?

So advancement of medical technology and medical need utterly fail to justify multiple scarce organ transplants. Their defense would have to invoke either of two much more difficult explanations. One is a direct, jolting challenge to the moral relevance of numbers at all in these kinds of acute care situations: there simply is no obligation to save the greater number. Such a position gets a foothold in our thinking through the claim that each and every individual deserves an equal chance of being saved. We should therefore flip coins to determine whether we will save the one or the four, not save the four right off because they are the greater number. Regardless of the merits of this view in academic philosophical terms,[1] however, it hardly fits the transplant setting. We continually strive to expand the organ pool. Why? To save more lives, obviously. If with that expanded supply we end up saving no more people than before because we use up enough of our organ bank on multiple organ recipients, what has been the point of our supply expansion efforts?

A second difficult explanation is at least anchored in some actual social reactions. Little objection to the occasional practice of using up multiple scarce organs on one recipient comes from competing single organ patients, patients' families, or their representatives. The reason, I suspect, is that the context of waiting together on a queue is already transparently and pervasively infused with luck—the luck of the right organ and a good match arriving at the right time for one candidate, but not for another. Living continually with such grave unknowns may lead people to celebrate unselfishly when anyone gets saved. No patient begrudges another's sheer luck: all understand there is no rhyme, reason, or desert in the outcome anyhow. Once in that laudable mindset, people may not even attend to the numbers. The many cast no challenging glance into the eyes of the few. Challenge, defense, claim—here, all are out of court. It's as if the many even consent to their own lack of rescue as long as someone is saved.

I am intrigued by this possibility of consent,[2] but I suspect that our surmisals here about the empathetic consent of organ failure patients who wait unsuccessfully on the queue are romantic and quite distort their actual feelings. Most of the real competitor potential recipients out there somewhere on the queue do not sit together in a transplant center's waiting room, directly sharing one another's fortune. In any case, why should those in society who manage the process of organ procural and disbursement not empathize sequentially with *all* who might be saved, thereby letting the numbers of real, equally invaluable rescuable persons build up to turn their decision? Again, in terms of persuasive justifications, multiple scarce organ transplants strike out.

Surgeons, the press, and the public need to face up to these considerations in cases like Laura Davies. How can transplant centers justify ultimately letting two or more persons somewhere down the queue likely die because they have drawn so much out of the organ bank to save one? And why should the press play along with this lifesaving delusion and publicize appeals to unknowing financial donors without telling them the morally relevant facts? If donors knew, why should they feel good about having contributed to a net *non-lifesaving* project? In the whole situation, only Laura Davies' parents, in their attachment to their child, come out clean.

Worse yet, the essential problem in multiple scarce organ cases portends bigger trouble. It has ominous implications for the distributions of other scarce health care resources. If in multiple organ transplants we are blind to the real lives of competing potential beneficiaries, where they too are acutely ill, how much more blind will we be in typical contexts of distributing scarce monies where the competing beneficiaries are more distant, and certainly not on any queue of named individuals?

Let's count before we cut.

QUESTIONS FOR CONSIDERATION

1. How do the cases of Laura Davies and Governor Casey illustrate the problem of multiple organ transplants?
2. How does Menzel critique the possible defense of multiple organ transplants?
3. What are Menzel's arguments supporting the moral relevance of numbers?
4. How does he react to the acceptance of multiple organ transplants by competing patients needing single organs?
5. What are Menzel's criticisms of transplant centers and the press regarding multiple organ transplants?

NOTES

1. Frances M. Kamm, *Morality, Mortality: Death and Whom to Save From It*, vol. 1 (New York: Oxford University Press, 1993), pp. 75–122. See also J. Taurek, "Should the Numbers Count?" *Philosophy and Public Affairs* 6, no. 4 (1977): 293–316; and Derek Parfit, "Innumerate Ethics," *Philosophy and Public Affairs* 7, no. 4 (1978): 285–301.

2. The attempt to discern the implications of consent to risk drove most of the author's reasoning in *Strong Medicine: The Ethical Rationing of Health Care* (New York: Oxford University Press, 1990).

Baruch Brody

Public Goods and Fair Prices: Balancing Technological Innovation with Social Well-Being

The scope of bioethics has expanded over the years from its original emphasis on questions arising out of clinical encounters and biomedical research to an increasing emphasis on questions about health policy and health care reform. I have long been convinced, however, that even this expanded scope is still conceived far too narrowly. While few technological advances in medicine take place without public commentary by bioethicists, major structural changes in the delivery of health care or in the conduct of biomedical research often go unnoticed by the bioethics community, despite the fact that these changes often raise profound moral and social issues.

A splendid example of this neglect was the silence of the bioethics community about the announcement on 11 April 1995 by Harold Varmus, the director of the National Institutes of Health, that the NIH would no longer insist on a "reasonable pricing clause" in Cooperative Research and Development Agreements and in Exclusive License Agreements between industry and government in the process of technology transfer.[1] This decision reversed a policy adopted in 1989 as a result of a public outcry over the pricing by Burroughs-Wellcome of AZT, which had been developed in part by researchers at the National Cancer Institute. This was an issue much debated in the research and biotechnology community for six years, with two major meetings at the NIH in 1994 devoted to it. There was no bioethics input at either of those meetings, despite the fact that the issue raises many important questions to which both moral theory and political philosophy have much to contribute. It is time for the bioethics community to expand its focus and provide input to many more issues.

The Technology Transfer Background

In the 1980s, the U.S. Congress passed two major acts[2] designed to promote collaboration between the federal research effort and the development of useful technologies, the process that has come to be called technology transfer.[3] The thinking behind these statutes is clearly articulated in the following congressional statement explaining the second act:

> The United States can no longer afford the luxury of isolating its government laboratories from university and industry laboratories. Already endowed with the best research institutions in the world, this country is increasingly challenged in its military and economic competitiveness. The national interest demands that the federal laboratories collaborate with universities and industry to ensure continued advances in scientific knowledge and its translation into useful technology. The Federal laboratories must be more responsive to national needs.[4]

The first of the two acts was the Bayh-Dole Act of 1980. It addressed the ownership of inventions made by researchers using federal funds from contracts or grants. Since 1963, when President Kennedy issued a memorandum on this question, the patents were held by the government when the resulting products were to be used by the general public, when the research concerned public health or welfare, when the government was the principal developer in the field, or when the contractor was running a federally owned facility. There was a widespread conviction that this policy often resulted in potentially useful government-owned inventions not being developed into useful products. Those who might develop useful products, it was felt, did not do so because they didn't own the technology and couldn't be assured of an adequate and safe return on their investment.

The 1980 Bayh-Dole Act changed this situation. Contractors or grantees are now entitled to retain the patent to inventions discovered during research funded by the federal government. While the act originally applied only to researchers working for nonprofit organizations (such as universities, medical schools, or hospitals) or small businesses, it was expanded by President Reagan in 1983 to cover virtually all contractors or grantees. Owning the technology, they can be more assured of an adequate return from their investments in developing it. However, there are some limitations on ownership. Royalties from the patent must be shared with the inventor and they must be used for the support of research and education. The federal government retains the right to use the invention for its own purposes and the right to require sublicensing when that action is "necessary to alleviate health or safety needs which are not reasonably satisfied" by the contractor or grantee. Despite these limitations, researchers were given a financial incentive to make useful inventions and their institutions were given a financial incentive to develop those inventions.

These provisions of the Bayh-Dole Act applied only to discoveries made in private laboratories and did not in any way affect the ownership of inventions made in federal laboratories. The number of government-owned patents continued to grow as a result of inventions made in federal laboratories even while virtually no new inventions from private laboratories were entering the inventory of government-owned patents. How could these federal inventions be transferred to the private sector for development? The Bayh-Dole Act addressed this question by giving federal agencies the power to offer both nonexclusive and exclusive licenses to private organizations that wish to develop the technologies. An exclusive license, which grants the private organization a monopoly on the development of the invention, must be justified on the grounds that it provides the sufficient incentive for the required investment in the development that would not be provided by a nonexclusive license. About 14 percent of the more than 11,000 government-owned patents obtained between 1981 and 1990 were licensed, with about 4 percent being exclusively licensed. The federal government received royalties on those licenses. That income came to 963.5 million between 1981 and 1990, primarily from the Health and Human Services patents on an AIDS test kit and on hepatitis B vaccines.[5] Even when an exclusive license is issued, the federal government still has the right to use the invention and to require that those receiving the license grant sublicenses when public health or safety requires it.

The Federal Technology Transfer Act, passed in 1986, supplements the Bayh-Dole Act by authorizing federal agencies to enter into CRADAs with private laboratories. Under these agreements, the government can contribute personnel, facilities, and equipment (but not funds) to a joint research and development program with a private laboratory that can contribute funds as well as these other resources. These agreements can give the private laboratory exclusive or nonexclusive licenses in inventions discovered by federal employees working under these agreements and can give them ownership of any invention made by their employees working under these agreements.

Two major themes emerge in these acts. The first is that social well-being is served if inventions discovered by federally funded research are developed by private organizations that are given the financial incentive of patent ownership of, or an exclusive license to, the developed invention. The second is that the public, even if served by these technology transfer arrangements, must still have its needs protected. When patents are obtained by the private laboratories on the results of federally funded research, the federal government still retains march-in rights if public need requires compulsory licensing of the patent. When exclusive licenses are issued for the development of federally owned patents, the exclusivity of the license can be withdrawn if required by public needs.

A continued attempt to balance these two themes was found in the proposed 1994 Technology Commercialization Act,[6] an act which did not pass. On the one hand, it would have furthered the transfer of technology to the private organizations entering into CRADAs by giving them first refusal of an exclusive license. As things currently stand, the government decides whether an exclusive license is justified. On the other hand, it would have continued to protect public needs by continuing the government's authority to require its collaborator to issue a license to use the invention to someone else when health and safety needs are not being reasonably satisfied by the collaborator.

Although both themes are stressed in the statement of the laws, the main emphasis seems to be on serving the public well-being by promoting technological development through technology transfer. Deciding which theme to emphasize certainly calls for moral and social reflection. The need for this reflection was further emphasized by the AZT pricing controversy and the resulting reasonable price clause controversy.

Reasonable Prices for the Products of Technology Transfer

In April of 1984, human immunodeficiency virus was identified as the cause of acquired immunodeficiency syndrome. Although skeptical that a traditional drug screening program would work to identify drugs active against a retrovirus, the NIH developed such a program and asked drug companies to send in drugs in their stock for screening. Burroughs Wellcome sent in AZT, a drug that had been developed through NCI funding in 1964 for use against cancer but had proved ineffective for that purpose. By February of 1985, the NCI determined that AZT worked against HIV in vitro. This led to an agreement with NIH, whereby Burroughs-Wellcome would supply the drug for clinical testing, using NCI-supplied thymidine to produce it while searching for a new supplier. By the fall of 1986, clinical testing through an NIH collaborative group had indicated that AZT delayed death in patients with AIDS. This led to approval by the FDA in early 1987, a rapid approval that became a model for its soon-to-be announced Subpart E Accelerated Approval Program. In March of 1987, Burroughs-Wellcome received a seven-year exclusive marketing privilege under the Orphan Drug Act, because it was then believed that the market would be very small. In February of 1988, it also received a patent for the use of AZT to treat HIV disease until 2005. None of this directly involved either the Bayh-Dole Act or the Technology Transfer Act, but it certainly involved a corporation receiving the benefit of research (in the 1960s) funded by government grants and research (in the 1980s) performed in cooperation with a federal agency.[7]

The original pricing for AZT produced an annual cost at the dosage then used of $10,000 to $12,000. By 1993, the annual cost of AZT had declined to $2,500, in part because of price reductions made in response to a public outcry and in part because of the scientific recognition that lower dosages would be equally efficacious. The immediate public outcry over the original pricing is easy to understand. Why, it was argued, should the price be so high when the research was funded with public dollars? Was the public's need for the drugs being served by allowing drug companies to charge that much for drugs? Perhaps the theme of protecting the public's needs should take precedence over the theme of serving social well-being by promoting technology transfer? On the other hand, there were those who argued that such prices for successful development must be allowed if commercial companies are to take the risk of attempting to develop promising inventions. Think of all the drugs that were efficacious against HIV in vitro but had failed clinical tests. How can we expect companies to invest in risky development unless they can reap profits in successful cases? Isn't this support of technology transfer exactly what is needed to serve the long-term social interest both in the development of new therapies and in the support of economic growth in a competitive world?

To avoid similar controversies about CRADA-related technology, the NIH announced in 1989 that it would impose a reasonable pricing clause when it granted exclusive licenses to intellectual property it already owned or when such property was developed under a CRADA and was then exclusively licensed to the NIH partner:

> DHHS has responsibility for funding basic biomedical research, for funding medical treatment through programs such as Medicare and Medicaid, for providing direct medical care, and, more generally, for protecting the health and safety of the public. Because of these responsibilities and the public investment in research that contributes to a product licensed under a CRADA, DHHS has a concern that there be a reasonable relationship

between the pricing of a licensed product, the public investment in that product, and the health and safety needs of the public. Accordingly, exclusive commercialization licenses granted for the NIH/ADAMHA intellectual property rights may require that this relationship be supported by reasonable evidence.[8]

Six products have been developed under CRADAs since 1986 without being exclusively licensed. Perhaps the most important was taxol for the treatment of cancer. The taxol ADA with Bristol-Myers contains a reasonable pricing clause, but there has been considerable controversy about its price. In addition, the NIH is developing nine products under CRADA exclusive licensing agreements; didanosine (ddI), being developed collaboratively with Bristol-Myers, is perhaps the most important example.

Some sense of NIH's changing attitude toward its own pricing clause came in February of 1993 when Dr. Bernadine Healy, then head of the NIH, testified before the Senate Committee on the Aging. She described the difficulties of enforcing the reasonable pricing clause, claiming that (a) the NIH has no mechanism to compel its partners to divulge the needed information to evaluate the reasonableness of the price; (b) the NIH lacked the expertise to use the information, even if it had it, to evaluate the reasonableness of the price; and, most crucially, (c) there was no theoretical basis for the whole idea of a reasonable price.

In the meantime, the pharmaceutical/biotechnological corporations had expressed strong opposition to the reasonable pricing clause. This was no doubt part of their general opposition to any attempt to control the price of drugs, an issue that was very important to them in light of the various attempts made as part of the health care reform proposals to control the prices of pharmaceuticals in the U.S. Moreover, the research community suggested that there was increasing reluctance to enter into CRADAs because of concern about pricing issues. All of these concerns were expressed very forcefully at two hearings held by the NIH in 1994. While some patient advocacy groups supported a revised version of the policy, others opposed it out of the fear that it would limit new product development. Any decline in such development is "unacceptable to people with cancer whose lives are dependent on more effective and less debilitating therapies," said Ellen Stovall of the National Coalition for Cancer Survivorship.[9]

As late as September of 1994, there seemed to be considerable support for a variety of proposals to modify the pricing clause or to replace it with provisions that would (a) ensure needed access to the new products by those who could not afford the prices and (b) secure higher royalties for the government as a return on its investment. This support was reflected in a great difference between the two meetings held at NIH. The first, held in July, was clearly dominated by opponents of the reasonable pricing clause, while the second, in September, seemed to involve a more balanced group seeking to find a compromise.[10] The bioethics community was not represented at either meeting.

In April of 1995, however, Dr. Harold Varmus, the new head of the NIH, decided simply to eliminate the clause, stressing its dangers to the development of new products. This decision was no doubt also related to the new antiregulatory mood in Washington after the 1994 elections. As Representative Wyden, long known for his concerns about drug pricing issues, said to the *New York Times*, "No one is oblivious to the political climate."[11]

Disambiguating the Issues

This episode raises many different questions. Let me begin by differentiating three sets of questions that I think deserve the most attention:

(1) Even if the development of new technologies based upon advances in scientific research is important to social well-being, is it legitimate for the government to fund these efforts by granting to private organizations intellectual property rights for inventions developed with public funds? Should the government at least have the right to some direct economic benefit from these intellectual property rights?

(2) Should those who are in need of new forms of technology (for example, new drugs) be entitled to them at a cost they can afford, or should the price of these technologies be set in the marketplace? Does it make a difference whether these new technologies are developed at least in part by public funding? Does it make a difference whether the owners of these new technologies are protected from competition, which might lower the prices, by patents and exclusive licenses?

(3) Assuming that all of these goals are legitimate, how should we balance them? Must we make a choice between them, or can we find ways to satisfy all of them?

The NIH's original announcement of its reasonable pricing clause treated all of these issues together. It assumed that the government would receive a direct economic return in exchange for the intellectual property rights. It assumed that pricing responsive to the degree of social funding is the appropriate form of that economic return since it lessens the cost of the products to Medicare and Medicaid. It assumed that those in need of the new drugs developed through technology transfer should not be denied access because of the price and that pricing responsive to the health and safety needs of the public is the appropriate way of ensuring that access. Finally, it assumed that a reasonable pricing clause that responded to both of these factors would provide enough of a return to investors to ensure a continued long-term contribution of such innovation to social well-being. But pricing related to the degree of social funding may be radically different from pricing related to ensuring access. Moreover, there is no guarantee that either approach ensures an adequate enough return to the investors to promote continued technological innovation. Finally, alternative ways might be found to give a direct economic return to the government and to assure needed access if it is decided that these are appropriate goals. What was needed was an independent examination of each of these issues: Are these appropriate goals? What are the alternative ways of securing them? Which ways least discourage the investment in technological innovation we are trying to encourage by the technology transfer process?

The same failure to examine separately each of these issues characterizes Dr. Varmus's decision to drop the reasonable pricing clause without replacing it with any other provision. Even if one agrees with the assumption that the reasonable pricing clause excessively interfered with technology transfer, so that it should be dropped, many other questions need to be considered: Are the goals of assuring access to the products of technology transfer and of providing the government with a direct economic return on its investment legitimate goals? What are alternative ways of achieving those goals? Are any of them compatible with continued encouragement of technology transfer?

These are the broader questions I believe bioethics needed to address in the CRADA debate. They are moral and political questions about the appropriate roles of government in promoting social well-being through technological innovation, about the legitimate expectations of all citizens to have access to the products of technological innovation they helped to fund, and about the balancing of these goals and expectations.

Providing Public Goods

Political philosophies differ in their conception of the functions of governments. Libertarians confine the government to those activities (for example, police, army, courts) aimed at protecting the rights of individual citizens and redressing violations of those rights. Consequentialists add the role of furnishing goods that improve social well-being (for example, roads, schools). Redistributionists emphasize the role of meeting the basic needs of citizens (for example, income support programs).

Government support of basic scientific research represents an example of the government furnishing a good, scientific knowledge, that improves social well-being. Why can't that good provided by private groups (universities or corporations) who recover their costs and earn a return on their investment by charging a fee to those who benefit from it? The standard answer is that scientific knowledge is a public good, a good that cannot be sold because those who do not pay receive the benefits anyway. Once basic scientific knowledge is discovered and reported, others can use it without paying a fee for it. As for the rest, the amount of private investment in research is likely to be less than is warranted in terms of the contribution that the research makes to social well-being. Government funding of research and government participation in the research effort resolves the problem by providing the additional investment in research justified by the contribution to social well-being. All this explains why we have agencies such as the NIH that conduct research in their own laboratories and fund research performed by private groups.

The development of new technologies using the results of basic research also improves social well-being, but is importantly different. Technological development results in products that can be sold, and if those products are patented, the resulting secure flow of income enables those who invested in development to recover their costs and earn a return on their investment. That is why these same agencies transfer intellectual property rights such as patents and exclusive licenses to private groups. By giving those private groups these intellectual property rights, the government increases the economic return to the private groups by enabling them to receive fees from those who use the products. This encourages them to invest more in development, thereby lessening the need for direct government support of those efforts. The government can also help by cooperating in the development phase through CRADAs. The transfer of the property rights and the cooperation with the development effort is to encourage investment in development, not necessarily to reward past effort. So the answer to part of our first question is that it may be very appropriate for the government to transfer property rights as called for by the Bayh-Dole Act and the Technology Transfer Act. In particular, forming CRADAs and transferring property rights to their results lessens the need for direct government funding of technological development.

The other half of that first question was whether the government should receive a direct economic return for its investment. That return, as was pointed out at the second NIH meeting, could come in the form of a royalty payment derived from sales of the product instead of in the form of Medicare and Medicaid savings from a reasonable pricing clause. One immediate observation is in place. The call for a direct economic return often seems to be based upon a misunderstanding that the government is cheated unless it gets a direct economic return. This misses the whole point of the government's support of public goods such as research and development; the true return is the promotion of the social well-being through the increased production of the public good.

Putting this misunderstanding aside, should there be a direct economic return? It is clear that insisting on such a return may actually be counterproductive. It certainly lessens, by the amount of the royalty, the return to the private group from the development effort. If the resulting return is insufficient, the private group would fail to conduct enough technological development. We just don't know if the resulting level of private investment would be adequate to actualize the full potential of social well-being from technological advances. Congress left this question open since it provided for both royalty-free and royalty-paying technology transfers, and I know of no empirical analysis that answers this question. A December 1994 Government Accounting Office report on the benefit of CRADAs[12] is typical of what exists. It documents for a set of ten CRADAs how technology was transferred and how that transfer resulted in beneficial commercial products. At no point does it discuss what level of governmental support was really needed to ensure the socially desirable private investment in comparison to what level of governmental support was actually provided.

This is likely to become very controversial in at least one case: the CRADA between Genetic Therapy Incorporated and the NIH for retroviral mediated ex vivo gene therapy. In March of 1995, the company, which had an exclusive license from the NIH, received a very broad patent that seems to cover all ex vivo gene therapy. The economic potential of this patent is very high. Is this the level of support needed? In answering this question, however, it is important not to focus on individual cases with the potential for major windfalls; these cases may well be balanced by many cases in which private organizations invest in technological development but secure no return. The important question is whether, in general, granting licenses without royalties is the level of support needed, or whether insisting on royalties in at least some cases is compatible with providing sufficient encouragement for needed technological development.

In short, we have good reasons for providing public support to private development activities. CRADAs and resulting intellectual property transfers enable us to provide public support for technology development without the direct public funding involved in supporting research. The reasonable pricing clause was not justified on the grounds that a direct return for the government investment in technology development was necessary. Still, some royalty payments might be appropriate. Resolution of this issue requires that we quantify the level of public support needed for private development efforts and compare that level with the level of actual support through CRADAs and royalty-free intellectual property transfers.

Barriers to Accessing Life-Prolonging Technologies

Supporters of the original reasonable pricing clause are likely to be unpersuaded by the analysis just presented. After all, they were concerned about the prices of AZT and other products of technological development serving as a barrier to access to new technologies, and the above analysis does not address that concern. What is the point of public support for technological development if those who need the resulting products cannot afford them? In what way is the development of unaffordable advances a public good?

While rhetorically powerful, this objection as it stands is ultimately unpersuasive. Even if highly priced, the resulting technologies do become available to many who have access to them because of their public or private insurance coverage. Moreover, their development also results in economic advances for the national economy, another good resulting from technology transfer. All of this makes these technological advancements deserving of public support through technology transfer.

Nevertheless, a number of legitimate issues cannot be ignored. One has to do with the pricing of product such as drugs that result from technological development. The other has to do with access to life-prolonging interventions.

In my recent book on the issue of drug pricing,[13] I argued for a number of conclusions about the pricing of drugs that I can only reiterate here and then apply to our controversy. They are:

(1) The United States is unique in the developed world in allowing the market to set the price of drugs.

(2) There are at least two good reasons why this approach is mistaken. Because of patent protection, drug manufacturers can attain monopoly prices and excessive profits for at least some of their drugs for a period of time while they lack real competitors. Moreover, the choice of drugs is usually made by physicians, who have had at least until recently few incentives to consider pricing, lessening the need for manufacturers to compete on pricing even when competing drugs are available.

(3) European pricing is not a model we ought to adopt because it fails to provide adequate economic incentives for research and development; there is reason to believe that the Europeans are free riding on the U.S. support of research and development through U.S. pricing.

(4) We need to develop a system of drug pricing that provides adequate economic incentives for drug research and development, taking into account the uncertainties and length of time involved, while limiting excessive promotional costs and profits. The British have done that in a way that makes sense in a system that is primarily a single-payer system; we need to do that in a way that fits into our multiple-payer system.

On the assumption that these conclusions are correct, a number of observations about the AZT and the CRADA pricing controversies seem appropriate. To begin with, AZT was a good example of a drug that at the time of its introduction lacked any competitors. This is just the type of case in which excessive monopoly prices are possible, illustrating why the current U.S. pricing scheme is unacceptable. Secondly, and more importantly, the anger at the pricing of AZT was inappropriately directed. The problem is not with the unreasonable pricing of drugs developed under some particular technology transfer scheme (the Orphan Drug Act or CRADAs), but with the lack of any social mechanism for generally controlling unreasonable prices for new drugs. Thirdly, and most importantly, we need to resist the claim that we must choose between controlling prices and giving adequate incentives for research and development. If we avoid the excesses of most of the European schemes, there is no reason why we cannot do both. The resulting system will not produce the lowest drug prices; British drug prices are among the highest in Europe. But it will give us the best balance between these two goals, especially if we can find a way to make the other developed countries pay for their share of drug research and development. Finally, in the meantime, mechanisms are available under the Bayh-Dole Act for dealing with the worst cases. The most important to my mind is the right of the granting federal agency under the Bayh-Dole Act to require that the private organization to which the technology was originally transferred grant a license to some other group to produce and sell the drug if this "action is necessary to alleviate health or safety needs not reasonably satisfied" by the private organization. If the price of the new drug is too high, the health needs of those who need the drug are not "reasonably satisfied."

Suppose that these policies were adopted and that the prices of new drugs developed through technological innovation were set under some general social mechanism. The prices might still be too high for some who are currently uninsured but in need of the drug to prolong their life. What then? This is, of course, the other crucial issue raised by the controversy.

This issue is obviously part of the broader issue of what degree of access to health care should be guaranteed. For those who accept the view that equal access means equal access to some appropriate level of care but not to every form of care, justifiably expensive new life-prolonging drugs raise the usual issue of the extent to which costs should determine the forms of health care that are part of that appropriate level of care. But several features of the cases arising out of technology transfer deserve special attention.

The first is that it is easy to avoid directly confronting the issue. Many drug companies were quite willing to consider programs that would provide these drugs for free to those who had no insurance and couldn't afford them. In general, the drug companies have actively promoted these programs as a way of avoiding price controls. Such programs are often funded by raising the price to insured users, thereby indirectly socially funding the drug without any explicit decision that this drug should be part of the appropriate level of care to which all are entitled. This type of subterfuge, however well intended, avoids rational discussion and decisionmaking and is a bad process for making important social decisions.

The other is that a good process has to consider the symbolic significance of some choices. What is the symbolic meaning of a decision that a new life-prolonging drug developed through technology transfer to promote social well-being is to be denied to some because of price? Isn't it that they are not part of the social order whose well-being is to be promoted? If the people in question already perceive themselves as being treated as social outcasts (as in the AZT case), this symbolic statement, even if unintended, may be unacceptable. Choices about coverage for the products of technology transfer need to consider the implications of symbolic meaning.

The CRADA reasonable pricing controversy should not have been just a technical discussion of a detail in government contracts. It raised fundamental questions about the role of government in promoting technological advances, about the pricing of those advances, and about access to their benefits. The voice of bioethics must advocate the discussion of those more fundamental issues.

QUESTIONS FOR CONSIDERATION

1. What was the significance of the Bayh-Dole Act of 1980 and the Federal Technology Transfer Act of 1986 on technology transfer? What were the two major themes that developed from these acts according to Brody?

2. How does the example of AZT illustrate the need for "reasonable prices for the products of technology transfer" in CODAs (cooperative research and development agreements)?

3. Do you believe that it is possible to find a balance between providing adequate incentives for research and development and controlling prices so that those who need the products can afford them?

4. How is technology transfer part of a larger social issue of access to health care?

NOTES

1. The announcement, and the background to it, received modest attention in the national press; the best coverage of it was Warren E. Leary, "Government Gives up Right to Control Prices of Drugs It Helps Develop" *New York Times*, 12 April 1995. Much more information is contained in a release from the NIH, *NIH News*, with an accompanying *Backgrounder*, both dated 11 April 1995.

2. The two acts are the Bayh-Dole Act (P.L. 9517) and the Technology Transfer Act (P.L. 94502). The relevant regulations for them are found in 37 *CFR* 401404.

3. The best introduction to these laws and their implications is J. V. Lacy, B. C. Brown, and M. R. Rubin, "Technology Transfer Laws Governing Federally Funded Research and Development," *Pepperdine Law Review* 19 (1991): 1–28. Another very useful account, with much background material, is chapter 9 of the OTA report, *Pharmaceutical Research and Development* (Washington: U.S. Government Printing Office, 1994).

4. Senate Report 283, 99th Congress, second session (1986).

5. This data comes from a GAO report entitled Technology Transferral Agencies Patent Licensing Activities (Washington: Government Accounting Office, 1991).

6. Senate Bill 1537, 103 Congress, second session.

7. Three excellent articles exploring this case and the resulting controversy are: Evan Ackiron, "Patents for Critical Pharmaceuticals," *American Journal of Law and Medicine* 17 (1991): 145–80; Mary T. Griffin, "AIDS Drugs and the Pharmaceutical Industry: A Need for Reform," *American Journal of Law and Medicine* 17 (1991): 363–410; S. R. Salbu, "AIDS and Drug Pricing: In Search of a Policy," *Washington University Law Quarterly* 71 (1993): 691–734.

8. Cited in the *NIH Backgrounder* referenced in footnote 1.

9. Quoted in S. Jenks, "Is the 'Reasonable Pricing' Clause Unreasonable" *Journal of the National Cancer Institute* 86 (1994): 1445–47.

10. An excellent account of the differences and of the attitude at the NIH in September is to be found in the 13 September issue of the Life Sciences version of the *Washington Fax*.

11. Quoted in Leary, "Government Gives up Right to Control Prices of Drugs."

12. GAO, *Technology Transfers: Benefits of Cooperative R&D Agreements* (Washington: Government Accounting Office, 1995).

13. Baruch A. Brody, *Ethical Issues in Drug Testing, Approval, and Pricing* (New York: Oxford University Press, 1995). The data supporting the claims about the European and the British systems can be found in chapter 4.

PART III: Biomedicine, Rights, and Responsibilities

ALEXANDER MORGAN CAPRON
The Burden of Decision

JOHN HARDWIG
What About the Family

JEFFREY BLUSTEIN
The Family in Medical Decisionmaking

Individual autonomy—the right of the competent individual to make intelligent and informed decisions about his own health and well-being—has long stood atop the list of values ethicists and health care providers bring to difficult bioethical questions. But advances in medical technologies have forced a rethinking of responsible decisionmaking: quite often, extraordinary measures are now successful in maintaining the "life" of the critically ill or seriously injured. These individuals are kept alive, but are often incompetent or have limited capacity in making autonomous decisions regarding their health care. Even those individuals who remain competent in their decisionmaking may find their interests in conflict with the interests of family members, medical staffs, or society in general. In such cases, the interests or rights of individuals seemingly must be balanced with their responsibilities, as well as with the rights and responsibilities of family members, health care providers, and society as a whole.

Mrs. Helga Wanglie, an eighty-six-year-old woman, broke her hip and was treated for the injury. Subsequently, she was returned to the hospital to be treated for respiratory failure. While on the respirator, Mrs. Wanglie suffered a cardiopulmonary arrest. She was diagnosed as having severe and permanent brain damage. Although her treatment continued, the medical staff concluded that Mrs. Wanglie was in a persistent vegetative state and that further treatment, including the use of the respirator, would not benefit her. Her husband, Oliver Wanglie, and his family refused to agree to removing the respirator. Her medical bills over seventeen months totaled $800,000 and were paid by a private insurance company.

The *Wanglie* case raises a number of interesting questions. How should treatment decisions be made? Who holds the greatest claim over this decision-making process? The now incapacitated individual? The prior expressed wishes of the individual? The family faced with great emotional and financial costs? Health care professionals who oversee the allocation of increasingly limited resources? What role does public policy—the concrete principles and programs by which government acts—play in these decisions?

This section will focus on responsibility in decisionmaking: that is, who should make these decisions rather than how such decisions should be made. The readings for this discussion will include:

- Alexander Morgan Capron's **The Burden of Decision** warns against the shifting burden of decisionmaking in bioethics cases produced by recent judicial intervention.
- John Hardwig's **What About the Family** argues for the importance of family interests in contrast to those of patient autonomy and public policy.
- Jeffrey Blustein's **The Family in Medical Decisionmaking** defends patient autonomy against the arguments of Hardwig regarding family interests and against communitarian visions of interests.

ALEXANDER MORGAN CAPRON

The Burden of Decision

Over the past three decades the courts have been a major forum not merely for resolving bioethical disputes but for acquainting the public with the hard choices that modern medicine so often poses. The courtroom has become such a familiar setting in this context that we seldom ask: what are we doing here? And yet a hard look at that issue is essential if we are going to preserve and enhance the very values articulated in such landmark opinions as *Cobbs v. Grant*,[1] In re *Quinlan*,[2] and *Barber v. Superior Court*.[3] Ironically, the groundwork laid in those cases now requires that judges be more reluctant to become involved in the disputes about medical interventions brought before them, lest in the process they subtly erode the high view of human dignity and liberty established in these cases on informed consent, patient autonomy, and the limits of medicine.

Of course, no one can deny the importance of the landmarks themselves. The full force of judicial authority and eloquence was needed to shake physicians from their predisposition to hold onto knowledge, conceal uncertainty, and reserve decision-making power to themselves. In opinion after opinion, judges made clear that before treating a patient, a physician must not merely obtain consent but must disclose the information the patient needs to make a decision about whether and how to proceed.

Some commentators have been skeptical that the judges ever meant what they said, so many have been the impediments they placed in the way of patients actually enforcing their rights by collecting damages for violations of their right to choose.[4] Yet the medical profession—along with patients and their advocacy groups—has apparently believed the ringing phrases in the judicial opinions, as have the rising corps of bioethicists who take the legal doctrine of informed consent as bedrock.

Indeed, only now, after twenty years of debate, are bioethicists seriously struggling with integrating concepts like community into an analysis that has focused almost entirely on autonomy and self-determination. Thus, informed consent has had an effect on physicians' attitudes, probably on their behavior, and certainly on how prominent physicians and ethicists describe the ideal physician-patient relationship that is far out of proportion to the doctrine's actual significance as a basis for recovery. It has been an influence for good of which the law can be proud, even if judges—like the rest of us—need some time getting used to the full implications of what they have written.

As manifested by the leading cases on informed consent, good reasons certainly exist for courts to become involved in some bioethics cases. When circumstances change in important ways—as in medicine over the past several decades—and existing doctrines seem inadequate or of unclear import, the courts perform a vital law-making function through their opinions in landmark cases. What I find to be troubling, however, is both our increasing proclivity to turn to the courts routinely, especially in treatment-termination cases, and judges' greater willingness "to yield to spasmodic sentiment, to vague and unregulated benevolence," in the trenchant phrase of Judge Cardozo.[5]

In this article, I will initially take the typical bioethics case to involve a disagreement about the recommended medical intervention (though later I will attempt to generalize some conclusions to a more diverse group of cases). The clear implication of the informed consent cases is that when disagreements occur, a patient's refusal of recommended treatment will be respected. Formally, courts have supported the notion of informed refusal. Yet the courts have been less robust in support of patient choice when the issue is not liability for inadequate disclosure but disagreement over the refusal itself. My concern is not just that the doctrine of informed consent will be undetermined by judicial failure to back up patient choices, but that physicians (along with health care administrators) will seek to transfer to judges the very paternalistic powers that thirty years of bioethical analysis and court cases have aimed to banish.

Here Comes the Judge

On what grounds, then, have courts sought to justify and explain their intervention in bioethical disputes? The first is protecting patients from harm. Although clearly problematic when applied to competent patients, the concept of protecting patients is a traditional (and appropriate) role for the judiciary. But that does not end concerns about transferred paternalism (from physicians to judges), it simply shifts the nature of the concern. It makes central an issue that has received too little attention, namely proper standards and procedures for the determination of incompetency. And it opens up the question: how is protection to be achieved?

A second major reason for involving the judiciary is to protect health care professionals from liability, both civil and criminal. If a physician turns off a respirator, might she find herself later defending a tort action brought by a disgruntled relative or, even worse, a criminal action brought by the district attorney? Frankly, this fear seems greatly exaggerated. As to the first, if informed decision making has occurred—whether by the patient directly or by whoever has authority to act on the patient's behalf—there is little likelihood of a suit being brought and even less of its succeeding. As to the risk of criminal prosecution, physicians are never convicted for carrying out decisions mutually made with qualified surrogates, much less with patients. Thus, there should be little cause for judges to intervene simply to dispense advance absolution for health care providers.

What about protection of third parties? Here the rationale for intervention is very dependent upon the facts at hand. In the case of life-sustaining treatment, for example, the argument that a mother with young children should not be permitted to forgo treatment that might lengthen her life was once persuasive with courts, but in recent years has been notable for its omission. More weighty, and—indeed—often decisive, is the judicial role in protecting third parties from harm that could come to them directly and palpably from a patient's choice, such as a refusal to be vaccinated when a contagion is loose.

The fourth reason cited to invoke judicial intervention—protection of societal interests—has the vice, or virtue, of great vagueness. The primary collective concern on which reliance is placed is the sanctity of human life. The central problem with this appeal is that it is so powerful as to overwhelm all others. In a system truly prepared to let the communal trump the individual, this would pose no problem. But even if greater attention is lately being paid to collective interests in bioethical discussions—such as the recognition that the need to stem the spread of HIV infection may justify certain limitations on individual privacy—our legal and philosophical framework in the end continues to favor personal liberty and diversity over conformity to a single norm, especially one that smacks of religious dogma. Thus, when societal interests are invoked to justify intervention, they are typically framed in a way that keeps them from trumping other interests.

Society's interest in respecting and protecting the norms of the medical profession has been much less influential with courts in recent years, for several reasons. Many judges have realized that too great respect for this interest is inherently inconsistent with the doctrine of informed consent. A patient should be under no greater obligation to accede to an intervention on the ground that it reflects "the norms of the profession" than because the attending physician favors it. Even more telling, the courts have come to see that professional norms are either nonexistent regarding a particular point (such as when life begins) or that current norms (as articulated, say, by the AMA's Council on Ethical and judicial Affairs) now firmly espouse respect for patient choice, not medical paternalism.

These five factors—protection of the patient, protection of professionals from liability, protection of third parties, protection of societal interests, and respect for the norms of the profession—might all be described as grounds for *societal* intervention, rather than uniquely for *judicial* intervention. The two get lumped together because, in a system that respects due process of law, exercise of the state's coercive power usually involves prior approval by a court. A sixth and final factor—resolution of disputes among the parties— is more narrowly relevant to judicial intervention, and is especially relevant in situations in which the dispute essentially involves private rather than collective interests.

As a general matter, we take it to be a mark of a civilized society that it provides forums where disagreements can be resolved in an orderly, principled, and unbiased fashion. Yet as courts have long recognized, there are good reasons for not exercising their potential jurisdiction, and a variety of doctrines—about justiciability, ripeness, and the like—exist to permit (and sometimes even to mandate) rejection of a request for judicial intervention. In bioethics cases, it is especially moot that courts heed basic principles about the need for a genuine controversy and for a question that is ripe for decision, while also being cautious in applying rules on mootness, since medical matters tend to move along a more rapid timetable and a strict bar of any case that is moot on its facts (the patient has died, for example) could lead many issues repeatedly to evade review.

Problems When Courts Do Intervene

Among the problems that arise when medical decision making is brought into the courtroom, I will mention half a dozen. First is the issue of time. Plainly, there are occasions when the legal system moves with a good deal of dispatch. But the strength of the system lies in its ability to deliberate carefully and thoughtfully about an issue, and especially in bioethics cases, there are plenty of issues, often rather unfamiliar ones for a judge, to deliberate about. The difference in sense of time between physicians and lawyers was crystallized for me by the statement of a physician who testified before the

President's Commission on Medical Ethics. She said that when her lawyer friends congratulate themselves on filing a brief on an emergency matter, they mean that they did it in a week or perhaps in several days, while when she has an emergency, she runs up the stairs in the hospital rather than waiting for an elevator.

A second problem with judicial intervention is the way these cases tend literally to dislocate judges: called to resolve cases that often involve bedbound patients, judges often hold their hearings in the hospital and even right at the patient's bedside. Judge J. Skelly Wright's trip to the Georgetown Hospital in an early Jehovah's Witness case may have been justified by his doubts about the patient's (fading) competence to refuse the blood transfusion,[6] but it provided no precedent for a similar maneuver a quarter century later by another District of Columbia judge who went to Angela Carder's hospital but never even spoke with her before ordering a cesarean section despite the objections of her family and attending physicians.[7] The trappings ought not be confused with the office, but there is something important for judicial decision making in the robe, the bench, the whole setting—and especially in the sense of security and propriety in decision making that the trappings give to the judge herself or himself. Of course, the robe and gavel may come along to the hospital. But everything about that alien environment conspires to tell the judge—and the parties and witnesses—that the men and women in white coats and green scrub suits, not the judge, are really in command.[8]

Third, judicial involvement in medical cases spawns communication difficulties. To begin with, the subject matter subverts the utility of the forum. This can, of course, occur in any highly complex and technical field in which the participants are used to communicating with each other through a shared vocabulary and, even more important, through shared knowledge and assumptions. It is not only time-consuming to spell out all the relevant information, but the participants are likely not always to know exactly what information is being correctly understood and when different presumptions are causing a point that they think means one thing to be heard differently in the "courtroom." Moreover, courtroom dramas lend themselves to false certainties. Even participants (such as patients and their families) normally inclined to feel ignorant or indecisive in a hospital setting are impelled by the nature of litigation to take firm stands and to paint the facts accordingly. The obverse problem also occurs: the forum subverts the task at hand. Since bioethics cases involve such personal matters and deeply felt values, everyone's discomfort at probing too aggressively poses a further impediment to clear and honest communication.

A further, more subtle communication problem arises when the parties merely want an imprimatur, not an independent resolution of a dispute—for example, in life-support cases when physicians do not seriously disagree with the family about stopping treatment of an incompetent patient and are in court at the insistence of the hospital's lawyer. The family may believe it is going along with what has been chosen by the physicians, who in turn think their medical judgment has been supported by the hospital, whose administrators are prepared to go ahead if approval can be obtained from the judge, who in turn thinks she is merely blessing what all the other parties agree to. Wouldn't the patient's interests be better served if the family and physician realized that the real decision rests with them, subject to later review (and, in an extreme case, even to sanctions) if they have not discharged this responsibility appropriately?

The lack of genuine controversy in many cases is also at odds with the traditional view of the adversarial system. Nor is this problem limited to cases about withdrawal of life-support. For example, in kidney transplant cases involving identical, minor twins, Massachusetts courts in the 1950s gave declaratory judgments on matters about which all participants—the twins, their parents, and the physicians—agreed.

Sometimes, when an incompetent person is involved, as in the landmark 1969 Kentucky sibling transplant case, *Strunk v. Strunk*,[9] an attempt is made to overcome this lack of controversy by appointing a guardian ad litem. Such a person seems to me to be in an awkward position, since it is expected that the guardian will oppose whatever motion has been made rather than do what a guardian should, that is, to exercise independent judgment about the incompetent's actual interests. Likewise, in some surrogate motherhood cases, the parties do not disagree with each other but rather join in asking the court for the same result; only the intervention of the state, into what are nominally private disputes, brings an element of genuine controversy.[10]

Assuming that these difficulties with judicial involvement are overcome, a fifth one goes to the heart of the effort to shift the burden of decision from medical to judicial shoulders, namely, the very difference in the mode of decision making in these two arenas. The hallmark of judicial decision making is its finality. Like Alexander facing the Gordian knot, the judge succeeds not by untangling a case but by cutting through contradictory facts and arguments and *resolving* the case. Once a final judgment has been entered, countless legal principles—from the standards applied by appellate courts in reviewing the facts found below, to the doctrines of estoppel and *stare decisis*—aim to avoid revisiting points already resolved. Judges may be left with a realization of the constructed, and highly fallible, nature of the reality that inheres in what they do. But to the outside world, it seems definite, fixed, and final—and to be honored not necessarily because one agrees with the outcome but because such respect for the judgments of courts is the linchpin of our legal system and indeed of civil order.

How far this seems from the uncertainty that inheres in matters medical! Are judges really ready for the job of surrogate physician, much less surrogate patient? For situations that do not just evolve over time but that may completely reverse themselves in a matter of minutes? For prospective rather than predominantly retrospective decisionmaking, in circumstances where the barrier to obtaining "the truth, the whole truth, and nothing but the truth" is not deceitful witnesses or crafty lawyers but the limits of current understanding of human functioning and a lack of time and resources to find out everything one might be able to know, much less want to know?

Faced with the pressures of decision making under conditions of extreme uncertainty, the impulse of judges called to decide bioethics cases is to temporize. I am not unsympathetic with this impulse. Indeed, I often wish physicians were *more* willing to employ it as a negotiating posture with their patients. But it fits poorly with many bioethics cases. When, in that famous *Georgetown College* case, judge Wright wrote that since "a life hung in the balance" and "[t]here was no time for research or reflection," he had authorized a blood transfusion for Mrs. Jones "to preserve the *status quo*,"[11] he actually denied the patient the one thing she wanted, which was to remain unsullied by a blood transfusion. By making a medical-type decision ("a blood transfusion is needed now to save this woman's life") he abdicated his real role of making and justifying a judicial decision ("the preservation of life, even involuntarily, is a higher value than a person's religious beliefs").

A sixth problem that occurs when bioethical issues end up in the courtroom is the inevitability of publicity. Most of us would like our medical care to be carried out in private. We probably think that we and our physicians would make better decisions in calmer and less contentious circumstances; moreover, our condition and treatment are simply no one else's business. Increasingly, however, medicine is like a three-ring circus. Not all of this results from the judicial process. Think, for example, of Barney Clark, the first recipient of the so-called permanent, totally implanted artificial heart, whose every breath was the subject of press releases from the University of Utah and whose urine output was reported on the nightly news from coast-to-coast. Perhaps Dr. Clark and his family gladly agreed to all this, but patients and families who are dragged into court typically do not give up their privacy so willingly.

Sometimes they may find cover as members of the ubiquitous Doe family. But in many other cases, for whatever reason—from Karen Quinlan to Nancy Cruzan, from Mary Beth Whitehead to Pamela Stewart Monson—the actual parties become familiar objects of national curiosity. The prospect of *People* magazine on the line for the judge in a bioethics case seems no more attractive—or conducive to good decision making—than tabloids replacing *The New England Journal of Medicine* as physicians' preferred venue for reporting their work.

Differences and Commonalities

Bioethics cases are a diverse lot, and the appropriate response for a judge faced with one will depend upon the category into which it falls. Let's consider three primary categories. First are "life support treatment decisions," the overwhelming majority of which involve competent or formerly competent persons. As lawyers and physicians become more accustomed to aiding their clients to execute durable powers of attorney and living wills, I suspect that the wishes of many—perhaps most—seriously ill patients regarding life-support will be available, either directly from them as competent patients or from their surrogate decision makers and explicit instructions. In such circumstances, judges should affirm that the decision rests with the patient. Except in extraordinary cases—involving perhaps a threat of contagion or the like—no substantial interests are arrayed against those of the patient, so there is no need for a judicial balancing act. The patient's choice may discomfort others, but that is often the consequence of an exercise of liberty, and a free society has to be able to function with that. The major concern is thus that the judicial process not interfere with good medical care and good communication between physician and patient or surrogate, including efforts to maintain or restore the patient's own decisionmaking capacity to the maximum extent.

If life support decisions ought to be characterized by maximal deference to the voice of the patient, judicial involvement with reproductive decisions-whether *in vitro* fertilization, artificial insemination, surrogate motherhood, or what-have-you—ought to be constantly attentive to interests that are not well represented by the loud voices of the adult parties to the transactions. This is not to suggest that courts should depart any further from the right of privacy than the U.S. Supreme Court or the law of a particular state requires. Yet, as the Michigan Court of Appeals has opined, "the welfare of the child [of the new reproductive techniques] must continue to be of paramount importance."[12] In this category of cases, judges may need to be pro-active to ensure that these children are treated as ends in themselves (with their own interests) and not merely as means to the ends of the adults involved.

The hardest cases are those—such as maternal-fetal cases—in which the exercise of one person's liberty squarely threatens the physical well-being of another. Here judges should remain firmly oriented in reality rather than abstraction. Frustrated by our inability to halt the epidemic of drug use, society will be tempted to look for easy and dramatic ways to protest the harmful consequences of this behavior. Punishing pregnant addicts is one such response. More helpful responses lie outside the courts' jurisdiction—with the legislature and the executive. But judges may be a force for improving society's response, as well as a protector of justice, if they insist that, if women are to be punished for actions that expose fetuses to harm, their actions must be truly "voluntary," in the sense that Justice Holmes used that term a century ago in his work on the common law, namely that the women had an opportunity to avoid the harm and unreasonably chose not to take it. For crack users and alcoholics, this means that before society tries to solve the problem of prenatal substance abuse with criminal prosecutions, it ought to make available to pregnant women drug detoxification and treatment programs appropriate to their circumstances.

Despite the differences among the categories of cases, several common threads also tie bioethics disputes together. We need to realize that in the majority of instances, courts do their jobs best when they try to ensure a fair and appropriate process rather than a particular outcome. Typically, this means that a court should be concerned with finding and empowering a competent decision maker, whether that be the patient or an appropriate surrogate.

One of the milestones in bioethics, the New Jersey Supreme Court's 1976 *Quinlan* decision, reveals problems in this regard. The justices are often praised for having suggested that cases of that type need not be routinely brought to court. Yet it should have been enough for the court to know that Joseph Quinlan was a knowledgeable, sincere, and careful spokesman for his daughter's interests, and that the choices he and her physician made would be reviewed by a hospital ethics committee. The court need not have put itself in the position of imagining what Karen would have decided if she "were herself miraculously lucid for an interval . . . and perceptive of her irreversible condition."[13]

Whether a surrogate is a natural guardian (as a parent for a child) or one appointed by the court, if the guardian's decision is challenged, the correct question is *not* whether the judge would make a different choice—for there will always be a range of choices rather than a single, correct choice, whether one is interpreting a patient's wishes under the "substituted judgment" doctrine or discerning the patient's "best interests" when his or her specific wishes are unknown. Instead, the question is whether the process by which choices were made reveals such lack of attention or devotion to the patient's welfare, such a conflict of interest, or such an inability to use relevant information to arrive at a decision, that the guardian should be replaced by someone else.

Complementing this basic principle is the desirability of courts preserving as much flexibility for decision making as possible, in the face of the uncertainty that characterizes so much of health care. A court that declines to make decisions itself can then focus on giving those who do have decisionmaking authority sufficient scope and reassurance to enable them to respond to the medical situation as it unfolds. Flexibility is most difficult to preserve exactly where it is most needed: when decisions are prospective, not retrospective, such as petitions to remove feeding tubes or to authorize a cesarean section on an unconsenting woman.

To the extent that checks on decision making are appropriate, courts would also do well to rely on consultants or advisors who are closer to the bedside. While few hospitals apparently responded to *Quinlan* by appointing hospital ethics committees, a majority—spurred by the so-called federal Baby Doe II regulations—now have such committees, though they are quite varied in composition, purpose, and actual functioning. Without giving such bodies *carte blanche*, the judiciary could do more to protect relevant interests by fostering and guiding the development of such close-to-the-bedside processes. If ethics committees are to possess the independence they need to provide necessary protection for incompetent patients, courts will have to give substance to what constitutes "reasonable" conduct by such a group.

Almost by rote, judges deciding difficult bioethical issues on unfamiliar points end by encouraging—often pleading for—a legislative response. While thoughtful legislation would be very welcome, experience has shown that serious problems can occur when judges' prayers for legislation are answered. The prime example is so-called living will legislation. Since the first one was passed in California in 1976, statutes on this topic have sown much confusion and have probably detracted as much from patients' real rights as they have added. I used to accept the notion that legislation, like sausage, is fine, one just does not want to watch it being made. I'm now much less sanguine about the products themselves, at least those that emerge from ordinary legislative processes, without the benefit of initial formulation by one of the state or national governmental bioethics panels.

Finally, and most fundamentally, the common thread I see for all bioethics cases is the desirability of holding off the eager willingness of others to shift the burden of decision onto the courts. Twenty four years ago, Justice Jacob Markowitz of the Supreme Court of New York had before him a petition brought by two of Sadie Nemser's three sons to be appointed her guardian for the purpose of consenting to an amputation of her gangrenous right ankle and foot. Her physicians wanted to operate but were reluctant to do so in the absence of judicial authorization because Mrs. Nemser's third son, a physician, refused to consent since he did not think his mother could survive the surgery or would benefit from it. From an investigation by a guardian ad litem and a psychiatrist, Justice Markowitz had no doubt that Mrs. Nemser was unable to understand the situation or to make an informed choice. Nevertheless, he declined to grant the petition. As he wrote, the physicians and hospitals were attempting to shift the burden of their responsibilities to the courts, to determine, in effect, whether doctors should proceed with certain medical procedures definitively found necessary or deemed advisable for the health, welfare, and perhaps even the life of a patient.

Rejecting their bid for immunity, which he found "incongruous" in light of the Hippocratic oath, the judge lamented "what an ultra-legalistic maze we have created." In its place, Judge Markowitz clearly favored "the exercise of sound medical judgment," to which I would add—in light of the subsequent elaboration of the informed consent doctrine—"in the context of mutual decision making by physician and patient (or surrogate) as informed partners." Judges would do well to follow the lead of the *Nemser* case and not to regard a refusal on their own part to intervene as indifference to patient's well-being. Instead, as Judge Markowitz demonstrated, it would be better for all concerned if courts reminded "those whose responsibility it actually is, to act appropriately, not arbitrarily, and without fear."[14]

QUESTIONS FOR CONSIDERATION

1. Capron indicates that recent judicial intervention has moved decision-making power from the physician to the patient. Is this shift justified? Are there problems with transferring responsibility from the medical expert to the patient?

2. Capron also expresses concern that judicial intervention may not shift decisionmaking responsibilities from paternalistic physicians to autono-

mous patients but from paternalistic physicians to paternalistic judges. What arguments would justify this concern?

3. What are the grounds that Capron indicates have led the courts to justify and explain their intervention in bioethical disputes? What are his criticisms of those grounds?

4. What are the six problems that Capron identifies whenever courts intervene in medical decisionmaking?

NOTES

1. *Cobbs v. Grant,* 8 Cal.2d 229, 502 P.2d 1 (1972). See also *Canterbury v. Spence,* 464 F.2d 772 (D.C. Cir.), *cert. denied,* 409 U.S. 1064 (1972); *Wilkinson v. Vesey,* 110 R.I. 606, 295, A.2d 676 (1972); *Natanson v. Kline,* 186 Kan. 393, 350 P.2d 1093 (1960); *Salgo v. Leland Stanford Etc. Bd. of Trustees,* 154 Cal. App. 2d 560, 317 P.2d 170 (1957).

2. *In re Quinlan,* 70 N.J. 10, 355 A.2d 647, *cert. denied,* 429 U.S. 922 (1976).

3. *Barber v. Superior Court,* 147 Cal. App. 3d 1006, 195 Cal. Rptr. 484 (1983).

4. Jay Katz, "Informed Consent—A Fairy Tale? Law's Vision," *University of Pittsburgh Law Review* 39 (1977), 137–74.

5. Benjamin N. Cardozo, *The Nature of the Judicial Process* (New Haven: Yale University Press, 1921), 141.

6. *Application of President and Directors of Georgetown College,* 331 F.2d 1000 (D.C. Cir), *cert. denied,* 377 U.S. 978 (1964).

7. *In re A.C.,* 533 A.2d 611 (D.C.C. App. 1987).

8. I find it hard to believe, for example, that the Indiana judge who in 1982 decided the original Baby Doe case in the wee hours of the night with "no judicial accoutrements whatsoever" in an unused storage closet on the top floor of that hospital in Bloomington deliberated on the matter exactly as he would have had it been heard during a regular workday at the courthouse. See Jeff Lyon, *Playing God in the Nursery* (New York: W.W. Norton & Co. 1985), 31.

9. *Strunk v. Strunk,* 445 S.W.2d 145 (Ky 1969).

10. See *Syrkowski v. Appleyard,* 122 Mich. App. 506, 333 N.W.2d 90 (1983) (refuses to issue order of filiation sought under Paternity Act to establish petitioner's status as natural father of fetus conceived pursuant to surrogate mother contract).

11. *Application of President and Directors of Georgetown College,* 331 F.2d 1000 (D.C.Cir.), *cert. denied,* 377 U.S. 978 (1964).

12. *Syrkowski v. Appleyard,* 122 Mich. App. 506, 333 N.W.2d 90, 93 (1983).

13. *In re Quinlan,* 70 N.J. 10, 355 A.2d 647, at 663.

14. *In re Nemser,* 273 N.Y.S2d 624, 629, 631 (Sup. Ct. 1966).

JOHN HARDWIG

What About the Family?

We are beginning to recognize that the prevalent ethic of patient autonomy simply will not do. Since demands for health care are virtually unlimited, giving autonomous patients the care they want will bankrupt our health care system. We can no longer simply buy our way out of difficult questions of justice by expanding the health care pie until there is enough to satisfy the wants and needs of everyone. The requirements of justice and the needs of other patients must temper the claims of autonomous patients.

But if the legitimate claims of other patients and other (non-medical) interests of society are beginning to be recognized, another question is still largely ignored: To what extent can the patient's family legitimately be asked or required to sacrifice their interests so that the patient can have the treatment he or she wants?

This question is not only almost universally ignored, it is generally implicitly dismissed, silenced before it can even be raised. This tacit dismissal results from a fundamental assumption of medical ethics: medical treatment ought always to serve the interests of the patient. This, of course, implies that the interests of family members should be irrelevant to medical treatment decisions or at least ought never to take precedence over the interests of the patient. All questions about fairness to the interests of family members are thus precluded, regardless of the merit or importance of the interests that will have to be sacrificed if the patient is to receive optimal treatment.

Yet there is a whole range of cases in which important interests of family members are dramatically affected by decisions about the patient's treatment; medical decisions often should be made with those interests in mind. Indeed, in many cases family members have a greater interest than the patient in which treatment option is exercised. In such cases, the interests of family members often ought to *override* those of the patient.

The problem of family interests cannot be resolved by considering other members of the family as "patients," thereby redefining the problem as one of conflicting interests among *patients*. Other members of the family are not always ill, and even if ill, they still may not be patients. Nor will it do to define the whole family as one patient. Granted, the slogan "the patient is the family" was coined partly to draw attention to precisely the issues I wish to raise, but the idea that the whole family is one patient is too monolithic. The conflicts of interests, beliefs, and values among family members are often too real and run too deep to treat all members as "the patient." Thus, if I am correct, it is sometimes the moral thing to do for a physician to sacrifice the interests of her patient to those of nonpatients—specifically, to those of the other members of the patient's family.

But what is the "family"? As I will use it here, it will mean roughly "those who are close to the patient." "Family" so defined will often include close friends and companions. It may also exclude some with blood or marriage ties to the patient. "Closeness" does not, however, always mean care and abiding affection, nor need it be a positive experience—one can hate, resent, fear, or despise a mother or brother with an intensity not often directed toward strangers, acquaintances, or associates. But there are cases where even a hateful or resentful family member's interests ought to be considered.

This use of "family" gives rise to very sensitive ethical—and legal—issues in the case of legal relatives with no emotional ties to the patient that I cannot pursue here. I can only say that I do not mean to suggest that the interests of legal relatives who are not emotionally close to the patient are always to be ignored. They will sometimes have an important financial interest in the treatment even if they are not emotionally close to the patient. But blood and marriage ties can become so thin that they become merely legal relationships. (Consider, for example, "couples" who have long since parted but who have never gotten a divorce, or cases in which the next of kin cannot be bothered with making proxy decisions.) Obviously, there are many important questions about just whose interests are to be considered in which treatment decisions and to what extent.

Connected Interests

There is no way to detach the lives of patients from the lives of those who are close to them. Indeed, the intertwining of lives is part of the very meaning of closeness. Consequently, there will be a broad spectrum of cases in which the treatment options will have dramatic and different impacts on the patient's family.

I believe there are many, many such cases. To save the life of a newborn with serious defects is often dramatically to affect the rest of the parents' lives and, if they have other children, may seriously compromise the quality of their lives, as well . . . The husband of a woman with Alzheimer's disease may well have a life totally dominated for ten years or more by caring for an increasingly foreign and estranged wife . . . The choice between aggressive and palliative care or, for that matter, the difference between either kind of care and suicide in the case of a father with terminal cancer or AIDS may have a dramatic emotional and financial impact on his wife and children. . . Less dramatically, the choice between two medications, one of which has the side effect of impotence, may radically alter the life a couple has together. . . The drug of choice for controlling high blood pressure may be too expensive (that is, requires too many sacrifices) for many families with incomes just above the ceiling for Medicaid. . .

Because the lives of those who are close are not separable, to be close is to no longer have a life entirely your own to live entirely as you choose. To be part of a family is to be morally required to make decisions on the basis of thinking about what is best for all concerned, not simply what is best for yourself. In healthy families, characterized by genuine care, one wants to make decisions on this basis, and many people do so quite naturally and automatically. My own grandfather committed suicide after his heart attack as a final gift to his wife—he had plenty of life insurance but not nearly enough health insurance, and he feared that she would be left homeless and destitute if he lingered on in an incapacitated state. Even if one is not so inclined, however, it is irresponsible and wrong to exclude or to fail to consider the interests of those who are close. Only when the lives of family members will not be importantly affected can one rightly make exclusively or even predominantly self-regarding decisions.

Although "what is best for all concerned" sounds utilitarian, my position does not imply that the right course of action results simply from a calculation of what is best for all. No, the seriously ill may have a right to special consideration, and the family of an ill person may have a duty to make sacrifices to respond to a member's illness. It is one thing to claim that the ill deserve special consideration; it is quite another to maintain that they deserve exclusive or even overriding consideration. Surely we must admit that there are limits to the right to special treatment by virtue of illness. Otherwise, everyone would be morally required to sacrifice all other goods to better care for the ill. We must also recognize that patients too have moral obligations, obligations to try to protect the lives of their families from destruction resulting from their illnesses.

Thus, unless serious illness excuses one from all moral responsibility— and I don't see how it could—it is an oversimplification to say of a patient who is part of a family that "it's his life" or "after all, it's his medical treatment," as if his life and his treatment could be successfully isolated from the lives of the other members of his family. It is more accurate to say "it's their lives" or "after all, they're all going to have to live with his treatment." Then the really serious moral questions are not *whether* the interests of family members are relevant to decisions about a patient's medical treatment *or whether* their interests should be included in his deliberations or in deliberations about him, but how far family and friends can be asked to support and sustain the patient. What sacrifices can they be morally required to make for his health care? How far can they reasonably be asked to compromise the quality of their lives so that he will receive the care that would improve the quality of his life? To what extent can he reasonably expect them to put their lives "on hold" to preoccupy themselves with his illness to the extent necessary to care for him?

The Anomaly of Medical Decisionmaking

The way we analyze medical treatment decisions by or for patients is plainly anomalous to the way we think about other important decisions family members make. I am a husband, a father, and still a son, and no one would argue that I should or even responsibly could decide to take a sabbatical, another job, or even a weekend trip *solely* on the basis of what I want for myself. Why should decisions about my medical treatment be different? Why should we have even thought that medical treatment decisions might be different?

Is it because medical decisions, uniquely, involve life and death matters? Most medical decisions, however, are not matters of life and death, and we as a society risk or shorten the lives of other people—through our toxic waste disposal decisions, for example—quite apart from considerations of whether that is what they want for themselves.

Have we been misled by a preoccupation with the biophysical model of disease? Perhaps it has tempted us to think of illness and hence also of treatment as, something that takes place *within* the body of the patient. What happens in my body does not—barring contagion—affect my wife's body, yet it usually does affect her.

Have we tacitly desired to simplify the practice and the ethics of medicine by considering only the *medical* or health-related consequences of treatment decisions? Perhaps, but it is obvious that we need a broader vision of and sensitivity to all the consequences of action, at least among those who are not simply technicians following orders from above. Generals need to consider more than military consequences, businessmen more than economic consequences, teachers more than educational consequences, lawyers more than legal consequences.

Does the weakness and vulnerability of serious illness imply that the ill need such protection that we should serve only their interests? Those who are sick may indeed need special protection, but this can only mean that we must take special care to see that the interests of the ill are duly considered. It does not follow that their interests are to be served exclusively or even that their interests must always predominate. Moreover, we must remember that in terms of the dynamics of the family, the patient is not always the weakest member, the member most in need of protection.

Does it make *historical,* if not logical, sense to view the wishes and interests of the patient as always overriding? Historically, illnesses were generally of much shorter duration; patients got better quickly or died quickly. Moreover, the costs of the medical care available were small enough that rarely was one's future mortgaged to the costs of the care of family members. Although this was once truer than it is today, there have always been significant exceptions to these generalizations.

None of these considerations adequately explains why the interests of the patient's family have been thought to be appropriately excluded from consideration. At the very least, those who believe that medical treatment decisions are morally anomalous to other important decisions owe us a better account of how and why this is so.

Limits of Public Policy

It might be thought that the problem of family interests is a problem only because our society does not shelter families from the negative effects of medical decisions. If, for example, we adopted a comprehensive system of national health insurance and also a system of public insurance to guarantee the incomes of families, then my sons' chances at a college education and the quality of the rest of their lives might not have to be sacrificed were I to receive optimal medical care.

However, it is worth pointing out that we are still moving primarily in the *opposite* direction. Instead of designing policies that would increasingly shelter family members from the adverse impact of serious and prolonged illnesses, we are still attempting to shift the burden of care to family members in our efforts to contain medical costs. A social system that would safeguard families from the impact of serious illness is nowhere in sight in this country. And we must not do medical ethics as if it were.

It is perhaps even more important to recognize that the lives of family members could not be sheltered from all the important ramifications of medical treatment decisions by any set of public policies. In any society in which people get close to each other and care deeply for each other, treatment decisions about one will often and *irremediably* affect more than one. If a newborn has been saved by aggressive treatment but is severely handicapped, the parents may simply not be emotionally capable of abandoning the child to institutional care. A man whose wife is suffering from multiple sclerosis may simply not be willing or able to go on with his own life until he sees her through to the end. A woman whose husband is being maintained in a vegetative state may not feel free to marry or even to see other men again, regardless of what some revised law might say about her marital status.

Nor could we desire a society in which friends and family would quickly lose their concern as soon as continuing to care began to diminish the quality of their own lives. For we would then have alliances for better but not for worse, in health but not in sickness, until death appears on the horizon. And we would all be poorer for that. A man who can leave his wife the day after she learns she has cancer, on the grounds that he has his own life to live, is to be deplored. The emotional inability or principled refusal to separate ourselves and our lives from the lives of ill or dying members of our families is not an unfortunate fact about the structure of our emotions. It is a desirable feature, not to be changed even if it could be; not to be changed even if the resulting intertwining of lives debars us from making exclusively self-regarding treatment decisions when we are ill.

Our present individualistic medical ethics is isolating and destructive. For by implicitly suggesting that patients make "their own" treatment decisions on a self-regarding basis and supporting those who do so, such an ethics encourages each of us to see our lives as simply our own. We may yet turn ourselves into beings who are ultimately alone.

Fidelity or Fairness?

Fidelity to the interests of the patient has been a corner-stone of both traditional codes and contemporary theories of medical ethics. The two competing paradigms of medical ethics—the "benevolence" model and the "patient autonomy" model—are simply different ways of construing such fidelity. Both must be rejected or radically modified. The admission that treatment decisions often affect more than just the patient thus forces major changes on both the theoretical and the practical level. Obviously, I can only begin to explore the needed changes here.

Instead of starting with our usual assumption that physicians are to serve the interests of the patient, we must build our theories on a very different assumption: The medical and nonmedical interests of both the patient and other members of the patient's family are to be considered. It is only in the special case of patients without family that we can simply follow the patient's wishes or pursue the patient's interests. In fact, I would argue that we must build our theory of medical ethics on the presumption of equality: the interests of patients and family members are morally to be weighed equally; medical and nonmedical interests of the same magnitude deserve equal consideration in making treatment decisions. Like any other moral presumption, this one can, perhaps, be defeated in some cases. But the burden of proof will always be on those who would advocate special consideration for any family member's interests, including those of the ill.

Even where the presumption of equality is not defeated, life, health, and freedom from pain and handicapping conditions are extremely important goods for virtually everyone. They are thus very important considerations in all treatment decisions. In the majority of cases, the patient's interest in optimal health and longer life may well be strong enough to outweigh the conflicting interests of other members of the family. But even then, some departure from the treatment plan that would maximize the patient's interests may well be justified to harmonize best the interests of all concerned or to require significantly smaller sacrifices by other family members. That the patient's interests may often outweigh the conflicting interests of others in treatment decisions is no justification for failing to recognize that an attempt to balance or harmonize different, conflicting interests is often morally required. Nor does it justify overlooking the morally crucial cases in which the interests of other members of the family ought to override the interests of the patient. Changing our basic assumption about how treatment decisions are to be made means reconceptualizing the ethical roles of both physician and patient, since our understanding of both has been built on the presumption of patient primacy, rather than fairness to all concerned. Recognizing the moral relevance of the interests of family members thus reveals a dilemma for our understanding of what it is to be a physician: Should we retain a fiduciary ethic in which the physician is to serve the interests of her patient? Or should the physician attempt to weigh and balance all the interests of all concerned? I do not yet know just how to resolve this dilemma. All I can do here is try to envision the options.

If we retain the traditional ethic of fidelity to the interests of the patient, the physician should excuse herself from making treatment decisions that will affect the lives of the family on grounds of a moral conflict of interest, for she is a one-sided advocate. A lawyer for one of the parties can not also serve as judge in the case. Thus, it would be unfair if a physician conceived as having a fiduciary relationship to her patient were to make treatment decisions that would adversely affect the lives of the patient's family. Indeed, a physician conceived as a patient advocate should not even *advise* patients or family members about which course of treatment should be chosen. As advocate, she can speak only to what course of treatment would be best for the patient, and must remain silent about what's best for the rest of the family or what should be done in light of everyone's interests.

Physicians might instead renounce their fiduciary relationship with their patients. On this view, physicians would no longer be agents of their patients and would not strive to be advocates for their patients' interests. Instead, the physician would aspire to be an impartial advisor who would stand knowledgeably but sympathetically outside all the many conflicting interests of those affected by the treatment options, and who would strive to discern the treatment that would best harmonize or balance the interests of all concerned.

Although this second option contradicts the Hippocratic Oath and most other codes of medical ethics, it is not, perhaps, as foreign as it may at first seem. Traditionally, many family physicians—especially small-town physicians who knew patients and their families well—attempted to attend to both medical and nonmedical interests of all concerned. Many contemporary physicians still make decisions in this way. But we do not yet have an ethical theory that explains and justifies what they are doing.

Nevertheless, we may well question the physician's ability to act as an impartial ethical observer. Increasingly, physicians do not know their patients, much less their patients' families. Moreover, we may doubt physicians' abilities to weigh evenhandedly medical and nonmedical interests. Physicians are trained to be especially responsive to medical interests and we may well want them to remain that way. Physicians also tend to be deeply involved with the interests of their patients, and it may be impossible or undesirable to break this tie to enable physicians to be more impartial advisors. Finally, when someone retains the services of a physician, it seems reasonable that she be able to expect that physician to be *her* agent, pursuing her interests, not those of *her* family.

Autonomy and Advocacy

We must also rethink our conception of the patient. On one hand, if we continue to stress patient autonomy, we must recognize that this implies that patients have moral responsibilities. If, on the other hand, we do not want to burden patients with weighty moral responsibilities, we must abandon the ethic of patient autonomy.

Recognizing that moral responsibilities come with patient autonomy will require basic changes in the accepted meanings of both "autonomy" and "advocacy." Because medical ethics has ignored patient responsibilities, we have come to interpret "autonomy" in a sense very different from Kant's original use of the term. It has come to mean simply the patient's freedom or right to choose the treatment he believes is best for himself. But as Kant knew well, there are many situations in which people can achieve autonomy and moral well-being only by sacrificing other important dimensions of their well-being, including health, happiness, even life itself. For autonomy is the *responsible* use of freedom and is therefore diminished whenever one ignores, evades, or slights one's responsibilities. Human dignity, Kant concluded, consists in our ability to refuse to compromise our autonomy to achieve the kinds of lives (or treatments) we want for ourselves.

If, then, I am morally empowered to make decisions about "my" medical treatment, I am also morally required to shoulder the responsibility of making very difficult moral decisions. The right course of action for me to take will not always be the one that promotes my own interests.

Some patients, motivated by a deep and abiding concern for the well-being of their families, will undoubtedly consider the interests of other family members. For these patients, the interests of their family are part of their interests. But not all patients will feel this way. And the interests of family members are not relevant *if* and *because* the patient wants to consider them; they are not relevant because they are part of the patient's interests. They are relevant *whether or not* the patient is inclined to consider them. Indeed, the *ethics* of patient decisions is most poignantly highlighted precisely when the patient is inclined to decide without considering the impact of his decision on the lives of the rest of his family.

Confronting patients with tough ethical choices may be part and parcel of treating them with respect as fully competent adults. We don't, after all, think it's right to stand silently by while other (healthy) adults ignore or shirk their moral responsibilities. If, however, we believe that most patients, gripped as they often are by the emotional crisis of serious illness, are not up to shouldering the responsibility of such decisions or should not be burdened with it, then I think we must simply abandon the ethic of patient autonomy. Patient autonomy would then be appropriate only when the various treatment options will affect only the patient's life.

The responsibilities of patients imply that there is often a conflict between patient autonomy and the patient's interests (even as those interests are defined by the patient). And we will have to rethink our understanding of patient advocacy in light of this conflict: Does the patient advocate try to promote the patient's (self-defined) *interests?* Or does she promote the patient's *autonomy* even at the expense of those interests? Responsible patient advocates can hardly encourage patients to shirk their moral responsibilities. But can we really expect health care providers to promote patient autonomy when that means encouraging their patients to sacrifice health, happiness, sometimes even life itself?

If we could give an affirmative answer to this last question, we would obviously thereby create a third option for reinterpreting the role of the physician: The physician could maintain her traditional role as patient advocate without being morally required to refrain from making treatment decisions whenever interests of the patient's family are also at stake if patient advocacy were understood as promoting patient autonomy and patient autonomy were understood as the responsible use of freedom, not simply the right to choose the treatment one wants.

Much more attention needs to be paid to all of these issues. However, it should be clear that absolutely central features of our theories of medical ethics—our understanding of physician and patient, and thus of patient advocacy as well as patient dignity, and patient autonomy—have presupposed that the interests of family members should be irrelevant or should always take a back seat to the interests of the patient. Basic conceptual shifts are required once we acknowledge that this assumption is not warranted.

Who Should Decide?

Such basic conceptual shifts will necessarily have ramifications that will be felt throughout the field of medical ethics, for a host of new and very different issues are raised by the inclusion of family interests. Discussions of privacy and confidentiality, of withholding/withdrawing treatment, and of surrogate decisionmaking will all have to be reconsidered in light of the interests of the family. Many individual treatment decisions will also be affected, becoming much more complicated than they already are. Here, I will only offer a few remarks about treatment decisions, organized around the central issue of who should decide.

There are at least five answers to the question of who should make treatment decisions in cases where important interests of other family members are also at stake: the patient, the family, the physician, an ethics committee, or the courts. The physician's role in treatment decisions has already been discussed. Resort to either the courts or to ethics committees for treatment decisions is too cumbersome and time-consuming for any but the most troubling cases. So I will focus here on the contrast between the patient and the family as appropriate decisionmakers. It is worth noting, though, that we need not arrive at one, uniform answer to cover all cases. On the contrary, each of the five options will undoubtedly have its place, depending on the particulars of the case at hand.

Should we still think of a patient as having the right to make decisions about "his" treatment? As we have seen, patient autonomy implies patient responsibilities. What, then, if the patient seems to be ignoring the impact of his treatment on his family? At the very least, responsible physicians must caution such patients against simply opting for treatments because they want them. Instead, physicians must speak of responsibilities and obligations. They must raise considerations of the quality of many lives, not just that of the patient. They must explain the distinction between making a decision and making it in a self-regarding manner. Thus, it will often be appropriate to make plain to patients the consequences of treatment decisions for their families and to urge them to consider these consequences in reaching a decision. And sometimes, no doubt, it will be appropriate for family members to present their cases to the patient in the hope that his decisions would be shaped by their appeals.

Nonetheless, we sometimes permit people to make bad or irresponsible decisions and excuse those decisions because of various pressures they were under when they made their choices. Serious illness can undoubtedly be an extenuating circumstance, and perhaps we should allow some patients to make some self-regarding decisions, especially if they insist on doing so and the negative impact of their decisions on others is not too great.

Alternatively, if we doubt that most patients have the ability to make treatment decisions that are really fair to all concerned, or if we are not prepared to accept a policy that would assign patients the responsibility of doing so, we may conclude that they should not be empowered to make treatment decisions in which the lives of their family members will be dramatically affected. Indeed, even if the patient were completely fair in making the decision, the autonomy of other family members would have been systematically undercut by the fact that the patient alone decided.

Thus, we need to consider the autonomy of all members of the family, not just the patient's autonomy. Considerations of fairness and, paradoxically, of autonomy therefore indicate that the *family* should make the treatment decision, with all competent family members whose lives will be affected participating. Many such family conferences undoubtedly already take place.

On this view, however, family conferences would often be morally *required*. And these conferences would not be limited to cases involving incompetent patients; cases involving competent patients would also often require family conferences.

Obviously, it would be completely unworkable for a physician to convene a family conference every time a medical decision might have some ramifications on the lives of family members. However, such discussion need not always take place in the presence of the physician; we can recognize that formal family conferences become more important as the impact of treatment decisions on members of the patient's family grows larger. Family conferences may thus be morally *required* only when the lives of family members would be dramatically affected by treatment decisions.

Moreover, family discussion is often morally *desirable* even if not morally required. Desirable, sometimes, even for relatively minor treatment decisions: After the family has moved to a new town, should parents commit themselves to two-hour drives so that their teenage son can continue to be treated for his acne by the dermatologist he knows and whose results he trusts? Or should he seek treatment from a new dermatologist?

Some family conferences about treatment decisions would be characterized throughout by deep affection, mutual understanding, and abiding concern for the interests of others. Other conferences might begin in an atmosphere charged with antagonism, suspicion, and hostility but move toward greater understanding, reconciliation, and harmony within the family. Such conferences would be significant goods in themselves, as well as means to ethically better treatment decisions. They would leave all family members better able to go on with their lives.

Still, family conferences cannot be expected always to begin with or move toward affection, mutual understanding, and a concern for all. If we opt for joint treatment decisions when the lives of several are affected, we need to face the fact that family conferences will sometimes be bitter confrontations in which past hostilities, anger, and resentments will surface. Sometimes, too, the conflicts of interest between patient and family, and between one family member and another will be irresolvable, forcing families to invoke the harsh perspective of justice, divisive and antagonistic though that perspective may be. Those who favor family decisions when the whole family is affected will have to face the question of whether we really want to put the patient, already frightened and weakened by his illness, through the conflict and bitter confrontations that family conferences may sometimes precipitate.

We must also recognize that family members may be unable or unwilling to press or even state their own interests before a family member who is ill. Such refusal may be admirable, even heroic; it is sometimes evidence of willingness to go "above and beyond the call of duty," even at great personal cost. But not always. Refusal to press one's own interests can also be a sign of inappropriate guilt, of a crushing sense of responsibility for the well-being of others, of acceptance of an inferior or dominated role within the family, or of lack of a sense of self-worth. All of these may well be mobilized by an illness in the family. Moreover, we must not minimize the power of the medical setting to subordinate nonmedical to medical interests and to emphasize the well-being of the patient at the expense of the well-being of others. Thus, it will often be not just the patient, but also other family members who will need an advocate if a family conference is to reach the decision that best balances the autonomy and interests of all concerned.

The existing theory of patient autonomy and also of proxy decisionmaking has been designed partly as a buttress against pressures from family members for both overtreatment and undertreatment of patients. The considerations I have been advancing will enable us to understand that sometimes what we've seen as undertreatment or overtreatment may not really be such. Both concepts will have to be redefined. Still, I do not wish to deny or minimize the problem of family members who demand inappropriate treatment. Treatment decisions are extremely difficult when important interests of the other members of the family are also at stake. The temptation of family members simply to demand the treatment that best suits *their* interests is often very real.

I do not believe, however, that the best safeguard against pressures from family members for inappropriate treatment is to issue morally inappropriate instructions to them in the hope that these instructions will prevent abuses. Asking a family member to pretend that her interests are somehow irrelevant often backfires. Rather, I think the best safeguard would be candidly to admit the moral relevance of the interests of other members of the family and then to support the family through the excruciating process of trying to reach a decision that is fair to all concerned.

Acknowledging the interests of family members in medical treatment decisions thus forces basic changes at the level of ethical theory and in the moral practice of medicine. The sheer complexity of the issues raised might seem a sufficient reason to ignore family interests in favor of the much simpler ethic of absolute fidelity to the patient. But that would be the ostrich approach to the complexities of medical ethics. We must not abandon our patients' families to lives truncated by an over-simplified ethic, for that would be an unconscionable toll to exact to make our tasks as ethicists and moral physicians easier.

Reconstructing medical ethics in light of family interests would not be all pain and no gain for ethicists and physicians. Acknowledging family members' interests would bring benefits as well as burdens to medical practitioners, for the practice of medicine has rarely been as individualistic as codes and theories of medical ethics have advocated. Indeed, much of what now goes on in intensive care nurseries, pediatricians' offices, intensive care units, and long-term care institutions makes ethical sense *only* on the assumption that the interests of other members of the family are also to be considered.

Contemporary ethical theory and traditional codes of medical ethics can neither help nor support physicians, patients, and family members struggling to balance the patient's interests and the interests of others in the family. Our present ethical theory can only condemn as unethical any attempt to weigh in the interests of other family members. If we would acknowledge the moral relevance of the interests of the family we could perhaps develop an ethical theory that would guide and support physicians, patients, and families in the throes of agonizing moral decisions.

Acknowledgments

I wish to thank Mary Read English, Michael Lavin, Gary Smith, Joanne Lynn, and Larry Churchill for valuable suggestions.

QUESTIONS FOR CONSIDERATION

1. Do you agree with Hardwig that medical treatment should not always serve the interests of the patient?
2. Give some examples of cases that Hardwig believes the interests of family members should override the interests of the patient. Do you agree with these examples?
3. How does Hardwig define the "family"? Should the family interests related to the patient's care be restricted to close relatives?
4. Do you agree with Hardwig that the seriously ill should have a right to special consideration? When, if ever, should that special consideration be overridden by family interest?

5. What other considerations should be made in medical decision making than the physical consequences of the illness alone?

6. Why does Hardwig contend that public policy changes would not adequately shelter family members from the negative effects of medical decisions? Are there public policy changes that would reduce such negative effects?

7. Do you agree with Hardwig that, ". . . the interests of patients and family members are morally to be weighed equally;"? Does this statement contradict his acknowledgment of special consideration for the seriously ill patient? Why does Hardwig say that considering the interests of all is not a utilitarian approach?

8. Why does Hardwig question the ability of physicians to be impartial advisors on the medical and nonmedical interests of all concerned? Do you agree?

9. How does Hardwig associate patient autonomy with Kant's emphasis upon responsibility? What implications would such responsibility have toward considering the interest of family members?

10. What role does Hardwig see for family conferences in making decisions regarding the interests of all family members? Do you believe such conferences would be practical and beneficial?

JEFFREY BLUSTEIN

The Family in Medical
Decisionmaking

Families have traditionally exercised, and continue to exercise, considerable
control overmedical treatment of minor children. In both law and morality,
families (or more specifically, parents) are regarded not just as interested
parties whose views should be solicited and taken into consideration, but
rather as rightful surrogate decisionmakers to whose judgment the physician
normally ought to defer. When the patient is an incompetent adult, physicians
often consult with family members (that is, children or siblings of the patient,
parents, spouse, etc.) about specific medical interventions and even about
continuation of treatment, and many physicians are guided by the family's
decision if it is not obviously unreasonable and if it does not contradict any
previously expressed wishes of the patient. Family involvement is also sought
when the patient is a competent adult, not, of course, because the family is
given the authority to decide for the patient, but because it is thought that
patients may need the emotional support of family members during times
of crisis.

The role of the family in treatment decisions for young children has been
extensively discussed in the bioethics literature; I will not rehearse the familiar
arguments for this general parental authority nor the reasons for preferring
families as proxies for noncompetent adults. I want instead to turn to the
case of competent adult patients and critically examine the current system of
medical decisionmaking and its legitimating ethos in the light of the fact that
patients are often cared for in the context of the family. I want to ask whether,
in view of certain features of the relationship between patients and their
families, the principle of patient self-determination at the core of contemporary
medical ethics is in need of some serious rethinking. Might it be that family
members, by virtue of their closeness to the patient, should not only have
some special authority to speak on behalf of patients who are incompetent,
but should also share decisional authority with patients who are competent?

A recent proposal that speaks to the family's role in medical decisionmaking has been advanced by John Hardwig. In his provocative essay, "What About the Family?"[1] he contemplates far-reaching changes in medical practice based on a critique of our prevailing patient-centered ethos. My discussion of his proposal is chiefly designed to pave the way for what I call a communitarian account of the role of the family in acute care decisionmaking. This account—which, I hasten to add, I do not endorse—has not to my knowledge been taken seriously as a theoretical possibility in the bioethics literature. Since the label "communitarian" is liable to be misunderstood, I should note at the outset that I am not interested in communitarianism as a political theory. Rather, I want to focus on the family as communitarian political writers sometimes think of it, namely, as a model for their conception of the larger society, and on the basis of this understanding of the family, to mount a challenge to the dominant patient-centered ethos that parallels the communitarian critique of liberal political philosophy. This communitarian position resembles Hardwig's proposal in that it does not regard the competent patient as the ultimate decisionmaker, but takes it as morally significant for the attribution of decisional authority that his or her life is intimately intertwined with the lives of close others. However, as we will see, the communitarian account is philosophically more radical than Hardwig's challenge to the dominant patient-centered medical ethos.

My own position is that the locus of decisional authority should remain the individual patient, but I also argue that family members, by virtue of their closeness to and intimate knowledge of the patient are often uniquely well qualified to shore up the patient's vulnerable autonomy and assist him or her in the exercise of autonomous decisionmaking. Families, in other words, can be an important resource for patients in helping them to make better decisions about their care. Recognition of this fact leads to a broader understanding of the duty to respect patient autonomy than currently prevails in acute care medicine.

Family Decisionmaking and Competent Patients

According to Hardwig, even when the patient is a competent adult, it may be quite appropriate to empower the family to "make the treatment decision, with all competent family members whose lives will be affected participating" (p. 9). This is so because family members have legitimate interests of their own that are likely to be affected in dramatic and profound ways by whatever treatment plan is chosen by or for the patient. Their interests may be affected in these ways because "family," by definition, consists of "those who are close to the patient" and "there is no way to detach the lives of patients from the lives of those who are close to them" (p. 6). Since family members must often revise their own priorities and significantly alter their life plans to accommodate the needs of sick or dying relatives, and since the nature and extent of the adjustment depends on the treatment plan that is followed for the patient, it would be wrong categorically to deny family members a role in determining what the treatment will be, how it will be administered, where, and so forth. For one thing, there is a presumption that "the interests of patients and family members are morally to be weighed equally" (p. 7), and family decisionmaking may be necessary to ensure that treatment decisions are fair to all concerned. Even when this is not necessary, the autonomy of other family members would be seriously undermined if the authority to make decisions that cut so deeply into their own lives belonged to the patient alone.

The interests of family members might be self-regarding or other-regarding. Particular choices about treatment can seriously affect the lives of family members in many ways, interfering not only with their own personal projects and individual lifestyles, but with their commitments to other family members as well. In any case, they are "separate" in the sense that they diverge from and possibly conflict with patient interests: they are not to be understood as interests in the interests of patients. Of course, those who love the patient also have a direct interest in the protection and promotion of the patient's interests, assuming that the patient has interests that can be protected and promoted. Indeed, this is part of the very meaning of love. But for Hardwig, there can be closeness without love, and even when there is love, there will usually be other interests of family members as well. When all of these interests are taken into account, it may turn out that what is best for the family as a whole is not what is best for the individual patient.

These other interests may be, and frequently are, quite legitimate, and treatment decisions should not be judged morally better or worse solely from the patient's perspective. Indeed, departures from optimal patient care may be justified "to harmonize best the interests of all concerned or to require significantly smaller sacrifices by other family members" (p. 7). Moreover, and very importantly, Hardwig expresses misgivings about the effectiveness of exhorting the patient to consider the impact of his or her decision on the lives of the rest of the family. Patients who seem to be ignoring their family's stake in the outcome of their decisionmaking process may sometimes respond appropriately to appeals from the physician or other family members, but many patients will be too self-involved to give the interests of others proper consideration or will use their illness as a kind of trump card to dominate the rest of the family. Because of this, Hardwig maintains, we must consider a more radical measure to ensure adequate protection of legitimate family interests, namely, rejection of the prevalent medical ethos according to which the competent patient is always the decisive moral agent. Under this ethos, it is certainly permissible for family members to offer information, counsel, and suasion to patients who must make treatment decisions. But the authority to make the decisions still resides with the competent patient alone, and this Hardwig finds untenable.[2]

The "ethic of patient autonomy" (p. 5) allows the competent patient, and the patient alone, to set the terms and conditions of care. Patients may be frightened and distracted by illness and hence in no position to give careful thought to the interests of others, but if their decisionmaking capacity is judged sufficient for the decision at hand, their wishes prevail. This troubles Hardwig because it amounts to giving patients permission to neglect or slight their moral responsibilities to other family members. Seriously ill patients tend to be self-absorbed and to make exclusively self-regarding choices about care, and in those cases where "the lives of family members would be dramatically affected by treatment decisions" Hardwig suggests that family conferences be "required" (pp. 9–10). These conferences would not merely have an advisory or supportive function: they would be decisionmaking forums. Patients and other family members would seek to reach a consensus that harmonizes the autonomy and interests of all concerned parties. Failing this, families would be forced "to invoke the harsh perspective of justice, divisive and antagonistic though that perspective might be" (p. 10).

Hardwig's proposal for greater family involvement in medical decisionmaking, however, runs up against the problem of patient vulnerability: joint family decisionmaking provides too many opportunities for the exploitation of patient vulnerability. Serious constraints on patient autonomy, such as anxiety, depression, fear, and denial, are inherent in the state of being ill.[3] Illness is also frequently disorienting in that patients find themselves thrust into unfamiliar surroundings, unable to pursue customary routines or to enjoy any significant degree of privacy. For these reasons, the ability of patients to assess their medical needs accurately and protect their own interests effectively is limited and precarious. But if those who are ill and those who are healthy already confront each other on an unequal psychological footing, then family conferences, as Hardwig conceives of them, seem especially ill advised. Weakened and confused by their illness, patients are easy prey to manipulation or coercion by other family members and may capitulate to family wishes out of guilt or fear. (Given that Hardwig would allow even hateful or resentful family members to be included in family conferences, this is not an idle worry.) Family members will understandably not want to be seen by the physician as opposing the wishes of the patient, and so they might exert pressure on the patient to concur with their opinions about treatment. Of course, even as matters now stand, with decisionmaking not generally thought to belong to the family as a whole, what seems like a patient's autonomous choice often only implements the choice of the others for him or her. But joint family decisionmaking is likely only to exacerbate this problem and to make truly independent choice even more dubious.

Hardwig, it should be noted, does acknowledge that a seriously weakened patient may well need an "advocate" (p. 10), or surrogate participant from outside the family, to take part in the joint family decision. However, this hardly resolves all the difficulties his proposal presents. The presence of an outsider in what is supposed to be a deeply personal and private conference might only create (further) hostility and suspicion among family members. And if consensus in the conference cannot be achieved, the rest of the family could simply overrule the patient's proxy participant, just as it could overrule the patient himself.

From a theoretical point of view, we should, I think, agree with Hardwig about the inadequacy of any view that denies or overlooks the essential interplay between rights and responsibilities. But the practical moral problem as I see it is how to design procedures and structures of decisionmaking that achieve an acceptable balance between rights and responsibilities, between the important values of a patient-centered ethos and the legitimate claims of other family members. If alternative approaches to medical decisionmaking are judged in this light, as Hardwig wants them to be, and not solely in terms of over-all happiness or preference satisfaction or the like, then family decisionmaking for competent patients confronts serious moral objections. For indications are that it will often result not in a mutual accommodation of the autonomy and interests of all affected parties, but rather in a serious erosion of patient autonomy and a subordination of patient interests to the competing interests of other family members.

The Communitarian Defense of Family Decisionmaking

I have focused on the problems that nonideal, less than fully harmonious families pose for Hardwig's proposal. Critics of the patient-as-primary-agent model might instead restrict their attention to those (admittedly infrequent) cases in which patients belong to close-knit and harmonious families, and with this as their conception of the family, offer a defense of family decisionmaking that challenges the patient-centered model in a more radical way than Hardwig does. In ideal families, suspicions, resentments, disagreements, and the like, if they exist, are muted and do not set the tone of family life. But more importantly, it may be claimed, the conception of the person that underlies the theory of patient autonomy is patently inappropriate here. The patient is not, as this theory presupposes, an atomic entity, a free and rational chooser of ends unencumbered by communal and other allegiances. On the contrary, his or her identity is constituted by family relationships, and he or she is united with other family members through common ends and mutual understanding. In these circumstances, the patient is too enmeshed in a network of relations to others to be properly singled out as the one to make treatment decisions.

I call this the communitarian argument for family decisionmaking to distinguish it from the argument from fairness and autonomy discussed in the previous section. When I refer below to what "communitarians" say about medical decisionmaking, I am not thinking of any particular authors who have advanced this position.[4] Rather, I am suggesting that elements of the communitarian view can be taken out of their political context and that a challenge to the prevailing patient-centered ethos can be constructed on the basis of a communitarian conception of the ideal family. Let us look at this challenge more closely.

In acute care settings, the relationship between patients and physicians is, if not exactly adversarial, at least one in which patients should not normally suppose that they and their physicians are participants in a common enterprise with common values and goals. The values involved in medical decisionmaking are by no means exclusively medical values, but also largely normative ones about which patients and physicians frequently disagree. In these circumstances, physicians may attempt to coerce compliance with their wishes, which they are in an advantageous position to do, or to control patient decisions by selective disclosure or nondisclosure of information. In recognition of normative diversity and in the face of various threats to patient autonomy in the caregiving relationship, we invoke the notion of patients' rights. Rights accord patients a protected space in which to make their own choices and pursue their ends free of inappropriate interference from others. Having rights, patients can confront caregivers with the demand that their (possibly conflicting) ends be respected.

Communitarian critics of the traditional ethos of patient autonomy need not deny that patients' rights and patient self-determination play an important role in the caregiving relationship. But, they note, the patient is not always to be thought of simply as the one who is sick or in need of medical attention. If the patient belongs to a close-knit and harmonious family, for example, it is the family as a whole whose values and goals may diverge from those of professional caregivers because such a family is a genuine community, not a mere collection of separate individuals with their own private and possibly conflicting interests. Members of a community have common ends, and these are conceived of and valued as common ends by the members. United by common ends and a common identity, the threats that work against the autonomy of some work against the autonomy of all. Moreover, in these cases the patient would not need to be protected from family pressures for inappropriate treatment. Rather, the family would act as advocate for the patient vis-a-vis the physician, and family decisionmaking would put patients on a much more equal footing with caregivers.

For communitarians the ethics of acute care, focusing as it does on the individual who is the subject of treatment, rests on a conception of the self that is at odds with how persons define and understand themselves in a community. This is a conception for a world of strangers, where the content of each person's good is, to quote Michael Sandel, "largely opaque" to others, where persons have divergent and possibly conflicting plans and interests, and where their capacity for benevolence is extremely limited.[5] But in the community of a close and harmonious family these conditions do not obtain. Rather, the defining features of such a family are mutual sympathy, common ends, a shared identity, love, and spontaneous affection. Of course, it is sheer wishful thinking, and cavalier as well, to assume that all families are like this. Family life may instead be fraught with dissension and interests may diverge and conflict. In these situations questions of justice come to the fore and the importance of individual rights (and individual patient rights) is enhanced. But within the context of a more or less ideal family, the circumstances that make personal autonomy both an appropriate and a pressing concern prevail to a relatively small degree.

For communitarian philosophers, individual rights have no place in intimate harmonious communities. Charles Taylor, for example, suggests that "the whole effort to find a background for the arguments which start from rights is misguided,"[6] and according to Michael Sandel, in "a more or less ideal family situation . . . individual rights and fair decision procedures are seldom invoked, not because injustice is rampant but because their appeal is preempted by a spirit of generosity in which I am rarely inclined to claim my fair share."[7] Rights, as communitarians understand them, are conflict notions, and if they play any role in intimate communities, it is remedial only.[8]

Unlike Hardwig's argument for family decisionmaking, the communitarian view I have constructed does not claim that families should make treatment decisions because this solves the problem of fairness or because this protects the autonomy of all those individual family members who have a stake in the outcome of treatment decisions. Rather, the argument proceeds from a picture of the family as a community of love where, it is alleged, questions of fairness and individual autonomy normally do not arise and are of minor importance. In the ideal family, there isn't enough of a distinction to begin with between self and others for these concerns to loom large. And this absence of a sharp line separating self and others is not a cause for alarm or a basis for moral criticism of family decisionmaking, but intrinsic to the nature of community, the experience of which, plainly, is an important good for humans.

The close-knit, harmonious family is a paradigm of community. Here the well-being of one family member does not just have an impact on the well-being of others, for this can happen in families that are no more than associations of individuals (like the ones Hardwig describes). Rather, in families that are genuine communities individuals identify with one another, such that the well-being of one is *part of* the well-being of the other. This being so, the communitarian maintains, decisions that importantly affect the well-being of one family member are the province of the entire family. To be sure, in the medical cases there is only one family member, the patient, who literally bears the decision in his or her flesh and bones. But this fact alone, it is believed, does not confer upon the patient a unilateral decisionmaking right. The right to make the decision is still a right of the family in ideal circumstances—a group right rather than a right of individuals.

However, since the communitarian argument for family decisionmaking applies only to families that are communities and not to those that are just collections of individuals whose lives affect each other in major ways, its implications for the practice of medicine will not be as significant as those of Hardwig's proposal. Many families, to acknowledge the obvious again, are not ideal. In addition, physicians frequently have only passing acquaintance with the patient's family and no reliable basis for judging the quality of the patient's relationship with other family members. Even if communitarians reveal genuine inadequacies in the prevalent ethos of patient autonomy and patient rights, physicians will often not be in a position to tell whether, in the particular case at hand, the family is harmonious enough to be entrusted with the authority to make decisions for one of its own. On the other hand, physicians will often have enough information to know that the lives of family members will be seriously affected by treatment decisions, and it is on this fact, not on the existence of a harmonious family, that Hardwig premises the case for joint family decisionmaking.

Still, the communitarian critique of the dominant medical ethos of patient autonomy and individual patients' rights raises interesting and important philosophical issues. Practical implications aside, the theoretical challenge it poses deserves a response. In what follows, I will try to indicate why I think this challenge fails.

How the Communitarian Challenge Fails

Even in families that are true communities of love, the harmony that exists among their members may not be so thoroughgoing that invocation of individual decisionmaking rights loses its point. It is not necessary for community that there be complete identity of all ends and unanimity on all matters of value or the good. On the contrary, there is room for significant disagreement about how to rank different components of a common conception of the good, about the proper means and strategies for achieving it, and about whether certain risks are worth taking to achieve common goals. Even if the members of a family are in broad agreement about what is of most importance in life, for example, this does not ensure that they will assess the costs and benefits of particular medical treatments similarly. Indeed, given the diversity of human nature and experience, such disagreements are not just possible but to be expected. Absolute harmony in decisionmaking and thoroughgoing convergence of values are only found in quite extraordinary communities. And this being the case, individual rights can be seen to have an importance the communitarian fails to acknowledge. They are not just claims we fall back on in the unhappy situation where community is lacking or faltering. Additionally, they serve to secure recognition of the diverse values and ends that persist even in intact and well-functioning communities. This lack of homogeneity is glossed over by talk of family rights.

Individual rights have an important place in community because the existence of community does not eradicate serious disagreement about ends, about the relationship between particular choices and shared ends, and so forth. Individual rights are needed because a significant degree of diversity may exist even in a group united by a common conception of the good. But what if, hard to imagine though it might be, there were a community without such diversity? Would individual rights have much importance in a perfectly homogeneous community like this? Would there be any point in ascribing rights to individual patients, rather than to families, if patients and their family members were in complete agreement about all matters pertaining to the good for themselves? Here if nowhere else, the communitarian would surely argue, individual rights are useless and irrelevant.

This is the conclusion we come to if we adopt a particular conception of rights. We find a clear and succinct statement of this conception in an earlier paper by Hardwig titled, "Should Women Think in Terms of Rights?" The thrust of this essay, unlike that of "What about the Family?" is communitarian:

> Thinking in terms of rights rests on a picture, first sketched by Hobbes and then made more palatable by Locke, of the person as atomistic, primarily egoistic, and asocial—only accidentally and externally related to others. If we are lucky our independent interests may coincide or happily divide in a symbiotic relationship . . . but we should not expect this to be the normal state of affairs.[9]

The normal state of affairs in a genuine community is quite different, however. Here persons are not just "accidentally and externally related" to each other, but understand themselves as participants in a common enterprise and regard the wellbeing of others as part of their own. No wonder then that rights should seem alien or antithetical to community and, more specifically, ideal familial love.

But communitarians who think of rights only in these familiar legalistic terms underestimate the complexities and possibilities inherent in individual lights. To be sure, rights sometimes function to protect the individual in the pursuit of his or her independent self-interest. But this hardly exhausts their significance. Consider these remarks by Neera Badhwar:

> An ideal family or friendship may wipe out all differences of ends, both final and intermediate, but it cannot wipe out "the separateness of life and experience." *Au contraire,* it would seem that it is precisely ideal familial love and friendship that will appreciate the "distinction of persons," recognizing the interest of each individual in *pursuing* a shared good, and her right to do so within the constraints of justice.[10]

On this view, rights are important even in the most closely knit and harmonious community. Even if the lives of persons are inextricably intertwined and their conceptions of the good agree in every respect, they remain numerically distinct persons with their own distinct perspectives on the world and an interest in expressing them. This interest in exercising one's agency in the pursuit of one's ends is not the same as an interest in seeing one's ends realized, for one's ends might be realizable quite independently of the operation of one's own agency. Nor is this interest contingent on one's ends being different from or in conflict with the ends of others.

By linking rights to this fundamental interest in one's own agency, we can explain what is wrong with the communitarians antipathy to rights. Thinking in terms of rights, on the present account, does not rest either directly or by implication on a picture of the person as atomistic, egoistic, and asocial. It rests rather on a picture of the person as a separate being, with a distinctive personal point of view and an interest in being able securely to pursue his or her own conception of the good. This by itself entails neither that one's relationships to others are intrinsic to one's identity nor that one is only accidentally and externally related to others. In ascribing rights to individuals, we are responding to these basic and universal features of persons.

It may help here to distinguish between having a right and insisting upon or demanding it. The language of demands does seem ill suited to harmonious families. If family members need to insist against one another that they have a right to make their own decisions, then we are probably dealing with a divided and quite antagonistic family. But these observations do not suffice to banish individual rights from harmonious families because the underlying supposition—that rights must always be linked to demands—is false. Rights can be expressed in different ways, and what is divisive and antagonistic to community is not the concept of rights, but only a certain way of expressing them. In harmonious families, rights are typically expressed "as reminders— gentle or forceful, matter-of-fact or emotional—of legitimate expectations and entitlements,"[11] and as such they play a vital role in the moral lives of families.

The implications of these remarks for a communitarian defense of family medical decisionmaking are clear. Even in extremely close families, patients may have different priorities from their loved ones and assess life choices in disparate ways, and these differences may surface in disagreements about how and even whether patients should be treated. Patients need their own rights regarding choice of treatment not just because family members cannot always be trusted to have the patient's best interests at heart, but because, even in families where trust is not an issue and there is a remarkable measure of agreement on ends and deep mutual affection, other family members may not always concur with the wisdom of the patient's choices. Rights protect patient autonomy and patient interests in these circumstances.

Further, rights for patients would be appropriate and useful even in those quite unusual families where the minimal sort of disagreement just mentioned is absent. For decisions about treatment often have dramatic and far-reaching consequences for the shape, quality, and duration of a patient's life, and individuals have an interest in determining for themselves the course their lives take. The interest in directing how one's life will go in accordance with one's values and preferences exists whether these values and preferences are uniquely one's own or shared with other family members, and it calls for recognition even when there is no disagreement between patient and family over the correct treatment decision. This is why patients have rights as individuals even under the unlikely conditions of absolute intrafamilial harmony: they protect the interests that patients have in exercising their agency.

Important questions remain about how belonging to a harmonious intimate community creates a new identity for the parties involved and about the interplay, for those who belong to such communities, between their interests as single individuals and their interests as members of community. But I believe enough has been said to establish the following, and this is all that is required for my purposes: community does not undermine the normative significance of the individual self nor does it render individual rights otiose.

Family Involvement in the Process of Decisionmaking

These responses to the communitarian position do not show that patient choices about treatment always trump the choices of family members, and they do not cut against Hardwig's argument for joint medical decisionmaking by all affected family members. What they show is only that the dominant patient-centered medical ethos cannot be refuted by the sort of all-out attack on the notion of individual rights the communitarian launches. To be sure, an adversarial and legalistic conception of individual rights is ill suited to those cases where family relationships are nonadversarial and there are no deep conflicts of interests, preferences, or values among family members. But if this is the basis for the communitarian claim that community renders individual rights (including patient rights) useless or of minor importance, the communitarian betrays a distorted and incomplete understanding of rights.

Should the choices of competent patients trump the choices of family members, except in the rarest of circumstances? "It is an oversimplification to say of a patient who is part of a family," Hardwig notes, that "it's his life" or "after all, it's his medical treatment" (p. 6). Plainly, this by itself hardly shows that patient choices take priority over the choices of others, for when lives are so intertwined that one life cannot be shaped without also shaping the lives of others, it's *their* lives too. Another approach is to argue for a unilateral decisionmaking right for patients on the ground that patients have more to lose than their family members. That is, when we measure the sacrifices that family members must make for a patient's health care and the costs to the patient of not receiving the treatment that, other family members aside, he or she would select, the patient's sacrifices almost always outweigh the family's. Of course, the reverberations of patients' self-regarding choices can be so shattering to the lives of other family members that a calculation of relative costs favors the family instead. But familial hardship from this source is usually less of a burden than serious illness, and this difference would be sufficient to establish at least a presumption in favor of patient decisionmaking.

But if the ethos of patient autonomy survives the challenges I have considered in this paper, it is nevertheless the case that current medical practice and medical ethics can be faulted for not giving the family a more prominent place in medical decisionmaking for competent patients, and that both family members and patients suffer as a result. For one thing, as we learned from our discussion of Hardwig, because treatment decisions often do have a dramatic impact on family members, procedures need to be devised, short of giving family members a share of decisional authority, that acknowledge the moral weight of their legitimate interests. For another, though patients might well benefit from family involvement in the process of formulating views about medical treatment, under the regime of patient autonomy patients tend to be treated for the most part as if they were solitary decisionmakers, isolated from intimate others.

The ethos of patient autonomy rightly understood takes seriously the impairments of autonomy that affect us when we are ill. Patients are not ideally autonomous agents but anxious, fearful, depressed, often confused, and subject to ill-considered and mistaken ideas. If we are genuinely concerned about ensuring patient self-determination, we will take these factors into account. Here it is necessary to distinguish, as Jay Katz does, between "choices" and "thinking about choices."[12] According to the dominant medical ethos, choices properly belong to the patient alone. At the same time, patients' capacities for reflective thought and effective action are limited and precarious, obliging them to converse and consult with supportive and caring others if they are to make their best choices. Patients' psychological capacities for autonomy can be enhanced by searching conversations with their physicians— the main point of Katz's book—and (I would add) by conversations with other family members.

To explain why this is so, we may turn to a characterization of the family found in Nancy Rhoden's influential law review article, "Litigating Life and

Death."[13] Her argument, which focuses on decisionmaking for incompetent patients, finds within family life features that warrant a legal presumption in favor of family choice. Family members are typically the best decisionmakers partly because of their special epistemic qualifications: they ordinarily have deep and detailed knowledge of one another's lives, characters, values, and desires. This knowledge might be based on specific statements made by one family member to another, for the intimacy of family life encourages and is partly constituted by the unguarded disclosure of one's most private thoughts and deepest feelings. But there may be nothing specific that was said or done to which family members can point as evidence of another member's preferences. Indeed, their knowledge, acquired through long association and the sharing of intense life experiences, is characteristically of the sort that "transcends purely logical evidence." In addition, family members are the best candidates to act as surrogates for an incompetent patient because of their special emotional bonds to the patient. This is important because possessing deep and detailed knowledge of another can put one in an especially good position to frustrate no less than fulfill this person's desires. Family members, however, can be presumed to have a deep emotional commitment to one another, and this makes it likely that they will put their knowledge to the right use—that is, that they will decide as the patient would have wanted.

Those features of families that, in Rhoden's view, justify a legal presumption in favor of family decisionmaking for incompetent patients—intimate knowledge, caring, shared history—also provide good reasons for family involvement in the competent patients' thinking about choices. Family members would have no veto power over a patient's decision and would have to honor the choice ultimately made, no matter how foolish or idiosyncratic. But in family conferences, where the process of making a decision is shared, they could encourage the patient to evaluate different treatment options in terms of their impact on the interests of other family members, and could attempt to persuade the patient that the best choice is one that is fair to all affected parties. In some cases, understanding what a particular treatment decision would cost other family members might give the patient a compelling reason to alter an initial choice.

For the physician, the duty to respect patient autonomy has as its corollary a duty to engage in conversation with patients and to encourage and facilitate conversation between patients and other persons to whom they are close (including family members), unless the physician has reason to think that such conversation will not in fact assist the patient in making autonomous decisions. Current medical practice does not in general reflect a commitment to foster this sort of conversation as an integral part of the physician's professional responsibility. But if, as Katz suggests, genuine respect for patient autonomy is shown not merely in accepting patients' yes or no response to a proposed intervention, but rather in facilitating patients' opportunities for serious reflection on their choices, then promoting discussion and dialogue between patient and family is an important part of the physician's duty to satisfy the patient's right of self-determination.

A useful parallel can be drawn here with a central tenet of family medicine. Family physicians stress the importance of adopting a systems approach to health and disease in which the patient is seen as part of a family system. It is the individual patient, not the family unit, that is the primary focus of care, most family physicians will say, but since poor family dynamics can predispose to or cause disease and illness, effective treatment of the patient requires sensitivity to the multiple roles of faulty family relationships in the etiology of disease. In other words, to use language familiar to family physicians, if the physician is to treat "the patient in the family" appropriately, the physician must be cognizant of "the family in the patient."[14] My remarks about promoting and facilitating family involvement in the process of decisionmaking make a similar point about the importance of physicians' generally extending their attention beyond the individual patient. Only now the rationale for doing so is not that family relationships may contribute to the illness the physician is trying to treat, but that family communication may assist patients in making autonomous decisions about how or whether to treat their illness. The family is the center of most people's lives, for better or for worse, and this means both that the health of individuals is most profoundly influenced by family relationships and that such relationships can play a vital role in restoring the autonomous functioning that illness undermines.

Acknowledgments

I want to thank John Arras, John Hardwig, Jonathan Moreno, Jim and Hilde Nelson, and several anonymous referees for the *Hastings Center Report* for comments on earlier drafts of this paper.

QUESTIONS FOR CONSIDERATION

1. What are the arguments upon which Blustein would agree with Hardwig regarding the role of the family in medical decisionmaking? In what areas

would Blustein disagree with Hardwig? What problems did Blustein identify with Hardwig's position?

2. What does Blustein mean by the "ethic of patient autonomy"?

3. How did Blustein characterize the communitarian position regarding the role of family decisionmaking? How does the communitarian position differ from Hardwig's viewpoint?

4. What are Blustein's objections to the communitarian account of the role of the family in medical decisionmaking?

5. How does Blustein account for the role of the family in medical decision-making in relation with the "ethic of patient autonomy"?

NOTES

1. John Hardwig, "What About the Family," *Hastings Center Report 10,* no. 2 (1990): 5–10.

2. Hardwig's proposal to "reconstruct medical ethics in light of family interests" (p. 10) is novel in that it rejects the model of patient-as-primary-agent for acute care. Others have argued, along lines similar to Hardwig's, that this is not the appropriate model for home care, where family members share heavily in the burdens of care on an ongoing basis. In the view of Bart Collopy, Nancy Dubler, and Connie Zuckerman, for example, "the ethical problem for home care becomes one of gauging the interplay of agents, the relative weight to be granted to the autonomy and interests of the family vis-à-vis those of the elderly recipient of care." While not disputing the value if the patient-centered model in acute care, these writers argue that decisionmaking in home care should be "an interactive process, involving negotiation, compromise, and the recognition of reciprocal ties." See "The Ethics of Home Care: Autonomy and Accommodation," special supplement, *Hastings Center Report* 20, no. 2 (1990): 1–16, at 9, 10.

3. See Terrence R. Ackerman, "Why Doctors Should Intervene," *Hastings Center Report* 12, no. 4 (1982): 14–17.

4. One author who has advanced something like a communitarian position is James Lindemann Nelson. See his "Taking Families Seriously," Hastings *Center Report* 22, no. 4 (1992): 6–12.

5. Michael Sandel, *Liberalism and the Limits of Justice* (Cambridge: Cambridge University Press, 1982), pp. 170–71.

6. Charles Taylor, "Atomism," in *Powers, Possession and Freedom,* ed. A. Kontos (Toronto: University of Toronto Press, 1979), p. 42.

7. Sandel, *Liberalism,* p. 33.

8. In a similar vein Alasdair MacIntyre, taking as his "moral starting point" the "fact that the self has to find its moral identity in and through its membership in communities," attacks the language of rights for its individualism and the ahistorical and asocial conception of the self it expresses. See *After Virtue* (Notre Dame, Ind.: University of Notre Dame Press, 1981), pp. 1–5, 64–67, 204–5.

9. John Hardwig, "Should Women Think in Terms of Rights?" *Ethics* 94, no. 3 (1984): 441–55, at 446.

10. Neera Badhwar, "The Circumstances of Justice: Liberalism, Community, and Friendship," forthcoming in *The Journal of Political Philosophy I* (1993).

11. Badhwar, "Circumstances of Justice."

12. Jay Katz, *The Silent World of Doctor and Patient* (New York: Free Press, 1984), p. 111.

13. Nancy Rhoden, "Litigating Life and Death," *Harvard Law Review* 102, no. 2 (1988): 375–446.

14. For a critical discussion of the distinctive orientation of family medicine, see Ronald J. Christie and C. Barry Hoffmaster, *Ethical Issues in Family Medicine* (New York: Oxford University Press, 1986), pp. 68–84.

PART IV: *Reproductive Freedom and Responsibility*

GILBERT MEILAENDER
Abortion: The Right to an Argument

MARY B. MAHOWALD
Is There Life After Roe v. Wade?

EDWARD A. LANGERAK
Abortion: Listening to the Middle

In 1973, an unmarried pregnant woman (using the fictitious name "Jane Roe") brought suit against the Texas state law that prohibited abortions except in cases in which the mother's life is in danger. The Supreme Court, in its now famous *Roe v. Wade* decision, ruled in favor of Roe's right to abortion based upon her "right to privacy." But Justice Harry A. Blackmun, in the majority opinion, stated that "the right of personal privacy includes the abortion decision, but that this right is not unqualified." Blackmun added that the state might intervene to "proscribe abortion" after fetal viability.

In *Webster v. Reproductive Health Services* (1989), the Supreme Court upheld a Missouri state law that prohibited the use of state funding, state employees, and public facilities in the performance of abortion. This decision moved beyond the *Roe* decision by inviting states to set their own abortion restrictions. Likewise, The *Webster* decision updated the *Roe* definition of fetal viability (24 weeks) to 20 weeks, reflecting newer medical technologies.

Are earlier abortions less problematic than later abortions? Is viability the "magic moment" by which the state acquires a compelling interest in protecting the life of the fetus? Will changing technologies require the courts to continually revisit the issue of fetal viability? Is it possible to find compromises that would lead to a consensus on public policy regarding abortions? What are the central moral questions that individuals continue to struggle with in the abortion debate? These questions will be the focus of this section.

The readings for this section include the following:

- Gilbert Meilaender's **Abortion: The Right to an Argument** criticizes both the "personhood argument"—that only rational, conscious beings are human persons—and the "bodily support argument"—that a woman has complete choice over what happens within her body.

- Mary B. Mahowald's **Is There Life After** *Roe v. Wade?* is critical of the emotional and misleading rhetoric of both "pro-choice" and "pro-life" activists. She attempts to examine the morally relevant factors that make the abortion decision a very complex issue.

- Edward A. Langerak's **Abortion: Listening to the Middle** proposes a "middle of the road" approach to abortion that he believes represents strong public consensus. He combines a "potentiality principle"—that a potential being already has a certain claim to life—with a societal "conferred claims approach"—society bestows a strong claim to life upon the fetus—that focuses upon the status of the fetus and the problems of late abortion.

GILBERT MEILAENDER

Abortion: The Right to an Argument

The call for "middle ground"—at least when the moral stakes really are high, as in the argument over abortion—must be seen for what it is: one substantive moral position among others, not the voice of sweet reason perched somewhere above the battle. Naturally, in the course of any good argument there is give-and-take, but to ask from the outset, "How little of what I believe would I be willing to settle for?" is a question whose corrupting possibilities ought to be resisted. We need to reengage the arguments about abortion as a people and thereby help to determine what sort of people we wish to be.

A Public Matter

Abortion is an issue that will not go away and, indeed, should not go away. Daniel Callahan has suggested that most of us respond on two levels to this issue. As a "public self" we take positions in public argument, express views to pollsters, perhaps even vote for candidates on the basis of their stance on the issue. But less public is the "shadow self" who experiences "a more troubled private cauldron of jumbled beliefs, cross-cutting emotions, and easily triggered, raw-end sensibilities." Speaking at least for himself, Callahan asserted that events of recent years had "raised . . . [his] uneasiness a notch or two" and led him to believe that he and his pro-choice allies needed to demonstrate a willingness to "concede the moral uncertainty of abortion decisions."[1]

Perhaps it is because of our collective "shadow self" that the issue has not gone away and, indeed, is returning to the center of public debate. I am not persuaded, however, that professions of uncertainty are what is needed, nor am I so certain that the "shadow self" has become increasingly uneasy. A little over ten years ago the *Hastings Center Report* published a case study with commentaries that was titled: "Can the Fetus Be an Organ Farm?"[2] I remember that I used it once as a discussion starter in class but found it singularly unsuccessful. It didn't really generate much discussion. No one was willing to answer "yes" to the question—and this among students almost all of whom would have called themselves pro-choice.

Times change. A decade later, John A. Robertson, a very respected figure in the medical ethics world, also writing in the *Hastings Center Report*, suggested that careful analysis of the question of conception and abortion for tissue procurement "is more ethically complicated than generally assumed."[3]

I doubt that the moral issues at stake have become more complicated in a decade or that we are keener analysts than our predecessors. The difference, in fact, may be a simple one that ought not to be blurred with talk of uncertainty or ethical complexity: What once seemed morally beyond the pale no longer seems so. A decade has encouraged us to think differently about the status of the fetus—differently enough that we argue soberly the pros and cons of fetal tissue transplantation and even conception and abortion for tissue procurement, which not long ago we would have regarded as a moral abomination. The "shadow self" can be pacified. And the language of uncertainty and complexity functions chiefly to make *us* rather than fetuses the victims. For it is, after all, *we* who must struggle and agonize over these decisions, we who are victimized by the need for such choices. And, in a way, we are victims. Guilt laden, we seek some means by which to wrest benefit from abortions too numerous for us any longer to count. It should be no surprise then, or even cause for particular complaint, that some will reject such ethical complexity as specious and turn to direct action in what is becoming the largest movement of civil disobedience in our nation's history.

But there must also continue to be room for argument and discussion, if only because that is at least part of what it means to call abortion a public issue. I have no special confidence that the argument would end in ways I approve, nor do I even know exactly what side of different arguments would be mine. I am, for example, far more certain that abortion for "genetic defect" is wrong than I am that an individual human life begins at conception. The central problems in the debate have remained remarkably stable over the years, and they are closely related problems. Two early and widely anthologized articles about abortion staked them out with a clarity that in many ways remains unsurpassed yet today. Mary Anne Warren's "On the Moral and Legal Status of Abortion" argued that fetuses, lacking personhood, were not entitled to protection against being killed.[4] Call this the "personhood" argument. Judith Jarvis Thomson's essay, "A Defence of Abortion," articulated (unforgettably!) the case for holding that, even were the personhood of the fetus established, women would not be obligated to use their bodies to support fetal life.[5] Call this the "bodily support" argument. There is, no doubt, a certain irony in the fact that these two arguments—so abstractly universal in scope—should dominate at a time when we have been taught by Carol Gilligan and her followers that women are more likely to contextualize difficult moral decisions.

But in any case, these remain the central moral issues, and they deserve our continued examination.

The Personhood Argument

The argument about the moral status of the fetus arises quite naturally and perhaps inevitably. The claim, "it's my body to do with as I wish," becomes more worrisome if that body is nourishing another human life equal in dignity. These two lives may be for a time inseparably joined, but if the fetus can claim a dignity like ours, we will surely have to worry about aborting it. In such a context the language of personhood has entered the debate. And it is important to note that this language, in the context of this debate, generally serves to exclude rather than include. The irony of our public debate is that the people labeled "conservative" are often those arguing for a more liberal and inclusive understanding of the meaning of human personhood. This language may once have served to include within our common humanity those whose skin color was not white. Now it increasingly serves as a language by which we mark off those human subjects who *cannot* lay claim to equal protection. This turn away from our liberal political heritage may yet prove cause for regret. As Philip Abbott has written:

> There are very few general laws of social science but we can offer one that has a deserved claim: the restriction of the concept of humanity in any sphere never enhances a respect for human life. It did not enhance the rights of slaves, prisoners of wars, criminals, traitors, women, children, Jews, blacks, heretics, workers, capitalists, Slavs, Gypsies. The restriction of the concept of personhood in regard to the fetus will not do so either.[6]

At issue here is not simply an important moral debate, but our understanding of the humanity we share.

If we do not wish to reduce our humanity to either its material or its spiritual dimension, we need a concept of the human person that does justice to the duality of our nature. But when we attempt to avoid the now dreaded Cartesian image of the "ghost in the machine," we often turn to an entirely functional understanding of the human being: A person is simply a body capable of intentional, self-aware action. And then what do we make of the "person" who lacks such capacities? Even if there are satisfactory ways to handle the old question whether a person sleeping is still a person, it will prove more difficult on this view to ascribe personhood to fetuses, infants and young children, and the senile.

Thus, for example, in an important work that gathers together many strands of this increasingly common view, H. Tristram Engelhardt asserts that persons are those who can be "concerned about moral arguments and . . . convinced by them. They must be self-conscious, rational, free to choose, and must possess moral concern."[7] It is clear that, judging on the basis of these criteria, many human beings will not qualify for personhood. And our obligations to them will be less stringent than to those—like ourselves—who are self conscious, rational, and in control. Engelhardt does not hesitate, for example, to speak of parents as owning their children, at least until such time as the children become self-conscious. We may argue at length whether it is helpful to use analogies from the history of our nation's struggle over slavery when thinking about abortion, but his language of ownership is surely striking. It is the almost certain result of restrictive and exclusivistic thinking about the meaning of personhood.

Having seen where the personhood argument leads, we often flinch a little and draw back. There is a scene in *Cymbeline*, one of Shakespeare's dramatic romances, in which the queen is gathering poisons. With her is Cornelius, an upright physician who suspects the evil deed she plans. She, however, claims to intend nothing more than a few experiments:

> *Queen*: I will try the forces
>   Of these thy compounds on such creatures as
>   We count not worth the hanging—but none human
>   To try the vigor of them and apply Allayments to their act, and by them gather
>   Their several virtues and effects.
> *Cornelius*: Your Highness
>   Shall from this practice but make hard your heart. (Act 1, scene V)

When we draw back from the full implications of the personhood argument, we often use versions of Cornelius's claim. Thus, for example, having claimed that infants are not persons and are therefore not entitled to protection and care equal to that which we owe each other, Engelhardt suggests that we might nonetheless wish to treat them as if they were. Doing so would support "virtues such as sympathy and care for human life, especially when that life is fragile and defenseless."[8] Mary Anne Warren used a similar argument to step back from the justification of infanticide to which her position seemed to lead. She suggested that as long as there were among us those whose hearts had not been made hard and who took pleasure in caring for infants (who are not yet persons)—as long, that is, as some remain who are not persuaded by the course of her argument—there will be reason enough not to kill such infants.[9] But we might just as easily suppose that, once we have clarified for

ourselves the distinction between personal and sub-personal forms of human
life, even the most cruel treatment of the latter need have no deleterious
effect on our respect for the former. There is certainly evidence to suggest
that such "doubling" is well within our capacities.[10]

If, for the moment, we still feel the force of such arguments, that is hard
to account for in terms of exclusivistic theories of personhood. We feel our
kinship with human beings who are neither rational nor self-conscious, feel
that what we do to them might begin to affect the way we treat each other,
because we share with them our embodied humanity. We too are not just
free, rational spirits, but are finite bodies, and we seek to discern in human
beings who lack capacities we take for granted the dignity we once had when
we were like them and will have if we should ever lose those capacities. At
stake is the development and enlargement of our concept of human community.
And surely the ability to sustain a bond of affection that unites us across
generations is as fundamental as "self-awareness" to our understanding of what
is integrally human.[11] Nor is this simply a point about private morality, which
can or should be separated from the public sphere. What sort of people we
wish to be, what the boundaries of our communities are, whether we want
ours to be a society, that defines membership chiefly in terms of cognitive
capacities—these are public, political questions not to be settled by scientific,
ethical, or legal experts. For them no answer can be given in advance, but
they cannot and should not be removed from the arena of public debate.

There may, in fact, be deeper theoretical difficulties with a narrow and
exclusivistic understanding of personhood. For there is a difference between
the characteristics that distinguish the human species, and the qualifications
for membership in the species. It may be that among the distinguishing
characteristics of humans are features like rationality, self-consciousness, and
moral concern. But one can be human without exercising (or even having
the capacity to exercise) such characteristics. To belong to humankind one
need only be begotten of human parents. Indeed, those who lack some of
these capacities are best described simply as the weakest and least advantaged
members of our community. There will be little point in advancing a morality
of "care" or in developing a theory of justice that gives pride of place to the
least advantaged if we systematically remove them from the scope of our
protection through some version of the personhood argument. When we do
so, we enclose the commons—we contract the scope of our concern to the
stronger and more gifted, those most like us. Perhaps we have not fully
exorcised from our thinking the ghost in the machine—the idea that the body
is only a vehicle for what really counts, the free, rational spirit. But the fetus
should be cared for and protected not because of any "personal" capacities,

but because weak and vulnerable humans—who, though lacking some of our qualities, do not lack equality with us—are the weakest members of the human community. This does not mean that abortion is never permissible, but it does make clear how heavy a burden the "bodily support" argument must carry: It will have to justify killing one who is equal in dignity to each of us. Granting, then, that the fetus is genuinely one of us, need a woman provide it with her bodily support?

The Bodily Support Argument

The practical assertion that, since pregnancy involves a woman's body, the choice of continuing that pregnancy must be hers alone, was first given powerful theoretical articulation and defense by Judith Thomson. And that claim has continued to play a central role in the moral argument and debate surrounding abortion. Stripped to its essentials, the argument asserts: We are embodied beings; thus the person is involved when the body is given or used. To require women to continue an unwanted pregnancy is, therefore, to ask of them personal sacrifice. Since men cannot become pregnant (and be required to make such sacrifice), prohibiting abortion is, in effect, the institutionalization of sexual inequality.

All three elements in the argument are necessary, though they are not always consistently developed. Thomson, for example, did not do full justice to the sense in which we are our bodies. She argued that it would never be unjust of a woman to abort, though there might be circumstances in which it would be indecent for her to do so. But then, discussing pregnancy resulting from rape, Thomson engaged in one too many thought experiments: She contemplated the possibility of abortion if the pregnancy were to last only an hour rather than nine months. In that case, Thomson held, although the woman would not act unjustly in aborting the fetus, it would be indecent of her not to carry it to "term." Yet surely this misses the reason why pregnancy resulting from rape constitutes a special case. Because the woman's body has been used and violated, her person has been assaulted—and this would be just as true if the pregnancy came to term within an hour. The argument needs a richer sense of our embodied personhood than Thomson herself offered.

That richer sense has been supplied by Patricia Beattie Jung, who argues that we should think of childbearing and organ donation as analogous activities.[12] Each offers a kind of bodily support, and each therefore involves a certain element of personal sacrifice. Since men haven't been required to serve as organ donors even when (because of tissue type) they could well do so Jung suggests that required childbearing does indeed mandate sexual inequality. A similar point has been made by Lawrence Tribe, who notes that "current law nowhere forces men to sacrifice their bodies and restructure their lives even in those tragic situations (of needed organ transplants, for example) where nothing less will permit their children to survive. . . ."[13]

We may well have doubts about the validity of the analogy. After all, current law also nowhere forces a *woman* to serve as an organ donor. Perhaps what the law would reflect (if abortion were regulated) is not institutionalized sexual inequality but some sense of an important difference between organ donation and abortion. When a man (or a woman) declines to serve as organ donor, and when we in turn decline to compel him or her to do so, what does *not* happen might be termed a kind of rescue operation. But potential donors, even if they are not required to rescue the imperiled person in need of an organ, are not permitted to aim at that person's death. That I decline to make the bodily and personal sacrifice of giving you my kidney does not entitle me to asphyxiate you, nor does it entitle me to stop others who might wish to offer you a kidney. If aborting a fetus meant only ceasing to carry it while permittng others to sustain its life—which, of course, it cannot mean, at least for the present—the analogy might seem more persuasive. Declining to donate a kidney and aborting a fetus may both be actions that result in death, but they differ in the important sense that only the latter can be said to aim at death. And if the day comes when it is medically possible to stop carrying a fetus without at the same time aiming at its death, we will be able to test the validity of the analogy more carefully in our actual practice.

One might, of course, redescribe abortion in a way that makes the analogy seem more plausible. Tribe proposes a thought experiment: If women automatically miscarried after conception unless they took a drug to prevent such a miscarriage, a law compelling them to take it would mandate a rescue operation calling for bodily sacrifice. Failing to take the drug would not be aiming to kill the fetus; it would only be failing to rescue. And since, unlike required organ donation, such a law could apply only to women, it would seem to institutionalize sexual inequality. What is striking about this thought experiment is the way in which—like so many of the brilliantly inventive analogies conceived by Judith Thomson—it invites us to alienate ourselves from the natural manner in which conception and birth take place.

We are invited to picture the fetus as an alien who may perhaps be invited in but who, if not welcomed, is essentially an invader. In pregnancies resulting from forcible intercourse, and perhaps also in other circumstances in which the woman's consent to intercourse has been greatly reduced, the thought experiment may well have merit. But that there are hard cases should not obscure the more general truth: that a fetus is not demanding access to some place it has no right to be; that it is simply seeking to survive in its natural environment. This is not to say, of course, that every fetus in its natural environment will at every moment be wanted or desired by its mother. But as Sidney Callahan has written, "morality also consists of the good and worthy acceptance of the unexpected events that life presents." And that is a principle which can and should be applied equally to fathers and mothers. Rather than adopting a position on abortion that "ratifies the view that pregnancies and children are a woman's private responsibility,"[14] we should do all in our power to encourage and require paternal responsibility. A fetus, being unwanted, does not thereby become an alien who may be destroyed. To justify that conclusion the "bodily support" argument would need considerable assistance from the "personhood" argument. Each feeds off the other; yet neither is adequate.

The Right to an Argument

As abortion returns again to the center of public debate, there is renewed interest in finding some "middle ground" upon which we can all agree, even if it requires that each of us "give" a little here or there. I doubt, however, that the answers to our moral puzzles are to be found in that direction. Talk of compromise or of a "middle ground" on which all can come together makes sense if it means that one should seek to understand sympathetically an argument with which one disagrees. Such sympathetic understanding and imagination are useful devices for achieving political compromise within a pluralistic society, but we should be clear that the call for middle ground is itself a substantive moral position—and possibly a very unsatisfactory one. Good politics may not be good ethics. What we need, therefore, is continued exploration of our moral disagreements, not consensus forged anywhere other than in the legislative sphere. We need to reconsider again the central moral issues at stake; for those issues go to the heart of how we understand ourselves as a people and how we define membership in this community.

QUESTIONS FOR CONSIDERATION

1. In the "personhood argument," what does Meilaender mean when he declares that the language of personhood serves to exclude rather than include?

2.   Why does Meilaender reject a criteria of personhood based upon self-consciousness, rationality, and free will? What kinship does he believe we have with humans who do not possess self-consciousness and rationality? Why does he believe the fetus should be cared for in spite of a lack of "personal qualities."

3.   How does Meilaender characterize the "bodily support argument"? What are his criticisms of this argument? What are the reasons he gives for rejecting the organ donation analogy?

4.   What are Meilaender's objections to the portrayal of the fetus as an alien in a place where it has no right to be? How do these objections relate to the concept of paternal responsibility?

5.   Why does Meilaender have reservations about the search for a "middle ground"? Why does he refer to such a compromise as a "substantive moral position"?

NOTES

1. Daniel Callahan, "How Technology Is Reframing the Abortion Debate," *Hastings Center Report* 16:1 (1986), pp. 33–42.

2. *Hastings Center Report* 8:5 (1978), pp. 23–25.

3. John Robertson, "Rights, Symbolism, and Public Policy in Fetal Tissue Transplants," *Hastings Center Report* 18:6 (1988), pp. 5–12.

4. *The Monist*, 57 (January, 1973), 43–61. Warren later added to the article a "Postscript on Infanticide." The article with postscript can be found in *Ethical Issues in Modern Medicine*, Roben Hunt and John Arras, eds., (Palo Alto, CA: Mayfield, 1977), pp. 159–77.

5. *Philosophy and Public Affairs* 1 (Fall, 1971), pp. 47–66.

6. Philip Abbott, "Philosophers and the Abortion Question," *Political Theory* 6:3 (1978), p. 329.

7. H. Tristram Engelhardt, Jr., *The Foundations of Bioethics* (New York: Oxford University Press, 1986), p. 105.

8. Engelhardt, *The Foundations of Bioethics*, p. 117.

9. See Warren, "Postscript on Infanticide."

10. Robert Jay Lifton, *The Nazi Doctors* (New York: Basic Books, 1986), pp. 418–465.

11. Abbott, "Philosophers," 332.

12. Patricia Beattie Jung, "Abortion and Organ Donation: Christian Reflections on Bodily Life Support," *Journal of Religious Ethics* 16:2 (1988), pp. 273–305.

13. Laurence H. Tribe, *Constitutional Choices* (Cambridge, MA: Harvard University Press, 1985), pp. 243–44.

14. Sidney Callahan, "Abortion and the Sexual Agenda," *Commonweal* (25 April 1986), pp. 232–238.

MARY B. MAHOWALD

Is There Life After Roe v. Wade?

It has been sixteen years since the landmark case *Roe v. Wade* was decided by a majority vote of the United States Supreme Court.[1] Sixteen years is enough time for humans and their laws to be conceived, embodied, and grow to maturity, but *Roe* still threatens to abort. In fact, by the time this article appears, it may have been overturned by a new decision that vitiates its main provisions.[2] Is there any way of saving its life? Is its life worth saving?

"Pro-life" activists would probably answer both questions negatively, and "pro-choice" activists would probably answer them affirmatively. For each side the answer to the second question is likely to be more definitive. Those whose views on the legality or morality of abortion are somewhere between absolute permissiveness and absolute condemnation, a position held by the majority of the American people,[3] may look for ways of saving what seems worth saving of *Roe*.

Why has the debate raged on without abatement for so long? Is it possible to find some areas of agreement that dissidents on the issue might acknowledge? While addressing these questions, I will also briefly sketch my own views on possible changes in *Roe* and the morality of abortion.

The Long Debate

Laws often have a settling as well as regulative influence on individuals. For example, legal enactments such as the Emancipation Proclamation and the Nineteenth Amendment granting women the vote eventually became settled opinion in American consciousness despite initial controversies. One might have thought, therefore, that by now the cool rationale of the Roe decision in 1973 would have quelled the heat of public debate about abortion. Instead, the heat has escalated from firey words to clinic bombings.

Intransigence on opposite sides of the issue, coupled with misleading and emotionally charged rhetoric, are partly to blame for prolongation of the controversy. Kristin Luker's account of the differences between "pro-life" and "pro-choice" activists suggests that both groups are basically closed to reconsideration of their positions.[4] For the most part, the rhetoric of abortion aims at different targets: "pro-lifers" focus on abortions for trivial reasons, performed even when the fetus is well-developed; "pro-choice" proponents tend to discuss abortions undertaken early for compelling reasons such as rape, or threat to a woman's health or life. One side refers to embryos as babies, and abortions as (therefore?) murder; the other describes a second trimester fetus as a blob of cells, and compares abortion to removal of a wart or tumor. The phrase "abortion on demand" is used prevalently to describe the current legal status of abortion; yet the text of the *Roe* ruling fails to support that interpretation.[5]

Beyond simplistic rhetoric and intransigence, thoughtful, well-developed arguments and openness to further consideration have helped to keep the debate constructively alive.[6] Increased knowledge of fetal development and advances in neonatology, along with the incidence of infertility and shortage of adoptable babies, have caused some to wane in their initial enthusiasm for *Roe*. Those whose main concern in legalizing safe abortions was to promote the health of poor women may be comforted by the reduction in morbidity and mortality related to abortions, but disturbed by the overall increase in the number of abortions performed.

Complexities of the Issue

Fortunately or unfortunately, I cannot honestly align myself with either "pro-choice" or "pro-life" activists.[7] Either side betrays, to me, the enormous complexity of the issue. This complexity is in part a function of the following features associated with abortion decisions: duration of gestation, circumstances of conception, age and competence of the pregnant woman, health status of the fetus, and health status of the pregnant woman. Regardless of the outcome of *Webster,* recognition of this complexity could be a beginning point for discussion between dissidents.

Duration of Gestation

For most people, abortion decisions become more difficult to justify as gestation progresses. For example, an intrauterine device, usually viewed as a contraceptive despite its abortifacient effect, is hardly controversial. RU 486, a drug that induces abortion very early in pregnancy, has evoked controversy because it allows a woman to abort herself; if the drug could be used effectively late in pregnancy its availability would surely be more disturbing to some individuals. Physicians who have no moral qualms about early abortions tend to avoid performing them during the second trimester.[8] Legal and emotional factors may trigger such avoidance more than moral concerns. In general, however, the more advanced the gestation, the more likely it is that significant moral factors are introduced, such as the onset of fetal brain activity (at about 8 weeks), and of fetal sentiency (probably during the second trimester).[9]

Roe maintains that fetal viability, "the ability (of the fetus) to survive ex utero, albeit with artificial aid," occurs during the third trimester, at which point the states may thereafter promote their interest in the "potentiality of human life" by proscribing abortion unless it is necessary for maternal health. Because of advances in perinatal and neonatal medicine, and greater availability of technology, the duration of gestation required for viability has been reduced since 1973.[10] Accordingly, the trimester breakdown by which abortion is permissible until the third trimester no longer provides an adequate guide to decisions based on fetal viability. Moreover, in a forty-week (full-term) gestation, just when second trimester ends and third trimester begins is unclear even to practicing physicians.[11]

Technically, abortion is no longer possible after viability, because termination of pregnancy, whether spontaneous or induced, is then clinically defined as premature birth.[12] However, Roe uses the term abortion to refer to termination of pregnancy both before and after viability, and many people, including practitioners, construe abortion as the termination of the fetus prior to birth, whether the fetus is viable or not. On that interpretation, if the fetus is considered viable or possibly viable, a method may be chosen to insure fetal demise in utero. If abortion is defined as termination of pregnancy rather than termination of the fetus, the method selected may be one that maximizes the chance of fetal survival.[13]

From a medical standpoint, the choice of method is partly determined by the duration of gestation: vacuum aspiration or suction curettage are appropriate during the first trimester, while induction methods (using saline, urea, or prostaglandin) or dilatation and evacuation (D&E) are appropriate during the second trimester. Roe says nothing about methods of abortion and their different effects on the fetus as well as the pregnant woman. Yet surely the possibility of fetal survival, of pain, and of risk to the pregnant woman's health are morally relevant factors influenced by the method selected.

Circumstances of Conception

Many opposed to legal abortion generally make exceptions for cases of rape or incest. Requiring a woman to maintain a pregnancy caused by rape imposes on her a constant reminder of the violence committed against her. Pregnancy due to incest may also have its origins in violence, and ordinarily entails social stigma and risk of birth defect.[14] Abortion in such circumstances is more likely to be morally justified than when intercourse occurs voluntarily in a nonincestuous relationship.

Voluntariness, as a crucial component of moral behavior, applies not only to intercourse but also to conception. Accordingly, we may wonder about responsibility for pregnancies that occur in spite of careful contraceptive practice, when intercourse is clearly voluntary but conception is not. The voluntariness of intercourse may imply responsibility for conception, at least on the part of those aware that contraception sometimes fails.[15] If contraception were faithfully practiced and fully reliable, neither pregnancy nor abortion could occur. When appropriate contraception fails, however, those who practice it are less responsible for the resultant pregnancy than those who don't.

Additional circumstances associated with abortion decisions include the marital and economic status of the pregnant woman, and responsibilities to others, such as a spouse, parents, or children already born. In most cases, however, the moral relevance of these circumstances rests on an assumption that commitment to parenthood is essentially linked with carrying a pregnancy to term. (I will return to this point later.) Moreover, different circumstances may influence the morality of the agent without altering the morality of the act. Abortion construed as the killing of an innocent person would thus be a morally wrong act, but mitigating circumstances would reduce the culpability of the agent committing the act.

Age and Competence of the Pregnant Woman

The age at which pregnancy occurs is relevant for medical as well as psychosocial reasons. Pregnancy and childbirth are not only particularly hazardous as discrete events for those who are not yet fully mature, but they also tend to impede such persons from reaching their full measure of development. Moreover, the younger the individual, the less likely it is that she has fully and freely consented to the pregnancy or to abortion.

Maternal age is also a risk factor for the fetus. The incidence of prematurity is greatest for the oldest and youngest age groups.[16] Women over thirty-five are often aware of their increased risk of conceiving a child with Down syndrome, and the incidence of medical complications for pregnant women as well as fetuses escalates as the age of the pregnant woman advances beyond the mid-thirties.[17] A forty-five-year-old woman whose children are already raised, may become pregnant when she fails to practice birth control because she mistakenly believes herself menopausal. Because of the risk factor, this suggests a morally different picture than the unplanned pregnancy of a twenty-five-year-old.

Competence, often related to age, is another morally relevant factor in abortion decisions. Partly because of laws against involuntary sterilization, incompetent and questionably competent adults sometimes become pregnant.[18] Here a pro-choice argument for abortion is hardly adequate. Here too, the possibility that the pregnant woman can or will be permitted to raise her offspring is remote. Competence thus applies not only to the capability for moral decisionmaking, but also to capability for parenthood.[19] So long as a child can be raised by others who are competent, the absence of competence for parenthood is not an adequate reason for abortion.

Health Status of the Fetus

In normal pregnancy, the health of the pregnant woman and of the fetus are interdependent. Nonetheless, early spontaneous abortions occur, sometimes before women realize they are pregnant, often because embryos or fetuses are abnormal.[20] Spontaneous abortions are thus a kind of natural eugenic event. Because of improvements in high-risk obstetrics, infertility treatment, and perinatology, some fetuses that would have previously succumbed in utero now survive. By means of prenatal diagnosis techniques we can detect fetal anomalies, some of which are treatable in utero and some ex utero.[21] Through legal access to safe abortions, an elective eugenic procedure is thus available.

Although clinicians may refer to elective abortion for fetal anomaly as "therapeutic," the procedure is not usually medically therapeutic for the pregnant woman. A rationale of fetal euthanasia may be applied to cases where the abnormality is so severe that survival seems worse than death (for example, Tay-Sachs disease or Lesch Nyhan syndrome). In most cases of abnormality, however, survival presents a greater burden to the family than to the child. It also entails a burden to society, which ordinarily subsidizes the treatment, education, and social supports necessary for disabled persons throughout their lifetimes. Down syndrome, a condition that is mentally debilitating but not generally emotionally or physically debilitating, is a clear example of a prenatally detectable anomaly that usually prompts abortion. The procedure may be defended as a means by which to avoid the psychological burdens that care for a person with Down syndrome entails; it can hardly be justified on the basis of the interests of the fetus.

Health Status of the Pregnant Woman

Some pregnancies are life threatening to some women. Since self-defense seems so basic a human right, few would argue that a woman is morally obliged to sacrifice her life for the sake of a fetus. However, some women in fact choose to risk their health for the sake of their fetuses, while others may decline to do so for unselfish reasons. Consider, for example, the following cases:

CASE A: A twenty-six-year-old married woman had Eisenmenger's syndrome, a condition that is life threatening in association with late pregnancy and childbirth. The cardiologist who had warned her against childbearing advised her to have an abortion when she became pregnant. The woman was aware that her chance of survival was about 50 percent, but insisted that she wanted to have the baby. Although her husband and parents preferred that she abort the fetus in order to maximize her own prospect of survival, she chose to continue the pregnancy. In conformity with the woman's wishes the infant was delivered by cesarean section. Despite aggressive efforts to support her throughout the medical crisis, she died four days later.

CASE B: A thirty-two-year-old woman with multiple sclerosis became pregnant despite use of a diaphragm. She and her husband had two children, four and six years old, for whom she was the principal caregiver. Although the couple were generally opposed to abortion, both were extremely concerned that continuation of the pregnancy would further compromise the woman's health. Previous pregnancies had resulted in permanent aggravation of her condition, to a point where she required a wheelchair. One week after learning she was pregnant the woman requested an abortion. She hoped, she said, to preserve her ability to care for the children she already had.

The woman described in Case A showed a heroic degree of self-sacrifice in behalf of the fetus. Poignant and appealing as it is, however, such self-sacrifice or virtue lies beyond the moral requirements of the law. Until and unless our society is willing to coerce some persons to risk their health for the sake of others—to donate bone marrow, blood, or a kidney, for example—we surely should not force pregnant women to do this for their fetuses.[22] Even then, the argument in behalf of those who are uncontroversially persons is more compelling than the argument made for fetuses. Accordingly, the woman who chose abortion in Case B may also be acting virtuously, pursuing an alternative that may in fact be the most loving and responsible course to follow.

Generally, the lesser the threat, the less convincing the self-defense rationale. At a certain point in the development process, the medical risk of elective abortion is equal to the risk of continuing the pregnancy to term and birth.[23] Psychological, social, and economic risks are also prevalently associated with pregnancy. Although these may influence the condition of the fetus, they directly affect the life of the pregnant woman. Unlike the fetus, however, she is able to communicate her priorities regarding her own interests or those of the fetus. In situations of conflict, whether or not her autonomy is socially supported depends on whether pro-choice or pro-life values prevail.

Possible Areas of Agreement

Should the values of one perspective prevail, or are there points of convergence that both sides might acknowledge? In addition to recognizing that abortion is a complex issue, I believe dissidents might agree on the following points.

Abortion Is a Bad Thing

Ordinarily, pregnancy represents a natural, healthy process that abortion interrupts. Elective abortion entails an actively invasive procedure for the woman undergoing the termination of her pregnancy. But whether the abortion is spontaneous or deliberate, the interruption signifies termination of a physiological relationship that has supported a developing human life, which is a positive human value. Unfortunately, *Roe* fails to acknowledge this "fact of life," confusing the philosophically controversial concept of person with the relatively simple biological concept of human life.

Often the circumstances that trigger abortion are themselves tragic, and the decision is an effort to minimize the harm done to those affected, including others besides the pregnant woman. It may of course be argued that the harm done to a fetus through abortion is always greater than that done to others by continuing an unwanted but healthy pregnancy. Nonetheless, one can acknowledge the harm of abortion while holding that in some circumstances it entails less harm than alternatives.

The term "pro-abortion" is a misleading label for those who argue for its permissibility only in certain circumstances. To limit those circumstances by providing alternatives to women is an appropriate objective of "pro-choice" as well as "pro-life" supporters. The Bush administration's proposal that adoption be more widely encouraged is an obvious possibility in this regard. Some argue, however, that adoption is more psychologically costly for pregnant women than abortion. More social supports for childrearing, especially when children are disabled, is another practical means of expanding the alternatives of pregnant women. Probably the most effective way to avoid abortions, however, is to improve the practice of contraception. If pregnancy were prevalently voluntary, the incidence of abortion would surely be reduced.

There Are Differences Between the Right to Terminate a Pregnancy, the Right to Terminate a Fetus, and Parental Responsibility

Neither morally nor practically is termination of pregnancy equivalent to termination of a fetus.[24] This is obviously true when the termination of pregnancy occurs through the birth of a live infant. It may also be true of procedures in which a nonviable fetus is removed for treatment of a condition that gravely threatens the life or health of a pregnant woman, such as ectopic pregnancy or cancer of the uterus. It is clearly not true when termination occurs because of fetal anomaly. In normal pregnancies, abortions may be elected with the intention of ending the pregnancy, terminating the fetus, and/or avoiding the responsibilities of motherhood. The last intention is also achievable by continuing the pregnancy, giving birth, and then surrendering the newborn into the care of others. *Roe* seems to ignore the latter possibility in arguing that "the problem of bringing a child into a family already unable, psychologically and otherwise, to care for it" provides grounds for abortion.

Several supporters of a woman's right to abortion explicitly limit their support to an understanding of abortion as termination of pregnancy rather than termination of a fetus.[25] In interpreting *Roe* with regard to survivors of legal "abortions," the states have assumed the same distinction. If termination of pregnancy occurs either spontaneously or electively after viability, a living survivor must be provided with the same medical care as is appropriate for any premature newborn. Even if the infant is nonviable, such terminations of pregnancy are technically considered live births rather than abortions.[26] As already mentioned, if the fetus in utero is considered viable or possibly viable, the practitioner may choose a procedure that will insure fetal or newborn demise, or a procedure that is most conducive to survival. At that point, the moral and practical difference between termination of pregnancy and termination of a fetus is inescapable.

Disclosure of Accurate Information Is as Morally Requisite Here as in Other Treatment Situations

Ordinarily, few people question the moral significance of full and accurate disclosure by caregivers presenting treatment options to competent, conscious patients. Free and informed consent is not possible without such disclosure. Nonetheless, communication is often influenced by the subjective biases of the communicator, and this is especially so in discussions of abortion. An important and obvious way of reducing bias is to use technically correct language rather than controversial terminology. For example, to refer to a pregnant woman as a mother is not technically correct unless she has already given birth; nor is the male whose sperm has fertilized a woman's ovum a father until the fertilized ovum produces a neonate. Neither embryos nor fetuses are yet babies, and should not therefore be characterized as such. Nor should fetuses be referred to as embryos, as in Luker's account,[27] because the term "embryo" understates the reality of fetal development, providing valid grounds for criticism by "pro-life" advocates.

But disclosure is not simply a matter of using correct terminology; it also involves selection of the content to be disclosed. Efforts to require disclosure of the developmental status of the fetus and alternatives to abortion (adoption, for example) have been rebuffed by Supreme Court decisions following *Roe.* In June 1986, the majority opinion in *Thornburgh* upheld a ruling of the Pennsylvania Court of Appeals on the unconstitutionality of requiring that certain information be provided to women seeking abortion. The information included the name of the physician who would perform the abortion, the probable gestational age of the fetus, a description of the medical risks associated with the procedure and with carrying the fetus to term, and an offer of materials to review regarding "the probable anatomical and physiological characteristics of the unborn child at two-week gestational increments from fertilization to full term, including any relevant information on the possibility of the unborn child's survival."[28]

In writing for the majority, Justice Blackmun argued that the above description of fetal characteristics was "overinclusive," that it is "not medical information that is always relevant to the woman's decision, and it may serve only to confuse and punish her anxiety, contrary to accepted medical practice." It is also possible that such information could lead to some women changing their mind about abortion. Selig Neubardt and Harold Schulman observed that when second trimester abortion patients were informed that the procedure (saline or prostaglandin infusion) would induce labor and delivery of a formed fetus, one fourth declined the procedure.[29]

In a dissenting opinion, Chief Justice Burger who voted with the majority in *Roe,* expressed concerns about "abortion on demand" as a practice he believes the Court never supported. *Roe,* he claimed, was based on the State's interest in preserving and protecting the health of the pregnant woman. Burger found it astonishing that the Court would deny that the state could "require that a woman contemplating an abortion be provided with accurate medical information concerning the risks inherent in the medical procedure which she is about to undergo and the availability of alternatives if she elects not to run those risks."[30] Ironically, his critique of the majority opinion is based on its failure to be sufficiently "pro-choice": denial of information pertinent to abortion decisions reduces the autonomy of pregnant women.

Pregnant Women Have Rights at Least Equivalent to Those of Non-pregnant People

Presumably, this claim is uncontroversial because the personhood of pregnant women is generally accepted. The fact of their pregnancy, whether deliberately undertaken or not, does not diminish their personhood. Accordingly, pregnant women ought not to be subjected to coercive treatment that others might effectively refuse, such as blood transfusion, surgery, or even hospitalization.[31] Even if treatment were imposed on an adult for the sake of minor children, further argument is needed to justify its imposition for the sake of fetuses. Minor children are uncontroversially persons, and fetuses are not.

With regard to induced abortion, a request for the procedure is not equivalent to refusal of treatment. Hence the request, while legally or morally legitimate, does not morally oblige a practitioner to perform the abortion. The pregnant woman's right to treatment, like the comparable right of nonpregnant persons, is contingent on the right of others to refuse to provide the treatment. To the extent that the pregnant woman's health or welfare is threatened by continuation of the pregnancy, her right to (the treatment of) abortion becomes stronger, and the right of others to refuse assistance becomes weaker.

Viability and Sentience of Fetuses Are Morally Relevant to Abortion Decisions

Viability allows others to care for the fetus after an abortion has been performed. The situation seems comparable to the obligation of someone who finds an abandoned newborn. When others can and are willing to care for the fetus-that-may-be-aborted the distinction between the right to terminate a pregnancy and the right to terminate a fetus is reintroduced. Even in cases of serious genetic defect, viable fetuses may be adopted after abortion. This provides prima facie grounds for requiring a method of terminating pregnancy that maximizes the chance of fetal survival.

Regarding sentience, the obligation to avoid inflicting pain on others, even animals or criminals who may legally be killed, is surely applicable to fetuses also. While little data are available concerning the capacity of the fetus to experience pain, it seems clear that the sentient capacity of a late gestation fetus resembles that of a neonate, and that the earlier the point of development, the more diminished that capacity.[32] Even the possibility of sentient capacity is morally relevant, and thus clearly has implications for decisions about techniques of abortion.

Legality and Morality Are Related but Not Equivalent

This may be the most telling point of all regarding the continuation of the abortion controversy. Although many of those who oppose abortion recognize that *Roe* takes no stand on the morality of abortion, their efforts have apparently concentrated on overturning the law rather than emphasizing their moral position. Yet their advocacy of moral decisionmaking about abortion entails the possibility that their position can and should be implemented regardless of whether the law is changed. A golden opportunity wrought by *Roe* has thus been missed, that of educating people more broadly about the fact that legality is not equivalent to morality, and about the morality of affirming life in all its forms and stages. Clearly, the moral force of a "pro-life" movement is weakened by failure to support other life-affirming efforts, such as opposition to a nuclear arms race or capital punishment.

The moral force of either "pro-life" or "pro-choice" arguments is weakened by failure on either side to expand the moral options of women who are or may be pregnant. Preoccupation with the legal status of abortion seems to have compromised efforts in this regard, strengthening the erroneous tendency to define morality in terms of legality. Admittedly, if women are legally coerced to continue pregnancies, the autonomy necessary for moral decisionmaking is thus reduced. But if *Roe* is substantially reaffirmed in *Webster,* the challenge to pro-choice advocates will remain what it has been all along: to insure that women's choices are not simply legal but morally informed and socially supported.

Possible Changes in Roe v. Wade

As the preceding account suggests, I don't consider *Roe* a model ruling. I believe the Court should retain certain features, such as its emphasis on viability of the fetus, implying certain obligations on the part of others, as well as its affirmation that women's health or life provides adequate reason for terminating pregnancy even in its later stages. But specification of trimesters, and of twenty-four weeks' gestation, as points for determining whether to honor women's requests for abortion, should be abandoned because of their ambiguity and inadequacy in establishing viability.

Although the majority opinion in Roe was based primarily on the pregnant woman's right to privacy, Justice Stewart argued in his concurring opinion that liberty rather than privacy should be emphasized. I agree with Stewart that personal liberty provides a clearer and more convincing rationale for women's right to choose abortion. In keeping with that rationale, instead of stating that "the abortion decision and its effectuation must be left to the medical judgment of the pregnant woman's attending physician,"[33] the Court should affirm the pregnant woman as primary decisionmaker, limiting the physician's role to medical aspects of the decision. If and when RU 486 is available, physicians will not be necessary for performance of safe early abortion. Support for state proscription of "any abortion by a person who is not a physician" therefore needs to be deleted from *Roe*.

Clarifications should be introduced regarding the distinction between controversial meanings of personhood and a living (human) embryo or fetus, as well as the difference (and relation) between a decision about pregnancy and a decision to raise a child. In addition, a number of points not addressed in *Roe* need to be articulated. These include acknowledgment that the right to terminate pregnancy is not necessarily equivalent to the right to terminate a fetus, and that a right to abortion applies to the former but not to the latter if the two are separable (as in cases of possible viability); recognition of obligations to a sentient fetus to reduce or eliminate pain unless the woman's health is thereby compromised; and affirmation that informed consent requirements should be satisfied, including full and accurate disclosure of pertinent information concerning the procedure.

These recommendations reflect in part my own moral point of view, but they do not represent it in its entirety. Consideration of the complexity of abortion decisions, and possible areas of agreement between dissidents leads me to articulate the following as a summary of that position.

1. Abortion is rarely if ever virtuous, sometimes morally justified, and sometimes immoral.
2. Such claims are neither negated nor affirmed by *Roe v. Wade,* that is, by the legality of abortion.
3. Our society is one in which the circumstances that occasion abortion are often immoral, sometimes more immoral than abortion, and one in which people do not now agree about the morality of abortion, nor do they appear likely to agree in the future.
4. The immoral conditions that sometimes occasion abortion include poverty, lack of social and medical supports for pregnancy and parent-

hood, stereotypic views of sex roles and biological parenthood, and a eugenic mentality that welcomes only "premium babies." Clearly, greater societal effort is needed to rectify these conditions. In addition, the following practices would facilitate moral decisions about pregnancy:

- broader education regarding the distinction between legality and morality, using pregnancy decisions as an example of but one area where the distinction is important;
- broader education concerning responsibility for contraception, encouragement of positive social attitudes toward and expansion of practical possibilities for adoption, information regarding the developmental status of the human embryo/fetus, and the various methods of abortion and their effects on pregnant women and fetuses;
- insistence that a pregnant woman's autonomy in decisions that affect her is as binding on others as is the autonomy of nonpregnant persons in decisions affecting them;
- broader regard for human life throughout the spectrum of development.

So long as societal disagreement about the morality of abortion remains, the law should not preempt the right and responsibility of individuals to make their own moral decisions. However, if the law were to become more restrictive (for example, by excluding late or second trimester abortions for nonmedical reasons), it might still reflect the moral sentiment of most people. If overturning *Roe* led to illegalization of abortions in extreme circumstances such as pregnancy due to rape and incest, or pregnancies that are life-threatening for women or fetuses, it would clearly betray the moral sentiment of most people.

I don't pretend to have developed all of the above points adequately, but most if not all have been well-developed elsewhere.[34] This account might serve as a springboard for further discussion among those who recognize not only that contradictory positions cannot both be true, but also that truth doesn't necessarily lie in the middle.

Acknowledgments

I wish to thank Lisa Cahill, Anthony Mahowald, Ann Patrick, and Mary Segers for helpful comments and suggestions; Maureen Hack and Patrick O'Grady for pertinent clinical information; and Carmen Guice for her assistance in preparing this article.

QUESTIONS FOR CONSIDERATION

1. Mahowald raises the question of why the debate over abortion continues to be intense and offers a partial answer by referring to the emotional and misleading rhetoric of abortion. How does she characterize the rhetoric of abortion by both the "pro-life" and "pro-choice" activists?

2. How does Mahowald maintain that the duration of gestation must be considered in order to clarify the issues of abortion? Why does she contend that moral problems are more significant with the advance of gestation?

3. What are her criticisms of Roe vs. Wade relative to viability? What does she mean by the statement "Technically, abortion is no longer possible after viability. . . ?" What are the morally relevant factors associated with the choice of method?

4. What are the circumstances of conception that Mahowald identifies as being morally relevant to an abortion decision? How does she differentiate between voluntariness related to conception and to intercourse?

5. According to Mahowald, what is the significance of the age and competence of the pregnant woman?

6. What are the morally relevant factors related to the health of the fetus and the health of the pregnant woman that Mahowald believes complicates the abortion decision?

7. What are the possible areas of agreement that Mahowald believes both sides of the abortion issue could compromise upon? What changes would she recommend in the Roe vs. Wade decision?

NOTES

1. *Roe v. Wade,* 410 U.S., 113.

2. The U.S. Supreme Court will issue its ruling in a Missouri case, *Webster v. Reproductive Health Services,* in the summer of 1989. The decision is widely expected to reaffirm, modify, or overturn *Roe.*

3. E. J. Dionne, Jr., "Poll on Abortion Finds the Nation is Sharply Divided," *New York Times* (26 April 1989), p. 1.

4. Kristin Luker, *Abortion and the Politics of Motherhood* (Berkeley: University of California Press, 1984), pp. 158–91.

5. Beverly Harrison, *Our Right to Choose* (Boston: Beacon Press, 1983), p. 232.

6. See Sidney Callahan and Daniel Callahan, eds. *Abortion: Understanding Differences* (New York: Plenum Press, 1984); Joel Feinberg, ed., *The Problem of Abortion* (Belmont, CA: Wadsworth, 1984); Rosalind Petchesky, *Abortion and Women's Choice* (Boston: Northeastern University Press, 1984); Harrison, *Our Right to Choose;* James T. Burtchaell, *Rachel Weeping* (San Francisco:

Harper and Row, 1982); L. W. Sumner, *Abortion and Moral Theory* (Princeton, NJ: Princeton University Press, 1981).

7. Mary B. Mahowald, "Abortion and Equality," in *Abortion: Understanding Differences,* pp. 178–96.

8. Jonathan Imber, *Abortion and the Private Practice of the Physician* (New Haven: Yale University Press, 1986), p. 57.

9. Nobuo Okado and Tokuzo Kojima, "Ontogeny of the Central Nervous System: Neurogenesis, Fibre Connection, Synaptogenesis and Myelination in the Spinal Cord," in *Continuity of Neural Functions from Prenatal to Postnatal Life,* Heinz F. R. Prechtl, ed. (Oxford: Blackwell Scientific Publications Ltd., 1984), pp. 31–42.

10. See Phillip G. Stubblefield, "Pregnancy Termination," in *Obstetrics: Normal and Problem Pregnancies,* Steven Gabbe, Jennifer Niebyl, and Joe Simpson, eds. (New York: Churchill Livingstone, 1986), p. 1072.

11. See *Williams Obstetrics,* 17th edition, Jack Pritchard, Paul MacDonald, and Norman Gant, eds., (Norwalk CT. Appleton-Century-Crofts, 1985), p. 246.

12. See *Williams Obstetrics,* 2, 745; Denise Main and Elliott Main, "Management of Preterm Labor and Delivery," in *Obstetrics,* 689. However, *Dorland's Medical Dictionary* (Philadelphia: W. B. Saunders Co., 1988), 27th edition, defines premature birth as the "birth of a premature infant" (p. 210) and premature infant as "one usually born after the twenty-seventh week and before full term, and arbitrarily defined as an infant weighing 1000 to 2499 grams at birth" (p. 833). Since *Dorland's* defines an abortus as "a fetus weighing less than 500 grams or being of less than 20 weeks' gestational age" this leaves neither designation (premature infant or abortus) applicable to the fetus expelled or removed from the uterus between twenty and twenty-seven weeks gestation.

13. For discussion of current methods of abortion, see *Williams Obstetrics,* 478–83, and Phillip G. Stubblefield, in *Obstetrics: Normal and Problem Pregnancies,* 1066–72.

14. Nathan M. Simon, "Psychological and Emotional Indications for Therapeutic Abortion," in *Abortion,* R. Bruce Sloane, ed. (New York: Grune and Stratton, 1971), pp. 86–87.

15. The "voluntariness" of intercourse may also be questioned on grounds of the sex-role stereotyping that limits the autonomy of women. See Catharine McKinnon, *Feminism Unmodified: Discourses on Life and the Law* (Cambridge: Harvard University Press, 1987), p. 94–95.

16. Robert K. Creasy, "Preterm Labor and Delivey" in *Maternal Fetal Medicine,* Robert K. Creasy and Robert Resnik, eds. (Philadelphia: W. B. Saunders Co., 1984), p. 416.

17. *Williams Obstetrics,* p. 801.

18. See *American Law Reports,* Cases and Annotations, Vol. 74 (San Francisco: Bancroft-Whitney Co., 1976), pp. 1211–30.

19. Mary B. Mahowald and Virginia Abernethy, "When a Mentally Ill Woman Refuses Abortion," *Hastings Center Report* 12 (1985), pp. 22–23.

20. *Williams Obstetrics,* p. 468.

21. Michael R. Harrison, Mitchell S. Golbus, and Roy A. Filly, "Management of the Fetus with a Correctible Congenital Defect" *Journal of the American Medical Association* 246:7 (1981), pp. 774–77; John C. Fletcher, "The Fetus as Patient: Ethical Issues," *Journal of the American Medical Association* 246:7 (1981), 772–73; Lawrence E. Karp, "Fetal Surgery," *American Journal of Medical Genetics* 13 (1982), pp. 357–58.

22. Mary B. Mahowald, "Beyond Abortion: Refusal of Caesarean Section," *Bioethics* 3:2 (1989), pp. 106–21.

23. *Williams Obstetrics,* p. 483 and *Roe v. Wade.*

24. Mary B. Mahowald, "Concepts of Abortion and Their Relevance to the Abortion Debate," *Southern Journal of Philosophy* 20 (Summer 1982), pp. 195–207.

25. Judith Jarvis Thomson, "A Defense of Abortion," in *The Problem of Abortion,* 187; Christine Overall, *Ethics and Human Reproduction* (Boston: Allen and Unwin, 1987), pp. 68–84.

26. *Williams Obstetrics,* p. 2.

27. Luker, *Abortion and the Politics of Motherhood,* p. 2.

28. *Thornburgh v. American College of Obstetrics and Gynecology* 476 U.S. 747.

29. Selig Neubardt and Harold Schulman, *Techniques of Abortion* (Boston: Little, Brown, 1977), p. 69.

30. *Thornburgh v. American College of Obstetrics and Gynecology* 476 U.S. 747.

31. Mary B. Mahowald, "Beyond Abortion: Refusal of Caesarean Section."

32. Okado and Kojima, "Ontogeny of the Central Nervous System."

33. *Roe v. Wade.*

34. Cf. note 6 above.

Edward A. Langerak

Abortion: Listening to the Middle

Says one critic of the philosophical debate on abortion: "Philosophers are not listened to because they do not listen."[1] Though I believe the charge is too strong, my own review of the literature makes it uncomfortably understandable. If there is any public consensus on abortion, as reflected in legal systems as well as in public opinion surveys, it is the middle-of-the-road view that some abortions are not permissible but that others are, and that some of the permissible abortions are more difficult to justify than others. But many of the most widely cited philosophical writings on abortion argue that the only coherent positions tend toward the extremes: all or most abortions are put into the same moral boat with either murder or, more frequently, elective surgery. In fact, proponents of the extremes tend to respect one another as at least being self-consistent, while joining in swift rebuttal of those who want it both ways and ignominiously try to be moderates on either murder or mandatory motherhood.

This reaction against the middle derives from some basic beliefs of those on the extremes. On the liberal side are those who believe that fetuses, and perhaps even very young infants, lack some necessary condition (say, self-consciousness) of personhood.[2] This view is often combined with the further assertion that the social consequences of society's conferring on the fetus a claim to life are such that the conferral should not be made until birth or shortly thereafter. On the conservative side there are those who believe that from conception (or very shortly thereafter) the fetus has as strong (or almost as strong) a claim to life as does any person. This claim resides either in some property thought sufficient for personhood (say, genetic endowment) that the fetus has in itself, or in the immediate conferral of personhood on the fetus by God or society.

Of course, as Schopenhauer said, arguments are not like taxicabs that you can dismiss when they become inconvenient; and the two extremes are quick to point out the problematic implications of each other's positions. The liberals are accused of courting infanticide and the conservatives of trivializing the moral category of murder. Such implications would be more damaging to the extremes were it not that most moderate positions have an equally problematic flaw—that of arbitrary line-drawing. My reading of the abortion literature suggests that there are two widely shared beliefs that moderate positions seek to incorporate in their approaches to the abortion issue. The first belief is that something about the fetus itself, not merely the social consequences of abortion, makes abortions (or at least many abortions) morally problematic. The second belief is that late abortions are significantly more morally problematic than early abortions. Not only are these beliefs widely shared by moderates, but I find that liberals and conservatives, whose positions implicitly reject one or both of these beliefs, often feel uncomfortable in rejecting them.

In accounting for these two beliefs, most middle positions maintain variations of what I call the "stage" approach and what its critics call the "magic moment" approach. The assertion is that at some point in the development of the fetus, say at the point of acquiring some vital sign, of sentience, of quickening, or of viability, the fetus suddenly moves from having no claim to life to having as strong (or almost as strong) a claim as an adult human. While the "stage" approach is consistent with the two beliefs underlying the moderate position, its difficulty has always been to explain the tremendous moral weight put on some specific point in what really amounts to a continuum in development. Critics on both extremes argue that, no matter what stage is picked as the "magic moment," the whole approach is prima facie arbitrary.

The implications of the liberal and conservative positions, including their denial of one or both of the moderate beliefs, and the prima facie arbitrariness of the stage positions, motivate consideration of an alternative that both is coherent and listens to the middle by accounting for the two beliefs.

Without examining all the alternatives. I will argue that the potentiality principle is plausible and accounts for the first belief—that something about the fetus itself makes abortion morally problematic—but that, by itself, it cannot account for the second belief—that late abortions are significantly more problematic than early abortions. I will then argue that a conferred claims approach is plausible, consistent with the potentiality principle, and accounts for the second belief though it cannot account for the first.

I will suggest that combining the potentiality principle with a conferred claims approach provides moderates with a coherent framework for thinking through the central questions of the abortion debate: (1) When does an individual human being attain either an inherent claim to life or such properties that society ought to confer on it a claim to life? (2) When do a person's or a group of persons' claims to life, physical or mental health, freedom, privacy, and self-actualization override another human being's claim to life? (3) When should answers to the first two question be incorporated into the law of a pluralistic society'?

The Potentiality Principle

I formulate the potentiality principle as follows: "If in the normal course of its development, a being will acquire a person's claim to life, then by virtue of that fact it already has some claim to life." To understand this principle, one must distinguish among "actual person," "a capacity for person-hood," "potential person," and "possible person." An *actual person* is a being that meets a sufficient condition (whatever that may be)[3] for personhood and thereby has as strong a claim to life as normal adult human beings. Roughly, a *capacity for personhood* is possessed by any being not currently exhibiting that capacity, but who has proceeded in the course of its development to the point where it could currently exhibit it (for example, a temporarily unconscious person). A *potential person* is a being, not yet a person, that will become an actual person in the normal[4] course of its development (for example, a human fetus). A *possible person* is a being that could, under certain causally possible conditions, become an actual person (for example, a human sperm or egg).[5]

This technical set of distinctions is important because the potentiality principle asserts that potential persons, but not possible persons, have a claim to life. Some attacks on the principle confuse these categories.[6] Also, the principle is consistent with granting full personhood to those with a capacity for personhood, a fact ignored by those who collapse "capacity" and "potentiality" and argue, for example, that the category of "potential person" endangers sleeping persons. Moreover, the distinctions can help us avoid sloppy language, such as that of the Supreme Court in *Roe v. Wade* when it asserted that at viability the state begins to have a compelling interest in "potential life." Clearly a fetus is actually alive and is even an actual human being, genetically defined; its unique status is that, given most criteria of personhood, it is neither an actual person nor a merely possible person—it is a potential person.

Potentiality and Temporality

The potentiality principle asserts that a potential person has a claim to life, albeit one that may be weaker than the claim of an actual person. Many people find this assertion intuitively plausible, but are unable to persuade those who challenge it. Here is my attempt to persuade.

It is clear that the unique status of the potential person has to do with its inherent "thrust" or predetermined tendency. A potential person is not simply a set of blueprints, it is an organism that itself will become the actual person toward which it is already developing. Controversial issues of personal identity arise here, but two points seem obvious. First, we cannot simply assume that its predetermined tendency already grants it the claims it will have in the future. To paraphrase H. Tristram Engelhardt, Jr., we must not lose the ability to distinguish between the claims of the future and those of the present;[7] or as S. I. Benn succinctly puts it, a potential president is not already commander-in-chief.[8] Second, those attracted to the potentiality principle do see some derivative relationship between the claims that a being will have in the normal course of its development and those that it has in the present.

I believe that the plausibility of the last point rests in perceiving humans as basically temporal beings. For actual persons this is true, first of all, from an internal point of view (a fact Heidegger uses for his entire ontology). Our self-consciousness so orients us to our past and our future that, in an important sense, we *are* our history and our projections as well as our present. A premedical student, for example, sees himself or herself as a future physician, not just as a science student. This temporal perception is also true from an external point of view, a point of view that extends to humans that are not yet persons. When we see a very young child, we see something of the adult it will, in the normal course of its development, become, as well as something of the baby that it once was. In this temporal perception lies, I believe, the respect we feel is due former persons (for example, respectful treatment of corpses) and, for that matter, former presidents. The respect we give former persons and presidents is not as great as that which we give actual ones, but that does not undermine the fact that some respect is due the former and that it is derivative from, indeed proportional to, the respect due to the latter.

Similarly, perceiving humans in a temporal context accounts for the respect many feel is due to humans by virtue of their potential. As an analogy, consider a potential president. Following my distinctions, such a person is not merely a possible president (something civics teachers used to say about every American child); he or she has already won the election but has not yet been inaugurated (on a somewhat arbitrarily selected date). The person is not yet commander-in-chief but, in the normal course, *will* (not *could*) be. Already that person receives some of the perquisites of the future office. The fact that the news media and others give the potential president more attention than the actual president, of course, may be the result of prudence, if not exploitation (the same derivation for much of the respect given actual presidents). But, at least in pre-Watergate times, some of the respect given actual presidents, and most of that given former presidents, derives from the high office that the person has or had, even when the person is not particularly deserving. Those who perceive a person in a temporal context and who, like myself, still respect an actual or former president by virtue of the office (apart from achievements in it), will derivatively have some respect toward a potential president by virtue of the office he or she will have.

Even those who deny that presidents ought to be respected simply by virtue of their office, should agree that some of the respect given persons derives from their "office" of personhood, apart from their achievements. In fact, traditionally the respect involving a claim to life derives from what persons are, rather than what they achieve or fail to achieve. If so, then perceiving humans in a temporal context should elicit some respect for former and potential persons, respect that is derivative from and proportional, though not identical, to the respect elicited by the actual persons they were or will become.

Temporality and Probability

Some may grant the strength of this argument as it applies to former persons, sensing that it accounts, for example, for our aversion to artificially keeping former persons "alive" in order to harvest their organs at a convenient time. However, whatever else we may say about former persons, they were certainly, at one time, actual persons. But the personhood of potential persons is still "outstanding" and there is no guarantee that it will be realized. The contingency of the "not yet" makes it asymmetrical with the "has been" even when we perceive humans in a temporal context.

This objection forces us to ask just what is the moral significance of the predetermined tendency of a potential person. Though the tendency does not guarantee personhood, it does distinguish the organism from possible persons by guaranteeing a dramatic shift in probabilities. This difference in probabilities is similar to that which distinguishes a potential president from a possible president. The potentiality principle asks us to respect a potential person by virtue not of what it *could* be, but of what it *will* be in the normal course of its development. Even those of us who refuse to mythologize the predetermined tendency in potential persons must agree that this tendency makes it highly likely that, without outside interference, they will become persons. Is this shift in probabilities of moral significance?

Consider the other end of the life-span. Those who believe that it is sometimes permissible to cease striving officiously to keep humans in an irreversible coma artificially alive, must agree that the irreversibility of the coma is seldom, if ever, absolutely guaranteed. But we believe it is morally irresponsible to allow the rare "miraculous recovery" to prevent acting on the best medical prognosis, when it indicates no reasonable hope of recovery. To shut off a respirator when there is a 50 percent chance of recovery, (or even a 5 percent chance, given our laudable bias toward erring in favor of personal life), is morally wrong, but not when the probability of recovery approaches (without reaching) zero. In an uncertain world, judgments of high probabilities are often the only kind we have. This makes dramatic shifts in probabilities morally significant.[9]

So I believe that the high probability of future personhood, inherent in a potential person, is of moral significance to those who perceive humans in a temporal context, and that this makes plausible the assertion of the potentiality principle. I hope I have at least shifted the burden of proof on to those who deny that the high probability of a fetus's becoming a person with a strong claim to life already grants it some (proportional) claim to life and respect.

Conferred Claims

Although the potentiality principle, as defended, accounts for the first belief—that something about the fetus itself makes abortion morally problematic—it leaves open the question of just how strong a claim to life should be attributed to the fetus. There are extreme liberals on the abortion issue who may grant the fetus some claim to life but simply argue that the claims of an actual person—claims to freedom and mental health—always override the claim to life of a fetus. Among those who use the potentiality principle, there will be intramural debates on how strong a claim to life it implies. I cannot argue the case here, but I believe that the most plausible use of it is one that allows the use of IUDs and "morning after" pills (both of which probably act as abortifacients), as well as abortions during the first trimester for such reasons as the woman's being too young for motherhood.[10] But then the claim to life attributed to the very early fetus cannot be very strong. The incidence of early spontaneous abortion is estimated[11] variously from 15 percent to over 50 percent, and second-trimester fetuses have a somewhat higher natural death rate than postviable fetuses. In other words, the probability of an older fetus becoming an actual person is perhaps double the probability of a zygote becoming a person. While this shift in probability is noteworthy, and marks implantation as a point of some moral significance, it is not nearly as significant as the difference in moral seriousness moderates see between a very early abortion and a late one. Consequently, if the inherent claim to life of a potential person is derived from and proportional to the probability of its becoming an actual person, one cannot in good faith allow the claim to life of a zygote to be easily overridden and then assert that the inherent claim to life of an older fetus is so vastly stronger that it all but cannot be overridden. Therefore, although the potentiality principle can account for the belief that something about the fetus itself makes abortion morally problematic, it cannot by itself account for the belief that late abortions are significantly more morally problematic than very early abortions.

However, the conferred claims approach can account for the second belief, although it cannot account for the first. Assume that, whatever moral claim to life an older fetus may have by virtue of its potentiality, the claim may not be strong enough to override the claim of a pregnant woman for an abortion. At what point should society confer a stronger claim to life on the fetus? At what point should society treat it as if it were a person?

The conferral approach to the status of the fetus is not an unusual one,[12] though it is sometimes thought incompatible with an approach that asserts an inherent claim in the fetus itself. But an approach that *confers* claims rubs an approach that *recognizes* inherent claims only if the inherent claim to life is thought to be as serious as an actual person's claim to life. In this case it would be futile (rather than contradictory) to ask what claims society ought to confer on it. However, when the recognized inherent claim is weaker than a normal adult's claim to life, as can be the case with the potentiality principle, one can coherently ask whether society ought, in addition, to confer on the fetus a stronger claim to life.

The argument in favor of such a conferral basically appeals to the social consequences of abortions and infanticide. For example, infants are so similar to persons that allowing them to be killed would generate a moral climate that would endanger the claim to life of even young persons. And older fetuses are so similar to infants that allowing them to be killed without due moral or legal process would endanger infants. Of course there must be a cutoff for this sort of argument. For example, most would agree that preventing the implantation of zygotes would have no discernible effect on our sympathetic capacities toward persons. At what point would abortions begin to have such effects, especially on medical personnel, that it is in society's interest to endow the fetus at that point with a stronger claim to life? This seems largely an empirical question and one not easily answered,[13] though I will suggest some guidelines below.

One difficulty with the conferral approach has always been that the relevant considerations are the interest and sympathies of actual persons, rather than moral claims inherent in the fetus itself. Indeed, the above argument is reminiscent of Kant's view that we ought not beat our dogs merely because beating our dogs might make us more inclined to beat people. Such arguments derive protection for some beings from the rather variable, even capricious, sympathies of other beings. Thus the conferral approach by itself does not account for the belief that something about the fetus itself makes abortion morally problematic; but this belief is accounted for by the potentiality approach.

Implantation, Quickening, Viability, and Birth

My combined approach escapes the problematic implications of the extremes but does it escape the flaw of arbitrary line-drawing that I attributed to those moderate positions that appeal to the stage or "magic moment" approach? Two related considerations show that it does. First, notice that the word "arbitrary" should not be used loosely. For example, there is a certain arbitrariness in making eighteen the age of majority rather than seventeen or nineteen. But the relevant criteria nonarbitrarily imply that, if a legally precise line must be drawn within the continuum of growth, the debate must focus on that time span rather than, say, the span between seven and nine.

Second, I submit that the two criteria I use—important shifts in probabilities and dangerous social consequences—nonarbitrarily suggest four spans (beyond that of conception) for moral and legal line-drawing in a potential person's continuum of growth. Although these criteria imply distinct spans for definite increments in the strength of the claim to life, at no stage does a potential person move from having no claim to having one as strong as an adult.

The first span, as we saw, is that of implantation, when the shift in probabilities of actual personhood signifies a somewhat stronger inherent claim to life, at least from the moral point of view. The recognition of this change is due apart from any consequentialist considerations about the difference between more or less unknowingly preventing implantation and knowingly detaching an implanted embryo. However, the remaining spans are suggested by consequentialist considerations about the psychological and social impact of abortions, considerations in favor of conferring an even stronger claim to life on the fetus.

The second span involves the traditional indicator of "quickening." When the fetus begins making perceptible spontaneous movements (around the beginning of the second trimester), its shape, its behavior, and even its beginning relationship with the mother and the rest of society (every father recalls when he first felt the fetus's movements) all suggest that abortions after this point will have personal and social consequences specifiably more serious than those of earlier abortions.

The third is that of viability, when a fetus is capable of living with simple medical care, outside the womb (around the end of the second trimester). Recall the "infanticide" trials of physicians who, claiming they were inducing abortions, were charged with participating in premature births and murders. This controversy is only one indication that killing potential persons after viability has social consequences (apart from legal ones) even more serious than abortions soon after quickening.

Finally, consider that allowing infanticide is generally regarded as a *reductio* of those positions that allow it. The aversion to infanticide is shared even by most of those whose criteria for personhood imply that a newborn is still only a potential person and not an actual one. This suggests that most people agree that at birth the potential person attains properties and relationships so close to those of actual persons that the consequences of killing at this point are practically the same as killing young persons.

If these observations are true, they justify conferring on newborns a claim to life as strong as that of adult persons. They also suggest partial wisdom in the Supreme Court's decision allowing states to grant a rather strong claim to life to postviable fetuses, a claim overridden only by the claim to life or health (I would specify "physical health") of the mother. But the court decision, in effect, mandates the allowing of abortion on demand for all previable fetuses. If my observations about quickening are correct, we should also draw an earlier line, conferring a claim to life on the fetus at the beginning of the second trimester, a claim less strong than that conferred at viability, but one overridden only by such serious claims as that of the mother to mental or physical health.[14] Probably the moral line drawn at implantation should remain outside the legal realm.

I admit the difficulties in legally implementing such an approach, but I doubt that they are insurmountable or as deep as the moral and legal difficulties of alternative approaches. Therefore I believe I have presented a plausible approach to the abortion issue that is coherent, is not arbitrary, and listens well to the considered intuitions of those in the middle.[15]

QUESTIONS FOR CONSIDERATION

1. What are the two elements of the "middle of the road" that Langerak identifies as the most likely view of public consensus? Do you agree?
2. How does Langerak characterize the "potentiality principle"? How does he distinguish this principle from "actual persons," "capacity for personhood", and "possible persons"?
3. Explain Langerak's description of potentiality as a temporal perception (Heidegger's "we are our possibilities")? How would he distinguish probability from possibility as a temporal perception?
4. In accounting for the view that late abortions are more problematic than earlier abortions, Langerak offers the "conferred claims" approach. Explain how he combines this approach with the "potentiality principle"?
5. How does Langerak attempt to avoid the "flaw of arbitrary line-drawing" in the stage or "magic moment" approach. What are the four distinct spans that he believes provides definite increments in the claim to life for the developing fetus. Where would he recommend that society draw the line in conferring a claim to life for the fetus? Do you agree?

NOTES

1. Roger Wertheimer, "Philosophy on Humanity," in *Abortion: Pro and Con,* ed. Robert L. Perkins (Cambridge: Schenkman Publishing Company), p. 127.

2. For brevity I use "fetus" in a generic sense to refer to unborn humans at any stage of development, including that of zygote, conceptus, and embryo. I assume the fetuses are human beings, genetically defined, and use "person" to refer to those human beings that have as strong a claim to life as a normal adult. I use "as strong a claim" rather than "same claim" because, if very young human beings are persons, their claim to life clearly involves the claim to be nurtured as well as the claim not to be killed, a feature that is not clearly true of a normal adult's claim to life. I use "claim" to life rather than "right" or "prima facie right" because my argument entails that a fetus's (though not a person's) claim to life can be held with varying degrees of strength, and I agree with Joel Feinberg *(Social Philosophy* [Englewood Cliffs: Prentice Hall, 1973], pp. 64–7) that this is a feature of claims rather than rights. Though Feinberg may object to my use of his distinction, I agree with him that the "right" or "valid claim" in a given instance is the strongest of competing claims. For an account of the relationship between claims and rights that I believe is consistent with my argument, see Bertram Bandman's "Rights and Claims" in *Bioethics and Human Rights,* eds. Elsie L. Bandman and Bertram Bandman (Boston: Little Brown and Company, 1978).

3. One advantage of the potentiality principle is that one need not specify the necessary or sufficient conditions for actual personhood; one need only note that, whatever they are, a potential person will acquire them in the normal course of its development. My own position is that self-consciousness is a necessary and perhaps a sufficient condition for personhood: "The fact that man can have the idea 'I' raises him infinitely above all the other beings living on earth. By this he is *a person"* (Immanuel Kant, *Anthropology from a Pragmatic Point of View,* trans.

Mary J. Gregor, The Hague: Martinus Nijhoff, 1947, p. 9). See also H. Tristram Engelhart, Jr. ("The Ontology of Abortion," *Ethics, 84/3* April, 1974, p. 230n): "Only self-conscious subjects can value themselves, and, thus, be ends in themselves, and, consequently, themselves make claims against us." While Joel Feinberg seems to object to thinking of personhood as a property, he does appeal to the fact that persons are "equally centers of experience, foci of subjectivity" (*op. cit.,* p. 93).

4. Although using the phrase "in the normal course of its development" rather than "in the normal course of events" emphasizes the teleological ("nature's aim") rather than the statistical probability aspect of "normal development," my later argument about probability and claims assumes that even a teleological notion of "normal" has statistical implications: if the natural end of (a) is to become (A) then it is highly probable that, without interference, (a) will become (A). I believe I am referring to what some Thomists call "active, natural potentiality," though I deny potential personhood is as claim-laden as actual personhood.

5. The class of potential and possible persons must be distinguished from the class (membership unknown) of future persons, namely the class of future actual persons who do not now exist but will in fact exist in the future. One must be careful with analogies between our duties to potential persons and our duties to future persons (for such an analogy, see Werner S. Pluhar, "Abortion and Simple Consciousness," *Journal of Philosophy,* 74/3 March, 1977, p. 167). If there are future persons (as is so likely as to be certain), they will be actual persons whose quality of life will be affected by actions we now perform, while it is debatable whether killing potential persons affects the quality of their lives as *persons.*

6. A point I argue in reply to Michael Tooley's "Abortion and Infanticide, " *Philosophy and Public Affairs* 2/4 (Summer, 1973), pp. 410–16.

7. Engelhart, p. 223.

8. "Abortion, Infanticide, and Respect for Persons," *The Problem of Abortion,* ed. Joel Feinberg (Belmont: Wadsworth Publishing Co., 1973), p. 103.

9. In this I agree with John T. Noonan, "An Almost Absolute Value in History," *The Morality of Abortion,* ed. John T. Noonan, Jr. (Cambridge: Harvard University Press, 1970), though he seems to argue wrongly that an abortion involves a high probability of killing a person. Instead, it kills a human that had a high probability of becoming a person.

10. Notice that if one uses the potentiality principle to attribute a very strong claim to life for the fetus, one has, in effect, denied the belief that late abortions are significantly more morally problematic than early abortions.

11. See Malcolm Potts, Peter Diggory, and John Peel, *Abortion* (Cambridge: Cambridge University Press, 1977), ch. 2. The highest estimate I have seen, at variance with most others, is 69 percent, by Harvard physiologist John D. Biggers *(Science,* vol. 202, October 13, 1978, p. 198).

12. See R. B. Brandt, "The Morality of Abortion" *(The Monist, Vol.* 56, 1972, pp. 504–26), for a quasi-Rawlsian development of this approach. See also Ronald M. Green, "Conferred Rights and the Fetus," *Journal of Religious Ethics,* 2/1 (1974), and Benn, *op. cit.*

13. See Magda Denes, *In Necessity and Sorrow: Life and Death in an Abortion Hospital* (New York: Penguin Books, 1977), for one description of the different social effects of abortions at different stages of pregnancy.

14. Notice that adding the conferred claims approach highly qualifies a possible implication of my defense of the potentiality principle, namely the implication that it is somewhat easier to justify aborting fetuses with defects that lower their probability of attaining personhood. Any arguments for conferring a stronger claim to life on fetuses at a given point would apply to most defective fetuses as well.

15. Patricia Fauser, James Gustafson, Gary Iseminger, Daniel Lee, and Frederick Stoutland gave me very helpful comments on an earlier draft of this essay.

PART V: Termination of Treatment

PART V:1: Setting Standards for Limiting Care

PART V:2: Terminating Treatment for the Terminally Ill

PART V:3: Treating Neonates with Birth Defects

PART V:4: *Active Voluntary Euthanasia and Physician-Assisted Suicide*

RICHARD DOERFLINGER
Assisted Suicide: Pro-Choice or Anti-Life

DAN W. BROCK
Voluntary Active Euthanasia

DANIEL CALLAHAN
When Self-Determination Runs Amok

New biomedical technologies, such as respirators, cardiac pacemakers, and kidney dialysis units, have greatly increased medicine's capacity to extend human life. In combination with a growing industry of long-term care, these advances are changing traditional notions of "old age" and "natural death." While some of these technologies clearly prolong the experience of life, others seem merely to extend the process of dying. Regardless of their life-extending or death-prolonging potentials, these advances are raising critical questions regarding the distribution of health care—especially long-term care—and what, if any, limitations should be placed on care.

Limiting Care and Terminating Treatment

In the early morning hours of 11 January 1983 a car driven by Nancy Cruzan slid off an icy Missouri road and rolled over. Cruzan was thrown from the car. Before medical assistance arrived, she suffered prolonged oxygen deprivation which led to massive, irreversible brain damage. Although a medical team restored Cruzan's breathing and heartbeat, she lay unconscious in a persistent vegetative state receiving nourishment through a gastric tube. After six years without any sign of recovery, Cruzan's parents sought to remove the feeding tube and allow Nancy to die. But the Supreme Court of Missouri refused their request, claiming there was insufficient evidence of Nancy Cruzan's wishes regarding the withdrawal of food and water. In 1990, the United States Supreme Court supported the Missouri decision by ruling that states could require "clear and convincing evidence" demonstrating a patient's choice before life-supporting benefits could be withdrawn. Four months after the decision, Cruzan's parents were able to offer witnesses that provided the "clear and convincing evidence" needed to convince the State of Missouri that she would wish that the feeding tube be withdrawn.

The *Cruzan* case illustrates the ethical dilemmas involved in withdrawing treatment from the terminally ill or permanently incapacitated. Are physicians ethically required to provide health care in all circumstances and at all times? Are there circumstances in which intense suffering or the total loss of "quality of life" would make termination of care (and the subsequent death of the patient) more humane than continued care? Does the medical community or the state have compelling reasons to restrict a patient's "right to die"? These issues—the obligation to resuscitate, the withholding of treatment, and doctor-assisted suicide—will provide the focus in the sections on "Setting Standards for Limiting Care" and "Terminating Treatment for the Terminally Ill."

Terminating Neonates with Birth Defects

On March 30, 1992, Theresa Pearson died due to complications of anencephaly. She was ten days old. Anencephaly is a fatal disorder in which an infant has developed only a brain stem; the higher cerebral brain is missing. At the time of her birth, Theresa's parents, Laura Campo and Justin Pearson, petitioned the court to have her declared "brain dead" so that her organs could be donated to infants waiting for tiny livers, lungs, hearts and kidneys. Florida courts refused such a declaration. By the time Theresa died several days later, her organs were not suitable for transplantation.

Theresa's case is repeated between 2000 and 3000 times annually in the United States. Anencephalic infants could provide an important source of organs for transplantation. This case raised questions concerning the status of neonates with severe defects. Do such infants have interests that should be protected? Should infants with severe defects be refused treatment? Does it alter society's concept of death or the purpose of medicine to declare infants like Theresa brain dead in order to help other infants? The articles in the section on "Treating Neonates with Birth Defects" will deal with such issues.

Active Voluntary Euthanasia and Physician-Assisted Suicide

Jack Miller, age 53, was dying of bone cancer and emphysema. Seeking to avoid the suffering associated with a terminal disease, he sought the assistance of Dr. Jack Kevorkian, a Michigan physician, in committing suicide. In an earlier instance, Janet Atkins, age 54, also sought the assistance of Dr. Kevorkian in committing suicide; however, Ms. Atkins was not a terminally ill patient, but rather was diagnosed with Alzheimer's disease.

Should physicians ever assist patients with suicide? Was Dr. Kevorkian justified in assisting Mr. Miller in avoiding the suffering of a terminal disease? Would the fact that Ms. Atkins was not terminal make a difference in whether Dr. Kevorkian should assist her in committing suicide? Should physicians ever practice active voluntary euthanasia? Do incompetent patients have a right to active nonvoluntary euthanasia? The articles in the section "Active Voluntary Euthanasia and Physician-Assisted Suicide" will focus upon these questions.

Part V:1: Setting Standards for Limiting Care

• John Hardwig's **Is There a Duty to Die?** explores various circumstances that might lead individuals to have a duty to die. He argues that medical technology enables people to survive longer than they are able to take care of themselves. They become a burden upon loved ones and threaten their health, savings, and careers.

• Daniel Callahan's **Terminating Treatment: Age As a Standard** offers principles for viewing age as a medical and "biographical" criterion for withholding treatment.

• Robert D. Truog's **Triage in the ICU** addresses the issue of terminating treatment for patients who have a poor prognosis, especially those utilizing scarce treatment such as found in the ICU. He notes that the treatment of such patients may prevent other patients with a higher "benefit index" from receiving therapy.

Part V:2: Terminating Treatment for the Terminally Ill

• Giles R. Scofield's **Is Consent Useful When Resuscitation Isn't?** focuses upon the need to maintain meaningful communications and respect for persons in light of the growing trend to withhold treatment. Such communications necessitate consent even when treatment is futile if we are to maintain our fundamental values.

• Kathleen Nolan's **In Death's Shadow: The Meaning of Withholding Resuscitation** points out that resuscitation (and its withholding) carries deep emotional and symbolic meaning for those involved in the decision to resuscitate or to withhold resuscitation. These meanings often outweigh rational considerations and demand special attention within the medical community.

• Joanne Lynn's and James F. Childress's **Must Patients Always Be Given Food and Water?** addresses permissible circumstances in which nutrition might be withheld from terminally ill patients.

Part V:3: Treating Neonates with Birth Defects

• Arthur L. Caplan's and Cynthia B. Cohen's **Standards of Judgment for Treatment** examines various standards for the treatment and nontreatment of infants with severe impairments. The emphasis is upon quality of life standards that include the "best interest of the child" and the "potential for human relations."

• Arthur L. Caplan's and Cynthia B. Cohen's **Deciding Not to Employ Aggressive Measures** analyzes the traditional distinction between withholding and withdrawing treatment. They also challenge the development of a public policy that would permit the killing of imperiled newborns and describe the kind of care that should be provided when the decision has been made to end aggressive measures.

• Alexander Morgan Capron's **Anencephalic Donors: Separating the Dead from the Dying** raises objections to proposals to change the Uniform Determination of Death Act and the Anatomical Gift Act to include anencephalics. He considers such proposals to be a radical alteration of the concepts of death and personhood.

Part V:4: Active Voluntary Euthanasia and Physician-Assisted Suicide

• Richard Doerflinger's **Assisted Suicide: Pro-Choice or Anti-Life?** investigates the arguments for and against doctor-assisted suicide for dying patients.

• Daniel Callahan's **When Self-Determination Runs Amok** characterizes the concept of self-determination in the context of social consequences. He observes the confusions that he believes occur over the difference between causality and culpability in euthanasia decisions.

• Dan Brock's **Voluntary Active Euthanasia** examines the potential bad consequences of voluntary active euthanasia. He also expresses concern over the possible slippery slope from voluntary to nonvoluntary euthanasia.

John Hardwig

Is There a Duty to Die?

Many people were outraged when Richard Lamm claimed that old people had a duty to die. Modern medicine and an individualistic culture have seduced many to feel that they have a right to health care and a right to live, despite the burdens and costs to our families and society. But in fact there are circumstances when we have a duty to die. As modern medicine continues to save more of us from acute illness, it also delivers more of us over to chronic illnesses, allowing us to survive far longer than we can take care of ourselves. It may be that our technological sophistication coupled with a commitment to our loved ones generates a fairly widespread duty to die.

When Richard Lamm made the statement that old people have a duty to die, it was generally shouted down or ridiculed. The whole idea is just too preposterous to entertain, or too threatening. In fact, a fairly common argument against legalizing physician-assisted suicide is that if it were legal, some people might somehow get the idea that they have a duty to die. These people could only be the victims of twisted moral reasoning or vicious social pressure. It goes without saying that there is no duty to die.

But for me the question is real and very important. I feel strongly that I may very well some day have a duty to die. I do not believe that I am idiosyncratic, morbid, mentally ill, or morally perverse in thinking this. I think many of us will eventually face precisely this duty. But I am first of all concerned with my own duty. I write partly to clarify my own convictions and to prepare myself. Ending my life might be a very difficult thing for me to do.

This notion of a duty to die raises all sorts of interesting theoretical and metaethical questions. I intend to try to avoid most of them because I hope my argument will be persuasive to those holding a wide variety of ethical views. Also, although the claim that there is a duty to die would ultimately require theoretical underpinning, the discussion needs to begin on the normative level. As is appropriate to my attempt to steer clear of theoretical commitments, I will use "duty," "obligation," and "responsibility" interchangeably, in a pretheoretical or preanalytic sense.[1]

Circumstances and a Duty to Die

Do many of us really believe that no one ever has a duty to die? I suspect not. I think most of us probably believe that there is such a duty, but it is very uncommon. Consider Captain Oates, a member of Admiral Scott's expedition to the South Pole. Oates became too ill to continue. If the rest of the team stayed with him, they would all perish. After this had become clear, Oates left his tent one night, walked out into a raging blizzard, and was never seen again.[2] That may have been a heroic thing to do, but we might be able to agree that it was also no more than his duty. It would have been wrong for him to urge—or even to allow—the rest to stay and care for him.

This is a very unusual circumstance—a "lifeboat case"—and lifeboat cases make for bad ethics. But I expect that most of us would also agree that there have been cultures in which what we would call a duty to die has been fairly common. These are relatively poor, technologically simple, and especially nomadic cultures. In such societies, everyone knows that if you manage to live long enough, you will eventually become old and debilitated. Then you will need to take steps to end your life. The old people in these societies regularly did precisely that. Their cultures prepared and supported them in doing so.

Those cultures could be dismissed as irrelevant to contemporary bioethics; their circumstances are so different from ours. But if that is our response, it is instructive. It suggests that we assume a duty to die is irrelevant to us because our wealth and technological sophistication have purchased exemption for us . . . except under very unusual circumstances like Captain Oates's.

But have wealth and technology really exempted us? Or are they, on the contrary, about to make a duty to die common again? We like to think of modern medicine as all triumph with no dark side. Our medicine saves many lives and enables most of us to live longer. That is wonderful, indeed. We are all glad to have access to this medicine. But our medicine also delivers most of us over to chronic illnesses and it enables many of us to survive longer than we can take care of ourselves, longer than we know what to do with ourselves, longer than we even are ourselves.

The costs—and these are not merely monetary—of prolonging our lives when we are no longer able to care for ourselves are often staggering. If further medical advances wipe out many of today's "killer diseases"—cancers, heart attacks, strokes, ALS, AIDS, and the rest then one day most of us will survive long enough to become demented or debilitated. These developments could generate a fairly widespread duty to die. A fairly common duty to die might turn out to be only the dark side of our life-prolonging medicine and the uses we choose to make of it.

Let me be clear. I certainly believe that there is a duty to refuse life-prolonging medical treatment and also a duty to complete advance directives refusing life-prolonging treatment. But a duty to die can go well beyond that. There can be a duty to die before one's illnesses would cause death, even if treated only with palliative measures. In fact, there may be a fairly common responsibility to end one's life in the absence of any terminal illness at all. Finally, there can be a duty to die when one would prefer to live. Granted, many of the conditions that can generate a duty to die also seriously undermine the quality of life. Some prefer not to live under such conditions. But even those who want to live can face a duty to die. These will clearly be the most controversial and troubling cases; I will, accordingly, focus my reflections on them.

The Individualistic Fantasy

Because a duty to die seems such a real possibility to me, I wonder why contemporary bioethics has dismissed it without serious consideration. I believe that most bioethics still shares in one of our deeply embedded American dreams: the individualistic fantasy. This fantasy leads us to imagine that lives are separate and unconnected, or that they could be so if we chose. If lives were unconnected, things that happened in my life would not or need not affect others. And if others were not (much) affected by my life, I would have no duty to consider the impact of my decisions on others. I would then be free morally to live my life however I please, choosing whatever life and death I prefer for myself. The way I live would be nobody's business but my own. I certainly would have no duty to die if I preferred to live.

Within a health care context, the individualistic fantasy leads us to assume that the patient is the only one affected by decisions about her medical treatment. If only the patient were affected, the relevant questions when making treatment decisions would be precisely those we ask: What will benefit the patient? Who can best decide that? The pivotal issue would always be simply whether the patient wants to live like this and whether she would consider herself better off dead.[3] "Whose life is it, anyway?" we ask rhetorically.

But this is morally obtuse. We are not a race of hermits. Illness and death do not come only to those who are all alone. Nor is it much better to think in terms of the bald dichotomy between "the interests of the patient" and "the interests of society" (or a third-party payer), as if we were isolated individuals connected only to "society" in the abstract or to the other, faceless members of our health maintenance organization.

Most of us are affiliated with particular others and most deeply, with family and loved ones. Families and loved ones are bound together by ties of care and affection, by legal relations and obligations, by inhabiting shared spaces and living units, by interlocking finances and economic prospects, by common projects and also commitments to support the different life projects of other family members, by shared histories, by ties of loyalty. This life together of family and loved ones is what defines and sustains us; it is what gives meaning to most of our lives. We would not have it any other way. We would not want to be all alone, especially when we are seriously ill, as we age, and when we are dying.

But the fact of deeply interwoven lives debars us from making exclusively self-regarding decisions, as the decisions of one member of a family may dramatically affect the lives of all the rest. The impact of my decisions upon my family and loved ones is the source of many of my strongest obligations and also the most plausible and likeliest basis of a duty to die. "Society," after all, is only very marginally affected by how I live, or by whether I live or die.

A Burden to My Loved Ones

Many older people report that their one remaining goal in life is not to be a burden to their loved ones. Young people feel this, too: when I ask my undergraduate students to think about whether their death could come too late, one of their very first responses always is, "Yes, when I become a burden to my family or loved ones." Tragically, there are situations in which my loved ones would be much better off—all things considered, the loss of a loved one notwithstanding—if I were dead.

The lives of our loved ones can be seriously compromised by caring for us. The burdens of providing care or even just supervision twenty-four hours a day, seven days a week are often overwhelming.[4] When this kind of caregiving goes on for years, it leaves the caregiver exhausted, with no time for herself or life of her own. Ultimately, even her health is often destroyed. But it can also be emotionally devastating simply to live with a spouse who is increasingly distant, uncommunicative, unresponsive, foreign, and unreachable. Other family members' needs often go unmet as the caring capacity of the family is exceeded. Social life and friendships evaporate, as there is no opportunity to go out to see friends and the home is no longer a place suitable for having friends in.

We must also acknowledge that the lives of our loved ones can be devastated just by having to pay for health care for us. One part of the recent SUPPORT study documented the financial aspects of caring for a dying member of a family. Only those who had illnesses severe enough to give them less than a 50 percent chance to live six more months were included in this study. When these patients survived their initial hospitalization and were discharged about one-third required considerable caregiving from their families; in 20 percent of cases a family member had to quit work or make some other major lifestyle change; almost one-third of these families lost all of their savings; and just under 30 percent lost a major source of income.[5]

If talking about money sounds venal or trivial, remember that much more than money is normally at stake here. When someone has to quit work, she may well lose her career. Savings decimated late in life cannot be recouped in the few remaining years of employability, so the loss compromises the quality of the rest of the caregiver's life. For a young person, the chance to go to college may be lost to the attempt to pay debts due to an illness in the family, and this decisively shapes an entire life.

A serious illness in a family is a misfortune. It is usually nobody's fault; no one is responsible for it. But we face choices about how we will respond to this misfortune. That's where the responsibility comes in and fault can arise. Those of us with families and loved ones always have a duty not to make selfish or self-centered decisions about our lives. We have a responsibility to try to protect the lives of loved ones from serious threats or greatly impoverished quality, certainly an obligation not to make choices that will jeopardize or seriously compromise their futures. Often, it would be wrong to do just what we want or just what is best for ourselves; we should choose in light of what is best for all concerned. That is our duty in sickness as well as in health. It is out of these responsibilities that a duty to die can develop.

I am not advocating a crass, quasi-economic conception of burdens and benefits, nor a shallow, hedonistic view of life. Given a suitably rich understanding of benefits, family members sometimes do benefit from suffering through the long illness of a loved one. Caring for the sick or aged can foster growth, even as it makes daily life immeasurably harder and the prospects for the future much bleaker. Chronic illness or a drawn-out death can also pull a family together, making the care for each other stronger and more evident.

If my loved ones are truly benefiting from coping with my illness or debility, I have no duty to die based on burdens to them.

But it would be irresponsible to blithely assume that this always happens, that it will happen in my family, or that it will be the fault of my family if they cannot manage to turn my illness into a positive experience. Perhaps the opposite is more common: a hospital chaplain once told me that he could not think of a single case in which a family was strengthened or brought together by what happened at the hospital.

Our families and loved ones also have obligations, of course. They have the responsibility to stand by us and to support us through debilitating illness and death. They must be prepared to make significant sacrifices to respond to an illness in the family. I am far from denying that. Most of us are aware of this responsibility and most families meet it rather well. In fact, families deliver more than 80 percent of the long-term care in this country, almost always at great personal cost. Most of us who are a part of a family can expect to be sustained in our time of need by family members and those who love us.

But most discussions of an illness in the family sound as if responsibility were a one-way street. It is not, of course. When we become seriously ill or debilitated, we too may have to make sacrifices. To think that my loved ones must bear whatever burdens my illness, debility, or dying process might impose upon them is to reduce them to means to my well-being. And that would be immoral. Family solidarity, altruism, bearing the burden of a loved one's misfortune, and loyalty are all important virtues of families, as well. But they are all also two-way streets.

Objections to a Duty to Die

To my mind, the most serious objections to the idea of a duty to die lie in the effects on my loved ones of ending my life. But to most others, the important objections have little or nothing to do with family and loved ones. Perhaps the most common objections are: (1) there is a higher duty that always takes precedence over a duty to die; (2) a duty to end one's own life would be incompatible with a recognition of human dignity or the intrinsic value of a person; and (3) seriously ill, debilitated, or dying people are already bearing the harshest burdens and so it would be wrong to ask them to bear the additional burden of ending their own lives.

These are all important objections; all deserve a thorough discussion. Here I will only be able to suggest some moral counterweights—ideas that might provide the basis for an argument that these objections do not always preclude a duty to die.

An example of the first line of argument would be the claim that a duty to God, the giver of life, forbids that anyone take her own life. It could be argued that this duty always supersedes whatever obligations we might have to our families. But what convinces us that we always have such a religious duty in the first place? And what guarantees that it always supersedes our obligations to try to protect our loved ones?

Certainly, the view that death is the ultimate evil cannot be squared with Christian theology. It does not reflect the actions of Jesus or those of his early followers. Nor is it clear that the belief that life is sacred requires that we never take it. There are other theological possibilities.[6] In any case, most of us—bioethicists, physicians, and patients alike—do not subscribe to the view that we have an obligation to preserve human life as long as possible. But if not, surely we ought to agree that I may legitimately end my life for other-regarding reasons, not just for self-regarding reasons.

Second, religious considerations aside, the claim could be made that an obligation to end one's own life would be incompatible with human dignity or would embody a failure to recognize the intrinsic value of a person. But I do not see that in thinking I had a duty to die I would necessarily be failing to respect myself or to appreciate my dignity or worth. Nor would I necessarily be failing to respect you in thinking that you had a similar duty. There is surely also a sense in which we fail to respect ourselves if in the face of illness or death, we stoop to choosing just what is best for ourselves. Indeed, Kant held that the very core of human dignity is the ability to act on a self-imposed moral law, regardless of whether it is in our interest to do so.[7] We shall return to the notion of human dignity.

A third objection appeals to the relative weight of burdens and thus, ultimately, to considerations of fairness or justice. The burdens that an illness creates for the family could not possibly be great enough to justify an obligation to end one's life—the sacrifice of life itself would be a far greater burden than any involved in caring for a chronically ill family member.

But is this true? Consider the following case:

An 87-year-old woman was dying of congestive heart failure. Her APACHE score predicted that she had less than a 50 percent chance to live for another six months. She was lucid, assertive, and terrified of death. She very much wanted to live and kept opting for rehospitalization and the most aggressive life-prolonging treatment possible. That treatment successfully prolonged her life (though with increasing debility) for nearly two years. Her 55-year-old daughter was her only remaining family, her caregiver, and the main source of her financial support. The daughter duly cared for her mother. But before her mother died, her illness had cost the daughter all of her savings, her home, her job, and her career.

This is by no means an uncommon sort of case. Thousands of similar cases occur each year. Now, ask yourself which is the greater burden:

a) To lose a 50 percent chance of six more months of life at age 87?
b) To lose all your savings, your home, and your career at age 55?

Which burden would you prefer to bear? Do we really believe the former is the greater burden? Would even the dying mother say that (a) is the greater burden? Or has she been encouraged to believe that the burdens of (b) are somehow morally irrelevant to her choices?

I think most of us would quickly agree that (b) is a greater burden. That is the evil we would more hope to avoid in our lives. If we are tempted to say that the mother's disease and impending death are the greater evil, I believe it is because we are taking a "slice of time" perspective rather than a "lifetime perspective."[8] But surely the lifetime perspective is the appropriate perspective when weighing burdens. If (b) is the greater burden, then we must admit that we have been promulgating an ethics that advocates imposing greater burdens on some people in order to provide smaller benefits for others just because they are ill and thus gain our professional attention and advocacy.

A whole range of cases like this one could easily be generated. In some, the answer about which burden is greater will not be clear. But in many it is. Death—or ending your own life—is simply not the greatest evil or the greatest burden.

This point does not depend on a utilitarian calculus. Even if death were the greatest burden (thus disposing of any simple utilitarian argument), serious questions would remain about the moral justifiability of choosing to impose crushing burdens on loved ones in order to avoid having to bear this burden oneself. The fact that I suffer greater burdens than others in my family does not license me simply to choose what I want for myself, nor does it necessarily release me from a responsibility to try to protect the quality of their lives.

I can readily imagine that, through cowardice, rationalization, or failure of resolve, I will fail in this obligation to protect my loved ones. If so, I think I would need to be excused or forgiven for what I did. But I cannot imagine it would be morally permissible for me to ruin the rest of my partner's life to sustain mine or to cut off my sons' careers, impoverish them, or compromise the quality of their children's lives simply because I wish to live a little longer. This is what leads me to believe in a duty to die.

Who Has a Duty to Die?

Suppose, then, that there can be a duty to die. Who has a duty to die? And when? To my mind, these are the right questions, the questions we should be asking. Many of us may one day badly need answers to just these questions.

But I cannot supply answers here, for two reasons. In the first place, answers will have to be very particular and contextual. Our concrete duties are often situated, defined in part by the myriad details of our circumstances, histories, and relationships. Though there may be principles that apply to a wide range of cases and some cases that yield pretty straightforward answers, there will also be many situations in which it is very difficult to discern whether one has a duty to die. If nothing else, it will often be very difficult to predict how one's family will bear up under the weight of the burdens that a protracted illness would impose on them. Momentous decisions will often have to be made under conditions of great uncertainty.

Second and perhaps even more important, I believe that those of us with family and loved ones should not define our duties unilaterally, especially not a decision about a duty to die. It would be isolating and distancing for me to decide without consulting them what is too much of a burden for my loved ones to bear. That way of deciding about my moral duties is not only atomistic, it also treats my family and loved ones paternalistically. They must be allowed to speak for themselves about the burdens my life imposes on them and how they feel about bearing those burdens.

Some may object that it would be wrong to put a loved one in a position of having to say, in effect, "You should end your life because caring for you is too hard on me and the rest of the family." Not only will it be almost impossible to say something like that to someone you love, it will carry with it a heavy load of guilt. On this view, you should decide by yourself whether you have a duty to die and approach your loved ones only after you have made up your mind to say good-bye to them. Your family could then try to change your mind, but the tremendous weight of moral decision would be lifted from their shoulders.

Perhaps so. But I believe in family decisions. Important decisions for those whose lives are interwoven should be made together, in a family discussion. Granted, a conversation about whether I have a duty to die would be a tremendously difficult conversation. The temptations to be dishonest could be enormous. Nevertheless, if I am contemplating a duty to die, my family and I should, if possible, have just such an agonizing discussion. It will act as a check on the information, perceptions, and reasoning of all of us. But even more importantly, it affirms our connectedness at a critical juncture in our lives and our life together. Honest talk about difficult matters almost always strengthens relationships.

However, many families seem unable to talk about death at all, much less a duty to die. Certainly most families could not have this discussion all at once, in one sitting. It might well take a number of discussions to be able to approach this topic. But even if talking about death is impossible, there are always behavioral clues about your caregiver's tiredness, physical condition, health, prevailing mood, anxiety, financial concerns, outlook, overall well-being, and so on. And families unable to talk about death can often talk about how the caregiver is feeling, about finances, about tensions within the family resulting from the illness, about concerns for the future. Deciding whether you have a duty to die based on these behavioral clues and conversation about them honors your relationships better than deciding on your own about how burdensome you and your care must be.

I cannot say when someone has a duty to die. Still, I can suggest a few features of one's illness, history, and circumstances that make it more likely that one has a duty to die. I present them here without much elaboration or explanation.

1. A duty to die is more likely when continuing to live will impose significant burdens—emotional burdens, extensive caregiving, destruction of life plans, and, yes, financial hardship—on your family and loved ones. This is the fundamental insight underlying a duty to die.

2. A duty to die becomes greater as you grow older. As we age, we will be giving up less by giving up our lives, if only because we will sacrifice fewer remaining years of life and a smaller portion of our life plans. After all, it's not as if we would be immortal and live forever if we could just manage to avoid a duty to die. To have reached the age of, say, seventy-five or eighty years without being ready to die is itself a moral failing, the sign of a life out of touch with life's basic realities.[9]

3. A duty to die is more likely when you have already lived a full and rich life. You have already had a full share of the good things life offers.

4. There is greater duty to die if your loved ones' lives have already been difficult or impoverished, if they have had only a small share of the good things that life has to offer (especially if through no fault of their own).

5. A duty to die is more likely when your loved ones have already made great contributions—perhaps even sacrifices—to make your life a good one.

Especially if you have not made similar sacrifices for their well-being or for the well-being of other members of your family.

6. To the extent that you can make a good adjustment to your illness or handicapping condition, there is less likely to be a duty to die. A good adjustment means that smaller sacrifices will be required of loved ones and there is more compensating interaction for them. Still, we must also recognize that some diseases—Alzheimer or Huntington chorea—will eventually take their toll on your loved ones no matter how courageously, resolutely, even cheerfully you manage to face that illness.

7. There is less likely to be a duty to die if you can still make significant contributions to the lives of others, especially your family. The burdens to family members are not only or even primarily financial, neither are the contributions to them. However, the old and those who have terminal illnesses must also bear in mind that the loss their family members will feel when they die cannot be avoided, only postponed.

8. A duty to die is more likely when the part of you that is loved will soon be gone or seriously compromised. Or when you soon will no longer be capable of giving love. Part of the horror of dementing disease is that it destroys the capacity to nurture and sustain relationships, taking away a person's agency and the emotions that bind her to others.

9. There is a greater duty to die to the extent that you have lived a relatively lavish lifestyle instead of saving for illness or old age. Like most upper middle-class Americans, I could easily have saved more. It is a greater wrong to come to your family for assistance if your need is the result of having chosen leisure or a spendthrift lifestyle. I may eventually have to face the moral consequences of decisions I am now making.

These, then, are some of the considerations that give shape and definition to the duty to die. If we can agree that these considerations are all relevant, we can see that the correct course of action will often be difficult to discern. A decision about when I should end my life will sometimes prove to be every bit as difficult as the decision about whether I want treatment for myself.

Can the Incompetent Have a Duty to Die?

Severe mental deterioration springs readily to mind as one of the situations in which I believe I could have a duty to die. But can incompetent people have duties at all? We can have moral duties we do not recognize or acknowledge, including duties that we never recognized. But can we have duties we are unable to recognize? Duties when we are unable to understand the concept of morality at all? If so, do others have a moral obligation to help us carry out this duty? These are extremely difficult theoretical questions. The reach of moral agency is severely strained by mental incompetence.

I am tempted to simply bypass the entire question by saying that I am talking only about competent persons. But the idea of a duty to die clearly raises the specter of one person claiming that another—who cannot speak for herself—has such a duty. So I need to say that I can make no sense of the claim that someone has a duty to die if the person has never been able to understand moral obligation at all. To my mind, only those who were formerly capable of making moral decisions could have such a duty.

But the case of formerly competent persons is almost as troubling. Perhaps we should simply stipulate that no incompetent person can have a duty to die, not even if she affirmed belief in such a duty in an advance directive. If we take the view that formerly competent people may have such a duty, we should surely exercise extreme caution when claiming a formerly competent person would have acknowledged a duty to die or that any formerly competent person has an unacknowledged duty to die. Moral dangers loom regardless of which way we decide to resolve such issues.

But for me personally, very urgent practical matters turn on their resolution. If a formerly competent person can no longer have a duty to die (or if other people are not likely to help her carry out this duty), I believe that my obligation may be to die while I am still competent, before I become unable to make and carry out that decision for myself. Surely it would be irresponsible to evade my moral duties by temporizing until I escape into incompetence. And so I must die sooner than I otherwise would have to. On the other hand, if I could count on others to end my life after I become incompetent, I might be able to fulfill my responsibilities while also living out all my competent or semicompetent days. Given our society's reluctance to permit physicians, let alone family members, to perform aid-in-dying, I believe I may well have a duty to end my life when I can see mental incapacity on the horizon.

There is also the very real problem of sudden incompetence—due to a serious stroke or automobile accident, for example. For me, that is the real nightmare. If I suddenly become incompetent, I will fall into the hands of a medical-legal system that will conscientiously disregard my moral beliefs and do what is best for me, regardless of the consequences for my loved ones. And that is not at all what I would have wanted!

Social Policies and a Duty to Die

The claim that there is a duty to die will seem to some a misplaced response to social negligence. If our society were providing for the debilitated, the chronically ill, and the elderly as it should be, there would be only very rare cases of a duty to die. On this view, I am asking the sick and debilitated to step in and accept responsibility because society is derelict in its responsibility to provide for the incapacitated.

This much is surely true: there are a number of social policies we could pursue that would dramatically reduce the incidence of such a duty. Most obviously, we could decide to pay for facilities that provided excellent longterm care (not just health care!) for all chronically ill, debilitated, mentally ill, or demented people in this country. We probably could still afford to do this. If we did, sick, debilitated, and dying people might still be morally required to make sacrifices for their families. I might, for example, have a duty to forgo personal care by a family member who knows me and really does care for me. But these sacrifices would only rarely include the sacrifice of life itself. The duty to die would then be virtually eliminated.

I cannot claim to know whether in some abstract sense a society like ours should provide care for all who are chronically ill or debilitated. But the fact is that we Americans seem to be unwilling to pay for this kind of long-term care, except for ourselves and our own. In fact, we are moving in precisely the opposite direction—we are trying to shift the burdens of caring for the seriously and chronically ill onto families in order to save costs for our health care system. As we shift the burdens of care onto families, we also dramatically increase the number of Americans who will have a duty to die.

I must not, then, live my life and make my plans on the assumption that social institutions will protect my family from my infirmity and debility. To do so would be irresponsible. More likely, it will be up to me to protect my loved ones.

A Duty to Die and the Meaning of Life

A duty to die seems very harsh, and often it would be. It is one of the tragedies of our lives that someone who wants very much to live can nevertheless have a duty to die. It is both tragic and ironic that it is precisely the very real good of family and loved ones that gives rise to this duty. Indeed, the genuine love, closeness, and supportiveness of family members is a major source of this duty: we could not be such a burden if they did not care for us. Finally, there is deep irony in the fact that the very successes of our life-prolonging medicine help to create a widespread duty to die. We do not live in such a happy world that we can avoid such tragedies and ironies. We ought not to close our eyes to this reality or pretend that it just doesn't exist. We ought not to minimize the tragedy in any way.

And yet, a duty to die will not always be as harsh as we might assume. If I love my family, I will want to protect them and their lives. I will want not to make choices that compromise their futures. Indeed, I can easily imagine that I might want to avoid compromising their lives more than I would want anything else. I must also admit that I am not necessarily giving up so much in giving up my life: the conditions that give rise to a duty to die would usually already have compromised the quality of the life I am required to end. In any case, I personally must confess that at age fifty-six, I have already lived a very good life, albeit not yet nearly as long a life as I would like to have.

We fear death too much. Our fear of death has lead to a massive assault on it. We still crave after virtually any life-prolonging technology that we might conceivably be able to produce. We still too often feel morally impelled to prolong life—virtually any form of life—as long as possible. As if the best death is the one that can be put off longest.

We do not even ask about meaning in death, so busy are we with trying to postpone it. But we will not conquer death by one day developing a technology so magnificent that no one will have to die. Nor can we conquer death by postponing it ever longer. We can conquer death only by finding meaning in it.

Although the existence of a duty to die does not hinge on this, recognizing such a duty would go some way toward recovering meaning in death. Paradoxically, it would restore dignity to those who are seriously ill or dying. It would also reaffirm the connections required to give life (and death) meaning. I close now with a few words about both of these points.

First, recognizing a duty to die affirms my agency and also my moral agency. I can still do things that make an important difference in the lives of my loved ones. Moreover, the fact that I still have responsibilities keeps me within the community of moral agents. My illness or debility has not reduced me to a mere moral patient (to use the language of the philosophers). Though it may not be the whole story, surely Kant was onto something important when he claimed that human dignity rests on the capacity for moral agency within a community of those who respect the demands of morality.

By contrast, surely there is something deeply insulting in a medicine and an ethic that would ask only what I want (or would have wanted) when I become ill. To treat me as if I had no moral responsibilities when I am ill or debilitated implies that my condition has rendered me morally incompetent. Only small children, the demented or insane, and those totally lacking in the capacity to act are free from moral duties. There is dignity, then, and a kind of meaning in moral agency, even as it forces extremely difficult decisions upon us.

Second, recovering meaning in death requires an affirmation of connections. If I end my life to spare the futures of my loved ones, I testify in my death that I am connected to them. It is because I love and care for precisely these people (and I know they care for me) that I wish not to be such a burden to them. By contrast, a life in which I am free to choose whatever I want for myself is a life unconnected to others. A bioethics that would treat me as if I had no serious moral responsibilities does what it can to marginalize, weaken, or even destroy my connections with others.

But life without connection is meaningless. The individualistic fantasy, though occasionally liberating, is deeply destructive. When life is good and vitality seems unending, life itself and life lived for yourself may seem quite sufficient. But if not life, certainly death without connection is meaningless. If you are only for yourself, all you have to care about as your life draws to a close is yourself and your life. Everything you care about will then perish in your death. And that—the end of everything you care about—is precisely the total collapse of meaning. We can, then, find meaning in death only through a sense of connection with something that will survive our death.

This need not be connections with other people. Some people are deeply tied to land (for example, the family farm), to nature, or to a transcendent reality. But for most of us, the connections that sustain us are to other people. In the full bloom of life, we are connected to others in many ways—through work, profession, neighborhood, country, shared faith and worship, common leisure pursuits, friendship. Even the guru meditating in isolation on his mountain top is connected to a long tradition of people united by the same religious quest.

But as we age or when we become chronically ill, connections with other people usually become much more restricted. Often, only ties with family and close friends remain and remain important to us. Moreover, for many of us, other connections just don't go deep enough. As Paul Tsongas has reminded us, "When it comes time to die, no one says, 'I wish I had spent more time at the office.' "

If I am correct, death is so difficult for us partly because our sense of community is so weak. Death seems to wipe out everything when we can't fit it into the lives of those who live on. A death motivated by the desire to spare the futures of my loved ones might well be a better death for me than the one I would get as a result of opting to continue my life as long as there is any pleasure in it for me. Pleasure is nice, but it is meaning that matters.

I don't know about others, but these reflections have helped me. I am now more at peace about facing a duty to die. Ending my life if my duty required might still be difficult. But for me, a far greater horror would be dying all alone or stealing the futures of my loved ones in order to buy a little more time for myself. I hope that if the time comes when I have a duty to die, I will recognize it, encourage my loved ones to recognize it too, and carry it out bravely.

Acknowledgments

I wish to thank Mary English, Hilde Nelson, Jim Bennett, Tom Townsend, the members of the Philosophy Department at East Tennessee State University, and anonymous reviewers of the *Report* for many helpful comments on earlier versions of this paper. In this paper, I draw on material in John Hardwig, "Dying at the Right Time; Reflections on (Un)Assisted Suicide" in *Practical Ethics*, ed. H. LaFollette (London: Blackwell, 1996), with permission.

QUESTIONS FOR CONSIDERATION

1. How does Hardwig argue that medical technology could lead to a widespread duty to die?
2. What does Hardwig mean by "the individualistic fantasy?"
3. What are the ways that Hardwig identifies that we can become a burden upon loved ones?
4. How does Hardwig respond to objections to having a duty to die?
5. What are the circumstances that Hardwig identifies as more likely to create a duty to die?
6. What is the relationship between the duty to die and competence?
7. How does Hardwig apply responsibility and meaning of life in support of a duty to die?

NOTES

1. Given the importance of relationships in my thinking, "responsibility"—rooted as it is in "respond"—would perhaps be the most appropriate word. Nevertheless, I often use "duty" despite its legalistic overtones, because Lamm's famous statement has given the expression "duty to die" a certain familiarity. But I intend no implication that there is a law that grounds this duty, nor that someone has a right corresponding to it.

2. For a discussion of the Oates case, see Tom L. Beauchamp, "What Is Suicide?" in *Ethical Issues in Death and Dying*, ed. Tom L. Beauchamp and Seymour Perlin (Englewood Cliffs, N.J.: Prentice-Hall, 1978).

3. Most bioethicists advocate a "patient-centered ethics"—an ethics which claims only the patient's interests should be considered in making medical treatment decisions. Most health care professionals have been trained to accept this ethic and to see themselves as patient advocates. For arguments that a patient centered ethics should be replaced by a family-centered ethics see John Hardwig, "What About the Family?" *Hastings Center Report* 20, no. 2 (1990): 5–10; Hilde L. Nelson and James L. Nelson, *The Patient in the Family* (New York: Routledge, 1995).

4. A good account of the burdens of caregiving can be found in Elaine Brody, *Women in the Middle: Their Parent-Care Years* (New York: Springer Publishing Co., 1990). Perhaps the best article-length account of these burdens is Daniel Callahan, "Families as Caregivers; the Limits of Morality" in *Aging and Ethics: Philosophical Problems in Gerontology*, ed. Nancy Jecker (Totowa N.J.: Humana Press, 1991).

5. Kenneth E. Covinsky et al., "The Impact of Serious Illness on Patients' Families," *JAMA* 272 (1994): 1839–44.

6. Larry Churchill, for example, believes that Christian ethics takes us far beyond my present position: "Christian doctrines of stewardship prohibit the extension of one's own life at a great cost to the neighbor. . And such a gesture should not appear to us as a sacrifice, but as the ordinary virtue entailed by a just, social conscience." Larry Churchill, *Rationing Health Care in America* (South Bend, Ind.: Notre Dame University Press, 1988), p. 112.

7. Kant, as is well known, was opposed to suicide. But he was arguing against taking your life out of self-interested motives. It is not clear that Kant would or we should consider taking your life out of a sense of duty to be wrong. See Hilde L. Nelson, "Death with Kantian Dignity," *Journal of Clinical Ethics* 7 (1996): 215–21.

8. Obviously, I owe this distinction to Norman Daniels. Norman Daniels, *Am I My Parents' Keeper? An Essay on Justice Between the Young and the Old* (New York: Oxford University Press, 1988). Just as obviously, Daniels is not committed to my use of it here.

9. Daniel Callahan, *The Troubled Dream of Life* (New York: Simon & Schuster, 1993).

Daniel Callahan

Terminating Treatment: Age as a Standard

Death, we are told, is no longer a hidden subject. That is at best a half-truth. The aged constitute the majority of those who die, some 70 percent, but a specific discussion of their dying is remarkably scant in legal, ethical, and medical writings. That omission is probably not accidental. The modernization of aging induces a sharp separation between aging and death. the latter is often treated as if it had little to do with the former, a kind of accidental conjunction. In medicine, the long-standing tradition of treating patients regardless of their age works against an open discussion, even though many physicians admit it is a consideration in their actual practice. The courts appear to follow a similar tradition. Despite the large number of decisions in recent years bearing on cases of elderly patients, that fact is typically not mentioned, though it is an obvious feature of the cases.

These inhibitions against explicit discussion of the elderly dying doubtless serve a valuable function. They reflect a sensible fear that the aged might be singled out for unfairly discriminatory treatment. They are a way of acknowledging the difficulty of sharply differentiating the medical conditions of the aged from those of other patients. Yet the pervasiveness of backstage debate about the care of the elderly dying among physicians and nurses, jurists and legislators, and the elderly themselves makes it imperative now to deal explicitly with the issue. There are also other reasons for having such a discussion. What is the proper goal of medicine for those who have already lived out a natural life span, by which I mean a full biographical, not a maximum biological life? That goal is, I believe, the relief of suffering rather than the extension of life. What are the practical implications of that position for the care of the critically ill, or elderly dying? If the goals of the aging ought to be service to the young and coming generations, what follows for their way of thinking about death? How does the ready availability of technology sway the making of decisions about the dying? I want to start with that last question.

Medical Technology: A House Divided

One of the hardy illusions of the past few decades has been the belief that with a few changes in law and attitudes, the dying can be spared excessive medical treatment and be allowed to die a "death with dignity." Yet the termination of treatment seems to remain almost as hard, if not harder, in practice now than in earlier times. That is true with the old as much as with the young. Despite the public debate and soothing words, both the public and physicians remain profoundly ambivalent about stopping the use of life-sustaining medical technologies. It is often and accurately said that the elderly do not want excessive and useless treatment. They greatly fear a death marked by technological oppressiveness, wrapped in a cocoon of tubes and machines. Yet they have also no less come—as we all have—to expect medicine whenever possible to extend their lives as well as alleviate or cure their diseases. These are not logically incompatible impulses, but they can be psychologically at odds.

Two fears seem to compete with each other among the elderly: on the one hand, that they will be abandoned or neglected if they become critically ill or begin to die and that few will care about their fate; or, on the other hand, that they will be excessively treated and their lives painfully extended. Death after a long, lingering illness marked by dementia and isolation in the back room of a nursing home similarly competes as a vision of horror with that of death in an intensive care unit, a dying constantly interrupted by painful and unwanted interventions. There is reason for such fears. Medicine steadily extends to the elderly the use of drugs, surgery, rehabilitation, and other procedures once thought suitable only for younger patients. Ever-more aggressive technological means are used to extend the life of the elderly. On the whole, the elderly welcome that development—even as they fear some of its consequences. They want, somehow, that most elusive of all goals: a steadily improving medical technology that will relieve their pain and illness while not leading to overtreatment and to a harmful extension of life.

The difficulty of making accurate prognoses is part of the problem. In all too many cases, technology is used because it is not known that a patient is dying or in irreversible decline. The prognosis of a terminal illness is always difficult to achieve. The problem is even greater, a recent Office of Technology Assessment (OTA) study concluded, when immediate decisions must be made about initiating treatment. Only for patients who have been fully diagnosed can estimates of survival probability be made. Even then, the probabilities are very likely to be insufficient for guiding decisionmaking about withholding or withdrawing treatment for an individual patient.[1]

The ordinary, almost instinctive, tendency of physicians faced with that uncertainty is then to use technology, to treat with vigor. For his or her part, the patient—who will ordinarily want to live, but may also be fearful of useless overtreatment—will be faced with a no less highly uncertain situation. How sick am I? What are my chances? Both patients and families are likely to have the same inclination as the physician, to treat. Given a normal desire to preserve life and to use available technologies, those impulses of both patients and physicians are understandable. The hard question, therefore, is not why technology is used so much by physicians, or why patients want it no less than doctors. We have to ask instead why it is so hard to stop using it, even when patient welfare and plain common sense appear to demand just that.

We should not see the question of terminating treatment as a sharply focused "yes" or "no" decision to treat vigorously or allow to die, a kind of binary "1" or "O" gateway to life or death. It is more realistically viewed as a continuum in which the odds of effective intervention slowly decline. At age sixty-five, a person (call him Mr. Smith) in otherwise good health who suffers a heart attack will be treated, and the available technology makes the odds of saving him good.[2] Then imagine Mr. Smith being diagnosed for an operable cancer of the colon at age seventy-five, with a 50 percent chance of full recovery. If he is still mentally alert and eager to live, both doctor and patient will most likely choose to go forward with the operation. Imagine still another phase: at eighty, he again suffers a heart attack of moderate severity, with the odds of complete recovery if vigorously treated at about 20 percent and partial recovery at about 60 percent. He will probably be treated. Then, at eighty-two, he suffers a moderately severe stroke, one from which his life can most likely be saved but which will almost certainly leave him semiparalyzed and probably only semicompetent thereafter (but amenable to rehabilitation efforts). Thereafter, he gradually declines and suffers a series of other strokes in his mid to late eighties, spending his last years debilitated and demented in a nursing home before dying at eighty-eight.

When, in that continuum, was he dying? There is no straightforward answer to that question, for he was—but for the technology—dying at many points. Each crisis presented the need to make a choice for or against initiating treatment. A familiar story then unfolded: since physicians generally aim to save life, and since patients ordinarily prefer to live rather than to die, and since at each point there was some realistic hope, treatment was undertaken. The good fight was fought.

Mr. Smith lived on because we expect medicine to continue to devise ever-more-ingenious ways to save our lives. That is why the annual budget of the National Institutes of Health (NIH) has always risen, budget crises or not. Few congressmen can resist the plea to appropriate funds to save lives through medical research. Why should anyone be astonished, much less indignant, that the other message many are trying to deliver—the need to stop treatment—has such a hard time getting through? Unrelenting "wars" against disease are being pursued by thousands of dedicated medical researchers and physicians at the same time that "natural death" legislation is being passed. The former campaigns are much more dedicated and powerful than the latter. We have been told endlessly—and truthfully, with the support of hard data— that more effective emergency care and the improvement of intensive-care units will save additional lives, and that better geriatric rehabilitation services (for which Mr. Smith was an ideal candidate at many points) will help restore the functioning of the lives thus saved. In the meantime, of course, physicians are being exhorted to stop trying so hard to perform technological miracles with those destined—assuming we can know that—to die. The double message is just about perfect, designed for maximum confusion. As a group the elderly dying are to be saved and those diseases which cause death eliminated. As individuals, however, the elderly dying should be allowed to die when it is right to do so and their diseases allowed to run their course.

Age as a Criterion

Could we not, however, turn to age as a criterion in order to know when to stop, when to say that no more should be done? I want to look first at one great source of confusion: the common failure to distinguish between age as a medical or technical criterion, pertinent to prognosis, and age as a person- or patient-centered criterion. By age as a medical criterion, I mean treating chronological age as if it were the equivalent of other physical characteristics of a patient—that is, as the equivalent of such typical medical indicators as weight, blood pressure, or white-cell count. Just as those characteristics would be reasonable considerations in treating a patient so also would age if it could be treated as a reliable technical consideration. Age as a person-centered characteristic, by contrast, would be understood as the relevance of a person's history and biography, his situation not as a collection of organs but as a person, to be taken into account when that personal situation could legitimately be considered. I will argue that age as a medical standard should be rejected, while age as a person-centered (what I will call a "biographical") standard can be used.

Age as a Medical Standard

The principal use of age as a medical standard would be in prognosis of treatment outcome: how well will an elderly person respond to and benefit from a treatment? In that respect, the main problem in using age as a standard is twofold. It is difficult to disentangle age from a wide range of other conditions that may coexist with old age. Do kidneys fail because a person is old, or simply because of the ravages of a disease that anyone could have, whatever his age? It is no less difficult to distinguish between the general characteristics of the aged as a group and the unique characteristics of any given aged person. The OTA report on aging and life-extending technology medicine notes the difficulties in making the necessary distinctions (which I have reordered slightly to bring out the underlying logic):

a. increasing age is associated with greater likelihood of physical decline, increased comorbidity, reduced physiological reserve, and cognitive impairment. Clinically, the probability of these decrements increases notably after age eighty-five; *but,*

b. chronological age turns out to be a poor predictor of the efficacy of a number of life-sustaining technologies (dialysis, nutritional support, resuscitation, mechanical ventilation, and antibiotics); *while,*

c. efficacy may be lessened for older patients in general; *but,*

d. improved medical assessment and care could improve that efficacy; *while,*

e. in any case very little is currently known about differences in treatment outcome that are due to age *per se* and those that are due to increased prevalence or severity of diseases in older ages; *but,*

f. in some classification systems (for the purposes of, say, admission to an ICU), chronological age functions as a proxy measure for age-associated factors that cannot be easily measured.[3]

I do not cite the OTA material with any intent to amuse. It is a careful set of distinctions based on the best empirical evidence available and makes perfectly clear why age alone is not a good predictor of medical outcome. It also nicely helps explain why physicians can also say that, in practice, they do make decisions based on the age of patients—but rarely can give a wholly defensible scientific account of themselves if pressed to do so. The puzzle, I think, is partially explained by the difference between (1) perceiving a patient as a whole person, whose combination, or gestalt, of characteristics makes it evident that he is old rather than young, which makes a difference in his future; and (2) perceiving and medically treating the person part by part, organ by organ. If we look at a person only as a collection of organs, any given characteristic may well be identical with that found in younger persons (some of whom have wrinkled skin, or failing kidneys, or are bald, or have osteoarthritis, for example). Moreover, even if in some cases, with some conditions, we know age to be generally relevant, we may not know where, on a continuum of characteristics of the aged as a group, any particular old person falls in terms of likely medical outcome. For all these reasons, age as a medical criterion is unreliable.

Age as a Biographical Standard

If we know someone's age, but nothing else about him, what do we know of significance? If the person is old—say, in his seventies (and certainly by his eighties)—we would know that most of his chronological life is in his past rather than his future, would not expect to find him playing football or climbing trees for recreation, might not be surprised to find that most of his friends are older rather than younger people, and might expect him to have two or more physical impairments, minor or major. Certain "age-associated" traits would almost invariably be present.

What makes him the person he is, and not someone else, is the combination of his age-associated traits and other, more idiosyncratic personal and social traits. That he was very old, with a statistically short life expectancy, would hardly be irrelevant to him as he thought about his life and his future or to the rest of us for many (even if not all) purposes. As Malcolm Cowley has noted, "we start by growing old in other people's eyes. Then slowly we come to share their judgment"[4] We would not make long-range plans with an elderly person the way we might with a younger person, nor would we likely invite him to take charge of strenuous long-term projects, even if he were highly talented. For his part, he would not be likely to undertake a total change in his way of life, such as immigrating to a new country, or undertaking extensive training for a new career. While age alone would not tell us whether he was lively or dour, bright or dull, we would most likely be far more impressed with great physical vitality in someone that age than in a teenager.

His age would, in other words, surely be a part of our overall understanding of him—not the whole story, but hardly of no consequence either. While many "age associated" facts will bear on the functioning of an elderly person, age as a biographical fact does not reduce to that. Age encompasses a relationship to time—less time statistically remains for an old person than a young person, and there is more personal history behind him as well. It encompasses a relationship to self-consciousness—life and its prospects will usually be thought about differently. And it encompasses a relationship to the passing of the generations—the old are next in line to pass as individuals. The old know they are old, and so does everyone else. Age is not an incidental trait of a person. Might the combination of age and other characteristics then be allowed to have a bearing on medical treatment, and particularly termination, decisions?

The Morality of Age as a Standard

Before attempting to answer that last question, it is necessary to inquire whether it is moral to make the attempt. Some would say no: age as a criterion for the termination of treatment should be ruled out of bounds altogether. A central strand of medical ethics holds that patients should be treated only on the basis of their strict medical needs, and that age should no more influence the way they are treated than should their race, sex, or ethnic background. Mark Siegler has pointed to one source of the objection, noting that a failure to retain "need-specific criteria with respect to elderly patients. . . . [would] undermine the traditions of clinical medicine, which are based upon medical need and patient preferences. . . . and [would] undermine the traditions of our society, which are based upon moral virtues of charity and compassion."[5] The immediate force of such objections is evident. While there has been some toleration in the medical-ethics literature for the idea of rationing by imposing external policy constraints on physicians, there has been little if any toleration for the idea of physician rationing at the bedside. Doctors are enjoined by medical morality to be unstinting advocates for the welfare of their individual patients and no less enjoined to use medical criteria only—"medical need"— in making their decisions. Yet it is precisely that tradition which my approach to limitation of health care for the aged calls into doubt. The high cost of health care, unrelenting technological developments, and the good of the elderly themselves require that it be examined afresh.

"Medical need," in the context of constant technological innovation, is inherently elastic and open-ended; as a guide to what is actually good for patients or what physicians are obliged to give them, it is highly unreliable. Experienced and conscientious physicians do in fact take age into account in termination decisions, and always have. Why should we therefore assume that age is not, and should not be, part of a responsible moral judgment? The problem in responding to this question is in distinguishing between a medical and a moral judgment. That an elderly person should be given a different drug dosage than a younger patient is ordinarily considered a purely medical judgment. By that statement is meant that if the aim is proper physical care of the patient in both cases, then different dosages may be indicated to achieve identical outcomes. A judgment of that kind can be based on scientific evidence. But the use of age as a "medical" indication is ambiguous. If it means that because of a person's age, medical treatment will be futile, do no good whatever, then it may properly be called a medical and not a moral judgment. It is a judgment about medical efficacy only. Yet if a judgment is also being passed about the worth of the life—that the treatment is futile not because it will fail technically but because the life saved is not worth saving because of age—then it has passed into the moral realm. According to the tradition of medical ethics, judgments about the social worth of a patient's life are unacceptable as grounds for terminating care. That is a solid and necessary tradition; but it does not touch the question of whether age as a standard might be defensible.

There is also another possibility for ambiguity. What is medical "need"? If understood as the needs of a patient's organs, or other physiological systems, treatment may (by ordinary standards) be required; otherwise they will fail. But if "need" is understood to be the needs of the patient as a person, not merely as an assemblage of deficient organs, no clear answer about the requirement of "medical need" may be forthcoming. Then the physician may have to make a moral judgment: will meeting the needs of the patent's organs meet his needs as a whole person? They are not necessary the same. It is not clear which need the tradition invoked by Siegler has in mind. More than that, the technological possibilities of medicine for organ sustenance, quite apart from overall patient welfare, mean that "medical need" can rarely if ever be kept free of moral evaluation and judgment. The good of organs is always subordinate to the good of the person. There is no such thing as pure "medical need"; it always presupposes some value judgment about the desirability of treatment.

Will it necessarily be the case, as James Childress has suggested, that the use of an age standard would symbolize "abandonment and exclusion from communal care"?[6] That would be likely only if it were widely believed or perceived that an age standard for exclusion from care came into use as a manifestation of society's rejection, denigration, or devaluation of elderly people. It would be a different matter if, instead, it emerged from a prudent effort to find an appropriate balance between the needs of the aged and those of younger generations, and from a conscientious effort to determine, in the face of potentially unlimited technological innovation in care for the aged, where a reasonable limit on care could be set. The "symbolic significance" of an age standard depends not on the mere fact of using age but on the meaning attributed to that fact; context, perceived motive, and articulated rationale determine that symbolic meaning. Childress would most likely be right if age were used as a standard in the present situation; but that would not necessarily be the case if its use were transformed so as to be seen as part of an affirmation of old age and not its denigration.

Age as a Biographical Standard for Terminating Treatment

How can a combination of age and other characteristics be allowed to have a bearing on the termination of treatment? How, I respond, can it not any longer? If "medical need" is too indeterminate and elastic a concept to be used by itself, then some use of age will be necessary to make a judgment about terminating care of the elderly. Since age is an important aspect of the patient as a person, someone who is not just a collection of organs, it falsifies the reality that is part of a person in his fullness to set it aside as irrelevant. Moreover, in addition to being a necessary part of a full and proper medical-moral judgment, age is a valuable and illuminating part telling us where the patient stands in relation to his own history. There are a large and growing number of elderly who are not imminently dying but who are feeble and declining, often chronically ill, for whom curative medicine has little to offer. That kind of medicine may still be able to do something for failing organs; it can keep them going a bit longer. But it cannot offer the patient as a person any hope of being restored to good health. A different treatment plan should be in order. That person's history has all but come to an end, and medical care needs to encompass that reality, not try to deny it.

For many people, beginning with the aged themselves, old age is a reason in itself to think about medical care in a different way, whether in forgoing its lifesaving powers when death is clearly imminent, or in forgoing its use even when death may be distant but life has become a blight rather than a blessing. The alternative is not, as some would have it, respect for life but an idolatrous enslavement to technology.

We should want to know not just what chronological age may tell us about the state of a person's body (as a technical criterion), but also what it morally and psychologically signifies for a person to have an old rather than a young body; or what it means for a person to be old rather than young when considering the prospect of painful treatment; or what it signifies to live life as an old person—or as a sick old person—who cannot expect to recapture the vitality of youth, or even of an earlier old age. When considered in those ways, age becomes a category of evaluation in its own right, something reasonable and proper to wonder and worry about. It bears not only on physical characteristics, but on a person's self-understanding, as something intrinsic (with varying degrees of intensity, to be sure) to a person's individuality and life story. The whole person—and it is that whole person who presents himself or herself for treatment—is a person of a certain chronological age: that determines many characteristics, and much of the coloring, of a person's life. That is the importance of the biographical point of view.

Principles for the Use of Age

How, from a biographical vantage point, should we formulate age as a criterion for the termination of treatment and make use of it in termination decisions? I will begin by proposing some general background principles for the termination of treatment of the aged, each meant to articulate themes developed earlier.

After a Person Has Lived Out a Natural Life Span, Medical Care Should No Longer Be Oriented to Resisting Death

No precise chronological age can readily be set for determining when a natural life span has been achieved—biographies vary—but it would normally be expected by the late seventies or early eighties. While a person's history may not be complete—time is always open-ended—most of it will have been achieved by that stage of life. It will be a full biography, even if more details are still to be added. Death beyond that period is not now, nor should it be, typically considered premature or untimely. Any greater precision than my "late seventies or early eighties" does not at present seem possible, and extended public discussion would be needed to achieve even a rough consensus on the appropriate age range. That discussion would also have to consider whether, for policy purposes, it would be necessary to set an exact age or a range only, and that would pose a classic policy dilemma. Too vague a standard of a "natural life span" would open the way for too great a flexibility of application to be fair or workable, while too specific a standard—one indifferent to the unique features of individual biographies—would preclude prudence and appropriate room for discretion.

Problems of that kind, however difficult, should not be used as an excuse to evade the necessity of setting some kind of age standard, or to conclude that any age standard must necessarily mean denying the value of the elderly.

The presumption against resisting death after a natural life span would not in any sense demean those who have lived that long or to suggest that their lives are less valuable than those of younger people. To come to the end of life in old age does not diminish the value of the life; that remains until the very end. This is not a principle, in short, for the comparison of lives. It reflects instead an acceptance of the inevitability of death in general and its acceptability for the individual after a natural life span in particular. Death will then take its proper place as a necessary link in the transition of generations.

Provision of Medical Care for Those Who Have Lived Out a Natural Life Span Will Be Limited to the Relief of Suffering

Medicine is not in a position to bring meaning and significance to the lives of the old. That only they can do for themselves, with the help of the larger culture. Yet medicine can help promote the physical functioning, the mental alertness, and the emotional stability conducive to this pursuit. These remain valuable goals, even when a natural life span has been attained. The difference at that point is that death should no longer be treated by medicine as an enemy. It may well be, of course, that medical efforts to relieve suffering will frequently have the unintended but foreseeable consequence of extending life expectancy. That is to be expected. A sharp line between relieving suffering and extending life will be on occasion difficult to draw, and under no circumstance would it be acceptable to fail to relieve suffering because of the possibility of life extension. The bias of the principle should be to stop resisting death after a certain age, but not when the price of doing so is unrelievable suffering. At the same time—the success of the hospice movement proves—it is perfectly possible to relieve suffering while not seeking to extend life.

The Existence of Medical Technology Capable of Extending the Lives of the Elderly Who Have Lived Out a Natural Life Span Creates No Presumption Whatever That the Technology Must Be Used for That Purpose

The uses of technology are always to be subordinated to the appropriate ends of medicine: that is, to the avoidance of premature death and to the relief of suffering. The alternative is slavery to the powers of technology— they, not we, will determine our end. Medicine should in particular resist the tendency to provide to the aged the life-extending capabilities of technologies developed primarily to help younger people avoid premature and untimely death. The use of those technologies should be subordinate to what is good for the elderly as individuals, good for them as members of society, good for them as a link in the passing of the generations, and good for the needs of other age groups.

The three principles detailed above are not so radical as they may first appear. They come close to actually articulating what many elderly express as their fears about aging and death. They indicate a wish that their life not be aggressively extended beyond a point at which they still possess a good degree of physical functioning and mental alertness, a life that has value and meaning for them; they are asking not for more years as such (though some would want just that), but for as many good years as possible; and that medical technology be limited in its use to those situations in which it will maintain or restore an adequate quality of life, not sustain and extend a deteriorating one.

QUESTIONS FOR CONSIDERATION

1. Do you agree with Callahan that the proper goal of medicine for those who have lived a full biographical life span should be "the relief of suffering rather than the extension of life"?

2. Callahan indicates that medical technology has created a contradiction for the elderly: a desire for improved medical technology that will extend their lives while relieving suffering and a fear that such technology will lead to excessive treatment and a painful extension of life. How can this contradiction be reduced?

3. Callahan describes the decision to end treatment as a continuum in which effective intervention declines with age. Do you agree?

4. What does Callahan mean by age as a medical criterion and age as person-centered or biographical standard? Do you agree that the former should be rejected while the latter should be a relevant factor in medical treatment and the decision to terminate treatment?

5. In examining the morality of age as a standard in medical treatment, Callahan contrasted using age as an assessment of the worth of a life and age as factor in meeting the needs of the whole person. Is this a valid moral distinction?

6. Do you agree with Callahan that old age is reason enough to either terminate treatment when death is imminent or end treatment when life has become unbearable?

NOTES

1. U.S. Congress Office of Technology Assessment, Biological Applications Program, *Life Sustaining Technologies and the Elderly* (Washington, DC: OTA, July 1987), 1–22ff.

2. I have adapted this description from a similar one developed by Jerome L. Avorn, "Medicine, Health, and the Geriatric Transformation," *Daedalus* 115 (Winter 1986), 215–17.

3. OTA, *Life-Sustaining Technologies*, 1–39–45.

4. Malcolm Cowley, *The View from Eighty* (New York: Penguin Books, 1982), p. 5. That line was quoted in G.C. Prado's remarkably interesting book *Rethinking How We Age* (Westport, CT: Greenwood Press, 1986), which analyzes psychological and social age, as distinguished from biological age.

5. Mark Siegler, "Should Age Be a Criterion in Health Care?" *Hastings Center Report* 14, no. 5 (October 1984): 27.

6. James F. Childress, "Ensuring Care, Respect, and Fairness for the Elderly," *Hastings Center Report* 14, no. 5 (October 1984): 29.

ROBERT D. TRUOG

Triage in the ICU

The United States has a seemingly limitless need for intensive care resources. More than 15 percent of our acute hospital beds are devoted to critical care, as compared with only 1 percent in Great Britain.[1] While some new technologies such as transluminal angioplasty have decreased the need for critical care beds, most are demanding ever more intense levels of care for longer periods of time. These dramatic changes in the demographics of hospital care have created new dilemmas for physicians and other caregivers.

Extracorporeal membrane oxygenation (ECMO) provides a case in point. ECMO is a form of cardiopulmonary bypass used primarily to support newborns with life-threatening respiratory failure. It is a truly "scarce" resource, available in few centers and requiring the presence of highly trained personnel around the clock. Patients can be supported with this technology for more than a month if necessary; but data from the National ECMO Registry indicates that over 99 percent of newborns who will survive ECMO therapy can be weaned off support in less than two weeks.[2] Nevertheless, some parents (and caregivers) believe that as long as there is "one chance in a million," their child should remain on ECMO. Continuation of this therapy despite a very poor prognosis is potentially wasteful of this expensive resource. More importantly, however, this practice can (and does) adversely affect the health and survival of other ill newborns. Infants who require ECMO frequently die if they cannot gain access to the therapy within several hours, and many are too ill to survive an extended transport to an alternate ECMO center. Should we withdraw ECMO from a newborn with a poor prognosis in favor of another newborn with a good prognosis if the child more likely to benefit needs the therapy to survive and cannot be safely transferred to another facility? This question is a concrete example of the kind of dilemmas increasingly encountered in many areas of critical care medicine.

The generally accepted answer to the question is straightforward. It is commonly considered ethically unacceptable to remove one patient from life-sustaining therapy to make room for another. Just as respect for a patient's autonomy requires consent before *initiating* therapy, so must we obtain consent before *withdrawing* it. In addition, the fiduciary relationship between physician and patient is commonly held to require physicians to be exclusively committed to the particular interests of their patients. "In caring for an individual patient, the doctor must act solely as that patient's advocate, against the apparent interests of society as a whole, if necessary."[3]

These considerations, however, are not absolute. The principle of respect for autonomy is only *prima facie,* and must be balanced against competing claims of justice. The mere fact that one patient needed ECMO sooner than another may not be a sufficient moral reason for giving it to that patient. "First come, first served" has been advocated as a method for allocating scarce resources between patients with similar needs, but it is less useful when the claims are not equal. Even if we assume that all patients have an *a priori* equal right to a scarce resource, a patient with a poor prognosis who has already consumed an appreciable part of that resource has less right to the continued use of it than someone with a better prognosis who has had no use of it at all. Simply because a patient is already receiving a benefit does not give that patient an ironclad right to further use of that benefit, nor does it imply that the caregivers have made a morally binding commitment to giving that benefit exclusively to him.

The fiduciary relationship between physicians and patients likewise does not commit physicians to tunnel vision in allocating scarce resources. Physicians routinely allocate resources among the patients under their care and between their patients and the rest of society. The surgeon who cancels her afternoon clinic because she is tied up with a complicated case in the operating room has allocated her limited time among her patients. The physician who agrees to put off a CT scan on his patient until tomorrow because other patients need the procedure more urgently is distributing a scarce resource between his patient and others in the community. Even when the therapy is life-sustaining, a physician's decision to shift the resource from one patient to another may be seen as a necessary exception to the general principle of exclusive commitment, as when a psychiatrist violates confidentiality to avoid putting another's life at risk. Fidelity to the covenant between patient and physician does not require physicians to be oblivious or unresponsive to the overall needs of others.

Can participation of a physician in the withdrawal of life-sustaining therapy be interpreted as abandonment of the patient? As a Hastings Center task force noted,

If explicit and ethical policies are developed by means of procedures that are open, informed, and fair, health care providers might be justified in limiting their treatments to patients in accordance with such policies. This would be in keeping with the long-standing concern of the health care professions with issues of justice and societal well-being, as well as with patient autonomy and well-being.[4]

The allocation decisions that may be made are constrained, however, by the principle of respect for autonomy and the special nature of the patient-physician relationship. The most important requirement is that patients must be aware of the conditions under which therapy may be discontinued *before* it is initiated. In other words, they must *prospectively* understand "the rules of the game." What is at issue here cannot be called "informed consent" since no meaningful choice is really being offered—the idea is, rather, that patients be forewarned. Since we currently do not inform patients or families of any restrictions on the continuation of ECMO or any other life-saving therapy, it is generally regarded as legally unacceptable to remove patients from therapy against their will, even to make room for others in need. In the example cited above, the child with the better prognosis must be denied the life-saving therapy in preference to the infant already receiving support.

The current approach, therefore, is to remove patients from life-sustaining therapy only when it is in *their* best interest, never when it is solely in the best interest of another. As noted above, however, there are compelling reasons for considering alternate methods of allocation. These would seek to maximize the benefits obtained from scarce resources by giving them to those most likely to respond to the therapy. In the case of ECMO, for example, newborns who could not be weaned from the therapy within a reasonable period (generally two weeks) would be removed from support if another child with a better prognosis needed it. Parents would be informed of this policy before being offered ECMO support. Such a policy would clearly maximize the benefits this technology has to offer.

Although ECMO is a dramatic example of a limited life-saving resource, all intensive-care therapies are fundamentally scarce, so this approach has similar relevance for virtually any form of intensive support. Adopting this strategy would therefore have a major impact on many aspects of ICU allocation. In considering these implications, it is helpful to borrow from the traditional concept of 'triage' and think of ICU patients as stratified in terms of their likelihood to benefit from ICU therapy. At one end are those patients admitted primarily for monitoring or nursing observation. These patients have a low likelihood of benefitting from ICU care since they probably will recover whether or not they are in the ICU. They have a low "benefit index," since they are too well to require all the technology and clinical skills that the ICU setting offers. At the other end of the spectrum are also patients with a low likelihood of benefitting from the ICU. In this case, however, the "benefit index" is low because these patients are too sick and likely to recover no matter how much care they receive. In the middle are those patients most likely to benefit from being in the ICU—those who truly require the high level of care available and who are expected to improve and ultimately recover.

Several reports have clearly documented that physicians *do* ration ICU resources under conditions of scarcity.[5] In all cases studied, however, these resources were denied or withdrawn *exclusively* from those patients on the "too well" end of the spectrum. In no case could it be determined that a patient who would clearly die without ICU care was removed from the ICU to make room for another patient with a better prognosis. ICU care is frequently withdrawn from terminal patients when this is believed to be in *that patient's* best interest, but none of the studies indicate that dying patients are discharged from the ICU when this is necessary to benefit *another* patient.

Is our current method of allocating ICU resources the best use of this scarce and expensive technology? First we must come to an understanding of what we mean by 'best use.' While there are many possible definitions, perhaps the most compelling is that which maximizes the health benefits that can be produced. Health benefits manifest as an increase in the quality as well as the longevity of individual lives. Does a system that denies or withdraws this resource only from those on the "too well" end of the spectrum result in the "best use" of this resource?

In most instances, optimal use of a medical resource requires that access be withheld from patients with a low likelihood of benefit on *both* ends of the spectrum. Our present system of favoring those on the "too sick" end of the spectrum can be justified only when the scarce resources are *temporarily* limited. Consider the case of a battlefield physician faced with the care of a large number of casualties after a landmine explodes in the middle of his platoon. If he knows that reinforcements are on the way and that sufficient help for evacuation and care of the wounded will be available within several hours, then his best course of action is to give preferential care to some of the more severely injured soldiers. Some of those who will surely die without immediate intervention may survive with prompt care, whereas those patients who are less severely injured probably will survive at least until additional help arrives. Under conditions of temporary scarcity, the choice of which patients to treat is shifted toward the "sicker" end of the spectrum, as this strategy maximizes the number of lives saved. On the other hand, if the platoon is isolated and the physician knows that help will not arrive for several days, he should direct his attention to those patients in the middle of the spectrum, and allow to die those who will place disproportionate demands on his attention. When scarcity is not temporary, the physician should allocate the available resources symmetrically around the middle of the spectrum, as in this case favoring the "too sick" not only fails to produce the best use of the scarce resources, but unfairly places all of the burden of allocation on those who are on the "too well" side of the spectrum.

Some shortages of ICU resources *are* temporary. If several nurses are out ill for the night shift, care should be preferentially directed toward the sicker patients in anticipation of full staffing in the morning. Most ICU limitations, however (like the scarcity of ECMO beds), are not temporary. In these circumstances, rational allocation demands the option of denying or withdrawing therapy from those on the "too sick" end of the spectrum.

An analogous approach has been widely adopted by organizations regulating the allocation of another scarce resource—transplantable organs.[6] Organ banks seek to maximize the benefits obtained from the limited number of available organs by choosing from among potential recipients those who are most likely to recover and sustain long-term organ function. This strategy means that patients who will certainly die without a transplanted organ may sometimes be passed over in favor of patients with a better prognosis. While similar in principle, organ allocation differs from ICU allocation in the way patients present for treatment. Transplantation programs are able to pick a candidate for a particular organ from among a group of qualified applicants. When an ICU bed becomes available, on the other hand, there is generally not a pool of candidates waiting for the bed. ICU patients make their claims sequentially, one at a time. Ethicists who have tried to draw analogies between organ transplantation and ICU allocation have not fully appreciated this fact, and have postulated contrived scenarios (such as simultaneous cardiac arrests)[7] to draw parallels with the transplantation situation. The important implication of this difference is that ICUs cannot exclusively rely on *withholding* care to assure delivery to those most likely to benefit. Since ICUs must allocate sequentially rather than at one point in time, it is also necessary to *withdraw* care if required to accommodate an individual with a greater potential for benefit.

Successful implementation of this approach requires that we resolve several important practical problems. First, we must arrive at an understanding of what constitutes 'benefit' and then develop accurate prognostic indicators that will enable us to assign individuals a position on the "benefit spectrum." The meaning of 'benefit' varies with the medical goals to be achieved as well as with the unique values of each patient. Robert Weir has pointed out the wide variety of medical meanings of the term 'beneficial':

1. the treatment is "beneficial" in the sense of making the *medical management* of the patient easier for the health care providers involved in the case;
2. the treatment is "beneficial" in the sense of providing *immediate, short-term relief* to the patient, without any long-term benefit;
3. the treatment is "beneficial" in the sense of *corrective therapy,* by improving an injurious or disabling condition without being curative;
4. the treatment is "beneficial" in the sense of *curing* a pathological condition "once and for all";
5. the treatment is "beneficial" in the sense of *maintaining the status quo condition* of the patient for an extended period of time;
6. the treatment is "beneficial" in the sense of *medical exprimentation,* with any actual benefits of the experimental procedure occurring to other patients in the future.[8]

Weir's third definition seems most appropriate to life-sustaining ICU therapy, with perhaps a reasonable goal being survival to hospital discharge with consciousness intact. Such a goal is in accord with several prominent consensus reports, which have concluded that permanently unconscious patients should generally not receive ICU care or deprive another patient of access to a scarce medical resource.[9]

Assessing prognosis for achieving this benefit is a notoriously difficult aspect of ICU care, but nevertheless one we routinely perform every day. We prognosticate when we recommend a liver transplant based on the likelihood of survival without one; we recommend toxic antibiotics by balancing their risks against the probability that the patient will die of an infection. Our uncertainty in making predictions about outcome and survival should not paralyze our allocation decisions any more than it does our medical decisions. Prognostic indicators have been developed for many types of ICU patients, such as those with severe neurologic dysfunction, multisystem organ failure, and hematologic malignancy, or those in respiratory failure secondary to AIDS or bone marrow transplantation.[10] Severity of illness scores such as the APACHE system may further assist our ability to characterize patients in terms of their likelihood to benefit from ICU therapy.[11]

In addition, we need to choose a threshold level of benefit that would justify withdrawing care from one patient to give it to another. If a patient receiving therapy has a 59 percent probability of benefit, and a newcomer patient's probability is 60 percent, should the patient receiving therapy give it up to the newcomer? If the probabilities are reversed the following day, should the therapy once again be switched? In an effort to avoid this type of chaos, previous allocation strategies have generally not attempted to reassess entitlement after the initial allocation. When access to hemodialysis was rationed in the late 1960s, for example, committees decided which patients were allowed access to the therapy, but once a patient was accepted into the program there was no attempt made to reassess suitability or consider withdrawing the therapy.[12] A reasonable way of preventing the confusion and turmoil that could result from continual reassessment would be to honor the principle of first come, first served[13] until the probability of benefit to the person receiving the therapy declined sufficiently far to justify withdrawal of the therapy in favor of another. Although it may seem excessively arbitrary to choose a cutoff of 1, 5, or 10 percent as a threshold for the probability of benefit, in actual practice there is usually a quantum transition from a reasonable likelihood of recovery to a situation where survival would be exceedingly unlikely. In only a minority of cases is the transition gradual and continuous; but even in these cases it would be fair to choose a reasonable (albeit arbitrary) threshold for the probability of benefit, provided it was applied uniformly to all patients in similar situations. Decisions based upon these probabilities should be founded upon clear institutional guidelines or reached through the work of a committee experienced in the clinical care of the critically ill patient. The tendency to continually expand the indications for scarce therapies and progressively shrink the category of patients too sick to benefit would have to be consciously resisted, otherwise the allocation problem would not really be resolved but only shifted to all of the patients now under the same category. Decisions should be regularly reviewed by referees not involved in the allocation system, and a well-defined mechanism for appeal should be available for patients or their advocates to question these deliberations.

This raises the issue of how therapy should be withdrawn once it is agreed that a patient has a benefit index below the threshold for entitlement. One option would be to remove therapy from these patients only when another patient in need of the therapy and with a higher benefit index presented for care. The other option would be to withdraw ICU care from anyone with a benefit index below the threshold value, regardless of whether another candidate was in need of the bed. The former strategy is advantageous in permitting the most continuous use of the resource, and in giving each patient the chance to prove the system wrong by mounting an unexpected or even miraculous recovery. The principal advantage of the latter approach is that it avoids the appearance of competition between patients. One can imagine the newcomer-patient being rolled into the ICU as the patient he has bumped is being removed from the unit. Such a policy might well induce guilt in the newcomer-patient, besides generating tremendous anxiety in those resident patients with low benefit indices as they wait for another candidate to arrive with a greater claim on the resource.

While each approach has its advantages and disadvantages, choosing a policy that withdraws care only when another patient actually requires the therapy permits our allocation decisions to be grounded in the needs of *real and particular* patients rather than in abstract considerations of probable benefit. This is crucial for preventing bedside allocation from becoming a faceless and impersonal technical task.

The model developed here is entirely dependent upon the assumption that the best use of ICU resources is that which maximizes the health benefits that can be obtained. It is plausible to argue that in matters of life and death we are seldom willing to accept an approach grounded purely in a standard of efficiency. Perhaps this is best illustrated by the fact that few would support a policy forcing the lethal donation of the heart, liver, and kidneys from a healthy citizen to save the lives of several other people dying from single-organ failure. Such a policy would certainly be considered unacceptable even though it would promote the best use of scarce transplantable organs. Stated more generally, perhaps the ICU is simply another place where individual rights should take precedence over the pursuit of the greatest good. In evaluating this claim, we must weigh the relative value of the individual rights that may be violated against the social good that is to be gained. In the transplant example, while saving lives is certainly an important social good, the right not to have one's body forcibly violated is generally held to be more important. In the case of scarce ICU resources, we must balance the value of maximizing the benefits from this socially owned and expensive resource against the right of patients and families to demand care from which they are very unlikely to benefit. Often these demands are based on the very understandable feelings of grief and despair that frequently surround the process of death, but we must decide how much weight the community should give to these feelings when they compromise the care of others who will suffer or die without access to the resource. A strategy that seeks to maximize the health benefits available from scarce ICU resources may therefore be justified in overriding the right of individuals to demand unlimited access to resources from which they are very unlikely to benefit.

Rationing is already a reality in the ICU. Studies indicate it is being performed without a clear idea of the principles and objectives that should underlie allocation decisions. Open discussion is necessary if we are to achieve strategies for allocation that are compatible with the moral requirements and health needs of our society. If we accept the model outlined above, then we have an obligation to remove some patients from life-sustaining therapy, even when it means their unavoidably imminent death. It is certainly tragic to tell a patient that we are removing him from life support and that he will now die. It is even worse, however, to tell someone that we are denying him a life-saving therapy because another has an unquestioned claim on that resource no matter how poor his prognosis. We cannot avoid making tragic decisions, but we can make them with the knowledge that we have done our best to be compassionate and fair.

QUESTIONS FOR CONSIDERATION

1.   Do you agree with Truog that the principle of autonomy must be balanced with the claims of justice? How does the example of a newborn on ECMO illustrate this point?

2.   Do you agree that, ". . . a patient with a poor prognosis who has already consumed an appreciable part of that resource has less right to the continued use of it than someone with a better prognosis . . ."?

3.   According to Truog, how would the traditional concept of "triage" be applied to patients with a high or low "benefit index"? What did he mean by the optimal use of medical resources?

4.   How would the procedure for the transplantation of organs be analogous to allocations in the ICU?

5.   What did Truog consider the advantages and disadvantages of removing therapy from a patient only when another patient with a higher benefit index needed the therapy, in contrast to always removing the therapy whenever a patient fell below the predetermined threshold?

6.   What did Truog mean by arguing that maximizing medical benefits must be balanced with the right to have access to unlimited medical resources that promise minimal benefits?

NOTES

1. Bryan Jennett, "Inappropriate Use of Intensive Care," *British Medical Journal* 289, no. 6460 (1984): 1709–11.

2. Data from Extracorporeal Life Support Organization, April 1989.

3. Norman G. Levinsky, "The Doctor's Master," *NEJM 31* 1, no. 24 (1984): 157375.

4. The Hastings Center, *Guidelines on the Termination of Life-Sustaining Treatment and the Care of the Dying* (Bloomington: Indiana University Press, 1987), p. 120.

5. Daniel E. Singer, Phyllis L. Carr, Albert G. Mulley, et al., "Rationing Intensive Care: Physician Responses to Resource Shortage," *NEJM* 309, no. 19 (1983): 115560; Michael J. Strauss, James P. LoGerfo, James A. Yeltatzie, et al., "Rationing of Intensive Care Unit Services: An Everyday Occurrence," *JAMA* 255, no. 9 (1986): 1143–46; Harry P. Selker, John L. Griffith, Frederick J. Dorey, et al., "How Do Physicians Adapt When the Coronary Care Unit Is Full? A Prospective Multicenter Study," *JAMA* 257, no. 9 (1987): 1181–85; Frederic L. Sax and Mary E. Charlson, "Utilization of Critical Care Units: A Prospective Study of Physician Triage and Patient Outcome," *Archives of Internal Medicine* 147, no. 5 (1987): 929–34; Paul E. Kalb and David H. Miller, "Utilization Strategies for Intensive Care Units," *JAMA* 261, no. 16 (1989): 2389–95; Nicholas G. Smedira, Bradley H. Evans, Linda S. Grais, et al., "Withholding and Withdrawal of Life Support from the Clinically Ill," *NEJM* 322, no. 5 (1990): 309–15.

6. Massachusetts Task Force on Organ Transplantation, "Patient Selection and Rationing Schemes," in *Report of the Massachusetts Task Force on Organ Transplantation* (Boston: Department of Public Health, 1984), pp. 71–86.

7. Kevin M. McIntyre, Robert C. Benfari and Margaret Pabst Battin, 'Two Cardiac Arrests, One Medical Team," *Hastings Center Report* 12, no. 2 (1982): 24–25.

8. Robert F. Weir, *Abating Treatment with Critically Ill Patients: Ethical and Legal Limits to the Prolongation of Life* (New York: Oxford University Press, 1989), p. 344.

9. President's Commission for the Study of Ethical Problems in Medicine and Biomedical and Behavioral Research, *Deciding to Forego Life-Sustaining Treatment: Ethical, Medical, and Legal Issues in Treatment Decisions* (Washington, D.C.: U.S. Government Printing Office, 1983), pp. 188–89; Hastings Center, *Guidelines on the Termination of Life-Sustaining Treatment;* Task Force on Ethics of the Society of Critical Care Medicine, "Consensus Report on the Ethics of Forgoing Life-Sustaining Treatments in the Critically Ill," *Critical Care Medicine* 18 (1990): 1435–39.

10. Michael S. Berger, Lawrence H. Pitts, Mary Lovely, et al., "Outcome from Severe Head Injury in Children and Adolescents, " *Journal of Neurosurgery 62,* no. 2 (1985): 194–99; William A. Knaus, Elizabeth A. Draper, Douglas P. Wagner, et al., "Prognosis in Acute Organ-System Failure," *Annals of Surgery* 202, no. 6 (1985): 685–93; Warwick Butt, Geoffrey Barker, Craig Walker, et al., "Outcome of Children with Hematologic Malignancy Who Are Admitted to an Intensive Care Unit," *Critical Care Medicine,* 16, no. 18 (1988): 761–64; Roland M. Schein, Margaret A. Fischl, Arthur E. Pitchenik, et al. "ICU Survival of Patients with the Acquired Immunodeficiency Syndrome," *Critical Care Medicine* 14, no. 12 (1986): 1026–27; Scott J. Denardo, Robert K. Oye, and Paul E. Bellamy, "Efficacy of Intensive Care for Bone Marrow Transplant Patients with Respiratory Failure," *Critical Care Medicine* 17, no. 1 (1989): 4–6.

11. James A. Kruse, Mary C. Thill Baharozian, and Richard W. Carlson, "Comparison of Clinical Assessment with APACHE II for Predicting Mortality Risk in Patients Admitted to a Medical Intensive Care Unit," *JAMA* 260, no. 12 (1988): 1739–42.

12. Shana Alexander, "They Decide Who Lives, Who Dies," in *Ethical Issues in Modern Medicine,* ed. R. Hunt and John Arras (Palo Alto, Calif.: Mayfield, 1977), pp. 409–24.

13. James E Childress, "Rationing of Medical Treatment" in *Encyclopedia of Bioethics,* vol. 4, ed. Warren T. Reich (New York: Free Press, 1978), pp. 1414–19.

GILES R. SCOFIELD

Is Consent Useful When Resuscitation Isn't?

At midnight
I pondered on the, beating of my heart;
One single pulse of anguish
Raged in my heart
At midnight.

—*Gustav Mahler*

Our increasing awareness that limitations of human knowledge, resources, and ingenuity impose finite horizons on medicine's ability to ward off disease, disability, and death has forced us to acknowledge that we must either limit medical interventions on a societal and individual basis or bankrupt ourselves.[1] Attaining a consensus about limiting treatment requires educating patients and society to understand that expectations once held about medicine no longer apply, or do so less categorically. Given our faith in medicine and its impact on personal well-being, adjusting ourselves to the realities of limited medical options will generate anxiety and a crisis in confidence, which will make shifting expectations even harder. How well we make this adjustment depends on how we make these decisions. If they occur or are perceived to occur in ways that generate suspicion and distrust, the ultimate decisions, no matter how fair or necessary they are, will prove unacceptable, and the process become paralyzed, protracted, fragmented, and counterproductive. We cannot avoid the effort reorientation involves or the disappointment unmet expectations create, but we can manage these difficulties and enhance the prospects for responsible deliberation by carefully framing the decisionmaking dialogue.

How we structure that dialogue depends on how we define consent, since that will determine both the character of the deliberation and the kind and quality of consensus we ultimately obtain. We need the model of consent most likely to insure that meaningful communication occurs, yet it must also be closely connected to our most fundamental social values as decisions to withhold treatment become more commonplace.[2]

In truth, decisions to withhold treatment are and always have been ubiquitous and frequent. They occur whenever a physician weighs and ultimately decides against offering or recommending that a patient be admitted, tested, treated, or referred. Such decisions are not necessarily invidious and often represent prudent restraint. Doctors are expected to use the professional expertise derived from their education, training, and experience to make judgments about what they believe should or should not be done in a given situation.

What is troublesome about a decision to withhold treatment is how it occurs. Because it is low-profile in nature, it does not have the inherent visibility that triggers consent when intervening or withdrawing are at issue. Thus, the fact that it has occurred may be known only to the doctor and those colleagues involved in the patient's care. Although affected by it, the patient may not know how, why, or even that the decision was made. Whether the proper criteria were correctly applied to a particular decision is unlikely to be examined beyond professional circles, which makes withholding especially problematic in terms of the values consent is supposed to serve.

Given the special nature of decisions to withhold treatment, we should not assume that the model of consent developed to provide accountability in an era of therapeutic relentlessness will do the job as medicine begins to rein itself in. Because greater justification is required to withhold than to withdraw treatment,[3] finding the right way to make these decisions becomes especially critical as we adjust individual and social expectations to the new realities setting limits creates. Theoretically, the order not to resuscitate a patient (DNR order) defies withholding's usual pattern. This decision requires express authorization and documentation reflecting the consent of the patient or the patient's surrogate, or, as in the case of emergency medical services, a physician's permission to withhold resuscitation. Because resuscitation, commonly known as CPR, is the expected response to sudden death, if it is not provided someone has to account for why.

Articles discussing consent to DNR orders have exposed thought processes usually confined to professional enclaves. This provides an opportunity to consider how such decisions ought to be made in light of the values consent serves. Due to CPR's ubiquitous, symbolic, and momentous nature—each of us may well face a decision about being resuscitated or allowed to die—how we decide to limit resuscitation is critical to developing a model of consent suited to making other decisions about limiting treatment.

CPR: In Like a Lion, Out Like a Lamb?

It is difficult now to imagine the enormous impact of the introduction of CPR. Catastrophic trauma, life-threatening surgery, and failed hearts no longer meant certain death. Medicine could reverse death's surest sign—the heart that had stopped beating. With its promise of life after death, CPR transformed medicine, society, and our expectations about mortality.

Society affirmed CPR's significance by declaring it an emergency procedure, which exempted it from consent prior to use. Public perceptions about CPR came largely from the media, which usually portrayed it and medicine in glowing, heroic terms. CPR rapidly proliferated into ICUs, general wards, and even the public domain, as emergency medical teams, police officers, firefighters, lifeguards, and concerned citizens learned to provide basic life support in the event of a cardiac arrest.

The emergency exception eventually evolved into presumed consent to CPR, making it society's standing order against death. This shielded CPR from patient and public scrutiny, hid its realities from all but those involved in administering or receiving it, fostered its indiscriminate use, and excused physicians from seeking anything other than grateful ratification when it worked or heartfelt solace when it did not.

Presumed consent freed physicians from disclosing that CPR's success, however defined, depends on a number of factors. The patient's condition and the presence of pathology are important determinants. Other noteworthy factors include: where the arrest occurs (in an ICU or elsewhere, for example); the nature of the arrest; whether the arrest is witnessed or not; the time elapsed between arrest and the commencement of resuscitative measures; the availability of the equipment and drugs needed to provide advanced life-support; whether the equipment works; how long resuscitative measures are employed; and the training, skill, experience, and collaborative ability of the code team.[4] Although some patients would have found such information germane to a decision about submitting to CPR and its sequelae, presumed consent obviated the need to secure real consent. Even where an arrest was "not unexpected," physicians who were unwilling or unable to talk to patients about resuscitation needed only to wait for an "emergency" to materialize in order to act. Presumed consent to CPR was medicine's license to intervene at will.

As time and experience brought balanced insight into CPR's benefits and limitations, perceptions about its life-saving powers yielded to the awareness that its effectiveness could no longer be categorically presumed nor its burdensomeness denied. Discussions about limiting CPR through DNR orders found their way into the literature and the courts.

Yet fast upon recognizing the need to make decisions about forgoing this not always beneficial treatment came attempts to exempt physicians from obtaining consent to a DNR order. Some contended that because consent prevents uninvited contact, there was no duty to secure consent not to commit a battery, a view that has been rejected.[5] Recent discussions concede that DNR orders require consent, but argue that there is no duty to secure a patient's consent when CPR is medically futile; when it would be futile to attempt resuscitation, consent to a DNR order may be presumed.

One need only translate presumed consent into its oxymoronic synonym— unilateral consent—to appreciate how radically it departs from the goal of collaborative decisionmaking. Although a DNR order is about *doing* nothing, it's not about nothing; nor is it about not doing something that no sensible physician would ever do. It reflects a physician's considered judgment that a patient is going to die and reverses society's standing order to preserve life against death. It has profound social, personal, and professional ramifications. To determine whether consent is useless when resuscitation is futile, we need to examine consent and futility more closely.

An Exercise in Futility

The argument that when CPR is futile consent is pointless rests on two prongs.[6] The first starts with the premise that what distinguishes physicians is the professional expertise that gives them the exclusive ability to make medical judgments. A physician's professional integrity lies in the ability to recognize and integrate what is known about a patient's medical condition with what medicine has to offer, and to exercise his or her best judgment about how or whether to proceed with treatment. That integrity and the value we place on such judgment are meaningless if patients may freely ignore or override it out of fear, irrationality, or ignorance. Because only physicians can evaluate whether an intervention is medically futile, they must have unilateral authority to make and act on judgments about matters that fall exclusively within the domain of their expertise.

The second prong analyzes futility according to the patient's autonomy interest. Without discounting autonomy's value, it argues that this interest is not unlimited. Patients may not demand treatment, especially treatment that would accomplish nothing. Similarly, physicians have no duty to provide and a patient may not successfully sue for the failure to provide futile treatment. Patient autonomy and consent are irrelevant to a decision about CPR when it offers no potential benefit.

Moreover, involving patients in deliberations about useless treatment confuses and upsets them. Some, believing that a discussion about CPR implies that it must be of some benefit (otherwise, why mention it?) will ask or insist that it be administered. Others will find such discussions disturbing because their hopeless condition has left them emotionally drained and vulnerable; they will think that seeking consent is cruel or demand CPR out of desperate fear. Instead of elevating form over substance, we should acknowledge that a patient's right to choose ends where futility begins.

These arguments seem so sensible, internally consistent, and authoritatively supported that their conclusion appears ineluctable. They seem to strike a reasonable balance between patient and physician autonomy and accommodate society's legitimate interest in not wasting resources. To suggest that decisions about futile treatment require consent sounds ludicrous; doctors have better things to do than discuss pointless therapy. Patient autonomy needs sensible limits, and authorizing doctors to enter DNR orders unilaterally when CPR is futile seems legally and ethically sound.

The apparent soundness of this conclusion evaporates upon close examination. In reality the futility exception is a dishonest solution to the tragic choice that decisions to limit treatment represent. It purports to respect, but in fact departs from the fundamental values consent is intended to serve. It will not generate the conversation we need if we are to attain a consensus about limiting treatment; nor will it make physicians sensitive in their dealings with patients, especially dying patients. It promotes a model of consent that is antithetical to setting limits in a democratic, caring manner.

The argument that physician expertise at judging futility justifies unilaterally entered DNR orders rests on several assumptions: agreement on what resuscitation means; a definition of what constitutes "futile" (and successful) treatment; concurrence that physicians can make such judgments accurately, reliably, and consistently; and agreement on what a DNR order means. Before empowering physicians to decide these matters unilaterally, we should analyze each of these assumptions.

The global pronouncement that resuscitation won't work obscures its subtle realities. Many people who stereotypically imagine resuscitation as a chest-thumping, bone-crushing, electrifying experience would be shocked to learn that depending on the clinical situation it defines a range of interventions.[7] Less invasive measures include drug support and fluid resuscitation. Thus, when a physician says that resuscitation is futile we cannot know what is meant, and will remain ignorant if nothing more is said. Even were we to agree that compression and defibrillation would be futile, pharmacological support with proper monitoring might be useful.

Implicit in the judgment that CPR is medically futile is a definition of medical success. Even assuming that physicians can predict whose CPR will succeed and whose won't, how they define success and whether their definition comports with the patient's, the family's, or the larger society's are legitimate questions. Presumed consent presupposes that only the physician's perspective matters.

Even if a physician's judgment that CPR won't work is sound and comports with the patient's perspective (difficult to accomplish if the patient is not involved in the decision), *why* it won't is significant, especially because CPR's success can depend on factors other than the patient's physiology or pathology. It's one thing to conclude that nothing more can be done, and something else to believe that we can do nothing more for you here. If patients might be better off elsewhere, presumed consent hides knowledge about that option from them.

The belief that physicians know futility when they see it is an illusion.[8] There is no set definition of medical futility, only suggested parameters that vary widely. Even if medicine could define medical futility, trusting physicians to make unilateral judgments assumes that they know what the definition is and can apply it accurately, consistently, and reliably. Medical judgment involves recognizing and integrating relevant data correctly, an uncertain process that inevitably involves false positives and negatives, erroneous judgments, and differing interpretations. The same doctor may view data about prognostically indistinguishable patients differently, and different doctors, depending on their specialty and experience, may assess the same patient's chances differently.[9] Presumed consent assumes a world of medical certainty that does not exist.

Moreover, futility is not some objective, value-free fact that jumps up and announces "Here I am." It is a concept, that is, a way of judging facts. We are concerned about futility precisely because we value not wasting resources. Whether it is futile "in fact" to attempt to keep someone alive may depend on whether that person is a potential organ donor, a potentially viable fetus, or worth salvaging for some socially or otherwise informed reason. Presumed consent assumes that in making medical decisions we can separate observer from observed, facts from values, and individuals from context, an assumption that is doubtful at best.[10] Among themselves physicians do not uniformly understand what a DNR order connotes,[11] putting aside whether their understanding agrees with the patient's. Some physicians equate a DNR order with a decision to withhold or withdraw other and sometimes all means of life support. A DNR order does not and was never meant to concern itself with anything other than resuscitative measures, but the fact that not all physicians know this, or that some who do nonetheless regard or treat a DNR order as authority to forgo other treatment argues against one-sided consent.

Finally, even if physicians *could* exercise judgment with the certainty they claim, that would not mean that they *should* make such decisions unilaterally. After all, if physicians cannot avoid the consent process where a treatment is "clearly" beneficial, why should they do so when it is "clearly" futile? And although a physician may not be held liable for failing to provide futile care, whether he or she actually exercised proper judgment in a given case is a question a court may decide.[12] A physician whose futility defense might ultimately prevail against the claim that CPR was wrongfully withheld must nonetheless defend against it, which should make even the most confident physician uneasy about presumed consent.

The second prong of the argument fares no better than the first. Its essential assumption—that because autonomy triggers the duty to secure consent, the absence of an autonomy interest excuses it—puts the ethical cart before the horse. Autonomy is important, but it is neither the sole nor the primary principle of medical ethics. It is derivative of and subordinate to the overarching obligation that we show respect for persons.[13] Respecting autonomy is simply one way of respecting persons. The futility exception ends its analysis where it ought to begin. By not asking whether excluding patients from deliberations about their fate demonstrates respect for them, presumed consent mistakenly equates ignoring persons with respecting them.

Presumed consent gives autonomy undue prominence because it erroneously assumes that autonomy is all there is to consent. Yet consent concerns itself with matters beyond autonomy. Among them: respecting human dignity; promoting rational decisionmaking; encouraging professional self-scrutiny; avoiding deceit and coercion; and educating the public.[14] Under this view of consent, futility looks different.

Given the variability, uncertainty, and biases that influence the physician, talking with patients forces a doctor to get clear on what lies beneath the judgment that resuscitation would be futile before giving this news to the person to whom it means the most. This fosters professional self-scrutiny and helps assure that the determination that CPR is medically futile does not become a sterilized way of unilaterally classifying patients as "pointless to treat," that is, not *worth* treating.

Presumed consent thwarts the legitimate goal of avoiding deceit and coercion. Unless physicians explain futility to patients we cannot determine if they do so accurately, deceptively, or manipulatively.[15] Imposing on patients consequences they have not assumed is a form of coercion. When what the patient believes and what the chart denotes do not reflect one another and the staff must act out the charade of hiding from the patient how close death is, deceit occurs.

Rational decisionmaking is a process of shared understanding and collaborative planning. It is not irrational to give patients the opportunity to agree with the assessment that CPR is futile; if anything, it is irrational *not* to afford them that chance. Decisions about CPR can open the door to other matters, assure the patient that "no code" does not mean "no treatment," and clarify to all concerned what DNR means, including that it can be reassessed. Rational decisionmaking cannot occur absent patient involvement, unless, of course, all decisions are to be made unilaterally.

Educating the public is an integral function of consent; as we educate patients we can educate and reorient society. Most patients and their families are unaware of medicine's recent change of heart about CPR. The best way to debunk the myths, fears, and misperceptions they may harbor from whatever source is by being candid with them in the course of making treatment decisions. Word will get around, and discussing beforehand why CPR won't work minimizes the chances for hurt feelings and possible recriminations if relatives later wonder why a loved one died without heroic efforts.

Respect for human dignity requires truth-telling. Most patients know something is wrong with them. They do not know how bad that something is and what, if anything, can be done about it. They are entitled to know that; presumably that is one reason they went to the doctor. Not acquainting patients with what is known and believed about their prospects and disenfranchising them from deliberations about their fate denigrates them.

Presumed consent's disrespect for personhood is reflected in its meager concept of autonomy, which it defines as a "negative right"—to be let alone. This simply repackages the already rejected view that consent to a DNR order is never required. It also suggests that patients need information only when medical choices need to be made. Nothing could be further from the truth.

Patients need medical information to make choices that have nothing to do with medicine, especially when no medical options exist. However commonplace DNR orders are to physicians, most patients cross this Rubicon only once, and need to know—in order to plan a funeral, say farewell to friends, try to hold on for the arrival of a new grandchild, or simply look out the window with the knowledge that time is drawing to a close. Patients are value systems, not organ systems, and consent serves a personal purpose even when it is medically useless.[16]

The futility exception's final arguments—that because patients will demand resuscitation or be so confused and upset by discussions about it they are best served by being excluded from such decisions—do not bear weight. Patients do not behave irrationally as frequently as some people fear, and the patient's first reaction may not last or be the last. Also, the idiosyncratic demands some patients may make do not justify a rule that excuses not talking with *all* patients. Finally, a doctor is always free to refrain from continuing to care for a patient whose demands for resuscitation violate his or her professional conscience, though separating from a patient at so critical a juncture should prod any physician to deep reflection. Similarly, the commonly invoked adage that candor hurts patients lacks the evidence to support the therapeutic privilege it creates. The truth is, many patients welcome and are relieved by the opportunity to be involved in such deliberations (which also gives those who want the chance to opt out).[17] The recommendation that physicians forgo consent when CPR is futile is usually based on studies in which patients were not adequately informed, or is made despite evidence that properly informed patients overwhelmingly agree with their doctor's recommendation. What these studies do establish is that physicians have trouble talking with patients. More silence is not the solution to that problem.

If a conversation intended to bring patients to a realistic understanding of their situation and of medicine's limited ability to postpone death confuses or hurts them (more so than silence bewilders or angers them), we should determine the cause and address it. Some patients will be upset because no one has ever been candid with them about their condition and prognosis; others because discussing death tongue-ties their doctor. The cure is not less, but more talk. Physicians need to converse more often, thoroughly, and carefully with their patients.

For such conversations to occur, physicians must regard them as integral to practicing good medicine. If they view consent as a form that patients must sign, instead of the ongoing process the form is supposed to substantiate, resuscitation decisions will elevate form over substance in a way that is insensitive and hurtful to patients. Physicians cannot pass patients along or avoid the responsibility for defusing situations their or their colleagues' silence creates. They need education, training, and support to ensure that these conversations occur appropriately and sensitively; which means learning how to converse candidly, comfortably, and sympathetically with patients about death and dying.[18]

Not conversing with patients about such matters should be the exception, not the rule. Indeed, if the expertise physicians gain from their knowledge and experience reveals anything, it is that there is rarely a good reason to wait until a crisis erupts or resuscitation is futile to determine what ought to be done. How often have physicians found their hands tied because they or one of their colleagues were too tongue-tied to plan ahead? If taking a patient's values history were as integral to clinical practice as the medical history is, physicians could establish early on in the relationship the foundation of knowledge and trust needed to discuss decisions concerning the sort of care and treatment patients want at the end of life.

Heads I Win, Tails You Lose

When viewed concretely, the futility exception loses much of the luster it generates in the abstract. It neither encourages advance planning nor discourages not talking with patients. It is unlikely to promote honest, shared decision-making or to demonstrate respect for persons and is antithetical to the values consent is supposed to serve. To appreciate the futility exception fully, however, we need to dig further.

The futility exception's latent significance appears when we compare it to its counterpart, the emergency exception. Whereas the futility exception arises partly out of solicitude for a patient's physical integrity, the emergency exception circumvents that integrity in theory and practice. What reconciles these contradictory exceptions is the doctrine of presumed consent, which each promotes. Presumed consent enables physicians "legally and ethically" to exclude patients from participating in decisions affecting them and to decide unilaterally whether to use or withhold resuscitation. What it protects is not a patient's physical integrity, but medicine's professional integrity. Lurking within the futility exception is the medical profession's desire to protect its autonomy against the threats posed by death and health care rationing.

Medicine's professional autonomy—its right to be let alone—rests on a belief in professional expertise that causes individuals and society to surrender to medical authority judgments about private and public health matters.[19] Among the most powerful sources of our faith in medicine is the belief that it can "do something" about death. Resuscitation, which transformed our view of medicine and death, symbolizes medicine's power and lies at the crux of its authority.[20]

For that authority to remain secure, medicine must maximize its control over how resuscitation is perceived and over decisions about when, where, how, and whether it will be used. Disclosing resuscitation's realities and permitting patients to participate in decisions about it diminishes that control and the professional power that comes with it. Because resuscitation decisions are about death, they are personally and professionally challenging. It is more attractive to gloss over or avoid conversations about death than to invite situations where physician or medical impotence is revealed through the overt confession, "There is nothing I (or we) can do."

The futility exception and presumed consent try to solve this problem in a way that does not seem to offend the values consent serves, thereby enabling medicine to retreat intact, as unaccountably as the emergency exception enabled it to advance. By completing the circle the emergency exception starts, the futility exception surrounds resuscitation with a model of consent that maximizes medicine's control over decisions about its use. With consent in favor of resuscitation already presumed, a physician who is unwilling or unable to talk to a patient about such matters need only delay determining a patient's DNR status until resuscitation is futile for the presumption to flip the other way. The decision gets made without the patient's ever knowing when, how, why, or even that it did. Between the emergency and futility exceptions, presumed consent gets patients coming and going.

The futility exception also enables medicine to control how resuscitation is perceived, and especially why it does not always work. Emphasizing the perception that some patients are simply "too far gone" for resuscitation to do any good helps hide the other truths about why and how often resuscitation fails. This preserves the heroic aura the emergency exception promotes. It also keeps the public from asking what all this suggests about whether prehospital use of CPR ought to remain unlimited; and whether cases such as Nancy Cruzan's raise as profound questions about CPR as they do about feeding tubes. For now, a conversation about an intervention that affects the public excludes it.

Additionally, the futility exception promotes the perception that physicians can (and therefore ought to) be trusted to limit medical resources unilaterally, especially to keep the health care system from being run into the ground by the demands of rapacious, irrational, idiosyncratic patients. Not only do doctors save lives, they save resources too. Setting limits, therefore, involves letting medicine set them for us.

The futility exception's suggestion of presumed consent will likely swallow the rule of actual consent in decisions to limit resuscitation, thereby enabling the medical profession to rein itself in unilaterally and unaccountably. It is medicine's license to withhold at will. It vests the profession whose accountability is at issue with the authority to determine when and whether that authority is properly exercised. It establishes a model of decisionmaking that purports to respect patients, when it actually rationalizes physician avoidance of death and legitimates medical authority.

If physicians are given the authority to enter DNR orders unilaterally when they believe resuscitation would be futile, nothing prevents their using the same reasoning to enter DNT (do-not-treat), DNH (do-not-hospitalize), or any other order denying treatment unilaterally when they believe it would be futile—whether 'futile' means not medically effective, not cost effective, or not worth it for this patient. The futility exception sets limits to everything and everyone except the medical profession's autonomy.

The decisionmaking model it promotes is undemocratic and uncaring. By vesting the medical profession with the authority to make decisions that should be the product of open discussion and shared deliberation, it forecloses the conversation we must have if we are to arrive at a genuine consensus about setting limits.[21] The legal fiction of presumed consent is no substitute for the solid work we all must do if we are to adjust ourselves to the new realities these limits impose. There is no such thing as presumed consensus.

The futility exception is uncaring because it legitimates and perpetuates the practice of isolating dying patients from their physicians. By placing a wall of silence between them, presumed consent severs the dying from the human community before death actually takes them from the world. It offers social death and exclusion at the one moment when we most need the consolation of our fellow men and women.[22] It limits respecting persons to the tissue-thin perspective conveyed by the right to be let alone (a pretty pathetic way of respecting patients we have no intention of touching) and ignores the deeper human values that make us who we are. The morally barren and impoverished ethics of indifference promoted by isolating, disenfranchising, and abandoning patients is no way to treat them as persons.[23]

Is Consent Futile?

Given the unacceptable consequences that result if we adopt the futility exception and presumed consent, we must ask what kind of consent will enable us to make decisions we need to make in a way that preserves our fundamental social values. To do that we must acknowledge what the decision not to resuscitate represents in the debate about how we set limits at the clinical and societal levels. It asks us, individually and collectively, to arrive at a consensus on how to integrate death and decisions about it into the legitimating values of our moral universe. Deciding what kind of life we want involves deciding what kind of death we can face.

To a society whose faith in medicine and whose commitment to the fundamental values of life and liberty has led it to declare that death, once a matter of fate, is now a matter of choice, how we want to allocate death represents the quintessential tragic choice.[24] It strikes at the heart of our strongest values—the Rule of Rescue, the presumption in favor of life—and at our deepest fears. Just when we most need to rely on our basic values to resolve this tragic choice, we find that death and decisions about it overwhelm medicine, life, and liberty. It is a choice we need, but do not want to make; it concerns values we want to hold onto absolutely, but cannot; and it forces us either to admit a truth that seems unbearable or hide it beneath illusions that preserve the moral foundations of social collaboration.

The futility exception is one such illusion. It preserves our faith in medicine, harmoniously reconciles a fundamentally irreconcilable clash of values, and cloaks a decision about allocating death behind a decision about resuscitation. As we have seen, it is a dishonest solution and unless those basic values change it is only a matter of time before it is exposed for illusion. When that happens, the tragic choice resurfaces, as it did in the *Wanglie* case, and we grope for other subterfuges we hope will do the trick, of which denying the personhood of the unconscious is one and leaving these decisions entirely to "patient self-determination" is another.

Because we cannot make death go away, we cannot keep the tragic choice from resurfacing. This means that we must either adopt subterfuge after dishonest subterfuge—and accept the moral erosion each illusion's failure causes—or decide to make these decisions openly and honestly. If we wish to remain true to the values served by consent and respect for persons, we must opt in favor of candor. Once we opt in favor of candor the answer to our question becomes ironically clear: consent is useful *because* resuscitation is futile.

Difficult though saying no to patients is, the dangers that flow from saying nothing at all are far worse. Obscuring the basis of decisionmaking will generate fear and misunderstanding and lead to abuse, especially of those groups within society traditionally subjected to neglect and mistreatment. Deciding to withhold or limit resuscitation asks us to accept the self-limiting condition of our mortality; deciding to forgo consent asks us to deny the basic values that define us as a society.

Forging a consensus about matters of clinical and social importance requires trust and honesty, and the current posture of the debate suggests that no one trusts anyone to make these decisions. The truth is, however, that we must trust ourselves to make them together, setting aside our fear and mistrust, and conversing openly and respectfully with each other.

For that conversation to occur, we will have to talk in ways we are unaccustomed to. Patients can no more marginalize the legitimate concerns physicians have about their integrity and the need to set reasonable limits than physicians can dismiss patients through the futility exception. Each must give up some autonomy to overcome the barriers that currently serve only to separate us from each other and prevent us from making decisions we need to make together. We must integrate a relational perspective into how we see ourselves and each other.[25] Thus, we must talk about rights in a different way. Instead of trumping them out as conversation-stoppers, we must use them—and the values they express—as the starting point for a conversation about how we can best reconcile our individual wants with our collective needs.

We might well turn a conversation about futility to a useful purpose, by deciding to place less emphasis on death-defying interventions and to put more effort into life-enhancing ones, such as preventive and public health measures, chronic and rehabilitative care, and improved access to care. Not only would this be attentive to patient well-being and autonomy, it might also generate renewed and more heartfelt respect for medicine and physicians.

The question is not whether we can, should, or must make caring and conversation integral to how we decide matters of clinical and social importance, but whether we will. If we do, the hour of our death need no longer be anguished, angry, or lonely.[26]

Acknowledgment

This article is dedicated to the memory of Shirley Katzenbach.

QUESTIONS FOR CONSIDERATION

1. What is the distinction that Scofield draws between the visibility of consent in withholding treatment in contrast to intervening or withdrawing treatment? How does the DNR order illustrate this distinction?

2. How does Scofield characterize the impact of CPR upon the expectations of medicine? Why has CPR's significance exempted it from prior consent?
3. What are the arguments that Scofield suggests would make consent pointless if CPR is futile? What are his criticisms of these arguments?
4. Characterize Scofield's concept of respect for persons. How would presumed consent express disrespect for persons?
5. What are the criticisms that Scofield makes against the medical profession for its use of the futility exception? Do you agree that these criticisms are fair?
6. What kind of consent would Scofield consider to be appropriate for meaningful communication?

NOTES

1. Robert H. Block, *Rationing Medicine* (New York: Columbia University Press, 1988); Daniel Callahan, *Setting Limits* (New York: Simon & Schuster, 1987); Larry R. Churchill, *Rationing Health Care in America* (Notre Dame, Ind.: University of Notre Dame, 1987).

2. Howard Brody, "Transparency: Informed Consent in Primary Care," *Hastings Center Report* 19, no. 5 (1989): 5–9; Marion Danis and Larry R. Churchill, "Autonomy and the Common Weal," *Hastings Center Report* 21, no. 1 (1991): 25–29.

3. Bernard Lo and Albert R. Jonsen, "Clinical Decisions to Limit Treatment," *Annals of Internal Medicine* 93, no. 5 (1980): 764–68; President's Commission for the Study of Ethical Problems in Medicine and Biomedical and Behavioral Research, *Deciding to Forego Life-Sustaining Treatment* (Washington, D.C.: U.S. Government Printing Office, 1983), pp. 73–77.

4. George E. Taffet, Thomas A. Teasdale, and Robert Luchi, "In-Hospital Cardiopulmonary Resuscitation," *JAMA* 260, no. 14 (1988): 2069–72; Peter Safar, "Resuscitation from Clinical Death: Pathophysiologic Limits and Therapeutic Potentials," *Critical Care Medicine* 16, no. 10 (1988): 923–41; Richard O. Cummins, Kaye Chesemore, Roger D. White et al., "Defibrillator Failures," *JAMA* 264, no. 8 (1990): 1019–25.

5. President's Commission, *Deciding to Forego Life-Sustaining Treatment*, pp. 231–58.

6. Donald J. Murphy, "Do-Not-Resuscitate Orders: Time for Reappraisal in Long-Term-Care Institutions," *JAMA* 260, no. 14 (1988): 2098–2101; Leslie I. Blackhall, "Must We Always Use CPR?" *NEJM* 317, no. 20 (1987): 1281–84; Tom Tomlinson and Howard Brody, "Ethics and Communication in Do-Not-Resuscitate Orders," *NEJM* 318, no. 1 (1988): 43–46; Tom Tomlinson and Howard Brody, "Futility and the Ethics of Communication," *JAMA* 264, no. 10 (1990):1276–80; J. Chris Hackler and Charles Hiller, "Family Consent to Orders Not to Resuscitate," *JAMA* 264, no. 10 (1990): 1281–83; Lawrence J. Schneiderman, Nancy S. Jecker, and Albert R. Jonsen, "Medical Futility: Its Meaning and Implications," *Annals of Internal Medicine* 112, no. 12 (1990): 949–54.

7. Peter Safar and Nicholas G. Bircher, *Cardiopulmonary Cerebral Resuscitation* (Philadelphia: Saunders, 1988); Jeffrey Hammond and C. Gillon Ward, "Decision Not to Treat: 'Do Not Resuscitate' Order for the Burn Patient in the Acute Setting," *Critical Care Medicine* 17, no. 2 (1989): 136–38.

8. John D. Lantos, Peter A. Singer, Robert M. Walker et al., "The Illusion of Futility in Clinical Practice," *American Journal of Medicine* 87, no. 1 (1989): 81–84; Lawrence J. Nelson,

"Primum Utilis Esse: The Primacy of Usefulness in Medicine, *Yale Journal of Biology and Medicine* 51, no. 6 (1978): 655–67; Donald J. Murphy and David B. Matchar, "Life-Sustaining Therapy: A Model for Appropriate Use," *JAMA* 264, no. 16 (1990):2103–8; AMA Council on Ethical and Judicial Affairs, "Guidelines for the Appropriate Use of Do-Not-Resuscitate Orders," *JAMA* 265, no. 14 (1991): 1869–71.

9. Robert M. Wachter, John M. Luce, Norman Hearst et al., "Decisions about Resuscitation: Inequities among Patients with Different Diseases but Similar Prognoses," *Annals of Internal Medicine* 111, no. 6 (1989): 525–32.

10. Daniel Callahan, "Values, Facts and Decisionmaking," *Hastings Center Report* 1 no. 1 (June 1971): 1.

11. John La Puma, Marc D. Silverstein, Carol B. Stocking et. al., "Life-Sustaining Treatment: A Prospective Study of Patients with DNR Orders in a Teaching Hospital," *Archives of Internal Medicine* 148, no. 10 (1988): 2193–98.

12. *Payne v. Marion General Hospital,* 549 N.E.2d 1043 (Ind. Ct. App. 1990).

13. The National Commission for the Protection of Human Subjects of Biomedical and Behavioral Research, *The Belmont Report* (Washington D.C.: U.S. Government Printing Office, 1978), pp. 4–6.

14. Jay Katz and Alexander M. Capron, *Catastrophic Diseases: Who Decides What?* (New Brunswick, N.J.: Transaction Books, 1982), pp. 82–90.

15. Theodore J. Schneyer, "Informed Consent and the Danger of Bias in the Formation of Medical Disclosure Practices," *Wisconsin Law Review* (1976): 124–70; Dennis H. Novack, Barbara J. Detering, Robert Arnold et al., "Physicians' Attitudes Toward Using Deception to Resolve Difficult Ethical Problems," *JAMA* 261, no. 20 (1989): 2980–85.

16. Stuart J. Youngner, "Who Defines Futility,", *JAMA* 260, no. 14 (1988): 2094–95; Stuart J. Younger, "Futility in Context," *JAMA* 264, no.10 (1990):1295–96; Susan M. Wolf, "Conflict between Doctor and Patient," *Law, Medicine & Health Care* 16, nos. 3–4 (1988): 197–203.

17. Ronald S. Schonwetter, Thomas A. Teasdale, George Taffet et al., "Educating the Elderly: Cardiopulmonary Resuscitation Discussions before and after Intervention," *Journal of the American Geriatrics Society* 39, no. 4 (1991): 372–77.

18. Bernard Lo, "Unanswered Questions about DNR Orders," *JAMA* 265, no, 14 (1991): 1874–75; Raanan Gillon, "Deciding Not to Resuscitate," *Journal of Medical Ethics* 15, no.4 (1989): 171–72; Giles R. Scofield, "Terminal Care and the Continuing Need for Professional Education," *Journal of Palliative Care* 5, no. 3 (1989): 32–36.

19. Paul Starr, *The Social Transformation of American Medicine* (New York: Basic Books, 1982), pp. 3–29; Eliot Freidson, *Professional Dominance: The Social Structure of Medical Care* (New York: Atherton, 1970).

20. Kathleen Nolan, "In Death's Shadow: The Meanings of Withholding Resuscitation," *Hastings Center Report* 17, no. 6 (1987): 9–14; Jay Katz, *The Silent World of Doctor and Patient* (New York: Free Press, 1984), pp. 213–25.

21. Eliot Freidson, *Profession of Medicine* (New York: Harper & Row, 1970), pp. 335–52; Michael Walzer, *Spheres of Justice* (New York: Basic Books, 1983), pp. 155–60, 284–90.

22. Michael Ignatieff, *The Needs of Strangers* (New York: Penguin Books, 1986), pp. 76–79.

23. Elizabeth V. Spelman, "On Treating Persons as Persons," *Ethics* 88, no. 2 (1978): 150–61.

24. Guido Calabresi and Philip Bobbit, *Tragic Choices* (New York: W.W. Norton & Co., 1978), pp. 17–28; Guido Calabresi, *Ideals, Beliefs, Attitudes and the Law* (Syracuse, N.Y.: Syracuse University Press, 1985), pp. 87–117; Peter L. Berger and Thomas Luckman, *The Social Construction of Reality* (New York: Doubleday, 1966), 101–2.

25. Daniel Callahan, "Autonomy: A Moral Good, Not an Obsession," *Hastings Center Report* 14, no. 5 (1984): 40–42; Martha Minow, *Making All the Difference* (Ithaca: Cornell

University Press, 1990); Robert N. Bellah, Richard Madsen, William Sullivan et al., *Habits of the Heart* (Berkeley and Los Angeles: University of California Press, 1985).

26. William F. May, "On Not Facing Death Alone," *Hastings Center Report* 18, no. 1 (1971): 2–3; Philip Aries, *The Hour of Our Death* (New York: Alfred A. Knopf, 1981), pp. 611–14.

KATHLEEN NOLAN

In Death's Shadow: The Meanings of Withholding Resuscitation

Death's permanence bounds life's transience and consists of irreversible losses of bodily functions. At the borders of irreversibility, however, lie shadowy regions where functions may be lost and regained, and where modern resuscitative skills interrupt cycles of functional loss that once led inevitably to death. The battle in the shadows appears to be with death itself, since until the advent of modern techniques of cardiopulmonary resuscitation, death's permanence was manifest in the absence of heartbeat and respiration.

Cardiac or respiratory arrest in a hospitalized patient generally initiates a swirl of activity. Doctors, nurses, and technicians, some wheeling carts equipped for electrical defibrillation, endotracheal intubation, and massive pharmacologic intervention, swarm to the bedside and immediately begin resuscitation. The patient, who appears dead, may yet be wrested from the shadows.

These portrayals of resuscitation and its withholding, like any others, reveal much more than just the events depicted. The description implies meanings beyond the mere actions, meanings implied in word choice and emphasis that suggest the character of the author and are partially created by the understanding of the audience.

None of this should be unexpected since language and meaning always intertwine. Words are symbols, their meanings "constituted by the ideas, images, and emotions" raised in the mind of the hearer.[1] "Language is the light of the emotions," and is "essentially symbolic." The obvious or literal meanings of words also point analogically to other, latent meanings, which linger almost subliminally in the etymologies, associations, interrelationships, and interdependence of words and other structures of language. The enigmatic quality of word-symbols makes them opaque to attempts at direct intellectual mastery, and enables them to manifest tensions, ambiguities, conflicts, and subconscious meanings. In an analogous sense, actions also carry symbolic meanings that are perceived and interpreted variously by observers with differing perspectives. Meanings, that is, are generated contextually. Because symbolic meanings are often "spontaneously formed and immediately significant," they have a uniquely revelatory character.[2]

Exploring the language and contexts of resuscitation and resuscitative decisionmaking illuminates some of the many controversies generated by the withholding of resuscitation. If resuscitation and its withholding have multiple, and sometimes conflicting meanings for patients, families, and clinicians, then recognizing this divergence is essential to communication and to decisionmaking. To understand a phenomenon, one must understand its language and its symbols.

A decision not to resuscitate short circuits this otherwise reflex-like response to cardiopulmonary arrest. In these cases, the arrest brings no summons to medical personnel, no rush of activity, no resuscitation. The patient's family and nurse wait gravely and quietly at the bedside for a doctor who will not resuscitate the patient but pronounce him dead. Unresisted, the shadows give way to darkness.

Symbolic Aspects of Resuscitation

In many ways resuscitation is similar to other treatments,[3] yet somehow it is experienced as dramatically different. Many clinicians find a decision not to resuscitate much more difficult than one to withhold chemotherapy or to forgo palliative surgery. Many patients and families also seem to find the decision to forgo resuscitation particularly troubling. Discussions of resuscitation rarely fail to generate strong emotions, some puzzling and unexpected.

The roots of these reactions may lie in the symbolic weightiness of the revival of a patient who appears and may be thought to be dead. Historically, loss of cardiac and respiratory function has defined, from the moment of its occurrence, an irreversible condition: death. A person whose heart no longer beat and who no longer breathed was dead.

The advent of modern resuscitative techniques changed this reality, giving resuscitation a curious and symbolically problematic kinship with death. The ability to succeed with resuscitation has forced definitions of death to incorporate the additional element of duration. "Death" no longer necessarily occurs at the instant the heart and lungs cease to function. In fact, the potential reversibility of loss of cardiopulmonary function makes it impossible ever to identify a precise moment of death. The pulseless and breathless patient appears dead, *is dead* at a symbolic level, if not in reality. Thus resuscitation seems to restore cardiopulmonary function in patients who have already "died." Were this true, it would indeed be "miraculous."

This underlying ambiguity about whether death has occurred generates subconscious conflicts that are revealed in the language of resuscitation. To resuscitate is to revive, to reanimate, to restore or to renew (life), to revitalize.[4] Note the conspicuous absence of "to resurrect" as a synonym. Scientific understanding combines with subconscious pressure to create a tacit prohibition on the use of the mythical or religious language of "resurrection" to describe the medical revival of a person thought to be dead. Here language protects against symbolism. In prohibiting the language of the miraculous, we deny the powerful and pervasive symbolism of resurrection embodied in every act of restoring circulation and respiration ("life") to one who was pulseless and breathless ("dead").

Language betrays itself, however, and the symbolism of miracles and magic surreptitiously insinuates itself into descriptions of resuscitation and related medical technologies. Consider the ubiquity of the phrase "the miracles of modern medicine" and the perception that doctors are "playing God." One of the pioneers in developing the modern defibrillator, Paul Zoll, expressed a curious queasiness about his "interference with destiny" when he kept a patient with partial heart-block alive (fully alert and responsive) by means of repeated external electrical stimulations.[5]

Medical terminology associated with resuscitation often compounds the confusion. Patients are said to be "brought back to life,"[6] and clinicians treat "recurrent sudden death."[7] What can it mean when clinicians claim to resuscitate "dead" patients?[8] On a symbolic level, resurrection subsists within these striking linguistic lapses.

The miracle of resuscitation lies in its symbolic control over death. This is dangerously potent symbolism, for it seemingly implies concomitant control over the illnesses causing death, that is, the ability to cure. Patients desperately wish for modern technology to extend clinicians' power over death and illness, and the symbolic features of resuscitation do little to dispel such hopes.

In resuscitative attempts, physicians probe death's interface with life, battle death close within its shadows, and having violated these taboos, casually ignore death's intimate embrace, whether the patient does or not. Physicians are taught to be comfortable in this role. Beginning with their anatomical dissections in medical school, they penetrate death's mysteries in ways forbidden to the uninitiated.[9] Their attitudes and actions subconsciously foster the mysteriousness of resuscitation.

When a hospitalized patient requires resuscitation, doors are closed, screens are placed, family and friends are ushered outside into a corridor or waiting room, and an emergency summons to other medical personnel is sounded over the hospital's public address system in the form of a "code."[10] These practices, ostensibly justified by desires not to flaunt one patient's possible death in front of others and not to offend the sensibilities of those unaccustomed to medicine's goriness and bodily invasiveness, are revealing. Resuscitative efforts take place within a context of secrecy and have a palpably violent quality.

Beneficent Violence

Much of medical and surgical practice displays a similar violent quality. Were it not for their beneficent purpose, many procedures and treatments would be perceived as brutal and violent assaults.[11] The moral meaning of these actions derives from their beneficent intent at the rational level, but the perception of violence may register at the symbolic level. A hospital-based resuscitation exhibits this tension at its worst. The distinctions between objective and subjective meanings, between reality and symbol, blur when medical personnel are called upon to insert tubes into the patient's nose, mouth, and assorted veins, to thump and then rhythmically pound the patient's chest, to administer sufficient electrical current to the patient's heart to jerk the rest of the body from the bed, to inject fluids, blood, and potent pharmaco-logic agents into the patient's vessels and heart, and in some instances to slice open the patient's chest and squeeze the heart's chambers directly. Nurses dispense drugs and equipment from a "crash" cart and the "code" brings assistance to the "arrest" as if to a request for help put out over a police frequency.

Another unnerving symbolism accompanies these violent images. A vague sexuality attends the rhythmic pressure against the patent's body, the insertion of tubes and instruments, and the mouth-to-mouth respiration often required. This symbolic intimacy parallels biblical accounts of miraculous revivals, where prayer, physical presence, and often embrace were needed for the expression and flow of resuscitative power:

> "He went in . . . and prayed to Yahweh. Then he climbed on the bed and stretched himself on top of the child, putting his mouth on his mouth, his eyes to his eyes, and his hands on his hands, and as he lowered himself on to him, the child's flesh grew warm . . . . Then the child sneezed and opened his eyes."[12]

Further confusion flows from the coping mechanisms required to defuse resuscitation's symbolic pressures. Although medical personnel can be persuaded that these procedures are justified in their attempt to save a patent's life, a natural aversion to engaging in violent or sexual attacks on patients presses them to cope by adopting a depersonalizing attitude toward the patient. Depersonalizing the patent during resuscitation, as during surgery, is desirable, and perhaps psychologically necessary, to facilitate provision of needed treatment. In the context of a resuscitative attempt this is aided by the corpse-like appearance of the patient. Unfortunately, it adds to the pre-existing confusion about whether the patient is, in fact, a corpse.

Resuscitation and the Meaning of Death

For nonprofessionals, the emotional response to resuscitative activities is more diffuse. To them, reviving such "corpses" is perceived as stealing from death its role as the natural end of life. "Dying nowadays is more gruesome in many ways, namely, more lonely, mechanical, and dehumanized; at times it is even difficult to determine technically when the time of death has occurred."[13] Resuscitation, in particular, can preempt the dramatic flourish of a dying person's last breath. A sense of anticlimax intrudes when the patient "breathes his last" and is then resuscitated. If death is an acceptable and sometimes desirable feature of life, resuscitation may be unwelcome. As Sir MacFarlane Burnet put it, "Doctors should not compel . . . people to die more than once."[14]

In all this resuscitation comes to mean interference. There is a nostalgic longing for a "normal" or "physiological" death, like that of Oliver Wendell Holmes's famous "one-hoss shay," where all tissues wear out at a harmonious rate.[15] Resuscitation conflicts with important meanings derived from a recognition of the value of so-called "death work" at the end of life. This death work involves a summing up, a leavetaking, a molding of one's death to fit one's identity and individuality—a desire to make one's death one's own.[16] The urge to set wrongs to right before dying may lead to important reconciliations, and subtle forms of saying farewell may cement for the dying person and survivors their shared relational identities. From this vantage, death meets defeat not at the hands of modern technology but at the hands of friendship or religious belief. The patient survives in family, friends, and perhaps God. Within this context, "death is no struggle, nor is it a state of indecision or fear. Instead it seems a desired state. . . ."[17]

Whether and when to cease the struggle against death is the implicit but rarely articulated question in resuscitative decisions. Implicit assumptions about the meaning of death coupled with unexamined responses to the underlying symbolic features of resuscitation probably account for many otherwise inexplicable attitudes and actions. Cardiopulmonary arrest, like extremely abnormal serum potassium or calcium levels, or uremia, can lead to death if uninterrupted, or can be treated, with function lost and then regained. Yet clinicians and families will sometimes withhold or partially withhold resuscitation when not withholding other treatments because they feel that in undergoing cardiopulmonary arrest the patient has *died* despite everything they could do. The concrete symbolism of death embodied in a now pulseless, immobile body sometimes triggers no or only token resuscitative attempts for patients whose electrolyte abnormalities would have been promptly corrected.

On the other hand, some clinicians purposefully ignore electrolyte or other abnormalities in dying patients, yet insist upon (token) attempts at resuscitation in the form of so-called "slow" or "light blue" codes.[18] In these cases, resuscitation serves as a subterfuge, protecting family members and medical personnel from experiencing fully their "failure" in having been unable to prevent the patient's death. The last minute flare of glory of an attempted resuscitation exorcises blame: death has its due only by defeating the best of medicine's technology, wielded by the most powerful of clinician-priests. Ultimately, everyone else "blames the victim" for dying. The patient alone has failed. Even a miracle was not enough.

Emotional Features of Resuscitation

Symbolic meanings invoke emotions without allowing easy access to intellectual resolution. Since the intellect sees only "reality," and actively attempts to strip away nonrational meanings, symbolically potent words and activities may arouse vaguely recognized and poorly understood tensions. Recognizing the symbolic dimension of resuscitation thus helps illuminate the often wrenching quality of emotions evoked by resuscitation in contrast to other potential therapies. For example, would a patient be said to risk "dying twice" if an emergency surgical procedure restarted failed kidneys?

Attempts at resuscitation, like "last ditch" surgical attempts, carry risks of the most fearful aspects of impending death: pain, isolation, violence, and loss of control. Beyond their bodily invasiveness, both carry an uncertainty of outcome that deprives the patient's death of any predictability. That family and friends must be excluded from the patient's presence precisely when death is most likely heightens the isolating and alienating aspects of both surgery and resuscitation.

These considerations underlie the historically well-accepted notion of surgical "inoperability." Many patients are not considered candidates for surgical intervention because their risk of dying during the procedure is seen as counterbalancing any good that could be accomplished. The patient's fear of "dying under the knife" parallels the surgeon's reluctance to assume what may appear to be a causal role in the death of an unstable patient. Hence, few debate the merits of withholding surgery from certain patients, and discussion of this issue seems fairly straightforward. Yet despite their similarities, deciding against resuscitation is much more difficult than deciding against surgery.

Here the importance of resuscitation's symbolic potency becomes clear. The threat of surgery exists only if a patient decides to "undergo the knife." Forgoing surgery therefore brings a certain comfort; the patient is spared the burden and the risk of incision and dissection, with its symbolism of a brutal attack on the body.

With resuscitation, on the other hand, there is no symbolically safe ground. Because it symbolically is a priestly function, patients and family can experience discussions of withholding resuscitation as threatening abandonment or excommunication. This is especially likely when the reasons for withholding are unclear, or if other more painful or less potentially effective treatment's have continued. Also, the emergency character of resuscitation conveys an urgency that the "elective" quality of proposed surgery lacks. If surgery is withheld, there is always a *risk* of death, while if resuscitation is withheld, there is a certainty of death.

These features make it extremely difficult for clinicians to discuss resuscitation with patients, even when they advocate patient decision-making. Many clinicians shrink from the task of educating the patient thoroughly in the nature of the procedures involved. How can clinicians articulate their experience of the events at the symbolic level? How can they be fair to their experience of the reality if they do not?

Resuscitation and the General Aims of Management

Failure to attend to the symbolic features of resuscitation directly also creates confusion in determining whether decisionmaking should focus on resuscitation as an issue separate from other aims of management. Proponents of such a separation seek to allay fears about potential withdrawal of other sorts of medical care.[19] They also see in such a separation the clearest protection of the patient's autonomy and decisionmaking right. Others are troubled by inconsistencies in treatment plans that result from isolating decisions about resuscitation from other decisions about care.[20] They suspect that considering resuscitation in isolation neither insures autonomy nor fosters good decision-making.

The temptation to focus narrowly on resuscitation arises from a failure to appreciate its pragmatic continuity with other forms of treatment. Although uniquely powerful on the symbolic level, resuscitation, like other medical interventions, is also a practical medical response to an altered physiologic state.

For most types of therapy a decision about the overall goal of therapy seems to imply certain attitudes toward component therapies. Thus, there is no need for separate attention to "Decisions to Withhold Steroids," "Decisions to Withhold Parenteral Nutrition," or "Decisions to Withhold Lymphocyte Transfusions." Such therapies are generally evaluated directly on the basis of their role in global management plans that define the overall goal(s) of treatment, usually stated in terms of curing or restoring function, prolonging survival, or maintaining comfort.[21] The appropriateness of any proposed therapeutic maneuver is defined by its ability to advance the identified management objectives. This is typical medical logic: the goal is specified first, and therapies are indicated if they serve as means to further the goal. Failure to place it in this framework leaves the clinician without a telos for resuscitation, and therefore without a pragmatic medical context to balance the symbolic.

Resuscitation can reasonably serve several different goals of medical management. Historically, resuscitation developed as a curative therapy; employed for persons previously healthy, it was a means to total cure. The first successful resuscitations were from near-drowning, and then from fibrillation caused by inhaled anesthetics or by electrocution.[22] In such settings, "resuscitation of the heart and lungs" was metonymous with "resuscitation of the entire person." Providing resuscitation in these settings has always seemed relatively unproblematic.

Resuscitation may also sustain life during a period of diagnosis or treatment of an underlying disease. Classic examples include patients resuscitated from drug overdoses or poisoning.[23] Here resuscitation may serve less as a treatment for the poisoning than as supportive therapy, insuring time for the natural resolution of the disease process or for institution of dialysis or other treatments. The use of resuscitation in the setting of coronary artery disease and myocardial infarction represents an extension of this principle. Although these patients may not be returned to full health, resuscitation is employed to serve an essentially curative goal.

In other settings, resuscitation functions less as a curative treatment than as a life-prolonging one. Like the surgical removal of only part of a deeply situated tumor, it temporizes, prolonging survival without improving the patient's underlying state of health. The main issue in withholding resuscitation, therefore, is not the "terminal" character of the illness, nor the "imminence" (by whatever definition) of death. Once resuscitation functions in the service of prolonged biologic function rather than of cure, its instrumental value shifts. If cure can be achieved, then pursuing this goal takes priority even if this entails major discomforts and risks, such as those that might accompany resuscitation. If curative therapies are unavailable or unacceptable to the patient, however, pursuing prolonged survival or comfort become the only options. Previously tacit understandings regarding risks and priorities must be explored critically because patients differ widely in their evaluations of the benefit of prolonged biologic survival and of the risks of potential life-prolonging treatments.

When not serving a curative goal, the usefulness of resuscitation must be assessed with attention to the patent's understanding of it on both an instrumental and a symbolic level. To do this well, clinicians must be willing to engage in a process of decisionmaking that stretches the notion of informed consent to the maximum.

Clinician and patient often share common understandings about the risks or side effects of many kinds of medical and surgical therapy, and understand the value of a treatment in terms of its instrumental utility, its ability to accomplish its intended goals. With resuscitation, on the other hand, the intrusion of idiosyncratic interpretations is virtually guaranteed, because for different patients, clinicians, and contexts, the meaning of resuscitation partakes to varying degrees in symbols of miracle, abandonment, brutality, isolation, and the separation of the soul from the body in death.

On the symbolic level, patients may have unique fears and desires that make resuscitation personally undesirable. A patient might fear resuscitation because it symbolizes abandonment at the time of death for example. On such grounds, it might be reasonable to include in the management plan all other major intensive care procedures, but to exclude resuscitation.[24]

In the majority of cases, however, emotional or symbolic grounds for decisionmaking are rarely explored. This may leave decisionmaking fragmented and inconsistent, and the patient's emotional needs neglected or misunderstood. If, for example, the basis for the decision is never articulated, the patient who rejected resuscitation out of fear that it would mean a death among strangers might still die in the intensive care unit at night with family never called in from the waiting room. A preferable approach would include frank discussion of the potential meanings of resuscitation on both the instrumental and symbolic levels so that its role in the patient's management meshes with other goals.

Involving Patients in Decisionmaking

Failure to recognize the potential symbolic meanings of resuscitation and to locate resuscitation clearly in a comprehensive management plan leads to great difficulty in discussions with patients. Lacking a means to articulate vaguely perceived distinctions between resuscitation and other interventions, a clinician may stumble haltingly through a confused and painful discussion. And he or she may end up presenting conclusions based on a sincere but slightly misguided intuition that this conversation concerns something more important than simply deciding about the use of steroids. Further, as the patient's condition and options, not to mention understanding and evaluations, are far from static, discussions must continue throughout a given hospitalization.

The need for continuing communication obviates any serious consideration of recent proposals to have all patients sign a form expressing decisions for or against resuscitation at the time of admission to the hospital.[25] Collapsing all the dialogue that should transpire over time into a single session, especially when focused on obtaining a signature on a piece of paper, mocks the essential sharing of information and values necessary to identify appropriate goals for this individual patient in these unique circumstances at this particular time. The delicate weighing of symbolic and other values required to develop a suitable management plan in situations where curative therapies are unavailable or unacceptable can hardly take place in an instant, and certainly cannot be communicated in one.

In addition, for most patients entering a hospital the issue of resuscitation is essentially vacuous, either because they are at small risk of cardiopulmonary arrest or because the nature of their treatment (elective surgery, for example) presupposes a willingness to accept emergency therapies necessary for their successful recovery. Of course, if a patient objects to the use of resuscitative techniques under any circumstances, then this must be announced at the outset. However, few patients object to resuscitation in settings where it has obvious curative value.

Discussions of resuscitation should use the clearest language possible. Because the goal is to understand each particular patient's goals and perspectives, clinicians should avoid summary terms such as "extraordinary measures" and "heroics." Both terms are fraught with ambiguity, and try to encapsulate too tidily extremely complicated concepts. Because the terms lack specific content, patients and clinicians may agree on "no heroics" or "no extraordinary means," only to discover later that each meant something quite different by the term. "Aggressive therapy" is another ambiguous term that frequently carries unintended connotations. "Aggressive" therapies would better be called "invasive" therapies since they range from surgery through cardiopulmonary resuscitation to nasogastric or intravenous feeding, and have in common *invasion* of the patient's bodily integrity. This may evoke images of aggression, but it does a disservice to medicine not to distinguish attack on the disease from attack on the patient. Here again, conscious and subconscious fears evoked by careless use of language may hinder the difficult, concrete evaluations of therapeutic worth that should be taking place.[26] Using language carefully is essential to advancing the "fundamental goal of allowing patents to participate in decisions about the circumstance of their death."[27]

Directions for the Future

When resuscitation broke from its historic roots as a specific treatment of a basic disease process and took on the additional roles of temporizing or palliative treatment, considerations of the relative values of life, death, mentation, biological survival, and comfort insinuated themselves into evaluations of the worth of the treatment. During the past quarter century, decisionmaking regarding resuscitation became necessary. Yet, resuscitation has not broken with its linguistic and symbolic roots as easily as it did from its historic roots. The symbolic power of resuscitation still looms large, and return from a pulseless and nonbreathing state will probably never fail to appear miraculous.

The importance of distinguishing symbolic or emotional concerns about resuscitation from more instrumental or pragmatic concerns suggests the possibility of a larger role for spiritual or psychological counseling as a part of or as a supplement to usual medical discussions of these issues. This may require expanding the care team, or expanding the individual clinician's concept of medical care.[28] At the very least, it involves suspending the quest for simple solutions or algorithms as substitutes for painstaking attention to the hopes and beliefs of individual patients.

In addition, awareness of the subliminal tensions and confusions associated with resuscitation and do-not-resuscitate decisions can ground more direct

•

examinations of unresolved substantive and procedural disputes. Clinicians should acknowledge the powerful emotional effects of discussing resuscitation, and should exercise care in the language they use to clarify their own and their patients' understandings of its relation to death and its potential role in therapy. Grounded in a common understanding and shared vocabulary, remaining controversies about resuscitation can proceed, not in the form of miscommunications and misconceptions, but in the form of true conflicts in values.

QUESTIONS FOR CONSIDERATION

1. Do you agree with Nolan that the symbolic association of resuscitation with miracles, magic and resurrection causes it to be experienced dramatically different by patients, family, and clinicians than other forms of therapy?

2. What did Nolan mean by the expression "beneficent violence" associated with resuscitation?

3. In what ways does Nolan characterize resuscitation as creating confusion over the meaning of death?

4. Nolan raises the question, how can clinicians articulate their experience of the events [resuscitation] at the symbolic level?" How would you answer that question?

5. Should resuscitation be evaluated separately from other therapies within a global management plan of treatment?

6. Nolan concludes by noting that symbolic or emotional concerns rather than pragmatic concerns regarding resuscitation suggest a larger role for spiritual or psychological counseling. Would such counseling be more appropriate for the clergy or psychologists than clinicians?

NOTES

1. Alfred N. Whitehead, *Symbolism: Its Meaning and Effect* (New York: Capricorn Books, 1972).

2. Paul Ricoeur, *The Symbolism of Evil* (Boston: Beacon, 1967).

3. "Standards and Guidelines for Cardiopulmonary Resuscitation (CPR) and Emergency Cardiac Care (ECC)," *Journal of the American Medical Association* 255:21 (June 6, 1986), 2905–84.

4. *Webster's New Collegiate Dictionary*, s.v. "resuscitate."

5. Paul M. Zoll, "The First Successful External Cardiac Stimulation and A-C Defibrillation," in *Advances in Cardiopulmonary Resuscitation*, ed. Peter Safar (New York: Springer-Verlag, 1977), 282.

6. J.W. Pearson, *Historical and Experimental Approaches to Modern Resuscitation* (Springfield, IL: Charles C. Thomas, 1965).

7. Elliot Rappaport, "Recurrent Sudden Death," *New England Journal of Medicine* 306: (1982), 1359–60.

8. D.K. Brooks, *Resuscitation* (London: Edward Arnold, 1967).

9. A.M. Kasper, "The Doctor and Death," in *The Meaning of Death,* ed. Herman Feifel (New York: McGraw-Hill, 1959).

10. Steven S. Spencer, "'Code' or 'No Code,' a Nonlegal Opinion," *New England Journal of Medicine* 300:3 (January 18, 1979), 138–40.

11. Talcott Parsons, *Social Structure and Personality* (Glencoe, IL: Free Press, 1964).

12. 2 Kings 4:29–35.

13. Elisabeth Kubler-Ross, *On Death and Dying* (New York: Macmillan, 1969), 8.

14. Ned H. Cassem, "Confronting the Decision to Let Death Come," *Critical Care Medicine* 2:3 (May–June, 1974), 113.

15. Lewis Thomas, "Notes of a Biology Watcher: The Deacon's Masterpiece," *New England Journal of Medicine* 292:2 (January 9, 1975), 93–95.

16. Elisabeth Kubler-Ross, *On Death and Dying.*

17. A.A. Hutschnecker, "Personality Factors in Dying Patients," in *The Meaning of Death,* ed. Herman Feifel (New York: McGraw-Hill, 1959), 246.

18. John Goldenring, "'Code' or 'No Code' Decision," *New England Journal of Medicine* 300:18 (May 3, 1979), 1058.

19. See, for example, Susanna E. Bedell, Denise Pelle, Patricia L. Maher, et al., "Do-Not-Resuscitate Orders for Critically Ill Patients in the Hospital: How Are They Used and What Is Their Impact?," *Journal of the American Medical Association* 256:2 (July 11, 1986), 233–37.

20. Robert M. Veatch, "Deciding against Resuscitation: Encouraging Signs and Potential Dangers," *Journal of the American Medical Association* 253:1 (January 4, 1985), 77–78.

21. Committee on Policy for DNR Decisions, Yale New Haven Hospital, "Report on Do Not Resuscitate Decisions," *Connecticut Medicine* 47:8 (August, 1983), 477–83.

22. D.K. Brooks, *Resuscitation.*

23. A. Barrington Baker, "Artificial Respiration, the History of an Idea," *Medical History* 15 (1971), 336–51.

24. Bernard Lo, Glenn Saika, William Strull, *et al.,* "'Do Not Resuscitate' Decisions: A Prospective Study at Three Teaching Hospitals," *Archives of Internal Medicine* 145 (June 1985), 115–17.

25. Ronald L. Stephens, "'Do Not Resuscitate Orders': Ensuring the Patient's Participation," *Journal of the American Medical Association* 255:2 (January 10, 1986), 240–41.

26. Robert J. Levine and Kathleen A. Nolan, "Do Not Resuscitate Decisions: A Policy," *Connecticut Medicine* 47:8 (August, 1983), 511–12.

27. David L. Jackson, Stuart J. Youngner, "Patient Autonomy and 'Death with Dignity': Some Clinical Caveats," *New England Journal of Medicine* 301:8 (Aug. 23, 1979), 404–408.

28. Eric J. Cassell, *The Healer's Art* (Cambridge, MA: M.I.T. Press, 1985).

JOANNE LYNN AND JAMES F. CHILDRESS

Must Patients Always Be Given Food and Water?

Many people die from the lack of food or water. For some, this lack is the result of poverty or famine, but for others it is the result of disease or deliberate decision. In the past, malnutrition and dehydration must have accompanied nearly every death that followed an illness of more than a few days. Most dying patients do not eat much on their own, and nothing could be done for them until the first flexible tubing for instilling food or other liquid into the stomach was developed about a hundred years ago. Even then, the procedure was so scarce, so costly in physician and nursing time, and so poorly tolerated that it was used only for patients who clearly could benefit. With the advent of more reliable and efficient procedures in the past few decades, these conditions can be corrected or ameliorated in nearly every patient who would otherwise be malnourished or dehydrated. In fact, intravenous lines and nasogastric tubes have become common images of hospital care.

Providing adequate nutrition and fluids is a high priority for most patients, both because they suffer directly from inadequacies and because these deficiencies hinder their ability to overcome other diseases. But are there some patients who need not receive these treatments? This question has become a prominent public policy issue in a number of recent cases. In May 1981, in Danville, Illinois, the parents and the physician of newborn conjoined twins with shared abdominal organs decided not to feed these children. Feeding and other treatments were given after court intervention, though a grand jury refused to indict the parents.[1] Later that year, two physicians in Los Angeles discontinued intravenous nutrition to a patient who had severe brain damage after an episode involving loss of oxygen following routine surgery. Murder charges were brought, but the hearing judge dismissed the charges at a preliminary hearing. On appeal, the charges were reinstated and remanded for trial.[2]

In April 1982, a Bloomington, Indiana, infant who had tracheoesophageal fistula and Down syndrome was not treated or fed, and he died after two courts ruled that the decision was proper but before all appeals could be heard.[3] When the federal government then moved to ensure that such infants would be fed in the future,[4] the Surgeon General, Dr. C. Everett Koop, initially stated that there is never adequate reason to deny nutrition and fluids to a newborn infant.

While these cases were before the public, the nephew of Claire Conroy, an elderly incompetent woman with several serious medical problems, petitioned a New Jersey court for authority to discontinue her nasogastric tube feedings. Although the intermediate appeals court has reversed the ruling,[5] the trial court held that he had this authority since the evidence indicated that the patient would not have wanted such treatment and that its value to her was doubtful.

In all these dramatic cases and in many more that go unnoticed, the decision is made to deliberately withhold food or fluid known to be necessary for the life of the patient. Such decisions are unsettling. There is now widespread consensus that sometimes a patient is best served by not undertaking or continuing certain treatments that would sustain life, especially if these entail substantial suffering.[6] But food and water are so central to an array of human emotions that it is almost impossible to consider them with the same emotional detachment that one might feel toward a respirator or a dialysis machine.

Nevertheless, the question remains: should it ever be permissible to withhold or withdraw food and nutrition? The answer in any real case should acknowledge the psychological contiguity between feeding and loving and between nutritional satisfaction and emotional satisfaction. Yet this acknowledgment does not resolve the core question.

Some have held that it is intrinsically wrong not to feed another. The philosopher G.E.M. Anscombe contends: "For wilful starvation there can be no excuse. The same can't be said quite without qualification about failing to operate or to adopt some courses of treatment."[7] But the moral issues are more complex than Anscombe's comment suggests. Does correcting nutritional deficiencies always improve patients' well-being? What should be our reflective moral response to withholding or withdrawing nutrition? What moral principles are relevant to our reflections? What medical facts about ways of providing nutrition are relevant? And what policies should be adopted by the society, hospitals, and medical and other health care professionals?

In our effort to find answers to these questions, we will concentrate upon the care of patients who are incompetent to make choices for themselves.

Patients who are competent to determine the course of their therapy may refuse any and all interventions proposed by others, as long as their refusals do not seriously harm or impose unfair burdens upon others.[8] A competent patient's decision regarding whether or not to accept the provision of food and water by medical means such as tube feeding or intravenous alimentation is unlikely to raise questions of harm or burden to others.

What then should guide those who must decide about nutrition for a patient who cannot decide? As a start, consider the standard by which other medical decisions are made: one should decide as the incompetent person would have if he or she were competent, when that is possible to determine, and advance that person's interests in a more generalized sense when individual preferences cannot be known.

The Medical Procedures

There is no reason to apply a different standard to feeding and hydration. Surely, when one inserts a feeding tube, or creates a gastrostomy opening, or inserts a needle into a vein, one intends to benefit the patient. Ideally, one should provide what the patient believes to be of benefit, but at least the effect should be beneficial in the opinions of surrogates and caregivers.

Thus, the question becomes: is it ever in the patient's interest to become malnourished and dehydrated, rather than to receive treatment? Posing the question so starkly points to our need to know what is entailed in treating these conditions and what benefits the treatments offer.

The medical interventions that provide food and fluids are of two basic types. First, liquids can be delivered by a tube that is inserted into a functioning gastrointestinal tract, most commonly through the nose and esophagus into the stomach or through a surgical incision in the abdominal wall and directly into the stomach. The liquids used can be specially prepared solutions of nutrients or a blenderized version of an ordinary diet. The nasogastric tube is cheap; it may lead to pneumonia and often annoys the patient and family, sometimes even requiring that the patient be restrained to prevent its removal.

Creating a gastrostomy is usually a simple surgical procedure, and, once the wound is healed, care is very simple. Since it is out of sight, it is aesthetically more acceptable and restraints are needed less often. Also, the gastrostomy creates no additional risk of pneumonia. However, while elimination of a nasogastric tube requires only removing the tube, a gastrostomy is fairly permanent, and can be closed only by surgery.

The second type of medical intervention is intravenous feeding and hydration, which also has two major forms. The ordinary hospital or peripheral

IV, in which fluid is delivered directly to the bloodstream through a small needle, is useful only for temporary efforts to improve hydration and electrolyte concentrations. One cannot provide a balanced diet through the veins in the limbs: to do that requires a central line, or a special catheter placed into one of the major veins in the chest. The latter procedure is much more risky and vulnerable to infections and technical errors, and it is much more costly than any of the other procedures. Both forms of intravenous nutrition and hydration commonly require restraining the patient, cause minor infections and other ill effects, and are costly, especially since they ordinarily require the patient to be in a hospital.

None of these procedures, then, is ideal; each entails some distress, some medical limitations, and some costs. When may a procedure be foregone that might improve nutrition and hydration for a given patient? Only when the procedure and the resulting improvement in nutrition and hydration do not offer the patient a net benefit over what he or she would otherwise have faced.

Are there such circumstances? We believe that there are; but they are few and limited to the following three kinds of situations: 1. The procedures that would be required are so unlikely to achieve improved nutritional and fluid levels that they could be correctly considered futile; 2. The improvement in nutritional and fluid balance, though achievable, could be of no benefit to the patient; 3. The burdens of receiving the treatment may outweigh the benefit.

When Food and Water May Be Withheld

Futile Treatment

Sometimes even providing "food and water" to a patient becomes a monumental task. Consider a patient with a severe clotting deficiency and a nearly total body burn. Gaining access to the central veins is likely to cause hemorrhage or infection, nasogastric tube placement may be quite painful, and there may be no skin to which to suture the stomach for a gastrostomy tube. Or consider a patient with severe congestive heart failure who develops cancer of the stomach with a fistula that delivers food from the stomach to the colon without passing through the intestine and being absorbed. Feeding the patient may be possible, but little is absorbed. Intravenous feeding cannot be tolerated because the fluid would be too much for the weakened heart. Or consider the infant with infarction of all but a short segment of bowel. Again, the infant can be fed, but little if anything is absorbed. Intravenous methods can be used, but only for a short time (weeks or months) until their complications, including thrombosis, hemorrhage, infections, and malnutrition, cause death.

In these circumstances, the patient is going to die soon, no matter what is done. The ineffective efforts to provide nutrition and hydration may well directly cause suffering that offers no counterbalancing benefit for the patient. Although the procedures might be tried, especially if the competent patient wanted them or the incompetent patient's surrogate had reason to believe that this incompetent patient would have wanted them, they cannot be considered obligatory. To hold that a patient must be subjected to this predictably futile sort of intervention just because protein balance is negative or the blood serum is concentrated is to lose sight of the moral warrant for medical care and to reduce the patient to an array of measurable variables.

No Possibility of Benefit

Some patients can be reliably diagnosed to have permanently lost consciousness. This unusual group of patients includes those with anencephaly, persistent vegetative state, and some preterminal comas. In these cases, it is very difficult to discern how any medical intervention can benefit or harm the patient. These patients cannot and never will be able to experience any of the events occurring in the world or in their bodies. When the diagnosis is exceedingly clear, we sustain their lives vigorously mainly for their loved ones and the community at large.

While these considerations probably indicate that continued artificial feeding is best in most cases, there may be some cases in which the family and the caregivers are convinced that artificial feeding is offensive and unreasonable. In such cases, there seems to be no adequate reason to claim that withholding food and water violates any obligations that these parties or the general society have with regard to permanently unconscious patients. Thus, if the parents of an anencephalic infant or of a patient like Karen Quinlan in a persistent vegetative state feel strongly that no medical procedures should be applied to provide nutrition and hydration, and the caregivers are willing to comply, there should be no barrier in law or public policy to thwart the plan.[9]

Disproportionate Burden

The most difficult cases are those in which normal nutritional status or fluid balance could be restored, but only with a severe burden for the patient. In these cases, the treatment is futile in a broader sense—the patient will not actually benefit from the improved nutrition and hydration. A patient who is competent can decide the relative merits of the treatment being provided, knowing the probable consequences, and weighing the merits of life under various sets of constrained circumstances. But a surrogate decision maker for a patient who is incompetent to decide will have a difficult task. When the situation is irremediably ambiguous, erring on the side of continued life and improved nutrition and hydration seems the less grievous error. But are there situations that would warrant a determination that this patient, whose nutrition and hydration could surely be improved, is not thereby well served?

Though they are rare, we believe there are such cases. The treatments entailed are not benign. Their effects are far short of ideal. Furthermore, many of the patients most likely to have inadequate food and fluid intake are also likely to suffer the most serious side effects of these therapies.

Patients who are allowed to die without artificial hydration and nutrition may well die more comfortably than patients who receive conventional amounts of intravenous hydration.[10] Terminal pulmonary edema, nausea, and mental confusion are more likely when patients have been treated to maintain fluid and nutrition until close to the time of death.

Thus, those patients whose "need" for artificial nutrition and hydration arises only near the time of death may be harmed by its provision. It is not at all clear that they receive any benefit in having a slightly prolonged life, and it does seem reasonable to allow a surrogate to decide that, for this patient at this time, slight prolongation of life is not warranted if it involves measures that will probably increase the patient's suffering as he or she dies.

Even patients who might live much longer might not be well served by artificial means to provide fluid and food. Such patients might include those with fairly severe dementia for whom the restraints required could be a constant source of fear, discomfort, and struggle. For such a patient, sedation to tolerate the feeding mechanisms might preclude any of the pleasant experiences that might otherwise have been available. Thus, a decision not to intervene, except perhaps briefly to ascertain that there are no treatable causes, might allow such a patient to live out a shorter life with fair freedom of movement and freedom from fear, while a decision to maintain artificial nutrition and hydration might consign the patient to end his or her life in unremitting anguish. If this were the case a surrogate decision maker would seem to be well justified in refusing the treatment.

Inappropriate Moral Constraints

Four considerations are frequently proposed as moral constraints on foregoing medical feeding and hydration. We find none of these to dictate that artificial nutrition and hydration must always be provided.

The Obligation to Provide "Ordinary" Care

Debates about appropriate medical treatment are often couched in terms of "ordinary" and "extraordinary" means of treatment. Historically, this distinction emerged in the Roman Catholic tradition to differentiate optional treatment from treatment that was obligatory for medical professionals to offer and for patients to accept.[11] These terms also appear in many secular contexts, such as court decisions and medical codes. The recent debates about ordinary and extraordinary means of treatment have been interminable and often unfruitful, in part because of a lack of clarity about what the terms mean. Do they represent the premises of an argument or the conclusion, and what features of a situation are relevant to the categorization as "ordinary" or "extraordinary"?[12]

Several criteria have been implicit in debates about ordinary and extraordinary means of treatment; some of them may be relevant to determining whether and which treatments are obligatory and which are optional. Treatments have been distinguished according to their simplicity (simple/complex), their naturalness (natural/artificial), their customariness (usual/unusual), their invasiveness (noninvasive/invasive), their chance of success (reasonable chance/futile), their balance of benefits and burdens (proportionate/disproportionate), and their expense (inexpensive/costly). Each set of paired terms or phrases in the parentheses suggests a continuum: as the treatment moves from the first of the paired terms to the second, it is said to become less obligatory and more optional.

However, when these various criteria, widely used in discussions about medical treatment, are carefully examined, most of them are not morally relevant in distinguishing optional from obligatory medical treatments. For example, if a rare, complex, artificial, and invasive treatment offers a patent a reasonable chance of nearly painless cure, then one would have to offer a substantial justification not to provide that treatment to an incompetent patient.

What matters, then, in determining whether to provide a treatment to an incompetent patient is not a prior determination that this treatment is "ordinary" per se, but rather a determination that this treatment is likely to provide this patient benefits that are sufficient to make it worthwhile to endure the burdens that accompany the treatment. To this end, some of the considerations listed above are relevant: whether a treatment is likely to succeed is an obvious example. But such considerations taken in isolation are not conclusive. Rather, the surrogate decision maker is obliged to assess the desirability to this patient of each of the options presented, including nontreatment. For most people at most times, this assessment would lead to a clear obligation to provide food and fluids.

But sometimes, as we have indicated, providing food and fluids through medical interventions may fail to benefit and may even harm some patients. Then the treatment cannot be said to be obligatory, no matter how usual and simple its provision may be. If "ordinary" and "extraordinary" are used to convey the conclusion about the obligation to treat, providing nutrition and fluids would have become, in these cases, "extraordinary." Since this phrasing is misleading, it is probably better to use "proportionate" and "disproportionate," as the Vatican now suggests,[13] or "obligatory" and "optional."

Obviously, providing nutrition and hydration may sometimes be necessary to keep patients comfortable while they are dying even though it may temporarily prolong their dying. In such cases, food and fluids constitute warranted palliative care. But in other cases, such as a patient in a deep and irreversible coma, nutrition and hydration do not appear to be needed or helpful, except perhaps to comfort the staff and family.[14] And sometimes the interventions needed for nutrition and hydration are so burdensome that they are harmful and best not utilized.

The Obligation to Continue Treatments Once Started

Once having started a mode of treatment, many caregivers find it very difficult to discontinue it. While this strongly felt difference between the ease of withholding a treatment and the difficulty of withdrawing it provides a psychological explanation of certain actions, it does not justify them. It sometimes even leads to a thoroughly irrational decision process. For example, in caring for a dying, comatose patient, many physicians apparently find it harder to stop a functioning peripheral IV than not to restart one that has infiltrated (that is, has broken through the blood vessel and is leaking fluid into surrounding tissue), especially if the only way to reestablish an IV would be to insert a central line into the heart or to do a cutdown (make an incision to gain access to the deep large blood vessels).[15]

What factors might make withdrawing medical treatment morally worse than withholding it? Withdrawing a treatment seems to be an action, which, when it is likely to end in death, initially seems more serious than an omission that ends in death. However, this view is fraught with errors. Withdrawing is not always an act: failing to put the next infusion into a tube could be correctly described as an omission, for example. Even when withdrawing is an act, it may well be morally correct and even morally obligatory. Discontinuing intravenous lines in a patient now permanently unconscious in accord with that patient's well-informed advance directive would certainly be such a case. Futhermore, the caregiver's obligation to serve the patient's interests through both acts and omissions rules out the exculpation that accompanies omissions in the usual course of social life. An omission that is not warranted by the patient's interests is culpable.

Sometimes initiating a treatment creates expectations in the minds of caregivers, patients, and family that the treatment will be continued indefinitely or until the patient is cured. Such expectations may provide a reason to continue the treatment as a way to keep a promise. However, as with all promises, caregivers could be very careful when initiating a treatment to explain the indications for its discontinuation, and they could modify preconceptions with continuing reevaluation and education during treatment. Though all patients are entitled to expect the continuation of care in the patient's best interests, they are not and should not be entitled to the continuation of a particular mode of care.

Accepting the distinction between withholding and withdrawing medical treatment as morally significant also has a very unfortunate implication: caregivers may become unduly reluctant to begin some treatments precisely because they fear that they will be locked into continuing treatments that are no longer of value to the patient. For example, the physician who had been unwilling to stop the respirator while the infant, Andrew Stinson, died over several months is reportedly "less eager to attach babies to respirators now."[16] But if it were easier to ignore malnutrition and dehydration and to withhold treatments for these problems than to discontinue the same treatments when they have become especially burdensome and insufficiently beneficial for this patient, then the incentives would be perverse. Once a treatment has been tried, it is often much clearer whether it is of value to this patient, and the decision to stop it can be made more reliably.

The same considerations should apply to starting as to stopping a treatment, and whatever assessment warrants withholding should also warrant withdrawing.

The Obligation to Avoid Being the Unambiguous Cause of Death

Many physicians will agree with all that we have said and still refuse to allow a choice to forego food and fluid because such a course seems to be a "death sentence." In this view death seems to be more certain from malnutrition and dehydration than from foregoing other forms of medical therapy. This implies that it is acceptable to act in ways that are likely to cause death, as in not operating on a gangrenous leg, only if there remains a chance that the patient will survive. This is a comforting formulation for caregivers, to be sure, since they can thereby avoid feeling the full weight of the responsibility for the time and manner of a patient's death. However, it is not a persuasive moral argument.

First, in appropriate cases discontinuing certain medical treatments is generally accepted despite the fact that death is as certain as with nonfeeding. Dialysis in a patient without kidney function or transfusions in a patient with severe aplastic anemia are obvious examples. The dying that awaits such patients often is not greatly different from dying of dehydration and malnutrition.

Second, the certainty of a generally undesirable outcome such as death is always relevant to a decision, but it does not foreclose the possibility that this course is better than others available to this patient.[17] Ambiguity and uncertainty are so common in medical decision making that caregivers are tempted to use them in distancing themselves from direct responsibility. However, caregivers are in fact responsible for the time and manner of death for many patients. Their distaste for this fact should not constrain otherwise morally justified decisions.

The Obligation to Provide Symbolically Significant Treatment

One of the most common arguments for always providing nutrition and hydration is that it symbolizes, expresses, or conveys the essence of care and compassion. Some actions not only aim at goals, they also express values. Such expressive actions should not simply be viewed as means to ends; they should also be viewed in light of what they communicate. From this perspective food and water are not only goods that preserve life and provide comfort; they are also symbols of care and compassion. To withhold or withdraw them—to "starve" a patient—can never express or convey care.

Why is providing food and water a central symbol of care and compassion? Feeding is the first response of the community to the needs of newborns and remains a central mode of nurture and comfort. Eating is associated with social interchange and community, and providing food for someone else is a way to create and maintain bonds of sharing and expressing concern. Furthermore, even the relatively low levels of hunger and thirst that most people have experienced are decidedly uncomfortable, and the common image of severe malnutrition or dehydration is one of unremitting agony. Thus, people are rightly eager to provide food and water. Such provision is essential to minimally tolerable existence and a powerful symbol of our concern for each other.

However, *medical* nutrition and hydration, we have argued, may not always provide net benefits to patients. Medical procedures to provide nutrition and hydration are more similar to other medical procedures than to typical human ways of providing nutrition and hydration, for example, a sip of water. It should be possible to evaluate their benefits and burdens, as we evaluate any other medical procedure. Of course, if family, friends, and caregivers feel that such procedures affirm important values even when they do not benefit the patient, their feelings should not be ignored. We do not contend that there is an obligation to withhold or to withdraw such procedures (unless consideration of the patient's advance directives or current best interest unambiguously dictates that conclusion); we only contend that nutrition and hydration may be foregone in some cases.

The symbolic connection between care and nutrition or hydration adds useful caution to decision making. If decision makers worry over withholding or withdrawing medical nutrition and hydration, they may inquire more seriously into the circumstances that putatively justify their decisions. This is generally salutary for health care decision making. The critical inquiry may well yield the sad but justified conclusion that the patient will be served best by not using medical procedures to provide food and fluids.

A Limited Conclusion

Our conclusion—that patients or their surrogates, in close collaboration with their physicians and other caregivers and with careful assessment of the relevant information, can correctly decide to forego the provision of medical treatments intended to correct malnutrition and dehydration in some circumstances—is quite limited. Concentrating on incompetent patients, we have argued that in most cases such patients will be best served by providing nutrition and fluids. Thus, there should be a presumption in favor of providing nutrition and fluids as part of the broader presumption to provide means that prolong life. But this presumption may be rebutted in particular cases.

We do not have enough information to be able to determine with clarity and conviction whether withholding or withdrawing nutrition and hydration was justified in the cases that have occasioned public concern, though it seems likely that the Danville and Bloomington babies should have been fed and that Claire Conroy should not.

It is never sufficient to rule out "starvation" categorically. The question is whether the obligation to act in the patient's best interests was discharged by withholding or withdrawing particular medical treatments. All we have claimed is that nutrition and hydration by medical means need not always be provided. Sometimes they may not be in accord with the patient's wishes or interests. Medical nutrition and hydration do not appear to be distinguishable in any morally relevant way from other life-sustaining medical treatments that may on occasion be withheld or withdrawn.

QUESTIONS FOR CONSIDERATION

1. Lynn and Childress noted that prior to the development of intravenous lines and nasogastric tubes most dying patients experienced malnutrition and dehydration. Could such treatment be considered extraordinary care in some cases? How would artificially providing nutrition and hydration differ from the use of a dialysis machine?
2. Lynn and Childress offer three situations whereby medical intervention to provide food and water may be withheld: futile treatment, no possibility of benefit, and disproportionate burden. How would you evaluate these situations?
3. If patients who die without being provided with food and water do so more comfortably, would this justify withholding such intervention?
4. If it is not in the patient's best interest to initiate or continue artificial hydration and nutrition, should it be provided in order to fulfill the expectations of the family or to symbolically express care and compassion?
5. Do you agree with Lynn and Childress that withholding of artificial hydration and nutrition should be limited to only a few cases and that, "there should be a presumption in favor of providing nutrition and fluids"?

NOTES

1. John A. Robertson, "Dilemma in Danville," *The Hastings Center Report* 11 (October 1981), 5–8.
2. T. Rohrlich, "2 Doctors Face Murder Charges in Patient's Death," L.A. *Times,* August 19, 1982, A–1; Jonathan Kirsch, "A Death at Kaiser Hospital," *California* 7 (1982), 79ff; Magistrate's findings, *California v. Barber and Nejdl,* No. A 925586, Los Angeles Mun. Ct. Cal., (March 9, 1983); Superior Court of California, County of Los Angeles, *California v. Barber and Nejdl,* No. AO 25586, tentative decision May 5, 1983.
3. *In re Infant Doe,* No. GU 8204–00 (Cir. Ct. Monroe County, Ind., April 12, 1982), writ of mandamus dismissed sub nom. *State ex rel. Infant Doe v. Baker,* No. 482 S140 (Indiana Supreme Ct. May 27, 1982).
4. Office of the Secretary, Department of Health and Human Services, "Nondiscrimination on the Basis of Handicap," *Federal Register* 48 (1983), 9630–32. [Interim final rule modifying

45 C.F.R. #84.61]. See Judge Gerhard Gesell's decision, *American Academy of Pediatrics v. Heckler,* No. 83–0774, U.S. District Court, D.C., April 24, 1983; and also George J. Annas, "Disconnecting the Baby Doe Hotline," *The Hastings Center Report* 13 (June 1983), 14–16.

5. *In re Claire C. Conroy,* Sup Ct. NJ (Chancery Div-Essex Co. No. P-19083E) February 2, 1983; *In re Claire C. Conroy,* Sup Ct NJ (Appellate Div. No. 4-2483-82T1) July 8, 1983.

6. The President's Commission for the Study of Ethical Problems in Medicine and Biomedical and Behavioral Research, *Deciding to Forego Life-Sustaining Treatment* (Washington, D.C.: Government Printing Office, 1982).

7. G.E.M. Anscombe, "Ethical Problems in the Management of Some Severely Handicapped Children: Commentary 2," *Journal of Medical Ethics* 7 (1981), 117–124, at 122.

8. See e.g., the President's Commission for the Study of Ethical Problems in Medicine and Biomedical and Behavioral Research, *Making Health Care Decisions* (Washington, D.C.: Government Printing Office, 1982).

9. President's Commission, *Deciding to Forego Life-Sustaining Treatment,* pp. 171–96.

10. Joyce V. Zerwekh, "The Dehydration Question," *Nursing 83* (January 1983), 47–51, with comments by Judith R. Brown and Marion B. Dolan.

11. James J. McCartney, "The Development of the Doctrine of Ordinary and Extraordinary Means of Preserving Life in Catholic Moral Theology before the Karen Quinlan Case," *Linacre Quarterly* 47 (1980), 215ff.

12. President's Commission, *Deciding to Forego Life-Sustaining Treatment,* pp. 82–90. For an argument that fluids and electrolytes can be "extraordinary," see Carson Strong, "Can Fluids and Electrolytes be 'Extraordinary' Treatment?" *Journal of Medical Ethics* 7 (1981), 83–85.

13. The Sacred Congregation for the Doctrine of the Faith, *Declaration on Euthanasia,* Vatican City, May 5, 1980.

14. Paul Ramsey contends that "when a man is irreversibly in the process of dying, to feed him and to give him drink, to ease him and keep him comfortable—these are no longer given as means of preserving life. The use of a glucose drip should often be understood in this way. This keeps a patient who cannot swallow from feeling dehydrated and is often the only remaining 'means' by which we can express our present faithfulness to him during his dying." Ramsey, *The Patient as Person* (New Haven: Yale University Press, 1970), pp. 128–29. But Ramsey's suggestion would not apply to a patient in a deep irreversible coma, and he would be willing to disconnect the IV in the Quinlan case; see Ramsey, *Ethics at the Edges of Life: Medical and Legal Intersections* (New Haven: Yale University Press, 1978), p. 275. Bernard Towers describes an appropriate approach to comfort and dignity: "When a patient is conscious to even the smallest degree, and if he appears to be thirsty and to have a swallowing reflex, and if there is no contraindication to oral fluids, his comfort and dignity would surely demand that he be given nourishing liquids, or at least water. If he lapses into coma, good nursing practice has traditionally required sponging out the mouth and moistening the lips, Now, if he lapses into a deep coma and is on a dying trajectory, would we then try to 'push' fluids by mouth or nasogastric tube? If we did, dignity would surely suffer. The comfort of the patient would, of course, be unaffected if the coma were deep enough and irreversible." Towers, "Irreversible Coma and Withdrawal of Life Support: Is It Murder If the IV Line Is Disconnected?" *Journal of Medical Ethics* 8 (1982), 205.

15. See Kenneth C. Micetich, Patricia H. Steinecker, and David C. Thomasma, "Are Intravenous Fluids Morally Required for a Dying Patient?" *Archives of Internal Medicine* 143 (May 1983), 975–78.

16. Robert and Peggy Stinson, *The Long Dying of Baby Andrew* (Boston: Little, Brown and Company, 1983), p. 355.

17. A recent article discussed a hypothetical case of maintaining a dying, comatose patient on a respirator while withdrawing IV fluids. The authors contend that this approach is not ironic because withdrawal of the respirator "creates the immediate consequence of death for which we must take responsibility. It represents an extreme form of abandonment." Nevertheless, they were willing to stop IV fluids, knowing that death would occur before long. As the article's survey reported, other physicians would have provided nutrition and fluids. See Micetich, Steinecker, and Thomasma, "Are Intravenous Fluids Morally Required for a Dying Patient?"

EDITED BY ARTHUR CAPLAN AND CYNTHIA B. COHEN

Standards of Judgment for Treatment

As parents and clinicians evaluate specific strategies for responding to uncertainty, it is essential to ask how they should determine whether treatment is *ethically right* for a particular infant. The ethical questions can only be resolved by establishing reasonable standards of judgment against which to measure strategies and procedures.

"Sanctity of Life" Standards

Many critics of the practice of selective nontreatment argue that we must concentrate on the *sanctity* of life. But what does it mean to base our decisions on the sanctity of each child's life? Does it mean that caregivers may *never* forgo treatment, or that they may do so only for the most catastrophically afflicted newborns? Without further specification, the "sanctity of life" standard remains a vague slogan, rather than a meaningful guide to decisionmaking.

Vitalism

The most extreme sanctity of life position would hold that "where there is life, there is hope," and that so long as a child continues to cling to life, he or she must be treated. According to this view, which we shall call "vitalism," the mere presence of a heartbeat, respiration, or brain activity is a compelling reason to sustain all efforts to save the child's life. Only the moment of death relieves caregivers of their duty to treat. An adherent of this vitalist philosophy would accordingly hold that except in cases where the child has been declared dead, all withholding and withdrawal of treatment is ethically wrong.

This most extreme sanctity of life position has few advocates. Its major flaw is that it would insist upon aggressive treatments even for those children who are deemed to be in the process of dying. If responsible physicians have concluded that a particular child cannot be saved, that he will soon die, then it seems pointless and cruel to continue to treat the child with medical interventions that are by no means benign. By insisting on treatment even in such hopeless cases, the vitalist can justly be accused of worshipping an abstraction, "life," rather than focusing on the concrete good of the patient. As theologian Paul Ramsey has cogently argued, the appropriate response to a dying patient is not the futile imposition of painful medical treatments, but rather kind and respectful *care* designed to ease the child's passing.

The Medical Indications Policy

A more reasonable sanctity of life position has been proposed by Paul Ramsey and adopted (with some modifications) in various versions of the Department of Health and Human Services so-called "Baby Doe Rules." According to this standard, each child possesses equal dignity and intrinsic worth (i.e. "sanctity") and therefore no child should be denied life-sustaining medical treatments simply on the basis of his or her "handicap" or future quality of life. Such treatments must be provided to all infants, except (1) when the infant is judged to be in the process of dying, or (2) when the contemplated treatment is itself deemed to be "medically contraindicated." As Ramsey puts it, *treatments* may be compared in order to see which will be medically beneficial for a child, but abnormal *children* may not be compared with normal children in order to determine who shall live.

This policy is supported by two complementary ethical principles. First, the "nondiscrimination principle" states that children with impairments may not be selected for nontreatment solely on the basis of their "handicapping condition." If an otherwise normal child would receive a certain treatment— for example, surgery to repair an intestinal blockage—then a child with an abnormality must receive like treatment. Failure to do so discriminates unfairly against the child with impairments.

Second, the "medical benefit principle" states that caregivers are obliged to provide any and all treatments deemed, according to "reasonable medical judgment," to be "medically beneficial" to the patient. This means that if a certain medical or surgical procedure would be likely to bring about its intended result of avoiding infection or some other fatal consequence, then it must be provided to the child.

Although this medical indications policy was obviously well intended, insofar as it attempted to prevent instances of *unjust* discrimination against newborns with impairments, we believe that it is an overly rigid and inappropriate guide to decisionmaking. The first problem is that the nondiscrimination principle would have decisionmakers ignore, not just relatively mild handicaps of the sort encountered in most children with spina bifida and Down syndrome, but also impairments that are genuinely catastrophic.

Consider, for example, the child suffering from severe birth asphyxia who also happens to have a grave heart defect. Although surgeons would be willing to operate to fix the heart of an otherwise normal infant, the fact that this particular infant will never be sufficiently conscious to interact with his environment would appear to be a factor that the child's caretakers might permissibly take into consideration. Should the child be subjected to major and painful cardiac surgery only so that he might subsist in a permanently unconscious state? Even though treatment might be withheld from such a grievously afflicted infant "solely on the basis of his handicap," such a decision would in no way count as *unjust* discrimination precisely because the child's handicap is so severe that he can no longer meaningfully be compared to an "otherwise normal" infant.

The second problem with the medical indications policy lies in its "medical benefit" principle. Although this principle works well in many cases—for example, mild to moderate spina bifida—it does so because we think that the treatment confers a benefit, not merely upon the child's spine, but rather upon the whole child.

Quality of Life Standards

Although we conclude that quality of life judgments are ethically proper, and indeed inevitable, a great deal of care must be given to specifying why quality of life matters and what qualitative conditions might justify the denial of treatment. Merely invoking the phrase "quality of life" will get us no farther than invocations of the "sanctity of life."

The phrase "quality of life," as used in medical contexts, is ambiguous and frequently misunderstood. It is sometimes used to denote the social worth of an individual, the value that individual has for society. According to this interpretation, a person's quality of life is determined by utilitarian criteria, measured by balancing the burdens and benefits to others, especially family members. It is this meaning of the phrase that gives rise to the greatest worries about undertreatment of newborns with impairments.

This interpretation of quality of life has been defended on the grounds that external circumstances are crucially important in the outlook for certain newborns and because of the increased stress families undergo in raising children with disabilities. Despite the recognition that these external factors play a role in parental attitudes toward treatment, the consensus of this report is that "quality of life" should refer to the present or future characteristics of the infant, judged by standards of the infant's own well-being and not in terms of social utility.

Another way of understanding "quality of life" is as measured against a norm of "acceptable" life. Yet it is often noted that what would not be acceptable to some people, for themselves, is clearly acceptable to others. A danger lies in drawing the line too high, thereby ruling as "unacceptable" the life of a person with multiple handicaps or with mild-to-moderate mental retardation. When quality-of-life assessments are made for newborns with impairments, caution must be exercised to avoid this pitfall.

An example of drawing the line of "acceptable" life too high is "the ability to work or marry," a factor cited by the British pediatrician, John Lorber. An example of a very low standard is permanent coma, a criterion appearing in the 1984 Child Abuse Amendments. This threshold is so low as to be noncontroversial.

A subset of the quality of life standard and an alternative to a medical indications policy is the standard known as the "best interest of the child." Traditionally, this standard has been employed by courts in making child custody determinations and other decisions involving placement of an infant or child.

Unlike the medical indications policy, the "best interest" standard does incorporate quality of life considerations. This standard holds that infants should be treated with life-sustaining therapy except when (1) the infant is dying, (2) treatment is medically contraindicated (the two exceptions built into the medical indications policy), and (3) continued life would be worse for the infant than an early death. The third condition opens the door to quality of life considerations, but requires that such considerations be viewed from the infant's point of view. That is, certain states of being, marked by severe and intractable pain and suffering, can be viewed as worse than death. Thus, according to the best interest standard, there is room to consider the possibility that an infant's best interest can lie in withholding or withdrawing medical treatments, resulting in death.

Care must be taken, however, not to employ a standard based on the sensibilities of unimpaired adults; for example, one in which adult decisionmakers judge, from their own perspective, that they would not want to live a life with mental or physical disabilities. An infant-centered quality of life standard should be as objective as possible, in an attempt to determine whether continued life would be a benefit, from the child's point of view. An impaired child does not have the luxury of comparing his life to a "normal" existence; for such a child, it is a question of life with impairments versus no life at all.

The greatest merit of the best interest standard lies precisely in its child-centeredness. This focus on the individual child will aid decisionmakers in avoiding the twin evils of overtreatment, sanctioned by the medical indications policy, and undertreatment, which might result from allowing negative consequences for the family or society to determine what treatment is appropriate for the infant.

Although we believe the best interest of the infant should remain the primary standard for decisionmaking on behalf of newborns with impairments, it has limits. In addition to the undeniable problem of vagueness, there is the further question of the applicability of this standard to some of the most troubling dilemmas in the neonatal nursery. As one critic has noted about the standard suggested in the President's Commission report, *Deciding to Forego Life-Sustaining Treatment*:

> The fact that the child-based best-interest standard would mandate treatment even in the face of a prognosis bereft of any distinctly human potentiality reveals a feature of that standard that has so far gone unnoticed. In such extreme cases, the best-interest standard tends to view the absence of pain as the only morally relevant consideration. No matter that the infant is doomed to a life of very short duration, and lacks the capacity for any distinctively human development or activity; so long as the child does not experience any severe burdens, interpreted from her point of view, the fact that she can anticipate no distinctly human benefits is of no moral consequence.

In an article published in 1974, Father Richard McCormick explained and defended a quality of life viewpoint that differs from the best interest standard. Noting that modern medicine can keep almost anyone alive, he posed the question: "Granted that we can easily save the life, what kind of life are we saving?" McCormick admits this is a quality of life judgment, and holds that we must face the possibility of answering this question when it arises.

McCormick's guideline is "the potential for human relationships associated with the infant's condition." Translated into the language of "best interests," an individual who lacks any present capacity or future potential for human relationships can be said to have no interests at all, except perhaps to be free from pain and discomfort.

Our conclusion is that there is a need for two different standards embodying relational potential considerations. The prevailing "best interest" notion presupposes that all infants have interests, but for some, the burdens of continued life can outweigh the benefits. The alternative "relational potential" standard focuses on the potential of the individual for human relationships, and presumes that some severely neurologically impaired children cannot be said to have interests to which a best interest standard might apply. In employing these two standards, decisionmakers should first determine whether the best interest standard applies to the case at hand. For the large majority of infants this standard is applicable, and should be used to determine whether life-sustaining treatment should be administered. However, if an infant is so severely neurologically impaired as to render the best interest standard inapplicable, then the alternative standard, lack of potential for human relationships, becomes the relevant criterion, placing decisionmaking within the realm of parental discretion.

When the best interest standard is applicable, because the infant's best interest can be determined, decisionmakers are obligated either to institute or to forgo life-sustaining treatment. In contrast, the relational potential standard is nonobligatory: it permits the withholding or withdrawing of therapy from infants who lack the potential for human relationships, but it does not require that treatment be forgone. Continued treatment would not benefit such infants, but neither would it harm them. An example might be an infant born with trisomy 13. Most such infants do not survive beyond the first year of life, are severely or profoundly mentally retarded, and have multiple malformations. Their chances of being able to experience human interactions are minimal. Unlike the best interest standard, which is infant-centered, the relational potential standard allows the interests of others—e.g., family or society—to weigh in the decision about whether to treat.

Whereas the honest and informed application of these standards in the Baby Doe case should have yielded a clear mandate to treat a life-threatening condition, cases involving much more severe impairments may resist any straightforward application of normative standards. Although the precise medical facts in the celebrated Baby Jane Doe case remain mired in controversy, cases *resembling* that of Baby Jane regularly pose problems for decisionmakers attempting to apply either a "best interest" or a "relational potential" test.

Suppose an individualized decisionmaking strategy were combined with our preferred "best interest/relational potential" substantive standard. Clearly, the most important result would be a tendency to apply the substantive standard to a somewhat different category of child in settings removed from the exigencies of the delivery room. The strategy of waiting for evidence to accumulate on the prospects of individual children will have the practical effect of postponing decisionmaking, so decisions will be made for somewhat older infants. Waiting for the evidence to come in will also mean that the question of withholding or withdrawing treatment may have to be raised for many children who have bonded with their parents and caregivers and left the neonatal ICU for other settings, such as the general pediatrics service, a long-term care facility, or even the child's home.

Notwithstanding its evident merits, this particular conjunction of substantive standard and decisionmaking strategy will have its costs. First, it will tend to be more expensive than the statistical approach, since it will usually require the initiation of costly medical treatment for all children whose best interests and relational potential cannot be judged at delivery or in the neonatal ICU.

Second, it will most likely exacerbate the anguish and pain of parents and health care providers, because decisions will more often be made after the child's caregivers have bonded with the child and come to regard him or her as more than a mere bundle of possibilities. Once a child has achieved some sort of identity and entered into a well-defined social role, decisions to terminate life-sustaining treatments will no doubt be even more disturbing and anxiety-producing than they are at present. Still, considering what is at stake, perhaps a heightened sense of anxiety is appropriate for such exceedingly difficult decisions.

In spite of these difficulties, we conclude that a "best interest/relational potential" standard combined with a strategy of "individualized approach" is the best policy. Endorsing this combination does not answer in the abstract the question of how reliable predictions must be in order to justify withholding treatment in particular cases. Nor does it do away with the inevitable trade-offs entailed by these dilemmas. But the only way to avoid tragic results is to oversimplify these dilemmas. Because parents will be the ones who have to live with the result, whether it is fortunate or is something everyone concerned would rather have avoided, there must be some range within which parents can choose how much risk they can tolerate and how much pain they, and their baby, can bear.

QUESTIONS FOR CONSIDERATION

1. How does this article characterize "vitalism" as an extreme sanctity of life position?
2. According to this article, the "medical indications policy" serves as a standard of judgment for the non-treatment of certain infants. Why do the authors reject this approach?

3. How would the "best interest of the child" standard include a "quality of life" criteria? Do you agree that this is a better standard than "vitalism" or "medical indications"?

4. Explain Father McCormick's guideline of the "potential for human relationships" standard. Why would this standard serve as an alternative to the "best interest" standard in the case of a child with no interests and no potential interest? How would this approach serve the interests of others?

5. The authors of this article recommend the addition of an individualized decisionmaking strategy. What problems do they identify with this approach?

EDITED BY ARTHUR CAPLAN AND CYNTHIA B. COHEN

Deciding Not to Employ
Aggressive Measures

Once it has been determined that continued aggressive treatment is not in the interest of a particular infant, a new set of ethical issues arises. What treatments may be forgone? Is there a morally important difference between actively killing rather than merely allowing to die? Is active killing ever permissible? What care is due the infant for whom aggressive treatments are inappropriate? There are questions that must be addressed whether one holds to a "best interest" standard or some other substantive standard. They are as follows:

1. When a treatment is not morally indicated, does it make any difference if the treatment is not initiated or if it is stopped? This is commonly known as the distinction between *withholding and withdrawing*.
2. Should active intervention intended to hasten death ever be permitted?
3. Once aggressive measures to sustain life are forgone, what obligations do caregivers have?

Withholding versus Withdrawing Treatments

There is a broad consensus among scholars in medical ethics that in *the context of a physician-patient relationship, there is no moral difference between withholding and withdrawing a treatment.* If there is no good reason to employ a particular measure for a particular patient, then it is equally defensible to withhold it or to withdraw it. Conversely, if a treatment is morally indicated, it is as wrong to withhold it as it would be to withdraw it.

Many physicians, however, cling to the belief that stopping a treatment is less justified legally and morally than not starting it. This erroneous belief probably derives from equating withdrawing with acts and withholding with omissions, and then assuming that it is only acts that cause a death. Acts are then viewed as more morally wrong than omissions despite the fact that the same result is produced.

Evil seems more often to be a product of actions rather than omissions. Yet that is not always true. Allowing someone to be harmed when the harm could have easily been prevented can be wrong. While a number of factors influence the assessment of the wrongfulness of an omission, none is more important than the question of what *relationship* exists between the person in need of help and the person capable of providing it.

A physician usually is not obliged to accept someone as a patient. Once the physician does so, however, a relationship is established that imposes strict duties. Within the context of that relationship and the duties arising from it, the distinction between acts and omission loses whatever moral significance it might have.

In a physician-patient relationship, many things that are clearly omissions are just as clearly wrong. If an otherwise healthy patient begins to choke to death in front of her physician, who fails to attempt to relieve the choking, the physician is guilty of a wrongful omission. Likewise, if some medical or surgical therapy would almost certainly benefit a patient, yet the physician refuses to perform or mention it, that physician has wronged the patient.

Physicians are morally and legally obligated to do what is best for their patients. A plea that a failure to perform a life-saving therapy was merely an omission, and therefore not so serious as an action, would be absurd. Similarly, once it was determined that a treatment was no longer benefiting a patient, the claim that removing it would be worse than never having started it is equally untenable.

Concerned physicians and others sometimes argue that whatever the ethics of the matter, they cannot withdraw a treatment because it would lead to legal entanglements. This position appears to be based on either or both of two premises: (1) a false belief about what the law requires, and (2) an empirical prediction that withdrawing is more likely to draw unwanted legal scrutiny than withholding.

The President's Commission for the Study of Ethical Problems in Medicine and Biomedical and Behavioral Research had this to say about what the law requires:

> Little if any legal significance attaches to the distinction between with-holding and withdrawing. Nothing in law—certainly not in the context of the doctor-patient relationship—makes stopping treatment a more serious legal issue than not starting treatment. In fact, not starting treat-

ment that *might* be in a patient's interests is more likely to be held a civil or criminal wrong than stopping the same treatment when it has proved unavailing.

The second belief is more plausible: Whatever the law says in theory, as a practical matter withdrawing a treatment is more likely to attract attention and lead to civil or criminal proceedings than would withholding the same treatment. Proponents of this view may argue further that even if no formal legal sanctions follow, there are significant financial and emotional costs associated with merely becoming entrapped in the process.

While superficially plausible, there is no systematic evidence to support the belief that withdrawing is more likely than withholding to draw legal scrutiny. The two most publicized cases of forgone treatment of newborns— Baby Doe and Baby Jane Doe—were both instances of withholding rather than withdrawing. Nor does the fear of an unjust suit or prosecution constitute a compelling moral reason for physicians or others to deny infants the care that is most likely to be in their best interests. Until the public, including local legal officials, come to understand that withdrawing a treatment is not, simply for that reason, ethically different from withholding a treatment, the remote possibility of legal entanglement simply may be one of the risks of providing competent and ethical care. The specter of public confusion reinforces the need to educate the public and the professions on this matter.

The reluctance to withdraw treatments that are not in the infant's best interests would not be a matter for concern if that reluctance did not have such terrible consequences. First, the refusal to withdraw such treatments at times results in prolonging the deaths of children with great burdens in suffering to themselves and their families, as well as unnecessary economic costs. Second, it is often true that we cannot know whether or not a treatment will help a patient without giving it a trial. Decisions to withdraw can be based, then, on better information than decisions to withhold. Third, decisions to withdraw are more likely to be discussed with patients (or in the case of newborns, their parents) than decisions to withhold. To the extent that this is true, decisions to withdraw better conform to standards of sound medical decisionmaking than decisions to withhold. Fourth, there are numerous reports from the U.S. and abroad that some physicians are reluctant to initiate a treatment on an imperiled newborn out of fear that they will never be able to discontinue it. To avoid that possibility, they refuse to begin such treatments in broad classes of infants, some of whom might well benefit from it. In these instances, a philosophical confusion has become lethal.

To some degree, the reluctance to withdraw a treatment probably reflects psychological pressures. While withholding usually means that one has not commenced to hope for success, withdrawing means surrendering hope. To the physician, it may signify failure. It may necessitate a painful conversation with the family, whose faith in the physician's ability may be shaken. The more effort the physician invests in a patient, the harder it becomes to give up.

All these understandable psychological pressures may make it more difficult for physicians to withdraw treatments. Yet none of them change the ethics of the situation: If the treatment is not serving the patient's best interests, then the treatment need not be given and may be withdrawn. If it is causing harm to the patient (as invasive measures sometimes do), then it ought to be withdrawn.

Active Intervention to Hasten Death?

One remarkable feature of the discussions about treatment decisions for imperiled newborns has been several commentators' advocacy of active killing once a decision has been made not to prolong life. But should a public policy that permits active killing, even of dying infants, be created?

From the infant's point of view, an earlier death may mean less suffering, and hence be more desirable than a prolonged and perhaps pain-filled dying. Doing what is best for the infant might seem to require, then, actively killing that infant. If we are willing to forgo life-sustaining treatment, what reasons could we offer for not killing that infant? Is there even a meaningful distinction in such contexts between active killing and "letting die"—forgoing life-sustaining treatment?

It has already been noted that in the context of the relationship between physician and patient, where the physician has a moral obligation to do what is best for the patient, the distinction between acts and omissions is morally unimportant. If there is an ethically significant difference between active killing and forgoing treatment, it must lie somewhere other than in the unhelpful territory of acts versus omissions. The issues at stake in discussions of "killing v. letting die" can be stated more precisely:

1. For any particular contemplated *act* of medical killing, is it morally justifiable for a physician to intervene to cause the death of a patient, with the intention of causing that death?
2. Should society condone the *policy* of physicians intervening intentionally to cause the deaths of their patients?

The distinction between individual cases and general practices—between acts and policies—is important. In a specific case, one may believe that a speedier death is in that infant's interests, all things considered. Yet one may still refuse to sanction active medical killing on the grounds that a policy permitting such killing would have such morally bad consequences that it ought to be resisted.

It is possible to construct a hypothetical scenario in which active killing appears to be the only way to prevent prolonged and irremediable suffering. One example could be an infant born with Werdnig-Hoffman disease, a condition of progressive muscular degeneration. Those born with this disease may be fully conscious and sentient, with their receptiveness to pain intact. Once their respiratory muscles fail, they may be kept alive on a ventilator, though they eventually lose the ability to use any muscle in the body. Their capacities to feel pain and to perceive what is happening in their environment lead some caregivers to presume that they suffer, perhaps grievously. Whether active killing in such a case is morally justified will depend upon a contested moral theory, as well as a number of empirical assumptions about what consequences will flow from the act.

If, as some believe, acts should be judged solely by their consequences, then particular acts of intentional medical killing could, in principle, be morally justified. In this theory, the key moral assumption is that only the *consequences* of actions count in judging their morality (and not for example, intentions or the breaking of moral rules).

In contrast to this many people believe that there are at least a few *prima facie* moral rules, that is, rules that support moral assessments that are not completely reducible to consequences, and that ought to be obeyed unless other moral considerations compel us to take a different course of action. Examples of such *prima facie* rules may be those requiting us to honor a promise, or refrain from taking a human life.

In addition, there are reasons to doubt that the consequences of active medical killing are always clearly on balance positive. Seeing this requires examining the empirical assumptions behind permitting active euthanasia.

For active killing to be justified on the basis of consequences, it must result in the most favorable consequences overall for the infant *and* for everyone else concerned directly and indirectly, now and in the future. But can we know with confidence that a quicker death is better for an infant? Is it certain that a dying infant must suffer? Whether an infant is experiencing suffering may be very difficult to determine. More important, advances in pain management make it possible to relieve all or almost all pain, especially if one is

318 Part V: Termination of Treatment

willing to increase the risk of respiratoy or circulatory depression by using larger than normal doses of pain-relieving drugs.

The medical-empirical and the ethical issues are inextricably intertwined in the case of an infant for whom we have decided to forgo life-sustaining treatments, but who may require potentially life-threatening doses of drugs to assure relief from pain. Those who believe that consequences are all that matters will see no difference between giving life-threatening dosages of pain-relievers with two different intentions: either to treat the pain aggressively while accepting the increased risk of death; or to intend to cause the death in order to eliminate the pain. Those who believe that intentions are important in judging the morality of an act see a profoundly important difference in the two intentions.

Beyond the uncertainties about whether being killed is best for the infant lie other questionable empirical assumptions about the consequences to others. For example, there is the matter of remorse. If the parents, physicians or others involved in the decision to kill the infant suffered overwhelming remorse, these negative consequences might outweigh the benefits to the infant. They would either suffer with it, or else by denying or suppressing it so erode their consciences that they might become overly willing to kill again in a less clear case. If they experienced little or no remorse, they might participate too readily in additional active killings. While the same might be said about forgoing treatment, it seems that in most people the guilt associated with active killing is greater than the qualms they might feel about forgoing medical treatment.

The moral case against a general policy permitting the killing of imperiled newborns is even stronger than the case against particular acts of killing. Once we move from idealized hypothetical cases to a policy allowing such killing, we must acknowledge the likelihood of errors—errors of prognosis, as well as the possibility of misidentifications. These are familiar consequences of human fallibility, and not of maliciousness.

Abuses are also possible. Parents may advocate killing their infants to serve their own purposes rather than their infants' welfare. Physicians may have strong convictions about particular kinds of disabilities they believe are "worse than death." Hospitals may see opportunities to cut costs. Whether or not errors or abuses occur frequently, people may suspect that they do, and their trust in caregivers and in hospitals may be diminished.

Another reason to reject a policy allowing active killing by medical personnel is that it may reflect a narrow, technological view of medicine that is already too dominant in the contemporary hospital. This concept of medicine tends towards the belief that if we cannot "fix" a problem, it is beyond the scope of our responsibility. It ignores the long tradition of caring, receptiveness and the refusal to abandon persons in need reflected in the common roots of the words "hospital" and "hospitality." Active killing, at one level, may be an effort to sweep away the failures of technological medicine. In fact, families and professional caregivers have much to offer dying and suffering persons.

What Care Should Be Given When Aggressive Measures Are Foregone?

As we have seen, while we reject any policy permitting active killing, there are instances when aggressive treatment should not be continued. However, the duty to care for patients does not end once aggressive measures are abandoned. Parents, nurses and physicians can still play a major role in caring for the infant. They can offer comfort with whatever measures are available, including warmth, food, and touch.

For those infants capable of feeling pain, relieving that pain is a matter of the highest priority. Suffering, other than that chosen by the person in the service of some greater good, is an evil. Modern medicine has the ability to diminish greatly the pain or suffering of seriously ill newborns. Although there may be some dispute about whether the most premature infants possess the neurological capacities to experience pain, in the absence of clear and convincing evidence to the contrary, we should assume they can and act accordingly.

Rather than diminishing, the moral duties of medical caregivers take a different form once we accept that a patient is dying, and lies beyond the reach of our curative powers. Sophisticated treatments intended to provide comfort have an important role. But, as Paul Ramsey reminds us, care and companionship may be at least as important. He says we should care, but only care for the dying. Before aggressive therapies were available, nurses and physicians were more accustomed to caring for dying patients. That art needs to be renewed.

The interests of the dying infant's family also ought to be considered. Those interests need not conflict with doing what is best for the infant. Some hospitals have made provisions for parents to hold their infants once invasive therapies have ceased. This could benefit infants and their parents. Another measure has been to allow the families to see and hold their infants once they have died. Some hospitals have tried to adapt concepts of hospice care in their practices with dying infants and their families. These worthy efforts to accept the realities of death, and to provide institutional support for families, deserve to be implemented and developed further.

QUESTIONS FOR CONSIDERATION

1. Do you agree with the authors that the distinction between withholding treatment and withdrawing treatment is not morally valid? Why do they contend that physicians believe that refusing to initiate treatment is more likely to be morally and legally justified than terminating treatment?

2. What are the terrible consequences that this article describes as a result of the reluctance to withdraw treatment?

3. What are the justifications that the authors offer in drawing a distinction between particular cases of a physician causing the death of a patient and a general public policy allowing physicians to cause the death of a patient when it is in the interest of the patient to do so? Why would this distinction be different from withholding and withdrawing treatment?

4. According to this article, what duties remain when aggressive measures have been withdrawn? How would hospice care serve as a model for the care of dying patients?

Alexander Morgan Capron

Anencephalic Donors: Separating the Dead from the Dying

In biomedical ethics, some cases involving individuals present true dilemmas: choosing between two evils (shorter life or longer suffering). Others are perplexing in another way: choosing between two goods (one person's privacy or another's well-being). When biomedical ethics moves to the realm of law and public policy, we face even more complex challenges. Consider, for example, several recent bills that aim to facilitate organ transplantation in infants by allowing organs to be taken from other babies who are born with most of their brains missing. These proposals aim to do good, but they create the possibility of doing great harm.

The Need and the Technology

In the past few years, medical interest in pediatric organ transplantation has rapidly expanded. Extensive press coverage of developments in immunosuppression and refinement of surgical techniques—particularly cardiac replacement in newborns—has created hope for some parents whose children have otherwise fatal heart, kidney, and liver problems.

Before these transplant procedures move from experimental to therapeutic, they must improve technically. Yet an inadequate supply of usable cadaver organs poses an even more formidable impediment. Cadaver organs for transplantation in older patients come primarily from the victims of accidents, especially automobile and motorcycle collisions. Relatively few newborns and very young children die under these or other circumstances that would make them suitable organ donors. Present methods of identifying possible donors and receiving permission to harvest their organs provide only a small fraction of the estimated 400 to 500 infant hearts and kidneys and 500 to 1,000 infant livers that are needed in the U.S. each year.

_____ 321 _____

The supply is likely to increase somewhat as transplant techniques are perfected for newborns and infants. And some refinements now underway in the methods for obtaining organs generally—such as the development of a national computerized registry and more intensive local organ procurement efforts—may partially ameliorate the shortage. The chance to make "the gift of life" to another infant may in time become a source of solace commonly offered to the parents of dead infants as it is to relatives of older accident victims.

The present (and perhaps long-range) inadequacy of organ supply for infants has led to proposals that the law be altered to allow organs to be taken from another group of babies—those born with a fatal neurologic condition called anencephaly, the absence of all or most of the cerebral hemispheres. According to Godfrey Oakley of the Centers for Disease Control, approximately 2,000 to 3,000 such babies are born every year. The initiative comes from surgeons who are developing the techniques for infant transplants, but parents of anencephalic infants have also publicly supported the idea, as they search for some meaning and comfort in the face of the death of their newborn.

The legislation takes two forms. The first, illustrated by a proposal made but subsequently withdrawn in the California Senate, is to modify the statutory standards for determining human death set forth in the Uniform Determination of Death Act (UDDA) or similar state laws so that they will encompass anencephalic babies. The second, illustrated by New Jersey Assembly Bill No. 3367, is to permit parents of an anencephalic child to donate its organs even though the child does not meet the requirement set forth in the Uniform Anatomical Gift Act (UAGA) that organs may be removed only after a physician not involved in the transplant procedure determines that the organ donor has died.

Both these attempts are well-meaning but in my view misguided. They would create very substantial problems, as well as undermine the very goal they seek.

Amending the Determination of Death Act

For many years, death was "defined" by the law through judicial decisions which, following accepted medical and popular opinion, held that death occurs when all bodily functions, specifically heartbeat and breathing, cease.

With the development of technology to sustain circulation and respiration, medical and popular views diverged. Physicians knew that other functions besides heart and lung activity had to be measured when artificial ventilation and drugs might be causing observable cardiopulmonary activity. By the late 1960s, medical studies had verified that tests detecting the complete absence of brain functions provide an accurate alternative way to establish the *same* physiologic state of death as the heart and lung measurements that are done on persons not on artificial life supports.

Thus, although people frequently speak of new "definitions" of death, what was actually involved was merely an updating of the means for determining death. Beginning with Kansas in 1970, many states gave legal recognition to two standards for determining that death has occurred: the traditional one of irreversible cessation of circulatory and respiratory functions, and the new one-irreversible cessation of all functions of the entire brain, including the brain stem—which is relevant when respirators and other treatments render the traditional standard unreliable.

By the late 1970s, when Congress wrote the mandate for the President's Commission for the Study of Ethical Problems in Medicine and Biomedical and Behavioral Research, a consensus existed among public officials, as well as legal, medical, and ethical commentators, on the need for simple and uniform legislation recognizing the new (brain) standard for determining death alongside the old (heart and lungs). From the joint efforts of the National Conference of Commissioners on Uniform State Laws, the American Medical Association, the American Bar Association, and the President's Commission, the UDDA emerged in 1982. It has been adopted in sixteen states legislatively, and in two others through explicit judicial recognition; statutes with provisions similar to the UDDA have been enacted in twenty other states, and the highest courts in an additional four states have accepted neurological determinations of death, without explicitly recognizing the UDDA's formulation of the appropriate language to achieve this end.

In February 1986 California Senator Milton Marks introduced Senate Bill 2018. He was apparently moved by an article in the San Francisco *Chronicle* that recounted the frustration of a couple who were unable to donate the organs of their anencephalic baby for transplantation to an infant patient at the University of California Medical Center. As originally proposed, the bill would have amended the UDDA by adding the statement that "an individual born with the condition of anencephaly is dead." Sen. Marks subsequently modified his bill and proposed that a state health advisory board make recommendations about the care of infants with life-threatening conditions, including the "feasibility and necessity" of infant organ transplants, the donation of organs from infants born with anencephaly, and any "necessary changes" in the UAGA or the UDDA.

Adding anencephalics to the category of dead persons would be a radical change, both in the social and medical understanding of what it means to be dead and in the social practices surrounding death. Anencephalic infants may be dying, but they are still alive and breathing. Calling them "dead" will not change physiologic reality or otherwise cause them to resemble those (cold and nonrespirating) bodies that are considered appropriate for post-mortem examinations and burial. The amendment of the UDDA to include anencephalics is therefore unwise, for several reasons.

To begin with, the UDDA provides that determinations of death "must be made in accordance with accepted medical standards." In the case of anencephalics, this provision creates enormous difficulty because physicians do not consider anencephalic infants as dead, but as dying. Their perception is borne out by statistics. One study of liveborn infants with anencephaly, conducted over a thirty-year period, found an equal distribution among males and females. Significantly more males survived the first day of life, but none lived longer than seven days, while female survival was comparable to male after the first day. One female (1.1 percent) survived 14 days:

> The results of this study show that over 40 percent of anencephalic infants can be expected to survive longer than 24 hours (51% males; 34% females), and of these, 35 percent will still be alive on the third day and 5 percent on the seventh day.[1]

For most of the infants in this study, anencephaly was the only neural tube defect, and most of these had no anomalies in other organ systems. Among those infants who also had spina bifida or encephalocele (a protrusion of the brain substance through an opening in the skull), one third had defects in another major organ system.

The UDDA's requirement that determinations of death accord with "accepted medical standards" might be read in another way were anencephaly added to the statute. This would hold that the requirement is met if accepted medical standards *for determining anencephaly* are applied. Although the diagnosis is usually made accurately by neurologists, authors of the thirty-year study just mentioned found that in "conducting this study, it became obvious that it is important to verify the diagnosis of anencephaly." They describe several cases of long survival:

> One infant initially coded as anencephaly, who survived over 4 months, had hydranencephaly rather than anencephaly, and another who lived for 12 days actually had amniotic band syndrome mimicking anencephaly.

Misdiagnosis by itself would not appear to be a great enough risk to preclude the use of anencephaly as a category to trigger further action (such as declaration of "death"). But the observed relationship to—or even overlapping with—other congenital neurological defects underlines the problems that the proposal would create. For example, hydranencephalics have normal brain development early in gestation; as a result of some event (such as an in utero infection) their cerebral hemispheres are destroyed and replaced with fluid. Like anencephalics, hydranencephalics survive depending upon the extent to which their brain stems are able to regulate vegetative functioning, but they usually survive somewhat longer because their skulls are intact and thus their brains are not open to infection.

To further complicate the picture, other neurological conditions, such as certain types of microcephaly, are also inconsistent with long-term survival. Microcephaly—literally, a small head—covers a spectrum of problems, including cases in which the hemispheres fail to form. Whatever their clinical differences from anencephalic babies, hydranencephalic and some microcephalic infants are conceptually indistinguishable if the characteristic separating anencephalics from normal children is their lethal neurological condition.

Because of the existence of these other diagnostic categories, decision makers will be pressured to expand the "definition" to sweep in other similarly situated "dead" neonates. Indeed, Dr. Alan Shewmon, a pediatric neurologist at UCLA, has pointed out that babies—such as hydranencephalics—who typically live a little longer than anencephalics are actually likely to be *more* attractive sources of organs because of the extra time for development. At present, the regional organ procurement association for California does not accept organs from infants younger than two months of age because of physiologic difficulties (such as the tendency of vessels to clot).

More important, these other diagnostic categories serve as a reminder that the proposals involve a variety of infants who are going to die in a relatively short time. Distinguishing those who will die within a day or two from those (including *some* microcephalics and hydranencephalics as well as the remaining anencephalics) who will die over the following two weeks is inevitably imprecise. The distinctions rest on clinical judgment, not moral principle.

What the Law Now Provides

Amending the UDDA would also open the door to other changes that the proponents of this particular amendment are unlikely to favor. Perhaps those who have proposed the change do not think it involves a major break with existing law because they are confused about what the law now provides.

Part of that confusion can be traced to the use of the term "brain death" to describe the newer standard for determining death. This terminology is misleading because it wrongly suggests that organs rather than organisms die, and because it implies that there are several *kinds* of death, when in fact death is a unitary concept that can be determined by several standards, each appropriate under particular circumstances.

"Defining" anencephalics as dead would place these patients into the same category as patients who lack the capacity to breathe on their own, which has always been taken as a basic sign of life. Perhaps the proponents of this change do not see this as a major alteration because they think the law already lumps together some people who are "more dead" (those whose hearts have stopped) with others who are merely "brain dead." But all persons found to meet the standards of the UDDA are equally dead; it is merely the means of measuring the absence of the integrated functioning of heart, lungs, and brain that differs between those who are and those who are not being treated by methods that can induce breathing and heartbeat.

Defining anencephalics as dead so that they may be used as organ donors could, ironically, actually decrease organ donation. Imagine the effect of the law on the process of seeking organ donations from the relatives of a deceased person. At present, when that situation arises, the person seeking permission can explain that the patient is dead; despite the heaving chest and other appearances of life, if the physicians were to cease the mechanical interventions, it would immediately be apparent that the body is in the same state that we have always recognized as dead. The next-of-kin are told that they do not face a difficult decision over whether to let the patient die; instead they face the reality that their loved one is now a corpse—albeit a corpse with artificially generated heartbeat and breathing—whose organs are still being maintained in a way that would make them useful for transplants. (Remember that only a fraction of persons declared dead on the basis of absence of brain functions are candidates for organ donation.[2])

If anencephalic babies were also regarded as dead bodies suitable for organ donation, this certainty would be lost. For in these cases, decisions about the extent of treatment remain—indeed, some parents may even wish to try heroic or experimental means to lengthen their child's life. The message to those involved in organ transplantation—both as relatives of potential donors and as physicians, nurses, and others seeking permission for donation—is thus likely to introduce new elements of uncertainty. Is *any* particular patient—

and not just an anencephalic baby—*really* dead? Or do the physicians mean only that the outlook for the patient's survival is poor, so why not allow the organs to be taken and bring about death in this (useful) fashion?

Alternatively, perhaps some who favor the anencephalic standard for death *do* mean to change the law radically. A few commentators have argued for many years that the statutes on death should move beyond new means for measuring the traditional state of death and should instead declare that persons who have lost only the higher (neocortical) functions of their brains are also dead.[3] These suggestions have been uniformly rejected by legislators across the country—as well as by most medical, ethical, and legal writers. Yet the inclusion of anencephalics in the "definition" of death would amount to the first recognition of a "higher brain" standard—and a first step toward a broader use of this standard—because these babies, despite the massive deficit in their brains, still have some functions (principally at the brain stem level).

To state that such patients are dead would be equivalent to saying that the late Karen Quinlan was "dead" for the more than ten years that she lived after her respirator was removed. Like the anencephalic babies, Ms. Quinlan and other patients in a persistent vegetative state lack the ability to think, to communicate, and probably even to process any sensations of pain and pleasure (at least in the way that we think of these phenomena). Some people may consider such a life as unrewarding, but that does not justify loose use of language about who is "dead." Emotionally, one may be tempted to say that a person in a permanent coma is "as good as dead" because he or she cannot participate in any of the activities that give life meaning. But such a breathing, metabolizing patient does not embody what we mean by dead and is not ready for burial—or organ donation.

A statute that labels anencephalics "dead" is a bad idea because either it will treat differently another group that is identical on the relevant criteria (the permanently comatose, who are dying and lacking consciousness) or it will lead to a further revision in medical and legal standards under which the permanently comatose would also be regarded as "dead" although many of them can survive for years with nothing more than ordinary nursing care.

For many people, the prospect of being in a permanent coma is unacceptable; if that occurred, they would want to be allowed to die without further treatment. But that is a separate problem to which society is already responding in other ways. It would be highly controversial—and, indeed, would be rejected by most people—to call people who are in a coma but who still breathe on their own "dead," especially when the purpose is to allow removal of their vital organs, which *would* then cause their death as that term is now used. This was the nightmarish scenario that took place in the Jefferson Institute in Robin Cook's novel *Coma*.

Amending the Anatomical Gift Act

Amending the UDDA would thus open up the possibility of an ever-increasing category of persons who are defined as "dead" because their organs might be useful in a legally sanctioned "Jefferson Institute." Moreover, the change in "definition" would apply far beyond transplantation to all contexts in which death arises, from burials to probate to criminal law. Amending the Anatomical Gift Act to permit organ harvesting from anencephalics might be subject to some of the same pressures for extension to other groups of dying, unconscious patients. But at least such a change in the law would be limited to organ donation and would thus avoid the conceptual problems that arise when dying is confused with death. Certainly, the need for infant organ donors requires serious consideration of proposals such as the one introduced in October 1986 by New Jersey Assemblyman Walter Kern, Jr.

Though the idea of living people choosing to give vital organs (as a better way of dying than simply getting old or sick) has been around for quite a while,[4] it has not been accepted. Anencephalic newborns should not be the opening wedge in such a revision of the organ donor process, for several reasons.

First, if society wants to adopt a policy of sacrificing living patients for their organs, it seems very strange—and a very bad precedent—to start with the most vulnerable patients. Unconsenting, incompetent patients who have never had a chance to express their views about whether, if near death but not yet dead, they would want their bodies cut up for purposes of organ donation, are the *least* suitable source. Moreover, how would one distinguish anencephalics from other possible candidates for involuntary sacrifice for organ donation, such as comatose, demented, or severely retarded patients?

Second, the argument that anencephalics are suitable because they *are* not living *persons* (since they are born with such profound mental defects that they will never be able to establish meaningful human interactions) is a radical redefinition of the accepted criterion for being considered a person, namely, live birth of the product of a human conception. If an anencephalic is not a living person for purposes of organ removal, what about for purposes of homicide, which might be justified on the same utilitarian grounds as organ removal (a greater benefit to the community) or even on the grounds that the death would be better for the parents or other members of the baby's family?

This concern raises the general issue of the justice of a proposal that would treat one being as a means of achieving a good for other beings (the grieving donor parents, the ailing recipient child). Certainly, one can imagine cases where there would be sufficient justification for sacrificing one child to save the life of another. For example, suppose that Siamese twins were joined by a six-chambered heart and the only chance of saving either one lay in performing an operation in which the twin with just a two-chambered heart was killed. But the agonizing process that would lead to a decision to proceed in such a rare case is very different from establishing a general rule that would be applied (inevitably, not always in such a conscientious fashion) to the thousands of anencephalic children born each year, to say nothing of other potential organ "donors" with other lethal conditions.

Third, even more than other potential involuntary organ "donors," the anencephalic opens the door to manipulation. The diagnosis of anencephaly is now often made prenatally. The parents are usually offered the option of abortion or of normal delivery, after which the child will die. If anencephalics come to be regarded as an attractive source of transplantable organs, women who would otherwise choose abortion may be pressured by physicians or others to carry the fetus to term and then perhaps to deliver by a riskier method (cesarian section) that would optimize the usefulness of the child as a source of organs.

Finally, amending the UAGA to allow organs to be removed from anencephalic babies seems likely to undermine, rather than reinforce, the public's support for, and confidence in, organ transplantation. Indeed, if the UAGA were to be amended in such a fashion, legislators might well insist on many protections. They would want to ensure the absolute reliability of the diagnosis and prognosis, for example, and to guard against any conflicting interests on the part of those seeking organs or consenting to organ removals from anencephalics. This could lead to the misguided addition of such safeguards for organ removal from dead bodies under the existing UAGA, thus undermining public confidence ("With safeguards like this, organ donation must be a bad or risky thing!") and diminishing the number of donated organs. At the very least it would unnecessarily encumber the process of organ retrieval, increasing its costs and reducing its yield. These would be ironic results for a measure with the well-intentioned purpose of increasing the organs available for transplantation.

Medical ingenuity should be directed toward finding ways to care for dying anencephalic (and other) babies so that when they become brain-dead, they can be organ donors (with their parents' permission). Medicine should not embark on a course of sacrificing living but incompetent patients for the admitted social good of transplanting organs.

QUESTIONS FOR CONSIDERATION

1. How does Capron characterize the inadequate supply of cadaver organs for transplantation? How would the use of anencephalic infants improve the supply of organs for children?

2. Why does Capron object to changing the Uniform Determination of Death Act to include anencephalic infants as "dead"? Do you agree with these objections?

3. Explain Capron's objection to the use of the term "brain dead" to characterize new criteria for determining death. How would the use of such terminology affect the identification of anencephalics?

4. What are Capron's objections to changing the Anatomical Gift Act to include anencephalics as organ donors? How would such a change radically alter the concept of personhood?

NOTES

1. P. A. Baird, and A. D. Sadovnick, "Survival in Infants with Anencephaly," *Clinical Pediatrics* 23 (1984), 268–72.

2. President's Commission for the Study of Ethical Problems in Medicine and Biomedical and Behavioral Research, *Defining Death* (1981), p. 23.

3. See, e.g., Robert M. Veatch, "The Whole-Brain Oriented Concept of Death: An Out-Moded Philosophical Formulation," *Journal of Thanatology* 3 (1975), 13.

4. Belding H. Scribner, "Ethical Problems of Using Artificial Organs to Sustain Human Life," *Transactions of American Society for Artificial Internal Organs* 10 (1964), 209, 211, stating personal preference, if ill with a fatal disease, to be able to have physician put him to sleep "and any useful organs taken prior to death."

*PART V:4: Active Voluntary Euthanasia
and Physician-Assisted Suicide*

Richard Doerflinger

*Assisted Suicide:
Pro-Choice or Anti-Life?*

The intrinsic wrongness of directly killing the innocent, even with the victim's consent, is all but axiomatic in the Jewish and Christian worldviews that have shaped the laws and mores of Western civilization and the self-concept of its medical practitioners. This norm grew out of the conviction that human life is sacred because it is created in the image and likeness of God, and called to fulfilment in love of God and neighbor.

With the pervasive secularization of Western culture, norms against euthanasia and suicide have to a great extent been cut loose from their religious roots to fend for themselves. Because these norms seem abstract and unconvincing to many, debate tends to dwell not on the wrongness of the act as such but on what may follow from its acceptance. Such arguments are often described as claims about a "slippery slope," and debate shifts to the validity of slippery slope arguments in general.

Since it is sometimes argued that acceptance of assisted suicide is an outgrowth of respect for personal autonomy, and not lack of respect for the inherent worth of human life, I will outline how autonomy-based arguments in favor of assisting suicide do entail a statement about the value of life. I will also distinguish two kinds of slippery slope arguments often confused with each other, and argue that those who favor social and legal acceptance of assisted suicide have not adequately responded to the slippery slope claims of their opponents.

Assisted Suicide versus Respect for Life

Some advocates of socially sanctioned assisted suicide admit (and a few boast) that their proposal is incompatible with the conviction that human life is of intrinsic worth. Attorney Robert Risley has said that he and his allies in the Hemlock Society are "so bold" as to seek to "overturn the sanctity of life principle" in American society. A life of suffering, "racked with pain," is "not the kind of life we cherish."[1]

Others eschew Risley's approach, perhaps recognizing that it creates a slippery slope toward practices almost universally condemned. If society is to help terminally ill patients to commit suicide because it agrees that death is objectively preferable to a life of hardship, it will be difficult to draw the line at the seriously ill or even at circumstances where the victim requests death.

Some advocates of assisted suicide therefore take a different course, arguing that it is precisely respect for the dignity of the human person that demands respect for individual freedom as the noblest feature of that person. On this rationale a decision as to when and how to die deserves the respect and even the assistance of others because it is the ultimate exercise of self-determination—"ultimate" both in the sense that it is the last decision one will ever make and in the sense that through it one takes control of one's entire self. What makes such decisions worthy of respect is not the fact that death is chosen over life but that it is the individual's own free decision about his or her future.

Thus Derek Humphry, director of the Hemlock Society, describes his organization as "pro-choice" on this issue. Such groups favor establishment of a constitutional "right to die" modeled on the right to abortion delineated by the U.S. Supreme Court in 1973. This would be a right to choose *whether or not* to end one's own life, free of outside government interference. In theory, recognition of such a right would betray no bias toward choosing death.

Life versus Freedom

This autonomy-based approach is more appealing than the straightforward claim that some lives are not worth living, especially to Americans accustomed to valuing individual liberty above virtually all else. But the argument departs from American traditions on liberty in one fundamental respect.

When the Declaration of Independence proclaimed the inalienable human rights to be "life, liberty, and the pursuit of happiness," this ordering reflected a long-standing judgment about their relative priorities. Life, a human being's very earthly existence, is the most fundamental right because it is the necessary condition for all other worldly goods, including freedom; freedom in turn makes it possible to pursue (without guaranteeing that one will attain) happiness. Safeguards against the deliberate destruction of life are thus seen as necessary to protect freedom and all other human goods. This line of thought is not explicitly religious but is endorsed by some modern religious groups:

> The first right of the human person is his life. He has other goods and some are more precious, but this one is fundamental—the condition of all the others. Hence it must be protected above all others.[2]

On this view suicide is not the ultimate exercise of freedom but its ultimate self-contradiction: a free act that by destroying life, destroys all the individual's future earthly freedom. If life is more basic than freedom, society best serves freedom by discouraging rather than assisting self-destruction. Sometimes one must limit particular choices to safeguard freedom itself, as when American society chose over a century ago to prevent people from selling themselves into slavery even of their own volition.

It may be argued in objection that the person who ends his life has not truly suffered loss of freedom, because unlike the slave he need not continue to exist under the constraints of a loss of freedom. But the slave does have some freedom, including the freedom to seek various means of liberation or at least the freedom to choose what attitude to take regarding his plight. To claim that a slave is worse off than a corpse is to value a situation of limited freedom less than one of no freedom whatsoever, which seems inconsistent with the premise of the "pro-choice" position. Such a claim also seems tantamount to saying that some lives (such as those with less than absolute freedom) are objectively not worth living, a position that "pro-choice" advocates claim not to hold.

It may further be argued in objection that assistance in suicide is only being offered to those who can no longer meaningfully exercise other freedoms due to increased suffering and reduced capabilities and lifespan. To be sure, the suffering of terminally ill patients who can no longer pursue the simplest everyday tasks should call for sympathy and support from everyone in contact with them. But even these hardships do not constitute total loss of freedom of choice. If they did, one could hardly claim that the patient is in a position to make the ultimate free choice about suicide. A dying person capable of making a choice of that kind is also capable of making less monumental free choices about coping with his or her condition. This person generally faces a bewildering array of choices regarding the assessment of his or her past life and the resolution of relationships with family and friends. He or she must finally choose at this time what stance to take regarding the eternal questions about God, personal responsibility, and the prospects of a destiny after death.

In short, those who seek to maximize free choice may with consistency reject the idea of assisted suicide, instead facilitating all choices *except* that one which cuts short all choices.

In fact proponents of assisted suicide do *not* consistently place freedom of choice as their highest priority. They often defend the moderate nature of their project by stating, with Derek Humphry, that "we do not encourage suicide for any reason except to relieve unremitting suffering." It seems their highest priority is the "pursuit of happiness" (or avoidance of suffering) and not "liberty" as such. Liberty or freedom of choice loses its value if one's choices cannot relieve suffering and lead to happiness; life is of instrumental value insofar as it makes possible choices that can bring happiness.

In this value system, choice as such does not warrant unqualified respect. In difficult circumstances, as when care of a suffering and dying patient is a great burden on family and society, the individual who chooses life despite suffering will not easily be seen as rational, thus will not easily receive understanding and assistance for this choice.

In short, an unqualified "pro-choice" defense of assisted suicide lacks coherence because corpses have no choices. A particular choice, that of death, is given priority over all the other choices it makes impossible, so the value of choice as such is not central to the argument.

A restriction of this rationale to cases of terminal illness also lacks logical force. For if ending a brief life of suffering can be good, it would seem that ending a long life of suffering may be better. Surely the approach of the California "Humane and Dignified Death Act"—where consensual killing of a patient expected to die in six months is presumably good medical practice, but killing the same patient a month or two earlier is still punishable as homicide—is completely arbitrary.

Slippery Slopes, Loose Cannons

Many arguments against sanctioning assisted suicide concern a different kind of "slippery slope": contingent factors in the contemporary situation may make it virtually inevitable in practice, if not compelling at the level of abstract theory, that removal of the taboo against assisted suicide will lead to destructive expansions of the right to kill the innocent. Such factors may not be part, of euthanasia advocates' own agenda; but if they exist and are beyond the control of these advocates, they must be taken into account in judging the moral and social wisdom of opening what may be a Pandora's box of social evils.

To distinguish this sociological argument from our dissection of the conceptual *logic* of the rationale for assisted suicide, we might call it a "loose cannon" argument. The basic claim is that socially accepted killing of innocent persons will interact with other social factors to threaten lives that advocates of assisted suicide would agree should be protected. These factors at present include the following:

The Psychological Vulnerability of Elderly and Dying Patients

Theorists may present voluntary and involuntary euthanasia as polar opposites; in practice there are many steps on the road from dispassionate, autonomous choice to subtle coercion. Elderly and disabled patients are often invited by our achievement-oriented society to see themselves as useless burdens on younger, more vital generations. In this climate, simply offering the *option* of "self-deliverance" shifts a burden of proof, so that helpless patients must ask themselves why they are *not* availing themselves of it. Society's offer of death communicates the message to certain patients that they *may* continue to live if they wish but the rest of us have no strong interest in their survival. Indeed, once the choice of a quick and painless death is officially accepted as rational, resistance to this choice may be seen as eccentric or even selfish.[3]

The Crisis in Health Care Costs

The growing incentives for physicians, hospitals, families, and insurance companies to control the cost of health care will bring additional pressures to bear on patients. Curt Garbesi, the Hemlock Society's legal consultant, argues that autonomy-based groups like Hemlock must "control the public debate" so assisted suicide will not be seized upon by public officials as a cost-cutting device. But simply basing one's own defense of assisted suicide on individual autonomy does not solve the problem. For in the economic sphere also, offering the option of suicide would subtly shift burdens of proof.

Adequate health care is now seen by at least some policymakers as a human right, as something a society owes to all its members. Acceptance of assisted suicide as an option for those requiring expensive care would not only offer health care providers an incentive to make that option seem attractive—it would also demote all other options to the status of strictly private choices by the individual. As such they may lose their moral and legal claim to public support—in much the same way that the U.S. Supreme Court, having protected abortion under a constitutional "right of privacy," has quite logically denied any government obligation to provide public funds for this strictly private choice. As life-extending care of the terminally ill is increasingly seen as strictly elective, society may become less willing to appropriate funds for such care, and economic pressures to choose death will grow accordingly.

Legal Doctrines on "Substituted Judgment"

American courts recognizing a fundamental right to refuse life-sustaining treatment have concluded that it is unjust to deny this right to the mentally incompetent. In such cases the right is exercised on the patient's behalf by others, who seek either to interpret what the patient's own wishes might have been or to serve his or her best interests. Once assisted suicide is established as a fundamental right, courts will almost certainly find that it is unjust not to extend this right to those unable to express their wishes. Hemlock's political arm, Americans Against Human Suffering, has underscored continuity between "passive" and "active" euthanasia by offering the Humane and Dignified Death Act as an amendment to California's "living will" law, and by including a provision for appointment of a proxy to choose the time and manner of the patient's death. By such extensions our legal system would accommodate nonvoluntary, if not involuntary, active euthanasia.

Expanded Definitions of Terminal Illness

The Hemlock Society wishes to offer assisted suicide only to those suffering from terminal illnesses. But some Hemlock officials have in mind a rather broad definition of "terminal illness." Derek Humphry says "two and a half million people alone are dying of Alzheimer's disease."[4] At Hemlock's 1986 convention, Dutch physician Pieter Admiraal boasted that he had recently broadened the meaning of terminal illness in his country by giving a lethal injection to a young quadriplegic woman—a Dutch court found that he acted within judicial guidelines allowing euthanasia for the terminally ill, because paralyzed patients have difficulty swallowing and could die from aspirating their food at any time.

The medical and legal meaning of terminal illness has already been expanded in the United States by professional societies, legislatures, and courts in the context of so-called passive euthanasia. A Uniform Rights of the Terminally Ill Act proposed by the National Conference of Commissioners on Uniform State Laws in 1986 defines a terminal illness as one that would cause the patient's death in a relatively short time if life-preserving treatment is *not* provided—prompting critics to ask if all diabetics, for example, are "terminal" by definition. Some courts already see comatose and vegetative states as "terminal" because they involve an inability to swallow that will lead to death unless artificial feeding is instituted. In the *Hilda Peter* case, the New Jersey Supreme Court declared that the traditional state interest in "preserving life" referred only to "cognitive and sapient life" and not to mere "biological" existence, implying that unconscious patients are terminal, or perhaps as good as dead, so far as state interests are concerned. Is there any reason to think that American law would suddenly resurrect the older, narrower meaning of "terminal illness" in the context of *active* euthanasia?

Prejudice against Citizens with Disabilities

If definitions of terminal illness expand to encompass states of severe physical or mental disability, another social reality will increase the pressure on patients to choose death: long-standing prejudice, sometimes bordering on revulsion, against people with disabilities. While it is seldom baldly claimed that disabled people have "lives not worth living," able-bodied people often say they could not live in a severely disabled state or would prefer death. In granting Elizabeth Bouvia a right to refuse a feeding tube that preserved her life, the California Appeals Court bluntly stated that her physical handicaps led her to "consider her existence meaningless" and that "she cannot be faulted for so concluding." According to disability rights expert Paul Longmore, in a society with such attitudes toward the disabled, "talk of their 'rational' or 'voluntary' suicide is simply Orwellian newspeak."[5]

Character of the Medical Profession

Advocates of assisted suicide realize that most physicians will resist giving lethal injections because they are trained, in Garbesi's words, to be "enemies of death." The California Medical Association firmly opposed the Humane and Dignified Death Act, seeing it as an attack on the ethical foundation of the medical profession.

Yet California appeals judge Lynn Compton was surely correct in his concurring opinion in the *Bouvia* case, when he said that a sufficient number of willing physicians can be found once legal sanctions against assisted suicide are dropped. Judge Compton said this had clearly been the case with abortion, despite the fact that the Hippocratic Oath condemns abortion as strongly as it condemns euthanasia. Opinion polls of physicians bear out the judgment that a significant number would perform lethal injections if they were legal.

Some might think this division or ambivalence about assisted suicide in the medical profession will restrain broad expansions of the practice. But if anything, Judge Compton's analogy to our experience with abortion suggests the opposite. Most physicians still have qualms about abortion, and those who perform abortions on a full-time basis are not readily accepted by their colleagues as paragons of the healing art. Consequently they tend to form their own professional societies, bolstering each other's positive self-image and developing euphemisms to blunt the moral edge of their work.

Once physicians abandon the traditional medical self-image, which rejects direct killing of patients in all circumstances, their new substitute self-image many require ever more aggressive effort to make this killing more widely practiced and favorably received. To allow killing by physicians in certain circumstances many create a new lobby of physicians in favor of expanding medical killing.

The Human Will to Power

The most deeply buried yet most powerful driving force toward widespread medical killing is a fact of human nature: Human beings are tempted to enjoy exercising power over others; ending another person's life is the ultimate exercise of that power. Once the taboo against killing has been set aside, it becomes progressively easier to channel one's aggressive instincts into the destruction of life in other contexts. Or as James Burtchaell has said: "There is a sort of virginity about murder; once one has violated it, it is awkward to refuse other invitations by saying, 'But that would be murder!'"[6]

Some will say assisted suicide for the terminally ill is morally distinguishable from murder and does not logically require termination of life in other circumstances. But my point is that the skill and the instinct to kill are more easily turned to other lethal tasks once they have an opportunity to exercise themselves. Thus Robert Jay Lifton has perceived differences between the German "mercy killings" of the 1930s and the later campaign to annihilate the Jews of Europe, yet still says that "at the heart of the Nazi enterprise . . . is the destruction of the boundary between healing and killing."[7] No other boundary separating these two situations was as fundamental as this one, and thus none was effective once it was crossed. As a matter of historical fact, personnel who had conducted the "mercy killing" program were quickly and readily recruited to operate the killing chambers of the death camps.[8] While the contemporary United States fortunately lacks the anti-Semitic and totalitarian attitudes that made the Holocaust possible, it has its own trends and pressures that may combine with acceptance of medical killing to produce a distinctively American catastrophe in the name of individual freedom.

These "loose cannon" arguments are not conclusive. All such arguments by their nature rest upon a reading and extrapolation of certain contingent factors in society. But their combined force provides a serious case against taking the irreversible step of sanctioning assisted suicide for any class of persons, so long as those who advocate this step fail to demonstrate why these predictions are wrong. If the strict philosophical case on behalf of "rational suicide" lacks coherence, the pragmatic claim that its acceptance would be a social benefit lacks grounding in history or common sense.

QUESTIONS FOR CONSIDERATION

1. In his criticism of the autonomy-based approach to assisted suicide, Doerflinger argued that, "safeguards against the deliberate destruction of life are thus seen as necessary to protect freedom and all other human goods." Do you agree?

2. Doerflinger states that life is a more basic right than freedom and that suicide (assisted or unassisted) is the ultimate self-contradiction of freedom. Can you think of any examples whereby life would be sacrificed for freedom?

3. In his "slippery slope" and "loose cannon" arguments, Doerflinger indicates that sanctioning suicide would lead to pressuring the elderly and disabled patients to die, making death decisions based upon economics, broadening the meaning of terminal illness, altering the commitment of the medical profession to preserve life, and encouraging human beings to exercise their power over the lives of others. Are these realistic probabilities resulting from sanctioning suicide or does Doerflinger commit the slippery slope fallacy?

NOTES

1. Presentation at the Hemlock Society's Third National Voluntary Euthanasia Conference, "A Humane and Dignified Death," 25–27 September, 1986, Washington, D.C. All quotations from Hemlock Society officials are from the proceedings of this conference unless otherwise noted.

2. Vatican Congregation for the Doctrine of the Faith, *Declaration on Procured Abortion* (1974), para. 11.

3. I am indebted for this line of argument to Dr. Eric Chevlen.

4. Denis Herbstein, "Campaigning for the Right to Die," *International Herald Tribune,* 11 September 1986.

5. Paul K. Longmore, "Elizabeth Bouvia, Assisted Suicide, and Social Prejudice," *Issues in Law & Medicine* 3:2 (1987), 168.

6. James T. Burtchaell, *Rachel Weeping and Other Essays on Abortion* (Kansas City: Andrews & McMeel, 1982), 188.

7. Robert Jay Lifton, *The Nazi Doctors: Medical Killing and the Psychology of Genocide* (New York: Basic Books, 1986), 14.

8. Yitzhak Rad, *Belzec, Sobibor, Treblinka* (Bloomington, IN: Indiana University Press, 1987), 11, 16–17.

Dan W. Brock

Voluntary Active Euthanasia

Since the case of Karen Quinlan first seized public attention fifteen years ago, no issue in biomedical ethics has been more prominent than the debate about forgoing life-sustaining treatment. Controversy continues regarding some aspects of that debate, such as forgoing life-sustaining nutrition and hydration, and relevant law varies some from state to state. Nevertheless, I believe it is possible to identify an emerging consensus that competent patients, or the surrogates of incompetent patients, should be permitted to weigh the benefits and burdens of alternative treatments, including the alternative of no treatment, according to the patient's values, and either to refuse any treatment or to select from among available alternative treatments. This consensus is reflected in bioethics scholarship, in reports of prestigious bodies such as the President's Commission for the Study of Ethical Problems in Medicine, The Hastings Center, and the American Medical Association, in a large body of judicial decisions in courts around the country, and finally in the beliefs and practices of health care professionals who care for dying patients.[1]

More recently, significant public and professional attention has shifted from life-sustaining treatment to euthanasia—more specifically, voluntary active euthanasia—and to physician-assisted suicide. Several factors have contributed to the increased interest in euthanasia. In the Netherlands, it has been openly practiced by physicians for several years with the acceptance of the country's highest court.[2] In 1988 there was an unsuccessful attempt to get the question of whether it should be made legally permissible on the ballot in California. In November 1991 voters in the state of Washington defeated a widely publicized referendum proposal to legalize both voluntary active euthanasia and physician-assisted suicide. Finally, some cases of this kind, such as "It's Over, Debbie," described in the *Journal of the American Medical Association*, the "suicide machine" of Dr. Jack Kevorkian, and the cancer patient "Diane" of Dr. Timothy Quill, have captured wide public and professional attention.[3]

Unfortunately, the first two of these cases were sufficiently problematic that even most supporters of euthanasia or assisted suicide did not defend the physicians' actions in them. As a result, the subsequent debate they spawned has often shed more heat than light. My aim is to increase the light, and perhaps as well to reduce the heat, on this important subject by formulating and evaluating the central ethical arguments for and against voluntary active euthanasia and physician-assisted suicide. My evaluation of the arguments leads me, with reservations to be noted, to support permitting both practices. My primary aim, however, is not to argue for euthanasia, but to identify confusions in some common arguments, and problematic assumptions and claims that need more defense or data in others. The issues are considerably more complex than either supporters or opponents often make out; my hope is to advance the debate by focusing attention on what I believe the real issues under discussion should be.

In the recent bioethics literature some have endorsed physician-assisted suicide but not euthanasia.[4] Are they sufficiently different that the moral arguments for one often do not apply to the other? A paradigm case of physician-assisted suicide is a patient's ending his or her life with a lethal dose of a medication requested of and provided by a physician for that purpose. A paradigm case of voluntary active euthanasia is a physician's administering the lethal dose, often because the patient is unable to do so. The only difference that need exist between the two is the person who actually administers the lethal dose—the physician or the patient. In each, the physician plays an active and necessary causal role.

In physician-assisted suicide the patient acts last (for example, Janet Adkins herself pushed the button after Dr. Kevorkian hooked her up to his suicide machine), whereas in euthanasia the physician acts last by performing the physical equivalent of pushing the button. In both cases, however, the choice rests fully with the patient. In both the patient acts last in the sense of retaining the right to change his or her mind until the point at which the lethal process becomes irreversible. How could there be a substantial moral difference between the two based only on this small difference in the part played by the physician in the causal process resulting in death? Of course, it might be held that the moral difference is clear and important—in euthanasia the physician kills the patient whereas in physician-assisted suicide the patient kills him- or herself. But this is misleading at best. In assisted suicide the physician and patient together kill the patient. To see this, suppose a physician supplied a lethal dose to a patient with the knowledge and intent that the patient will wrongly administer it to another. We would have no difficulty in morality or the law recognizing this as a case of joint action to kill for which both are responsible.

If there is no significant, intrinsic moral difference between the two, it is also difficult to see why public or legal policy should permit one but not the other; worries about abuse or about giving anyone dominion over the lives of others apply equally to either. As a result, I will take the arguments evaluated below to apply to both and will focus on euthanasia.

My concern here will be with *voluntary* euthanasia only—that is, with the case in which a clearly competent patient makes a full voluntary and persistent request for aid in dying. Involuntary euthanasia, in which a competent patient explicitly refuses or opposes receiving euthanasia, and nonvoluntary euthanasia, in which a patient is incompetent and unable to express his or her wishes about euthanasia, will be considered here only as potential unwanted side-effects of permitting voluntary euthanasia. I emphasize as well that I am concerned with *active* euthanasia, not withholding or withdrawing life-sustaining treatment, which some commentators characterize as "passive euthanasia." Finally, I will be concerned with euthanasia where the motive of those who perform it is to respect the wishes of the patient and to provide the patient with a "good death," though one important issue is whether a change in legal policy could restrict the performance of euthanasia to only those cases.

A last introductory point is that I will be examining only secular arguments about euthanasia, though of course many people's attitudes to it are inextricable from their religious views. The policy issue is only whether euthanasia should be permissible, and no one who has religious objections to it should be required to take any part in it, though of course this would not fully satisfy some opponents.

The Central Ethical Argument for Voluntary Active Euthanasia

The central ethical argument for euthanasia is familiar. It is that the very same two fundamental ethical values supporting the consensus on patients' rights to decide about life-sustaining treatment also support the ethical permissibility of euthanasia. These values are individual self-determination or autonomy and individual well-being. By self-determination as it bears on euthanasia, I mean people's interest in making important decisions about their lives for themselves according to their own values or conceptions of a good life, and in being left free to act on those decisions. Self-determination is valuable because it permits people to form and live in accordance with their own conception of a good life, at least within the bounds of justice and consistent with others doing so as well. In exercising self-determination people take responsibility for their lives and for the kinds of persons they become. A central aspect of human dignity lies in people's capacity to direct their lives in this way. The value of exercising self-determination presupposes some minimum of decisionmaking capacities or competence, which thus limits the scope of euthanasia supported by self-determination; it cannot justifiably be administered, for example, in cases of serious dementia or treatable clinical depression.

Does the value of individual self-determination extend to the time and manner of one's death? Most people are very concerned about the nature of the last stage of their lives. This reflects not just a fear of experiencing substantial suffering when dying, but also a desire to retain dignity and control during this last period of life. Death is today increasingly preceded by a long period of significant physical and mental decline, due in part to the technological interventions of modern medicine. Many people adjust to these disabilities and find meaning and value in new activities and ways. Others find the impairments and burdens in the last stage of their lives at some point sufficiently great to make life no longer worth living. For many patients near death, maintaining the quality of one's life, avoiding great suffering, maintaining one's dignity, and insuring that others remember us as we wish them to become of paramount importance and outweigh merely extending one's life. But there is no single, objectively correct answer for everyone as to when, if at all, one's life becomes all things considered a burden and unwanted. If self-determination is a fundamental value, then the great variability among people on this question makes it especially important that individuals control the manner, circumstances, and timing of their dying and death.

The other main value that supports euthanasia is individual well-being. It might seem that individual well-being conflicts with a person's self-determination when the person requests euthanasia. Life itself is commonly taken to be a central good for persons, often valued for its own sake, as well as necessary for pursuit of all other goods within a life. But when a competent patient decides to forgo all further life-sustaining treatment then the patient, either explicitly or implicitly, commonly decides that the best life possible for him or her with treatment is of sufficiently poor quality that it is worse than no further life at all. Life is no longer considered a benefit by the patient, but has now become a burden. The same judgment underlies a request for euthanasia: continued life is seen by the patient as no longer a benefit, but now a burden. Especially in the often severely compromised and debilitated states of many critically ill or dying patients, there is no objective standard, but only the competent patient's judgment of whether continued life is no longer a benefit.

Of course, sometimes there are conditions, such as clinical depression, that call into question whether the patient has made a competent choice, either to forgo life-sustaining treatment or to seek euthanasia, and then the patient's choice need not be evidence that continued life is no longer a benefit for him or her. Just as with decisions about treatment, a determination of incompetence can warrant not honoring the patient's choice; in the case of treatment, we then transfer decisional authority to a surrogate, though in the case of voluntary active euthanasia a determination that the patient is incompetent means that choice is not possible.

The value or right of self-determination does not entitle patients to compel physicians to act contrary to their own moral or professional values. Physicians are moral and professional agents whose own self-determination or integrity should be respected as well. If performing euthanasia became legally permissible, but conflicted with a particular physician's reasonable understanding of his or her moral or professional responsibilities, the care of a patient who requested euthanasia should be transferred to another.

Most opponents do not deny that there are some cases in which the values of patient self-determination and well-being support euthanasia. Instead, they commonly offer two kinds of arguments against it that on their view outweigh or override this support. The first kind of argument is that in any individual case where considerations of the patient's self-determination and well-being do support euthanasia, it is nevertheless always ethically wrong or impermissible. The second kind of argument grants that in some individual cases euthanasia may not be ethically wrong, but maintains nonetheless that public and legal policy should never permit it. The first kind of argument focuses on features of any individual case of euthanasia, while the second kind focuses on social or legal policy. In the next section I consider the first kind of argument.

Euthanasia Is the Deliberate Killing of an Innocent Person

The claim that any individual instance of euthanasia is a case of deliberate killing of an innocent person is, with only minor qualifications, correct. Unlike forgoing life-sustaining treatment, commonly understood as allowing to die, euthanasia is clearly killing, defined as depriving of life or causing the death of a living being. While providing morphine for pain relief at doses where the risk of respiratory depression and an earlier death may be a foreseen but unintended side effect of treating the patient's pain, in a case of euthanasia the patient's death is deliberate or intended even if in both the physician's ultimate end may be respecting the patent's wishes. If the deliberate killing of an innocent person is wrong, euthanasia would be nearly always impermissible.

In the context of medicine, the ethical prohibition against deliberately killing the innocent derives some of its plausibility from the belief that nothing in the currently accepted practice of medicine is deliberate killing. Thus, in commenting on the "It's Over, Debbie" case, four prominent physicians and bioethicists could entitle their paper "Doctors Must Not Kill."[5] The belief that doctors do not in fact kill requires the corollary belief that forgoing life-sustaining treatment, whether by not starting or by stopping treatment, is allowing to die, not killing. Common though this view is, I shall argue that it is confused and mistaken.

Why is the common view mistaken? Consider the case of a patient terminally ill with ALS disease. She is completely respirator dependent with no hope of ever being weaned. She is unquestionably competent but finds her condition intolerable and persistently requests to be removed from the respirator and allowed to die. Most people and physicians would agree that the patient's physician should respect the patient's wishes and remove her from the respirator, though this will certainly cause the patient's death. The common understanding is that the physician thereby allows the patient to die. But is that correct?

Suppose the patient has a greedy and hostile son who mistakenly believes that his mother will never decide to stop her life-sustaining treatment and that even if she did her physician would not remove her from the respirator. Afraid that his inheritance will be dissipated by a long and expensive hospitalization, he enters his mother's room while she is sedated, extubates her, and she dies. Shortly thereafter the medical staff discovers what he has done and confronts the son. He replies, "I didn't kill her, I merely allowed her to die. It was her ALS disease that caused her death." I think this would lightly be dismissed as transparent sophistry—the son went into his mother's room and deliberately killed her. But, of course, the son performed just the same physical actions, did just the same thing, that the physician would have done. If that is so, then doesn't the physician also kill the patient when he extubates her?

I underline immediately that there are important ethical differences between what the physician and the greedy son do. First, the physician acts with the patient's consent whereas the son does not. Second, the physician acts with a good motive—to respect the patent's wishes and self-determination—whereas the son acts with a bad motive—to protect his own inheritance. Third, the physician acts in a social role through which he is legally authorized to carry out the patent's wishes regarding treatment whereas the son has no such authorization. These and perhaps other ethically important differences show that what the physician did was morally justified whereas what the son did was morally wrong. What they do not show, however, is that the son killed while the physician allowed to die. One can either kill or allow to die with or without consent, with a good or bad motive, within or outside of a social role that authorizes one to do so.

The difference between killing and allowing to die that I have been implicitly appealing to here is roughly that between acts and omissions resulting in death.[6] Both the physician and the greedy son act in a manner intended to cause death, do cause death, and so both kill. One reason this conclusion is resisted is that on a different understanding of the distinction between killing and allowing to die, what the physician does is allow to die. In this account, the mother's ALS is a lethal disease whose normal progression is being held back or blocked by the life-sustaining respirator treatment. Removing this artificial intervention is then viewed as standing aside and allowing the patient to die of her underlying disease. I have argued elsewhere that this alternative account is deeply problematic, in part because it commits us to accepting that what the greedy son does is to allow to die, not kill.[7] Here, I want to note two other reasons why the conclusion that stopping life support is killing is resisted.

The first reason is that killing is often understood, especially within medicine, as unjustified causing of death; in medicine it is thought to be done only accidentally or negligently. It is also increasingly widely accepted that a physician is ethically justified in stopping life support in a case like that of the ALS patient. But if these two beliefs are correct, then what the physician does cannot be killing, and so must be allowing to die. Killing patients is not, to put it flippantly, understood to be part of physicians' job desciiption. What is mistaken in this line of reasoning is the assumption that all killings are *unjustified* causings of death. Instead, some killings are ethically justified, including many instances of stopping life support.

Another reason for resisting the conclusion that stopping life support is often killing is that it is psychologically uncomfortable. Suppose the physician had stopped the ALS patient's respirator and had made the son's claim, "I didn't kill her, I merely allowed her to die. It was her ALS disease that caused her death." The clue to the psychological role here is how naturally the 'merely" modifies "allowed her to die." The characterization as allowing to die is meant to shift felt responsibility away from the agent—the physician—and to the lethal disease process. Other language common in death and dying contexts plays a similar role; "letting nature take its course" or "stopping prolonging the dying process" both seem to shift responsibility from the physician who stops life support to the fatal disease process. However psychologically helpful these conceptualizations may be in making the difficult responsibility of a physician's role in the patient's death bearable, they nevertheless are confusions. Both physicians and family members can instead be helped to understand that it is the patent's decision and consent to stopping treatment that limits their responsibility for the patient's death and that shifts that responsibility to the patient.

Many who accept the difference between killing and allowing to die as the distinction between acts and omissions resulting in death have gone on to argue that killing is not in itself morally different from allowing to die.[8] In this account, very roughly, one kills when one performs an action that causes the death of a person (we are in a boat, you cannot swim, I push you overboard, and you drown), and one allows to die when one has the ability and opportunity to prevent the death of another, knows this, and omits doing so, with the result that the person dies (we are in a boat, you cannot swim, you fall overboard, I don't throw you an available life ring, and you drown). Those who see no moral difference between killing and allowing to die typically employ the strategy of comparing cases that differ in these and no other potentially morally important respects. This will allow people to consider whether the mere difference that one is a case of killing and the other of allowing to die matters morally, or whether instead it is other features that make most cases of killing worse than most instances of allowing to die. Here is such a pair of cases:

CASE 1. A very gravely ill patient is brought to a hospital emergency room and sent up to the ICU. The patient begins to develop respiratory failure that is likely to require intubation very soon. At that point the patient's family members and long-standing physician arrive at the ICU and inform the ICU staff that there had been extensive discussion about future care with the patient when he was unquestionably competent. Given his grave and terminal illness, as well as his state of debilitation, the patient had firmly rejected being placed on a respirator under any circumstances, and the family and physician produce the patient's advance directive to that effect. The ICU staff do not intubate the patient, who dies of respiratory failure.

CASE 2. The same as Case I except that the family and physician are slightly delayed in traffic and arrive shortly after the patient has been intubated and placed on the respirator. The ICU staff extubate the patient, who dies of respiratory failure.

In Case 1 the patient is allowed to die, in Case 2 he is killed, but it is hard to see why what is done in Case 2 is significandy different morally than what is done in Case 1. It must be other factors that make most killings worse than most allowings to die, and if so, euthanasia cannot be wrong simply because it is killing instead of allowing to die.

Suppose both my arguments are mistaken. Suppose that killing is worse than allowing to die and that withdrawing life support is not killing, although euthanasia is. Euthanasia still need not for that reason be morally wrong. To see this, we need to determine the basic principle for the moral evaluation of killing persons. What is it that makes paradigm cases of wrongful killing wrongful? One very plausible answer is that killing denies the victim something that he or she values greatly—continued life or a future. Moreover, since continued life is necessary for pursuing any of a person's plans and purposes, killing brings the frustration of all of these plans and desires as well. In a nutshell, wrongful killing deprives a person of a valued future, and of all the person wanted and planned to do in that future.

A natural expression of this account of the wrongness of killing is that people have a moral right not to be killed.[9] But in this account of the wrongness of killing, the right not to be killed, like other rights, should be waivable when the person makes a competent decision that continued life is no longer wanted or a good, but is instead worse than no further life at all. In this view, euthanasia is properly understood as a case of a person having waived his or her right not to be killed.

This rights view of the wrongness of killing is not, of course, universally shared. Many people's moral views about killing have their origins in religious views that human life comes from God and cannot be justifiably destroyed or taken away, either by the person whose life it is or by another. But in a pluralistic society like our own with a strong commitment to freedom of religion, public policy should not be grounded in religious beliefs which many in that society reject. I turn now to the general evaluation of public policy on euthanasia.

Would the Bad Consequences of Euthanasia Outweigh the Good?

The argument against euthanasia at the policy level is stronger than at the level of individual cases, though even here I believe the case is ultimately unpersuasive, or at best indecisive. The policy level is the place where the main issues lie, however, and where moral considerations that might override arguments in favor of euthanasia will be found, if they are found anywhere. It is important to note two kinds of disagreement about the consequences for public policy of permitting euthanasia. First, there is empirical or factual disagreement about what the consequences would be. This disagreement is greatly exacerbated by the lack of firm data on the issue. Second, since on any reasonable assessment there would be both good and bad consequences, there are moral disagreements about the relative importance of different effects. In addition to these two sources of disagreement, there is also no single, well-specified policy proposal for legalizing euthanasia on which policy assessments can focus. But without such specification, and especially without explicit procedures for protecting against well-intentioned misuse and ill-intentioned abuse, the consequences for policy are largely speculative. Despite these difficulties, a preliminary account of the main likely good and bad consequences is possible. This should help clarify where better data or more moral analysis and argument are needed, as well as where policy safeguards must be developed.

Potential Good Consequences of Permitting Euthanasia

What are the likely good consequences? First, if euthanasia were permitted it would be possible to respect the self-determination of competent patients who want it, but now cannot get it because of its illegality. We simply do not know how many such patients and people there are. In the Netherlands, with a population of about 14.5 million (in 1987), estimates in a recent study were that about 1,900 cases of voluntary active euthanasia or physician-assisted suicide occur annually. No straightforward extrapolation to the United States is possible for many reasons, among them, that we do not know how many people here who want euthanasia now get it, despite its illegality. Even with better data on the number of persons who want euthanasia but cannot get it, significant moral disagreement would remain about how much weight should be given to any instance of failure to respect a person's self-determination in this way.

One important factor substantially affecting the number of persons who would seek euthanasia is the extent to which an alternative is available. The widespread acceptance in the law, social policy, and medical practice of the right of a competent patient to forgo life-sustaining treatment suggests that the number of competent persons in the United States who would want euthanasia if it were permitted is probably relatively small.

A second good consequence of making euthanasia legally permissible benefits a much larger group. Polls have shown that a majority of the American public believes that people should have a right to obtain euthanasia if they want it.[10] No doubt the vast majority of those who support this right to euthanasia will never in fact come to want euthanasia for themselves. Nevertheless, making it legally permissible would reassure many people that if they ever do want euthanasia they would be able to obtain it. This reassurance would supplement the broader control over the process of dying given by the right to decide about life-sustaining treatment. Having fire insurance on one's house benefits all who have it, not just those whose houses actually burn down, by reassuring them that in the unlikely event of their house burning down, they will receive the money needed to rebuild it. Likewise, the legalization of euthanasia can be thought of as a kind of insurance policy against being forced to endure a protracted dying process that one has come to find burdensome and unwanted, especially when there is no life-sustaining treatment to forgo. The strong concern about losing control of their care expressed by many people who face serious illness likely to end in death suggests that they give substantial importance to the legalization of euthanasia as a means of maintaining this control.

A third good consequence of the legalization of euthanasia concerns patients whose dying is filled with severe and unrelievable pain or suffering. When there is a life-sustaining treatment that, if forgone, will lead relatively quickly to death, then doing so can bring an end to these patients' suffering without recourse to euthanasia. For patents receiving no such treatment, however, euthanasia may be the only release from their otherwise prolonged suffering and agony. This argument from mercy has always been the strongest argument for euthanasia in those cases to which it applies.[11]

The importance of relieving pain and suffering is less controversial than is the frequency with which patients are forced to undergo untreatable agony that only euthanasia could relieve. If we focus first on suffering caused by physical pain, it is crucial to distinguish pain that *could* be adequately relieved with modern methods of pain control, though it in fact is not, from pain that is relievable only by death.[12] For a variety of reasons, including some physicians' fear of hastening the patient's death, as well as the lack of a publicly accessible means for assessing the amount of the patient's pain, many patients suffer pain that could be, but is not, relieved.

Specialists in pain control, as for example the pain of terminally ill cancer patients, argue that there are very few patients whose pain could not be adequately controlled, though sometimes at the cost of so sedating them that they are effectively unable to interact with other people or their environment. Thus, the argument from mercy in cases of physical pain can probably be met in a large majority of cases by providing adequate measures of pain relief. This should be a high priority, whatever our legal policy on euthanasia—the relief of pain and suffering has long been, quite properly, one of the central goals of medicine. Those cases in which pain could be effectively relieved, but in fact is not, should only count significantly in favor of legalizing euthanasia if all reasonable efforts to change pain management techniques have been tried and have failed.

Dying patients often undergo substantial psychological suffering that is not fully or even principally the result of physical pain.[13] The knowledge about how to relieve this suffering is much more limited than in the case of relieving pain, and efforts to do so are probably more often unsuccessful. If the argument from mercy is extended to patients experiencing great and unrelievable psychological suffering, the numbers of patients to which it applies are much greater.

One last good consequence of legalizing euthanasia is that once death has been accepted, it is often more humane to end life quickly and peacefully, when that is what the patient wants. Such a death will often be seen as better than a more prolonged one. People who suffer a sudden and unexpected death, for example by dying quickly or in their sleep from a heart attack or stroke, are often considered lucky to have died in this way. We care about how we die in part because we care about how others remember us, and we hope they will remember us as we were in "good times" with them and not as we might be when disease has robbed us of our dignity as human beings. As with much in the treatment and care of the dying, people's concerns differ in this respect, but for at least some people, euthanasia will be a more humane death than what they have often experienced with other loved ones and might otherwise expect for themselves.

Some opponents of euthanasia challenge how much importance should be given to any of these good consequences of permitting it, or even whether some would be good consequences at all. But more frequently, opponents cite a number of bad consequences that permitting euthanasia would or could produce, and it is to their assessment that I now turn.

Potential Bad Consequences of Permitting Euthanasia

Some of the arguments against permitting euthanasia are aimed specifically against physicians, while others are aimed against anyone being permitted to perform it. I shall first consider one argument of the former sort. Permitting physicians to perform euthanasia, it is said, would be incompatible with their fundamental moral and professional commitment as healers to care for patients and to protect life. Moreover, if euthanasia by physicians became common, patients would come to fear that a medication was intended not to treat or care, but instead to kill, and would thus lose trust in their physicians. This position was forcefully stated in a paper by Willard Gaylin and his colleagues:

> The very soul of medicine is on trial . . . This issue touches medicine at its moral center; if this moral center collapses, if physicians become killers or are even licensed to kill, the profession—and, therewith, each physician—will never again be worthy of trust and respect as healer and comforter and protector of life in all its frailty.

These authors go on to make clear that, while they oppose permitting anyone to perform euthanasia, their special concern is with physicians doing so:

> We call on fellow physicians to say that they will not deliberately kill. We must also say to each of our fellow physicians that we will not tolerate killing of patients and that we shall take disciplinary action against doctors who kill. And we must say to the broader community that if it insists on tolerating or legalizing active euthanasia, it will have to find nonphysicians to do its killing.[14]

If permitting physicians to kill would undermine the very "moral center" of medicine, then almost certainly physicians should not be permitted to perform euthanasia. But how persuasive is this claim? Patients should not fear, as a consequence of permitting *voluntary* active euthanasia, that their physicians will substitute a lethal injection for what patients want and believe is part of their care. If active euthanasia is restricted to cases in which it is truly voluntary, then no patient should fear getting it unless she or he has voluntarily requested it. (The fear that we might in time also come to accept nonvoluntary, or even involuntary, active euthanasia is a slippery slope worry I address below.) Patients' trust of their physicians could be increased, not eroded, by knowledge that physicians will provide aid in dying when patients seek it.

Might Gaylin and his colleagues nevertheless be correct in their claim that the moral center of medicine would collapse if physicians were to become killers? This question raises what at the deepest level should be the guiding aims of medicine, a question that obviously cannot be fully explored here. But I do want to say enough to indicate the direction that I believe an appropriate response to this challenge should take. In spelling out above what I called the positive argument for voluntary active euthanasia, I suggested that two principal values—respecting patients' self-determination and promoting their well-being—underlie the consensus that competent patients, or the surrogates of incompetent patients, are entitled to refuse any life-sustaining treatment and to choose from among available alternative treatments. It is the commitment to these two values in guiding physicians' actions as healers, comforters, and protectors of their patients' lives that should be at the "moral center" of medicine, and these two values support physicians' administering euthanasia when their patients make competent requests for it.

What should not be at that moral center is a commitment to preserving patients' lives as such, without regard to whether those patients want their lives preserved or judge their preservation a benefit to them. Vitalism has been rejected by most physicians, and despite some statements that suggest it, is almost certainly not what Gaylin and colleagues intended. One of them, Leon Kass, has elaborated elsewhere the view that medicine is a moral profession whose proper aim is "the naturally given end of health," understood as the wholeness and well-working of the human being; "for the physician, at least, human life in living bodies commands respect and reverence—*by its very nature.*" Kass continues, "the deepest ethical principle restraining the physician's power is not the autonomy or freedom of the patient; neither is it his own compassion or good intention. Rather, it is the dignity and mysterious power of human life itself."[15] I believe Kass is in the end mistaken about the proper account of the aims of medicine and the limits on physicians' power, but this difficult issue will certainly be one of the central themes in the continuing debate about euthanasia.

A second bad consequence that some foresee is that permiting euthanasia would weaken society's commitment to provide optimal care for dying patents. We live at a time in which the control of health care costs has become, and is likely to continue to be, the dominant focus of health care policy. If euthanasia is seen as a cheaper alternative to adequate care and treatment, then we might become less scrupulous about providing sometimes costly support and other services to dying patients. Particularly if our society comes to embrace deeper and more explicit rationing of health care, frail, elderly, and dying patients will need to be strong and effective advocates for their own health care and other needs, although they are hardly in a position to do this. We should do nothing to weaken their ability to obtain adequate care and services.

This second worry is difficult to assess because there is little firm evidence about the likelihood of the feared erosion in the care of dying patents. There are at least two reasons, however, for skepticism about this argument. The first is that the same worry could have been directed at recognizing patients' or surrogates' rights to forgo life-sustaining treatment, yet there is no persuasive evidence that recognizing the right to refuse treatment caused a serious erosion in the quality of care of dying patients. The second reason for skepticism about this worry is that only a very small proportion of deaths would occur from euthanasia if it were permitted. In The Netherlands, where euthanasia under specified circumstances is permitted by the courts, though not authorized by statute, the best estimate of the proportion of overall deaths that result from it is about 2 percent.[16] Thus, the vast majority of critically ill and dying patents will not request it, and so will still have to be cared for by physicians, families, and others. Permitting euthanasia should not diminish people's commitment and concern to maintain and improve the care of these patients.

A third possible bad consequence of permitting euthanasia (or even a public discourse in which strong support for euthanasia is evident) is to threaten the progress made in securing the rights of patients or their surrogates to decide about and to refuse life-sustaining treatment.[17] This progress has been made against the backdrop of a clear and firm legal prohibition of euthanasia, which has provided a relatively bright line limiting the dominion of others over patients' lives. It has therefore been an important reassurance to concerns about how the authority to take steps ending life might be misused, abused, or wrongly extended.

Many supporters of the right of patients or their surrogates to refuse treatment strongly oppose euthanasia, and if forced to choose might well withdraw their support of the right to refuse treatment rather than accept euthanasia. Public policy in the last fifteen years has generally let life-sustaining treatment decisions be made in health care settings between physicians and patients or their surrogates, and without the involvement of the courts. However, if euthanasia is made legally permissible greater involvement of the courts is likely, which could in turn extend to a greater court involvement in life-sustaining treatment decisions. Most agree, however, that increased involvement of the courts in these decisions would be undesirable, as it would make sound decisionmaking more cumbersome and difficult without sufficient compensating benefits.

As with the second potential bad consequence of permitting euthanasia, this third consideration too is speculative and difficult to assess. The feared erosion of patients' or surrogates' rights to decide about life-sustaining treatment, together with greater court involvement in those decisions, are both possible. However, I believe there is reason to discount this general worry. The legal rights of competent patients and, to a lesser degree, surrogates of incompetent patients to decide about treatment are very firmly embedded in a long line of informed consent and life-sustaining treatment cases, and are not likely to be eroded by a debate over, or even acceptance of, euthanasia. It will not be accepted without safeguards that reassure the public about abuse, and if that debate shows the need for similar safeguards for some life-sustaining treatment decisions they should be adopted there as well. In neither case are the only possible safeguards greater court involvement, as the recent growth of institutional ethics committees shows.

The fourth potential bad consequence of permitting euthanasia has been developed by David Velleman and turns on the subtle point that making a new option or choice available to people can sometimes make them worse off, even if once they have the choice they go on to choose what is best for them.[18] Ordinarily, people's continued existence is viewed by them as given, a fixed condition with which they must cope. Making euthanasia available to people as an option denies them the alternative of staying alive by default. If people are offered the option of euthanasia, their continued existence is now a choice for which they can be held responsible and which they can be asked by others to justify. We care, and are right to care, about being able to justify ourselves to others. To the extent that our society is unsympathetic to justifying a severely dependent or impaired existence, a heavy psychological burden of proof may be placed on patients who think their terminal illness or chronic infirmity is not a sufficient reason for dying. Even if they otherwise view their life as worth living, the opinion of others around them that it is not can threaten their reason for living and make euthanasia a rational choice. Thus the existence of the option becomes a subtle pressure to request it.

This argument correctly identifies the reason why offering some patients the option of euthanasia would not benefit them. Velleman takes it not as a reason for opposing all euthanasia, but for restricting it to circumstances where there are "unmistakable and overpowering reasons for persons to want the option of euthanasia," and for denying the option in all other cases. But there are at least three reasons why such restriction may not be warranted. First, polls and other evidence support that most Americans believe euthanasia should be permitted (though the recent defeat of the referendum to permit it in the state of Washington raises some doubt about this support). Thus, many more people seem to want the choice than would be made worse off by getting it. Second, if giving people the option of ending their life really makes them worse off, then we should not only prohibit euthanasia, but also take back from people the right they now have to decide about life-sustaining treatment. The feared harmful effect should already have occurred from securing people's right to refuse life-sustaining treatment, yet there is no evidence of any such widespread harm or any broad public desire to rescind that right. Third, since there is a wide range of conditions in which reasonable people can and do disagree about whether they would want continued life, it is not possible to restrict the permissibility of euthanasia as narrowly as Velleman suggests without thereby denying it to most persons who would want it; to permit it only in cases in which virtually everyone would want it would be to deny it to most who would want it.

A fifth potential bad consequence of making euthanasia legally permissible is that it might weaken the general legal prohibition of homicide. This prohibition is so fundamental to civilized society, it is argued, that we should do nothing that erodes it. If most cases of stopping life support are killing, as I have already argued, then the court cases permitting such killing have already in effect weakened this prohibition. However, neither the courts nor most people have seen these cases as killing and so as challenging the prohibition of homicide. The courts have usually grounded patients' or their surrogates' rights to refuse life-sustaining treatment in rights to privacy, liberty, self-determination, or bodily integrity, not in exceptions to homicide laws.

Legal permission for physicians or others to perform euthanasia could not be grounded in patients' rights to decide about medical treatment. Permitting euthanasia would require qualifying, at least in effect, the legal prohibition against homicide, a prohibition that in general does not allow the consent of the victim to justify or excuse the act. Nevertheless, the very same fundamental basis of the right to decide about life-sustaining treatment—respecting a person's self-determination—does support euthanasia as well. Individual self-determination has long been a well-entrenched and fundamental value in the law, and so extending it to euthanasia would not require appeal to novel legal values or principles. That suicide or attempted suicide is no longer a criminal offense in virtually all states indicates an acceptance of individual self-determination in the taking of one's own life analogous to that required for voluntary active euthanasia. The legal prohibition (in most states) of assisting in suicide and the refusal in the law to accept the consent of the victim as a possible justification of homicide are both arguably a result of difficulties in the legal process of establishing the consent of the victim after the fact. If procedures can be designed that clearly establish the voluntariness of the person's request for euthanasia, it would under those procedures represent a carefully circumscribed qualification on the legal prohibition of homicide. Nevertheless, some remaining worries about this weakening can be captured in the final potential bad consequence, to which I will now turn.

This final potential bad consequence is the central concern of many opponents of euthanasia and, I believe, is the most serious objection to a legal policy permitting it. According to this "slippery slope" worry, although active euthanasia may be morally permissible in cases in which it is unequivocally voluntary and the patient finds his or her condition unbearable, a legal policy permitting euthanasia would inevitably lead to active euthanasia being performed in many other cases in which it would be morally wrong. To prevent those other wrongful cases of euthanasia we should not permit even morally justified performance of it.

Slippery slope arguments of this form are problematic and difficult to evaluate.[19] From one perspective, they are the last refuge of conservative defenders of the status quo. When all the opponent's objections to the wrongness of euthanasia itself have been met, the opponent then shifts ground and acknowledges both that it is not in itself wrong and that a legal policy which resulted only in its being performed would not be bad. Nevertheless, the opponent maintains, it should still not be permitted because doing so would result in its being performed in other cases in which it is not voluntary and would be wrong. In this argument's most extreme form, permitting euthanasia is the first and fateful step down the slippery slope to Nazism. Once on the slope we will be unable to get off.

Now it cannot be denied that it is *possible* that permitting euthanasia could have these fateful consequences, but that cannot be enough to warrant prohibiting it if it is otherwise justified. A similar *possible* slippery slope worry could have been raised to securing competent patients' rights to decide about life support, but recent history shows such a worry would have been unfounded. It must be relevant how likely it is that we will end with horrendous consequences and an unjustified practice of euthanasia. How *likely* and *widespread* would the abuses and unwarranted extensions of permitting it be? By abuses, I mean the performance of euthanasia that fails to safisfy the conditions required for voluntary active euthanasia, for example, if the patient has been subtly pressured to accept it. By unwarranted extensions of policy, I mean later changes in legal policy to permit not just voluntary euthanasia, but also euthanasia in cases in which, for example, it need not be fully voluntary. Opponents of voluntary euthanasia on slippery slope grounds have not provided the data or evidence necessary to turn their speculative concerns into well-grounded likelihoods.

It is at least clear, however, that both the character and likelihood of abuses of a legal policy permitting euthanasia depend in significant part on the procedures put in place to protect against them. I will not try to detail fully what such procedures might be, but will just give some examples of what they might include:

1. The patient should be provided with all relevant information about his or her medical condition, current prognosis, available alternative treatments, and the prognosis of each.
2. Procedures should ensure that the patient's request for euthanasia is stable or enduring (a brief waiting period could be required) and fully voluntary (an advocate for the patient might be appointed to ensure this).
3. All reasonable alternatives must have been explored for improving the patient's quality of life and relieving any pain or suffering.
4. A psychiatric evaluation should ensure that the patient's request is not the result of a treatable psychological impairment such as depression.[20]

These examples of procedural safeguards are all designed to ensure that the patient's choice is fully informed, voluntary, and competent, and so a true exercise of self-determination. Other proposals for euthanasia would restrict its permissibility further—for example, to the terminally ill—a restriction that cannot be supported by self-determination. Such additional restrictions might, however, be justified by concern for limiting potential harms from abuse. At the same time, it is important not to impose procedural or substantive safeguards so restrictive as to make euthanasia impermissible or practically infeasible in a wide range of justified cases.

These examples of procedural safeguards make clear that it is possible to substantially reduce, though not to eliminate, the potential for abuse of a policy permitting voluntary active euthanasia. Any legalization of the practice should be accompanied by a well-considered set of procedural safeguards together with an ongoing evaluation of its use. Introducing euthanasia into only a few states could be a form of carefully limited and controlled social experiment that would give us evidence about the benefits and harms of the practice. Even then firm and uncontroversial data may remain elusive, as the continuing controversy over what has taken place in The Netherlands in recent years indicates.[21]

The Slip into Nonvoluntary Active Euthanasia

While I believe slippery slope worries can largely be limited by making necessary distinctions both in principle and in practice, one slippery slope concern is legitimate. There is reason to expect that legalization of voluntary active euthanasia might soon be followed by strong pressure to legalize some nonvoluntary euthanasia of incompetent patients unable to express their own wishes. Respecting a person's self-determination and recognizing that continued life is not always of value to a person can support not only voluntary active euthanasia, but some nonvoluntary euthanasia as well. These are the same values that ground competent patients' right to refuse life-sustaining treatment. Recent history here is instructive. In the medical ethics literature, in the courts since *Quinlan,* and in norms of medical practice, that right has been extended to incompetent patients and exercised by a surrogate who is to decide as the patient would have decided in the circumstances if competent.[22] It has been held unreasonable to continue life-sustaining treatment that the patient would not have wanted just because the patient now lacks the capacity to tell us that. Life-sustaining treatment for incompetent patients is today frequently forgone on the basis of a surrogate's decision, or less frequently on the basis of an advance directive executed by the patient while still competent. The very same logic that has extended the right to refuse life-sustaining treatment from a competent patient to the surrogate of an incompetent patient (acting with or without a formal advance directive from the patient) may well extend the scope of active euthanasia. The argument will be, Why continue to force unwanted life on patients just because they have now lost the capacity to request euthanasia from us?

A related phenomenon may reinforce this slippery slope concern. In The Netherlands, what the courts have sanctioned has been clearly restricted to voluntary euthanasia. In itself, this serves as some evidence that permitting it need *not* lead to permitting the nonvoluntary variety. There is some indication, however, that for many Dutch physicians euthanasia is no longer viewed as a special action, set apart from their usual practice and restricted only to competent persons.[23] Instead, it is seen as one end of a spectrum of caring for dying patients. When viewed in this way it will be difficult to deny euthanasia to a patient for whom it is seen as the best or most appropriate form of care simply because that patient is now incompetent and cannot request it.

Even if voluntary active euthanasia should slip into nonvoluntary active euthanasia, with surrogates acting for incompetent patents, the ethical evaluation is more complex than many opponents of euthanasia allow. Just as in the case of surrogates' decisions to forgo life-sustaining treatment for incompetent patients, so also surrogates' decisions to request euthanasia for incompetent persons would often accurately reflect what the incompetent person would have wanted and would deny the person nothing that he or she would have considered worth having. Making nonvoluntary active euthanasia legally permissible, however, would greatly enlarge the number of patients on whom it might be performed and substantially enlarge the potential for misuse and abuse. As noted above, frail and debilitated elderly people, often demented or otherwise incompetent and thereby unable to defend and assert their own interests, may be especially vulnerable to unwanted euthanasia.

For some people, this risk is more than sufficient reason to oppose the legalization of voluntary euthanasia. But while we should in general be cautious about inferring much from the experience in The Netherlands to what our own experience in the United States might be, there may be one important lesson that we can learn from them. One commentator has noted that in The Netherlands families of incompetent patients have less authority than do families in the United States to act as surrogates for incompetent patients in making decisions to forgo life-sustaining treatment.[24] From the Dutch perspective, it may be we in the United States who are *already* on the slippery slope in having given surrogates broad authority to forgo life-sustaining treatment for incompetent persons. In this view, the more important moral divide, and the more important with regard to potential for abuse, is not between forgoing life-sustaining treatment and euthanasia, but instead between voluntary and nonvoluntary performance of either. If this is correct, then the more important issue is ensuring the appropriate principles and procedural safeguards for the exercise of decisionmaking authority by surrogates for incompetent persons in all decisions at the end of life. This may be the correct response to slippery slope worries about euthanasia.

I have cited both good and bad consequences that have been thought likely from a policy change permitting voluntary active euthanasia, and have tried to evaluate their likelihood and relative importance. Nevertheless, as I noted earlier, reasonable disagreement remains both about the consequences of permitting euthanasia and about which of these consequences are more important. The depth and strength of public and professional debate about whether, all things considered, permitting euthanasia would be desirable or undesirable reflects these disagreements. While my own view is that the balance of considerations supports permitting the practice, my principal purpose here has been to clarify the main issues.

The Role of Physicians

If euthanasia is made legally permissible, should physicians take part in it? Should only physicians be permitted to perform it, as is the case in The Netherlands? In discussing whether euthanasia is incompatible with medicine's commitment to curing, caring for, and comforting patents, I argued that it is not at odds with a proper understanding of the aims of medicine, and so need not undermine patients' trust in their physicians. If that argument is correct, then physicians probably should not be prohibited, either by law or by professional norms, from taking part in a legally permissible practice of euthanasia (nor, of course, should they be compelled to do so if their personal or professional scruples forbid it). Most physicians in The Netherlands appear not to understand euthanasia to be incompatible with their professional commitments.

Sometimes patients who would be able to end their lives on their own nevertheless seek the assistance of physicians. Physician involvement in such cases may have important benefits to patients and others beyond simply assuring the use of effective means. Historically, in the United States suicide has carried a strong negative stigma that many today believe unwarranted. Seeking a physician's assistance, or what can almost seem a physician's blessing, may be a way of trying to remove that stigma and show others that the decision for suicide was made with due seriousness and was justified under the circumstances. The physician's involvement provides a kind of social approval, or more accurately helps counter what would otherwise be unwarranted social disapproval.

There are also at least two reasons for restricting the practice of euthanasia to physicians only. First, physicians would inevitably be involved in some of the important procedural safeguards necessary to a defensible practice, such as seeing to it that the patient is well-informed about his or her condition, prognosis, and possible treatments, and ensuring that all reasonable means have been taken to improve the quality of the patient's life. Second, and probably more important, one necessary protection against abuse of the practice is to limit the persons given authority to perform it, so that they can be held accountable for their exercise of that authority. Physicians, whose training and professional norms give some assurance that they would perform euthanasia responsibly, are an appropriate group of persons to whom the practice may be restricted.

Acknowledgments

Earlier versions of this paper were presented at the American Philosophical Association Central Division meetings (at which David Velleman provided extremely helpful comments), Massachusetts General Hospital, Yale University School of Medicine, Princeton University, Brown University, and as the Brin Lecture at The Johns Hopkins School of Medicine. I am grateful to the audiences on each of these occasions, to several anonymous reviewers, and to Norman Daniels for helpful comments. The paper was completed while I was a Fellow in the Program in Ethics and the Professions at Harvard University.

QUESTIONS FOR CONSIDERATION

1. Brock indicates that in some bioethics literature physician-assisted suicide is viewed as acceptable while euthanasia is not. How does Brock criticize this distinction?
2. Describe the two values that Brock offers in support of voluntary active euthanasia.
3. How does Brock respond to the charge that "euthanasia is the deliberate killing of an innocent person"? How does the example of the greedy son illustrate his point?
4. Why does Brock indicate that euthanasia at the policy level is more problematic than on an individual level?
5. According to Brock, what are the potential good consequences of a public policy allowing euthanasia?
6. What are the potential bad consequences of a public policy allowing euthanasia and how does Brock respond to such concerns?
7. Do you agree with Brock that the policy procedures he listed would assure patients that their autonomy and well-being would be protected? Why would he wish to restrict euthanasia to the terminally ill? Why shouldn't a patient with a low quality of life have access to euthanasia?
8. Why does Brock express a concern for the possible slippery slope of voluntary active euthanasia into nonvoluntary active euthanasia? Why does he believe the United States is already on the slippery slope of nonvoluntary euthanasia?
9. Why does Brock believe performing euthanasia should be restricted to physicians?

NOTES

1. President's Commission for the Study of Ethical Problems in Medicine and Biomedical and Behavioral Research, *Deciding to Forego Life-Sustaining Treatment* (Washington, D.C.: U.S. Government Printing Office, 1983); The Hastings Center, *Guidelines on the Termination of Life-Sustaining Treatment and Care of the Dying* (Bloomington: Indiana University Press, 1987); *Current Opinions of the Council on Ethical and Judicial Affairs of the American Medical Association—1989:*

Withholding or Withdrawing Life-Prolonging Treatment (Chicago: American Medical Association, 1989); George Annas and Leonard Glantz, "The Right of Elderly Patients to Refuse Life-Sustaining Treatment," *Milbank Memorial Quarterly* 64, suppl. 2 (1986): 95–162; Robert F. Weir, *Abating Treatment with Critically Ill Patients* (New York: Oxford University Press, 1989); Sidney J. Wanzer et al. "The Physician's Responsibility toward Hopelessly Ill Patients," *NEJM* 310 (1984): 955–59.

2. M.A.M. de Wachter, "Active Euthanasia in the Netherlands," *JAMA* 262, no. 23 (1989): 3315–19.

3. Anonymous, "It's Over, Debbie," *JAMA* 259 (1988): 272; Timothy E. Quill, "Death and Dignity," *NEJM* 322 (1990): 1881–83.

4. Wanzer et al., "The Physician's Responsibility toward Hopelessly Ill Patients: A Second Look," *NEJM* 320 (1989): 844–49.

5. Willard Gaylin, Leon R. Kass, Edmund D. Pellegrino, and Mark Siegler, "Doctors Must Not Kill," *JAMA* 259 (1988): 2139–40.

6. Bonnie Steinbock, ed., *Killing and Allowing to Die* (Englewood Cliffs, N.J.: Prentice Hall, 1980).

7. Dan W. Brock, "Forgoing Food and Water: Is It Killing?" in *By No Extraordinary Means: The Choice to Forgo Life-Sustaining Food and Water,* ed. Joanne Lynn (Bloomington: Indiana University Press, 1986), pp. 117–31.

8. James Rachels, "Active and Passive Euthanasia," *NEJM* 292 (1975): 78–80; Michael Tooley, *Abortion and Infanticide* (Oxford: Oxford University Press, 1983). In my paper, "Taking Human Life," *Ethics* 95 (1985): 851–65, I argue in more detail that killing in itself is not morally different from allowing to die and defend the strategy of argument employed in this and the succeeding two paragraphs in the text.

9. Dan W. Brock, "Moral Rights and Permissible Killing," in *Ethical Issues Relating to Life and Death,* ed. John Ladd (New York: Oxford University Press, 1979), pp. 94–117.

10. P. Painton and E. Taylor, "Love or Let Die," *Time,* 19 March 1990, pp. 62–71; *Boston Globe*/Harvard University Poll, *Boston Globe,* 3 November 1991.

11. James Rachels, *The End of Life* (Oxford:Oxford University Press, 1986).

12. Marcia Angell, "The Quality of Mercy," *NEJM* 306 (1982): 98–99; M. Donovan, P. Dillon, and L. Mcguire, "Incidence and Characteristics of Pain in a Sample of Medical-Surgical Inpatients," *Pain* 30 (1987): 69–78.

13. Eric Cassell, *The Nature of Suffering and the Goals of Medicine* (New York: Oxford University Press, 1991).

14. Gaylin et al., "Doctors Must Not Kill."

15. Leon R. Kass, "Neither for Love Nor Money: Why Doctors Must Not Kill," *The Public Interest* 94 (1989): 25–46; cf. also his *Toward a More Natural Science: Biology and Human Affairs* (New York: The Free Press, 1985), chs. 6–9.

16. Paul J. Van der Maas et al., "Euthanasia and Other Medical Decisions Concerning the End of Life," *Lancet* 338 (1991): 669–74.

17. Susan M. Wolf, "Holding the Line on Euthanasia," Special Supplement, *Hastings Center Report* 19, no. 1 (1989): 13–15.

18. My formulation of this argument derives from David Velleman's statement of it in his commentary on an earlier version of this paper delivered at the American Philosophical Association Central Division meetings; a similar point was made to me by Elisha Milgram in discussion on another occasion. For more general development of the point see Thomas Schelling, *The Strategy of Conflict* (Cambridge, Mass.: Harvard University Press, 1960); and Gerald Dworkin, "Is More Choice Better Than Less?" in *The Theory and Practice of Autonomy* (Cambridge: Cambridge University Press, 1988).

19. Frederick Schauer, "Slippery Slopes," *Harvard Law Review* 99 (1985): 361–83; Wibren van der Burg, "The Slippery Slope Argument," *Ethics* 102 (October 1991): 42–65.

20. There is evidence that physicians commonly fail to diagnose depression. See Robert I. Misbin, "Physicians Aid in Dying," *NEJM* 325 (1991): 1304–7.

21. Richard Fenigsen, "A Case against Dutch Euthanasia," Special Supplement, *Hastings Center Report* 19, no. 1 (1989): 22–30.

22. Allen E. Buchanan and Dan W. Brock, *Deciding for Others: The Ethics of Surrogate Decisionmaking* (Cambridge: Cambridge University Press, 1989).

23. Van der Maas et al., "Euthanasia and Other Medical Decisions."

24. Margaret P. Battin, "Seven Caveats Concerning the Discussion of Euthanasia in Holland," *American Philosophical Association Newsletter on Philosophy and Medicine 89,* no. 2 (1990).

Daniel Callahan

When Self-Determination Runs Amok

The euthanasia debate is not just another moral debate, one in a long list of arguments in our pluralistic society. It is profoundly emblematic of three important turning points in Western thought. The first is that of the legitimate conditions under which one person can kill another. The acceptance of voluntary active euthanasia would morally sanction what can only be called "consenting adult killing." By that term I mean the killing of one person by another in the name of their mutual right to be killer and killed if they freely agree to play those roles. This turn flies in the face of a long-standing effort to limit the circumstances under which one person can take the life of another, from efforts to control the free flow of guns and arms, to abolish capital punishment, and to more tightly control warfare. Euthanasia would add a whole new category of killing to a society that already has too many excuses to indulge itself in that way.

The second turning point lies in the meaning and limits of self-determination. The acceptance of euthanasia would sanction a view of autonomy holding that individuals may, in the name of their own private, idiosyncratic view of the good life, call upon others, including such institutions as medicine, to help them pursue that life, even at the risk of harm to the common good. This works against the idea that the meaning and scope of our own right to lead our own lives must be conditioned by, and be compatible with, the good of the community, which is more than an aggregate of self-directing individuals.

The third turning point is to be found in the claim being made upon medicine: it should be prepared to make its skills available to individuals to help them achieve their private vision of the good life. This puts medicine in the business of promoting the individualistic pursuit of general human happiness and well-being. It would overturn the traditional belief that medicine should limit its domain to promoting and preserving human health, redirecting it instead to the relief of that suffering which stems from life itself, not merely from a sick body.

I believe that, at each of these three turning points, proponents of euthanasia push us in the wrong direction. Arguments in favor of euthanasia fall into four general categories, which I will take up in turn: (1) the moral claim of individual self-determination and well-being; (2) the moral irrelevance of the difference between killing and allowing to die; (3) the supposed paucity of evidence to show likely harmful consequences of legalized euthanasia; and (4) the compatibility of euthanasia and medical practice.

Self-Determination

Central to most arguments for euthanasia is the principle of self-determination. People are presumed to have an interest in deciding for themselves, according to their own beliefs about what makes life good, how they will conduct their lives. That is an important value, but the question in the euthanasia context is, What does it mean and how far should it extend? If it were a question of suicide, where a person takes her own life without assistance from another, that principle might be pertinent, at least for debate. But euthanasia is not that limited a matter. The self-determination in that case can only be effected by the moral and physical assistance of another. Euthanasia is thus no longer a matter only of self-determination, but of a mutual, social decision between two people, the one to be killed and the other to do the killing.

How are we to make the moral move from my right of self-determination to some doctor's right to kill me—from *my* right to *his* right? Where does the doctor's moral warrant to kill come from? Ought doctors to be able to kill anyone they want as long as permission is given by competent persons? Is our right to life just like a piece of property, to be given away or alienated if the price (happiness, relief of suffering) is right? And then to be destroyed with our permission once alienated?

In answer to all those questions, I will say this: I have yet to hear a plausible argument why it should be permissible for us to put this kind of power in the hands of another, whether a doctor or anyone else. The idea that we can waive our right to life, and then give to another the power to take that life, requires a justification yet to be provided by anyone.

Slavery was long ago outlawed on the ground that one person should not have the right to own another, even with the other's permission. Why? Because it is a fundamental moral wrong for one person to give over his life and fate to another, whatever the good consequences, and no less a wrong for another person to have that kind of total, final power. Like slavery, dueling was long ago banned on similar grounds: even free, competent individuals should not have the power to kill each other, whatever their motives, whatever the circumstances. Consenting adult killing, like consenting adult slavery or degradation, is a strange route to human dignity.

There is another problem as well. If doctors, once sanctioned to carry out euthanasia, are to be themselves responsible moral agents—not simply hired hands with lethal injections at the ready—then they must have their own *independent* moral grounds to kill those who request such services. What do I mean? As those who favor euthanasia are quick to point out, some people want it because their life has become so burdensome it no longer seems worth living.

The doctor will have a difficulty at this point. The degree and intensity to which people suffer from their diseases and their dying, and whether they find life more of a burden than a benefit, has very little directly to do with the nature or extent of their actual physical condition. Three people can have the same condition, but only one will find the suffering unbearable. People suffer, but suffering is as much a function of the values of individuals as it is of the physical causes of that suffering. Inevitably in that circumstance, the doctor will in effect be treating the patient's values. To be responsible, the doctor would have to share those values. The doctor would have to decide, on her own, whether the patient's life was "no longer worth living."

But how could a doctor possibly know that or make such a judgment? Just because the patient said so? I raise this question because, while in Holland at the euthanasia conference reported by Maurice de Wachter elsewhere in this issue, the doctors present agreed that there is no objective way of measuring or judging the claims of patients that their suffering is unbearable. And if it is difficult to measure suffering, how much more difficult to determine the value of a patient's statement that her life is not worth living?

However one might want to answer such questions, the very need to ask them, to inquire into the physician's responsibility and grounds for medical and moral judgment, points out the social nature of the decision. Euthanasia is not a private matter of self-determination. It is an act that reqiures two people to make it possible, and a complicit society to make it acceptable.

Killing and Allowing to Die

Against common opinion, the argument is sometimes made that there is no moral difference between stopping life-sustaining treatment and more active forms of killing, such as lethal injection. Instead I would contend that the notion that there is no morally significant difference between omission and commission is just wrong. Consider in its broad implications what the eradication of the distinction implies: that death from disease has been banished, leaving only the actions of physicians in terminating treatment as the cause of death. Biology, which used to bring about death, has apparently been displaced by human agency. Doctors have finally, I suppose, thus genuinely become gods, now doing what nature and the deities once did.

What is the mistake here? It lies in confusing causality and culpability, and in failing to note the way in which human societies have overlaid natural causes with moral rules and interpretations. Causality (by which I mean the direct physical causes of death) and culpability (by which I mean our attribution of moral responsibility to human actions) are confused under three circumstances.

They are confused, first, when the action of a physician in stopping treatment of a patient with an underlying lethal disease is construed as *causing* death. On the contrary, the physician's omission can only bring about death on the condition that the patient's disease will kill him in the absence of treatment. We may hold the physician morally responsible for the death, if we have morally judged such actions wrongful omissions. But it confuses reality and moral judgment to see an omitted action as having the same causal status as one that directly kills. A lethal injection will kill both a healthy person and a sick person. A physician's omitted treatment will have no effect on a healthy person. Turn off the machine on me, a healthy person, and nothing will happen. It will only, in contrast, bring the life of a sick person to an end because of an underlying fatal disease.

Causality and culpability are confused, second, when we fail to note that judgments of moral responsibility and culpability are human constructs. By that I mean that we human beings, after moral reflection, have decided to call some actions right or wrong, and to devise moral rules to deal with them. When physicians could do nothing to stop death, they were not held responsible for it. When, with medical progress, they began to have some power over death—but only its timing and circumstances, not its ultimate inevitability—moral rules were devised to set forth their obligations. Natural causes of death were not thereby banished. They were, instead, overlaid with a medical ethics designed to determine moral culpability in deploying medical power.

To confuse the judgments of this ethics with the physical causes of death— which is the connotation of the word *kill*—is to confuse nature and human action. People will, one way or another, die of some disease; death will have dominion over all of us. To say that a doctor "kills" a patient by allowing this to happen should only be understood as a moral judgment about the licitness of his omission, nothing more. We can, as a fashion of speech only, talk about a doctor *killing* a patient by omitting treatment he should have provided. It is a fashion of speech precisely because it is the underlying disease that brings death when treatment is omitted; that is its cause, not the physician's omission. It is a misuse of the word *killing* to use it when a doctor stops a treatment he believes will no longer benefit the patient—when, that is, he steps aside to allow an eventually inevitable death to occur now rather than later. The only deaths that human beings invented are those that come from direct killing—when, with a lethal injection, we both cause death and are morally responsible for it. In the case of omissions, we do not cause death even if we may be judged morally responsible for it.

This difference between causality and culpability also helps us see why a doctor who has omitted a treatment he should have provided has "killed" that patient while another doctor—performing precisely the same act of omission on another patient in different circumstance—does not kill her, but only allows her to die. The difference is that we have come, by moral convention and conviction, to classify unauthorized or illegitimate omissions as acts of "killing." We call them "killing" in the expanded sense of the term: a culpable action that permits the real cause of death, the underlying disease, to proceed to its lethal conclusion. By contrast, the doctor who, at the patient's request, omits or terminates unwanted treatment does not kill at all. Her underlying disease, not his action, is the physical cause of death; and we have agreed to consider actions of that kind to be morally licit. He thus can truly be said to have "allowed" her to die.

If we fail to maintain the distinction between killing and allowing to die, moreover, there are some disturbing possibilities. The first would be to confirm many physicians in their already too-powerful belief that, when patients die or when physicians stop treatment because of the futility of continuing it, they are somehow both morally and physically responsible for the deaths that follow. That notion needs to be abolished, not strengthened. It needlessly and wrongly burdens the physician, to whom should not be attributed the powers of the gods. The second possibility would be that, in every case where a doctor judges medical treatment no longer effective in prolonging life, a quick and direct killing of the patient would be seen as the next, most reasonable step, on grounds of both humaneness and economics. I do not see how that logic could easily be rejected.

Calculating the Consequences

When concerns about the adverse social consequences of permitting euthanasia are raised, its advocates tend to dismiss them as unfounded and overly speculative. On the contrary, recent data about the Dutch experience suggests that such concerns are right on target. From my own discussions in Holland, and from the articles on that subject in this issue and elsewhere, I believe we can now fully see most of the *likely* consequences of legal euthanasia.

Three consequences seem almost certain, in this or any other country: the inevitability of some abuse of the law; the difficulty of precisely writing, and then enforcing, the law; and the inherent slipperiness of the moral reasons for legalizing euthanasia in the first place.

Why is abuse inevitable? One reason is that almost all laws on delicate, controversial matters are to some extent abused. This happens because not everyone will agree with the law as written and will bend it, or ignore it, if they can get away with it. From explicit admissions to me by Dutch proponents of euthanasia, and from the corroborating information provided by the Remmelink Report and the outside studies of Carlos Gomez and John Keown, I am convinced that in The Netherlands there are a substantial number of cases of nonvoluntary euthanasia, that is, euthanasia undertaken without the explicit permission of the person being killed. The other reason abuse is inevitable is that the law is likely to have a low enforcement priority in the criminal justice system. Like other laws of similar status, unless there is an unrelenting and harsh willingness to pursue abuse, violations will ordinarily be tolerated. The worst thing to me about my experience in Holland was the casual, seemingly indifferent attitude toward abuse. I think that would happen everywhere.

Why would it be hard to precisely write, and then enforce, the law? The Dutch speak about the requirement of "unbearable" suffering, but admit that such a term is just about indefinable, a highly subjective matter admitting of no objective standards. A requirement for outside opinion is nice, but it is easy to find complaisant colleagues. A requirement that a medical condition be "terminal" will run aground on the notorious difficulties of knowing when an illness is actually terminal.

Apart from those technical problems there is a more profound worry. I see no way, even in principle, to write or enforce a meaningful law that can guarantee effective procedural safeguards. The reason is obvious yet almost always overlooked. The euthanasia transaction will ordinarily take place within the boundaries of the private and confidential doctor-patient relationship. No one can possibly know what takes place in that context unless the doctor chooses to reveal it. In Holland, less than 10 percent of the physicians report their acts of euthanasia and do so with almost complete legal impunity. There is no reason why the situation should be any better elsewhere. Doctors will have their own reasons for keeping euthanasia secret, and some patients will have no less a motive for wanting it concealed.

I would mention, finally, that the moral logic of the motives for euthanasia contain within them the ingredients of abuse. The two standard motives for euthanasia and assisted suicide are said to be our right of self-determination, and our claim upon the mercy of others, especially doctors, to relieve our suffering. These two motives are typically spliced together and presented as a single justification. Yet if they are considered independently—and there is no inherent reason why they must be linked—they reveal serious problems. It is said that a competent, adult person should have a right to euthanasia for the relief of suffering. But why must the person be suffering? Does not that stipulation already compromise the principle of self-determination? How can self-determination have any limits? Whatever the person's motives may be, why are they not sufficient?

Consider next the person who is suffering but not competent, who is perhaps demented or mentally retarded. The standard argument would deny euthanasia to that person. But why? If a person is suffering but not competent, then it would seem grossly unfair to deny relief solely on the grounds of incompetence. Are the incompetent less entitled to relief from suffering than the competent? Will it only be affluent, middle-class people, mentally fit and savvy about working the medical system, who can qualify? Do the incompetent suffer less because of their incompetence?

Considered from these angles, there are no good moral reasons to limit euthanasia once the principle of taking life for that purpose has been legitimated. If we really believe in self-determination, then any competent person should have a right to be killed by a doctor for any reason that suits him. If we believe in the relief of suffering, then it seems cruel and capricious to deny it to the incompetent. There is, in short, no reasonable or logical stopping point once the turn has been made down the road to euthanasia, which could soon turn into a convenient and commodious expressway.

Euthanasia and Medical Practice

A fourth kind of argument one often hears both in The Netherlands and in this country is that euthanasia and assisted suicide are perfectly compatible with the aims of medicine. I would note at the very outset that a physician who participates in another person's suicide already abuses medicine. Apart from depression (the main statistical cause of suicide), people commit suicide because they find life empty, oppressive, or meaningless. Their judgment is a judgment about the value of continued life, not only about health (even if they are sick). Are doctors now to be given the right to make judgments about the kinds of life worth living and to give their blessing to suicide for those they judge wanting? What conceivable competence, technical or moral, could doctors claim to play such a role? Are we to medicalize suicide, turning judgments about its worth and value into one more clinical issue? Yes, those are rhetorical questions.

Yet they bring us to the core of the problem of euthanasia and medicine. The great temptation of modern medicine, not always resisted, is to move beyond the promotion and preservation of health into the boundless realm of general human happiness and well-being. The root problem of illness and mortality is both medical and philosophical or religious. "Why must I die?" can be asked as a technical, biological question or as a question about the meaning of life. When medicine tries to respond to the latter, which it is always under pressure to do, it moves beyond its proper role.

It is not medicine's place to lift from us the burden of that suffering which turns on the meaning we assign to the decay of the body and its eventual death. It is not medicine's place to determine when lives are not worth living or when the burden of life is too great to be borne. Doctors have no conceivable way of evaluating such claims on the part of patients, and they should have no right to act in response to them. Medicine should try to relieve human suffering, but only that suffering which is brought on by illness and dying as biological phenomena, not that suffering which comes from anguish or despair at the human condition.

Doctors ought to relieve those forms of suffering that medically accompany serious illness and the threat of death. They should relieve pain, do what they can to allay anxiety and uncertainty, and be a comforting presence. As sensitive human beings, doctors should be prepared to respond to patients who ask why they must die, or die in pain. But here the doctor and the patient are at the same level. The doctor may have no better an answer to those old questions than anyone else; and certainly no special insight from his training as a physician. It would be terrible for physicians to forget this, and to think that in a swift, lethal injection, medicine has found its own answer to the riddle of life. It would be a false answer, given by the wrong people. It would be no less a false answer for patients. They should neither ask medicine to put its own vocation at risk to serve their private interests, nor think that the answer to suffering is to be killed by another. The problem is precisely that, too often in human history, killing has seemed the quick, efficient way to put aside that which burdens us. It rarely helps, and too often simply adds to one evil still another. That is what I believe euthanasia would accomplish. It is self-determination run amok.

QUESTIONS FOR CONSIDERATION

1. Characterize the three turning points in Western thought that Callahan believes are being pushed by advocates of euthanasia.
2. Callahan rejects the idea that the right of self-determination includes the right to give another the power to take life. How did he illustrate this objection with examples of slavery and dueling?
3. How does Callahan characterize the social nature of euthanasia in contrast to the view that it is a private matter of self-determination?
4. What are the confusions between causality and culpability that Callahan identifies with the notion that no moral difference exists between causing death and allowing it to occur? What are the "disturbing possibilities" he fears will occur if we fail to maintain the distinction between causing death and allowing it to occur?
5. What are the "adverse social consequences" that Callahan contends will occur with the legalization of euthanasia? How does Holland provide an example of such consequences?
6. Why does Callahan argue that a physician who assists in suicide abuses medicine? How would active voluntary euthanasia constitute an abuse of medicine in general, according to Callahan?

PART VI: Family, Parenthood, and New Reproductive Technologies

PART VI:1: Fertility, Parenthood, and Surrogacy

PART VI:2: The Care and Handling of Human Embryos

New reproductive technologies (NRTs), including *in vitro* fertilization, artificial insemination, embryo transfer, surrogacy, genetic diagnosis, and embryo freezing, are raising numerous moral and legal concerns. The very meaning of the family and parenthood is being called into question. What is a proper understanding of parenthood? Of reproduction? What reproductive technologies should be available to parents? Do the new reproductive technologies place special burdens on women and children? Do embryos have rights?

Fertility, Parenthood, and Surrogacy

In 1984, Karen Fereira-Jorge, wife of Alcino, of Johannesburg, South Africa, almost bled to death giving birth to her son. In emergency surgery, her uterus was removed. Both she and her husband (Alcino)—Roman Catholics— desired more children. They considered adoption and surrogacy.

Karen's mother, Pat Anthony, suggested an alternative. Karen's eggs would be fertilized with Alcino's sperm *in vitro* and then implanted Pat's uterus. In short, Pat would carry and give birth to her own biological/genetic granddaughter.

This case caused no problem with the South African government. Roman Catholic Church officials denounced the action, but a local priest promised to baptize the children. In late September of 1987, Pat gave birth to triplets: David, Paula, and Jose.

This case exemplifies both the benefits of new reproductive techniques as well as the moral and religious concerns of such techniques. Obviously, Karen and Alcino were given another opportunity to have their own genetic children; however, Pat gave birth to the children. In what sense could Pat be considered the "mother" of the children? Did Pat allow herself to be used as a "human incubator"? Are women exploited or liberated by the uses of these kinds of technologies?

The Care and Handling of Human Embryos

In the 1980's, a Tennessee couple, Mary Sue and Junior Lewis Davis, who were unable to conceive by natural means, turned to a Knoxville clinic for *in vitro* fertilization procedures. As a result of these procedures, seven embryos were produced and frozen for future implantation. But in the late 1980s, the marriage soured and the couple divorced. The courts were left to decide the fate of the frozen embryos as both parents vied for "custody" of the "pre-born children." In late 1989, Tennessee Circuit Court Judge W. Dale Young's decision startled the nation by holding that "human life begins at conception" and that the embryos should not be allowed to thaw (to be destroyed). Young proclaimed that it was in the "manifest best interest" of "the child or children *in vitro*" that they be preserved and thus made "available for implantation" in the future.

The *Davis* case illustrates the complex issues involved in the new prenatal technologies. *In vitro* fertilization and the transplantation of fetal tissue as a part of medical treatment have raised yet-to-be answered ethical questions. Do human embryos have rights? If so, who protects these rights? What are the obligations of parents to embryos created by *in vitro* fertilization? Under what conditions should fetal tissue be used in transplantation? Is a market in aborted fetal tissues a possibility? These questions—the relative rights and interests of parents and embryos, the "custody" of frozen embryos, and the transplantation of fetal tissue—will provide the focus of this discussion.

Readings for this section address such issues from a variety of perspectives:

Fertility, Parenthood, and Surrogacy

- Ruth Macklin's **Artificial Means of Reproduction and Our Understanding of the Family** is an analysis of the effects of artificial reproduction on the meaning of the concept of the family. She identifies a number of legal and ethical problems generated by new reproductive techniques.
- Janice G. Raymond's **Reproductive Gifts and Gift Giving: The Altruistic Woman** is an examination of what she calls the "altruistic ethic" in reference to surrogacy. While commercial surrogacy is often considered unacceptable, altruistic surrogacy is often endorsed by society. Raymond raises a number of challenges to altruistic surrogacy where "women are not only the gift givers but the gift as well."

The Care and Handling of Human Embryos

- Andrea Bonnicksen's **Genetic Diagnosis of Human Embryos** is an examination of the benefits of embryo screening over prenatal screening for couples at risk of having children with serious genetic disorders. She also examines the need for developing clinical policies for such screening and also for possible embryo therapy.
- Barbara Katz Rothman's **Not All That Glitters Is Gold** is a response to Bonnicksen's essay that focuses upon the costs of embryo diagnosis to individual women and to society as a whole.
- John A. Robertson's **Resolving Disputes Over Frozen Embryos** argues that, in light of the numerous legal disputes regarding embryos produced by *in vitro* fertilization, couples should specify in advance binding instructions for the disposition of unused embryos.
- David T. Ozar's **The Case Against Thawing Unused Frozen Embryos** states that, regardless of one's understanding of the rights (or lack of rights) of frozen embryos, these embryos ought to remain frozen as long as they are capable to survive implantation.

RUTH MACKLIN

Artificial Means of Reproduction and Our Understanding of the Family

It is an obvious truth that scientific and technologic innovations produce changes in our traditional way of perceiving the world around us. We have only to think of the telescope, the microscope, and space travel to recall that heretofore unimagined perceptions of the macrocosm and the microcosm have become commonplace. Yet it is not only perceptions, but also conceptions of the familiar that become altered by advances in science and technology. As a beginning student of philosophy, I first encountered problems in epistemology generated by scientific knowledge: If physical objects are really composed of molecules in motion, how is it that we perceive them as solid? Why is it that objects placed on a table don't slip through the empty spaces between the molecules? If the mind is nothing but electrical processes occurring in the brain, how can we explain Einstein's ability to create the special theory of relativity or Bach's ability to compose the Brandenburg Concertos?

Now questions are being raised about how a variety of modes of artificial means of reproduction might alter our conception of the family. George Annas has observed:

> Dependable birth control made sex without reproduction possible . . . . Now medicine is closing the circle . . . by offering methods of reproduction without sex; including artificial insemination by donor (AID), in vitro fertilization (IVF), and surrogate embryo transfer (SET). As with birth control, artificial reproduction is defended as life-affirming and loving by its proponents, and denounced as unnatural by its detractors.[1]

Opponents of artificial reproduction have expressed concerns about its effects on the family. This concern has centered largely but not entirely on surrogacy arrangements. Among the objections to surrogacy made by the

Roman Catholic Church is the charge that "the practice of surrogate mother-hood is a threat to the stability of the family."[2] But before the consequences for the family of surrogacy arrangements or other new reproductive practices can be assessed, we need to inquire into our understanding of the family. Is there a single, incontrovertible conception of the family? And who are the "we" presupposed in the phrase, "our understanding"? To begin, I offer three brief anecdotes.

The first is a remark made by a long-married, middle-aged man at a wedding. The wedding couple were both about forty. The bride had been married and divorced once, the groom twice. During a light-hearted discussion about marriage and divorce, the middle-aged man remarked: "I could never divorce my wife. She's family!"

The second is a remark made by a four-year-old boy. I had just moved to the neighborhood and was getting to know the children. The four-year-old, named Mikey, was being tormented by a five-year-old named Timmy. I asked Mikey, "Is Timmy your brother?" Mikey replied: "Not any more. Not the way he acts!"

The third story appears in a case study presented as part of a bioethics project on everyday dilemmas in nursing home life. A resident, Mrs. Finch, is a constant complainer who seeks more choices and independence than the nursing home allows. A social worker at the home talked to Mrs. Finch about her adaptation, suggesting that she think of the residents and staff group as a large family where "we all make allowances for each other" and "we all pull our weight." Mrs. Finch responded that she is in the nursing home because she needs health care. She already has a family and does not want another one.

In my commentary on the case of Mrs. Finch, I gave an analysis that suggests some of the complexities in understanding the concept of the family. I wrote:

> Mrs. Finch is quite right to reject the social worker's suggestion that the nursing home be viewed as "a large family." A family is a well-defined social and cultural institution. People may choose to "adopt" unrelated persons into their own family, and biologically related family members may choose to "disown" one of their members (which doesn't sever the kinship ties, though it may sever relations). But an organization or institution does not become a "family" because members or residents are exhorted to treat each other in the way family members should. The social worker's well-intended chat with Mrs. Finch is an exhortation to virtue rather than a proper reminder about the resident's obligations to her new "family."[3]

The Biological Concept of Family

It is possible, of course, to settle these conceptual matters simply and objectively by adopting a biological criterion for determining what counts as a family. According to this criterion, people who are genetically related to one another would constitute a family, with the type and degree of relatedness described in the manner of a family tree. This sense of *family* is important and interesting for many purposes, but it does not and cannot encompass everything that is actually meant by *family*, nor does it reflect the broader cultural customs and kinship systems that also define family ties.

What makes the first anecdote amusing is the speaker's deliberate use of the biological sense of *family* in a nonbiological context, that is, the context of being related by marriage. In saying that he could never divorce his wife because "she's family," he was conjuring up the associations normally connected with biologically related family and transferring those associations to a person related by the convention of marriage. In a society in which the divorce rate hovers around 50 percent, being a family member related by marriage is often a temporary state of affairs.

What makes the second anecdote amusing is Mikey's denial, based solely on Timmy's behavior, that his biologically related sibling was his brother. When two people are biologically related, they cannot wave away that kinship relation on grounds of their dislike of the other's character or conduct. They can sever their relationship, but not their genetic relatedness. Whether family members ought to remain loyal to one another, regardless of how they act, is an ethical question, not a conceptual one.

The third story also relies on the biological notion of family. Mrs. Finch construed the concept literally when she insisted that she already had a family and "didn't need another one." When I observed in my commentary that a family is a well-defined social and cultural institution, I meant to rebut the social worker's implication that anything one wants to call a family can thereby become a family. Yet considered from a moral perspective, our conception of the family does draw on notions of what members owe to one another in a functional understanding of the family:

> Families should be broadly defined to include, besides the traditional biological relationships, those committed relationships between individuals which fulfill the functions of family.[4]

It seems clear that we need a richer concept than that of biological relatedness to flesh out our understanding of the family. Although the biological concept is accurate in its delineation of one set of factors that determine what is a family, it fails to capture other significant determinants.

Newly developed artificial means of reproduction have rendered the term *biological* inadequate for making some critical conceptual distinctions, along with consequent moral decisions. The capability of separating the process of producing eggs from the act of gestation renders obsolete the use of the word *biological* to modify the word *mother*. The techniques of egg retrieval, in vitro fertilization (IVF), and gamete intrafallopian transfer (GIFT) now make it possible for two different women to make a biological contribution to the creation of a new life. It would be a prescriptive rather than a descriptive definition to maintain that the egg donor should properly be called the biological mother. The woman who contributes her womb during gestation—whether she is acting as a surrogate or is the intended rearing mother—is also a biological mother. We have only to reflect on the many ways that the intrauterine environment and maternal behavior during pregnancy can influence fetal and later child development to acknowledge that a gestating woman is also a biological mother. I will return to this issue later in considering how much genetic contributions should count in disputed surrogacy arrangements.

Additional Determinants of the Meaning of Family

In addition to the biological meaning, there appear to be three chief determinants of what is meant by *family*. These are law, custom, and what I shall call subjective intentions. All three contribute to our understanding of the family. The effect of artificial means of reproduction on our understanding of the family will vary, depending on which of these three determinants is chosen to have priority. There is no way to assign a priori precedence to any one of the three. Let me illustrate each briefly.

Law as a Determinant of Family
Legal scholars can elaborate with precision and detail the categories and provisions of family law. This area of law encompasses legal rules governing adoption, artificial insemination by donor, foster placement, custody arrangements, and removal of children from a home in which they have been abused or neglected. For present purposes, it will suffice to summarize the relevant areas in which legal definitions or decisions have determined what is to count as a family.

Laws governing adoption and donor insemination stipulate what counts as a family. In the case of adoption, a person or couple genetically unrelated to a child is deemed that child's legal parent or parents. By this legal rule, a new family is created. The biological parent or parents of the child never cease to be genetically related, of course. But by virtue of law, custom, and usually emotional tics, the adoptive parents become the child's family.

The Uniform Parentage Act holds that a husband who consents to artificial insemination by donor (AID) of his wife by a physician is the legal father of the child. Many states have enacted laws in conformity with this legal rule. I am not aware of any laws that have been enacted making an analogous stipulation in the case of egg donation, but it is reasonable to assume that there will be symmetry of reasoning and legislation.

Commenting on the bearing of family law on the practice of surrogacy, Alexander M. Capron and Margaret J. Radin contend that the "legal rules of greatest immediate relevance" to surrogacy are those on adoption. These authors identify a number of provisions of state laws on adoption that should apply in the case of surrogacy. The provisions include allowing time for a "change of heart" period after the agreement to release a child, and prohibition of agreements to relinquish parental rights prior to the child's birth.[5]

Capron and Radin observe that in the context of adoption, "permitting the birth mother to reclaim a child manifests society's traditional respect for biological ties."[6] But how does this observation bear on artificial reproduction where the biological tie can be either genetic or gestational?

Consider first the case of the gestational surrogate who is genetically unrelated to the child. Does society's traditional respect for biological ties give her or the genetic mother the right to "reclaim" (or claim in the first place) the child? Society's traditional respect is more likely a concern for genetic inheritance than a recognition of the depth of the bond a woman may feel toward a child she has given birth to.

Secondly, consider the case of egg donation and embryo transfer to the wife of the man whose sperm was used in IVF. If the sperm donor and egg recipient were known to the egg donor, could the donor base her claim to the child on "society's traditional respect for biological ties"? As I surmised earlier, it seems reasonable to assume that any laws enacted for egg donation will be similar to those now in place for donor insemination. In the latter context, society's traditional respect for biological ties gave way to other considerations arising out of the desire of couples to have a child who is genetically related to at least one of the parents.

Custom as a Determinant of Family

The most telling examples of custom as a determinant of family are drawn from cultural anthropology. Kinship systems and incest taboos dictated by folkways and mores differ so radically that few generalizations are possible.

Ruth Benedict writes: "No known people regard all women as possible mates. This is not in an effort, as is so often supposed, to prevent inbreeding in our sense, for over great parts of the world it is an own cousin, often the daughter of one's mother's brother, who is the predestined spouse."[7] In contrast, Benedict notes, some incest taboos are

> extended by a social fiction to include vast numbers of individuals who have no traceable ancestors in common . . . . This social fiction receives unequivocal expression in the terms of relationship which are used. Instead of distinguishing lineal from collateral kin as we do in the distinction between father and uncle, brother and cousin, one term means literally "man of my father's group (relationship, locality, etc.) or his generation.". . . Certain tribes of eastern Australia use an extreme form of this so-called classificatory kinship system. Those whom they call brothers and sisters are all those of their generation with whom they recognize any relationship.[8]

One anthropologist notes that "the family in all societies is distinguished by a stability that arises out of the fact that it is based on marriage, that is to say, on socially sanctioned mating entered into with the assumption of permanency."[9] If we extend the notion of socially sanctioned mating to embrace socially sanctioned procreation, it is evident that the new artificial means of reproduction call for careful thought about what should be socially sanctioned before policy decisions are made.

Subjective Intention as a Determinant of Family

This category is most heterogeneous and amorphous. It includes a variety of ways in which individuals—singly, in pairs, or as a group—consider themselves a family even if their arrangement is not recognized by law or custom. Without an accompanying analysis, I list here an array of examples, based on real people and their situations.

- A homosexual couple decides to solidify their relationship by taking matrimonial vows. Despite the fact that their marriage is not recognized by civil law, they find an ordained minister who is willing to perform the marriage ceremony. Later they apply to be foster parents of children with AIDS whose biological parents have died or abandoned them. The foster agency accepts the couple. Two children are placed in foster care with them. They are now a family.

- A variation on this case: A lesbian couple has a long-term monogamous relationship. They decide they want to rear a child. Using "turkey-baster" technology, one of the women is inseminated, conceives, and gives birth to a baby. The three are now a family, with one parent genetically related to the child.
- Pat Anthony, a forty-seven-year-old grandmother in South Africa, agreed to serve as gestational surrogate for her own daughter. The daughter had had her uterus removed, but could still produce eggs and wanted more children. The daughter's eggs were inseminated with her husband's sperm, and the resulting embryos implanted in her own mother. Mrs. Anthony gave birth to triplets when she was forty-eight. She was the gestational mother and the genetic grandmother of the triplets.
- Linda Kirkman was the gestational mother of a baby conceived with a sister's egg and destined to live with the infertile sister and her husband. Linda Kirkman said, "I always considered myself her aunt." Carol Chan donated eggs so that her sister Susie could bear and raise a child. Carol Chan said: "I could never regard the twins as anything but my nephews." The two births occurred in Melbourne within weeks of each other."[10]

My point in elucidating this category of heterogeneous examples is to suggest that there may be entirely subjective yet valid elements that contribute to our understanding of the family, family membership, or family relationships. I believe it would be arbitrary and narrow to rule out all such examples by fiat. The open texture of our language leaves room for conceptions of family not recognized by law or preexisting custom.

Posing the question, Who counts as family? Carol Levine replies: "The answer to this apparently simple question is by no means easy. It depends on why the question is being asked and who is giving the answer."[11] Levine's observation, made in the context of AIDS, applies equally well to the context of artificial means of reproduction.

The Gestational versus the Genetic Mother

One critical notion rendered problematic by the new technological capabilities of artificial reproduction is the once-simple concept of a mother. The traditional concept is complicated by the possibility that a woman can gestate a fetus genetically unrelated to her. This prospect has implications both for public policy and our understanding of the family. The central policy question is, How much should genetic relatedness count in disputed surrogacy arrangements?

A Matter of Discovery or Decision?

Which criterion—genetic or gestational—should be used to determine who is the "real" mother? I contend that this question is poorly formulated. Refering to the "real" mother implies that it is a matter of discovery, rather than one calling for a decision. To speak of "the real x" is to assume that there is an underlying metaphysical structure to be probed by philosophical inquiry. But now that medical technology has separated the two biological contributions to motherhood, in place of the single conjoint role provided by nature, some decisions will have to be made.

One decision is conceptual, and a second is moral. The conceptual question is: Should a woman whose contribution is solely gestational be termed a mother of the baby? We may assume, by analogy with our concept of paternity, that the woman who makes the genetic contribution in a surrogacy arrangement can properly be termed a mother of the baby. So it must be decided whether there can be only one mother, conceptually speaking, or whether this technological advance calls for new terminology.

Conceptual decisions often have implications beyond mere terminology. A decision not to use the term *mother* (even when modified by the adjective *gestational*) to refer to a woman who acts in this capacity can have important consequences for ethics and public policy. As a case in point, the Wayne County Circuit Court in Michigan issued an interim order declaring a gamete donor couple to be the biological parents of a fetus being carried to term by a woman hired to be the gestational mother. Upon birth, the court entered an order that the names of the ovum and sperm donors be listed on the birth certificate, rather than that of the woman who gave birth, who was termed by the court a "human incubator."[12]

The ethical question posed by the separation of biological motherhood into genetic and gestational components is, Which role should entitle a woman to a greater claim on the baby, in case of dispute? Since the answer to this question cannot be reached by discovery, but is, like the prior conceptual question, a matter for decision, we need to determine which factors are morally relevant and which have the greatest moral weight To avoid begging any ethical questions by a choice of terminology, I use the terms *genetic mother* and *gestational mother* to refer to the women who make those respective contributions. And instead of speaking of the "real" mother, I'll use the phrase primacy mother when referring to the woman presumed to have a greater claim on the child.

Morally Relevant Factors

The possibilities outlined below are premised on the notion that surrogacy contracts are voidable. I take this to mean that no legal presumption is set up by the fact that there has been a prior contract between the surrogate and the intended rearing parents. From an ethical perspective, that premise must be argued for independently, and convincing arguments have been advanced by a number of authors.[13] If we accept the premise that a contractual provision to relinquish a child born of a surrogacy agreement has no legal force, the question then becomes, Is there a morally relevant distinction between the two forms of surrogacy with respect to a claim on the child? Who has the weightiest moral claim when a surrogate is unwilling to give the baby up after its birth? Where should the moral presumption lie? The question may be answered in one of three ways.

1. Gestation. According to this position, whether a woman is merely the gestational surrogate, or also contributes her genetic material, makes no difference in determining moral priorities. In either case, the surrogate is the primary mother because the criterion is gestation.

The gestational position is adopted by George Annas and others who have argued that the gestational mother should be legally presumed to have the right and responsibility to rear the child. One reason given in support of this presumption is "the greater biological and psychological investment of the gestational mother in the child."[14] This is referred to as "sweat equity." A related yet distinct reason is "the biological reality that the mother at this point has contributed more to the child's development, and that she will of necessity be present at birth and immediately thereafter to care for the child."[15]

The first reason focuses on what the gestational mother deserves, based on her investment in the child, while the second reason, though mentioning her contribution, also focuses on the interests of the child during and immediately after birth. Annas adds that "to designate the gestational mother, rather than the genetic mother, the legal or 'natural mother' would be protective of children."[16]

2. Genetics. In surrogacy arrangements, it is the inseminating male who is seen as the father, not the husband of the woman who acts as a surrogate. This is because the genetic contribution is viewed as determinative for fatherhood. By analogy, the woman who makes the genetic contribution is the

primary mother. This position sharply distinguishes between the claim to the child made by the two different types of surrogate. It makes the surrogate who contributes her egg as well as her womb the primary (or sole) mother. But now recall the fact that in AID, the law recognizes the husband of the inseminated woman as the father—proof that laws can be made to go either way.

This position was supported by the court in *Smith & Smith v. Jones & Jones,* on grounds of the analogy with paternity. The court said: "The donor of the ovum, the biological mother, is to be deemed, in fact, the natural mother of this infant, as is the biological father to be deemed the natural father of this child."[17]

Legal precedents aside, is there a moral reason that could be invoked in support of this position? One possibility is "ownership" of one's genetic products. Since each individual has a unique set of genes, people might be said to have a claim on what develops from their own genes, unless they have explicitly relinquished any such claims. This may be a metaphorical sense of ownership, but it reflects the felt desire to have genetically related children— the primary motivation behind all forms of assisted reproduction.

Another possible reason for assigning greater weight to the genetic contribution is the child-centered position. Here it is argued that it is in children's best interest to be reared by parents to whom they are genetically related. Something like this position is taken by Sidney Callahan. She writes:

> The most serious ethical problems in using third-party donors in alternative reproduction concern the well-being of the potential child . . . . A child who has donor(s) intruded into its parentage will be cut off from its genetic heritage and part of its kinship relations in new ways. Even if there is no danger of transmitting unknown genetic disease or causing physiological harm to the child, the psychological relationship of the child to its parents is endangered—with or without the practice of deception and secrecy about its origins.[18]

Additional considerations lending plausibility to this view derive from data concerning adopted children who have conducted searches for their biological parents, and similar experiences of children whose birth was a result of donor insemination and who have sought out their biological fathers. In the case of gestational surrogacy, the child is genetically related to both of the intended rearing parents. However, there is no data to suggest whether children born of gestational mothers might someday begin to seek out those women in a quest for their "natural" or "real" mothers.

3. Gestation and genetics. According to this position, the surrogate who contributes both egg and womb has more of a claim to being the primary mother than does the surrogate who contributes only her womb. Since the first type of surrogate makes both a genetic and a gestational contribution, in case of a dispute she gets to keep the baby instead of the biological father, who has made only one contribution. But this does not yet settle the question of who has a greater moral claim to the infant in cases where the merely gestational surrogate does not wish to give up the baby to the genetic parents. To determine that, greater weight must be given either to the gestational component or the genetic component.

Subsidiary Views

One may reject the notion that the only morally relevant considerations are the respective contributions of each type of surrogate. Another possible criterion draws on the biological conception of family, and thus takes into account the contribution of the genetic father. According to this position, two genetic contributions count more than none. This leads to three subsidiary views, in addition to the three main positions outlined above.

4. Gestational surrogates have less of a moral claim to the infant than the intended parents, both of whom have made a genetic contribution. This is because two (genetic) contributions count more than one (gestational) contribution. This view, derived from "society's traditional respect for biological ties," gives greatest weight to the concept of family based on genetic inheritance.

5. A woman who contributes both egg and womb has a claim equal to that of the biological father, since both have made genetic contributions. If genetic contribution is what determines both "true" motherhood and fatherhood, the policy implications of this view are that each case in which a surrogate who is both genetic and gestational mother wishes to keep the baby would have to go to court and be settled in the manner of custody disputes.

As a practical suggestion, this model is of little value. It throws every case of this type of surrogacy—the more common variety—open to this possibility, which is to move backwards in public policy regarding surrogacy.

6. However, if genetic and gestational contributions are given equal weight, but it is simply the number of contributions that counts, the artificially inseminated surrogate has the greater moral claim since she has made two contributions—genetic and gestational—while the father has made only one, the genetic contribution.

What can we conclude from all this about the effects of artificial means of reproduction on the family and on our conception of the family? Several conclusions emerge, although each requires a more extended elaboration and defense than will be given here.

A broad definition of family is preferable to a narrow one. A good candidate is the working definition proposed by Carol Levine: "Family members are individuals who by birth, adoption, marriage, or declared commitment share deep personal connections and are mutually entitled to receive and obligated to provide support of various kinds to the extent possible, especially in times of need."[19]

Some of the effects of the new reproductive technologies on the family call for the development of public policy, while others remain private, personal matters to be decided within a given family. An example of the former is the determination of where the presumptions should lie in disputed surrogacy arrangements, whose rights and interests are paramount, and what procedures should be followed to safeguard those rights and interests. An example of the latter is disclosure to a child of the facts surrounding genetic paternity or maternity in cases of donor insemination or egg donation, including the identity of the donor when that is known. These are profound moral decisions, about which many people have strong feelings, but they are not issues to be addressed by public policy.

It is not at all clear that artificial modes of reproduction threaten to produce greater emotional difficulties for family members affected, or pose more serious ethical problems, than those already arising out of longstanding practices such as adoption and artificial insemination. The analogy is often made between the impact on women who serve as surrogates and those who have lost their biological offspring in other ways.

Warning of the dangers of surrogacy, defenders of birth mothers have related the profound emotional trauma and lasting consequences for women who have given their babies up for adoption. One such defender is Phyllis Chesler, a psychologist who has written about the mother-infant bond and about custody battles in which mothers have lost their children to fathers. Dr. Chesler repolis that many women never get over having given up their child for adoption. Their decision "leads to thirty to forty years of being haunted."[20] Chesler contends that the trauma to women who have given up their babies for adoption is far greater than that of incest, and greater than that felt by mothers who have lost custody battles for their children.

Additional evidence of the undesirable consequences for birth mothers of adoption is provided by Alison Ward, a woman who serves as an adoption reform advocate. Having given up her own daughter for adoption in 1967, she found and was reunited with her in 1980. Ms. Ward said to an audience assembled to hear testimony on surrogacy:

> I think that you lack the personal experience I have: that of knowing what it is like to terminate your parental rights and go for years not knowing if your child is dead or alive. All the intellectual and philosophical knowledge in the world cannot begin to touch having to live your life as a birthparent. Last Sunday was Mother's Day. It seems ironic, as our country gives such lip service to the values of motherhood and the sanctity of the bond between mother and child, that we even consider legalizing a process [surrogacy] which would destroy all that.[21]

The effects of these practices on children are alleged to be equally profound and damaging. Scholarly studies conducted in recent years have sought to evaluate the adjustment of children to adoption. One expert notes that "the pattern emerging from the more recent clinical and nonclinical studies that have sampled widely and used appropriate controls, generally supports the view that, on the average, adopted children are more likely to manifest psychological problems than nonadopted children."[22] The additional fact that numerous adopted children have sought to find their biological parents, despite their being in a loving family setting, suggests that psychological forces can intrude on the dictates of law or custom regarding what counts as a family. Although it is easier to keep secret from a child the circumstances surrounding artificial insemination and egg donation, such secrets have sometimes been revealed with terrible emotional consequences for everyone involved.

Alison Ward compares the impact of surrogacy on children to both situations:

> There will always be pain for these children. just as adoptive parents have learned that they cannot love the pain of their adopted children away, couples who raise children obtained through surrogacy will have to deal with a special set of problems. Donor offspring . . . rarely find out the truth of their origins. But, some of them do, and we must listen to them when they speak of their anguish, of not knowing who fathered them; we must listen when they tell us how destructive it is to their self esteem to find out their father sold the essence of his lineage for $40 or so, without ever intending to love or take responsibility for them. For children born of surrogacy contracts, it will be even worse: their own mothers did this to them.[23]

Phyllis Chesler paints a similarly bleak picture of the effect on children of being adopted away from their birth mothers. She contends that this has "dramatic, extreme psychological consequences." She cites evidence indicating that adopted children seem more prone to mental and emotional disorders than other children, and concludes that "children need to know their natural origins."[24]

These accounts present only one side, and there is surely another, more positive picture of parents and children flourishing in happy, healthy families that would not have existed but for adoption or artificial insemination. Yet the question remains, What follows in any case from such evidence? Is it reasonable to conclude that the negative consequences of these practices, which have altered traditional conceptions of the family, are reasons for abolishing them? Or for judging that it was wrong to institute them in the first place, since for all practical purposes they cannot be reversed? A great deal more evidence, on a much larger scale, would be needed before a sound conclusion could be reached that adoption and artificial insemination have had such negative consequences for the family that they ought never to have been socially sanctioned practices.

Similarly, there is no simple answer to the question of how artificial means of reproduction affect our understanding of the family. We need to reflect on the variety of answers, paying special attention to what follows from answering the question one way rather than another. Since there is no single, univocal concept of the family, it is a matter for moral and social decision just which determinants of "family" should be given priority.

QUESTIONS FOR CONSIDERATION

1. How does Macklin use the examples of the middle-aged man, the four-year old boy and the woman in the nursing home to illustrate the diversity of meaning in the concept of family?
2. Explain Macklin's contention that new reproductive techniques render the term "biological" inadequate for certain conceptual distinctions and moral decisions. How does she indicate that the term "mother" becomes obsolete with such reproductive techniques?
3. How does Macklin describe the effects of artificial reproduction on the legal determination of the meaning of family? What are some legal issues raised when the biological connection can be genetic or gestational?
4. What social sanctions does Macklin believe will be affected by artificial reproduction?

5. How do the examples of subjective intention illustrate ways that artificial means of reproduction will affect family associations not sanctioned by law or custom?

6. Explain Macklin's characterization of the concept of "mother" in the conflict between gestation and genetic. What are the public policy implications that she identifies in this conflict? What are the arguments that support the definition of mother by gestation and by genetics?

7. What analogy does Macklin draw between surrogacy and adoption? What are the effects of adoption on women and children?

NOTES

1. George J. Annas, "Redefining Parenthood and Protecting Embryos," in *Judging Medicine* (Clifton, N.J.: Humana Press, 1988), p. 59. Reprinted from the *Hastings Center Report 14*, no. 5 (1984).

2. William E. Bolan, Jr., Executive Director, New Jersey Catholic Conference, "Statement of New Jersey Catholic Conference in Connection with Public Healing on Surrogate Mothering," Commission on Legal and Ethical Problems in the Delivery of Health Care, Newark, N.J., 11 May 1988.

3. Ruth Macklin, "Good Citizen, Bad Citizen: Case Commentary," in *Everyday Ethics: Resolving Dilemmas in Nursing Home Life*, ed. Rosalie A. Kane and Arthur L. Caplan (New York: Springer, 1990), p. 65.

4. Cited in Carol Levine, "AIDS and Changing Concepts of Family," *Milbank Quarterly* 68, supp. I (1990): 37.

5. Alexander M. Capron and Margaret J. Radin, "Choosing Family Law over Contract Law as a Paradigm for Surrogate Motherhood," *Law, Medicine & Health Care* 16 (Spring-Summer 1988): 35.

6. Capron and Radin, "Choosing Family Law over Contract Law," p. 35.

7. Ruth Benedict, *Patterns of Culture* (New York: Mentor Books, 1934), p. 29.

8. Benedict, *Patterns of* Culture, p. 30.

9. Melville J. Herskovits, *Cultural Anthropology* (New York: Alfred A. Knopf, 1955), p. 171.

10. R. Alta Charo, "Legislative Approaches to Surrogate Motherhood," *Law, Medicine & Health Care* 16 (Spring-Summer 1988): 104.

11. Levine, "AIDS and Changing Concepts of Family," p. 35.

12. O.T.A. report "Infertility: Medical and Social Choices," p. 284; case cited *Smith & Smith v. Jones & Jones*, 85-532014 DZ, Detroit MI, 3rd Dist. (15 March 1986), as reported in *BioLaw*, ed. James F. Childress, Patricia King, Karen H. Rothenberg, et al. (Frederick, Md.: University Publishers of America, 1986). See also George J. Annas, "The Baby Broker Boom," *Hastings Center Report* 16, no. 3 (1986): 30–31.

13. See, e.g., George J. Annas, "Death without Dignity for Commercial Surrogacy: The Case of Baby M," *Hastings Center Report,* 18, no. 2 (1988): 21–24; and Bonnie Steinbock, "Surrogate Motherhood as Prenatal Adoption," in *Surrogate Motherhood: Politics and Privacy, ed.* Larry Gostin (Bloomington: Indiana University Press, 1990), pp. 123–35.

14. Sherman Elias and George J. Annas, "Noncoital Reproduction," *JAMA* 255 (3 January 1986): 67.

15. Annas, "Death without Dignity," p. 23.

16. Annas, "Death without Dignity," p. 24.

17. Annas, "The Baby Broker Boom," p. 31.

18. "The Ethical Challenge of the New Reproductive Technology," presentation before the Task Force on New Reproductive Practices; published in John E. Monagle and David C. Thomasma, eds., *Medical Ethics: A Guide for Health Care Professionals* (Frederick, Md.: Aspen Publishers, 1987).

19. Levine, "AIDS and Changing Concepts of Family," p. 36.

20. This statement and subsequent ones attributed to Phyllis Chesler are taken from her unpublished remarks made at a public hearing on surrogacy conducted by the New Jersey Bioethics Commission, Newark, N.J., II May 1988, in which the author was a participant.

21. Written testimony, presented orally at the New Jersey Bioethics Commission's public hearing on surrogacy, 11 May 1988.

22. David M. Brodzinsky, "Adjustment to Adoption: A Psychosocial Perspective," *Clinical Psychology Review* 7 (1987): 29.

23. Ward, written testimony from New Jersey public hearing.

24. Chesler, oral testimony at New Jersey public hearing.

JANICE G. RAYMOND

Reproductive Gifts and Gift Giving: The Altruistic Woman

In the aftermath of the "Baby M" case, the surrogacy debate has mostly left the media forum and entered the state legislatures. Many of these legislatures are now debating the legal status of surrogate contracts. Where legislative committees have opposed commercial contracts, they have tended to view alternative non-commercial surrogate parenting arrangements as ethically and legally permissible. An underlying theme here is that noncommercial arrangements are seen as altruistic. This article examines the implications of an altruistic ethic, particularly in reference to surrogacy, and highlights its problems for women in reproductive realm.

Gifts and Gift Giving

In his well-known study, *The Gift Relationship: From Human Blood to Social Policy*, Richard Titmuss opposed commercial systems of blood supply to non-commercial and altruistic systems of blood giving. Titmuss's concern was to shore up the spirit of altruism and voluntarism which he saw declining in western societies. His analysis is, in the main, a positive assessment of the possibilities of altruistic blood donation. But Titmuss also understood that giving was influenced by "the relationships set up, social and economic, between the system and the donor," and that these relationships are "strongly determined by the values and cultural orientations permeating the donor system and the society in general."[1] The dialectic between the values and structural factors emerges strongly in his work. We must ask, he wrote, if there is truly "no contract of custom, no legal bond, no functional determinism, no situations of discriminatory power, domination, constraint of compulsion, no sense of shame or guilt, no gratitude imperative and no need for the penitence of a

Chrysostom" (239). The role of cultural values and constraints in shaping gift-giving arrangements is vital.

In the case of many new reproductive practices, and surrogacy especially, "the donor system" mainly depends on women as the gift givers—women who donate the use of their bodies and the fruit of their wombs. Those who endorse altruistic surrogacy as an alternative to commercial surrogacy accept, without comment or criticism, that it is primarily women who constitute the altruistic population called upon to contribute gestating capacities.[2] The questions that Titmuss raised about "contract of custom," "functional determinism," "situations of discriminatory power," "domination, constraint or compulsion," as well as possible "shame or guilt" and a "gratitude imperative" form part of the unexamined hallowing of altruistic surrogacy.

This unexamined acceptance of women as reproductive gift givers is very much related to a longstanding patriarchal tradition of giving women away in other cultural contexts—for sex and in marriage, for example. Following Titmuss, we must continually in these discussions of altruism ask: who gives and why? But further, who has been given away historically and why? In this sense, women are not only the gift givers but the gift as well. The pervasiveness of women's personal and social obligation to give shapes the contexts of reproductive gifts and gift giving. We see this most clearly in the situation of so-called altruistic surrogacy.

Altruism versus Commercialism

Those critical of commercial surrogacy often contrast it to noncommercial or altruistic surrogacy. The New Jersey Supreme Court, in its appellate judgment, *In the Matter of Baby M*, found surrogate contracts contrary to the law and public policy of the state. Nonetheless, it concluded that there were no legal impediments to arrangements "when the surrogate mother volunteers, without any payment, to act as a surrogate."[3] Many state legislative committees are taking action to prohibit commercial surrogacy but are leaving untouched the whole area of noncommercial surrogate practices. Altruism and voluntarism emerge as moral virtues in opposition to commercialism. George Annas, who has opposed commercial surrogacy, is sympathetic to the view that "one can distinguish between doing something out of love and doing it for money. As long as existing adoption laws are followed, voluntary relinquishment of a child to a close relative (such as an infertile sister) seem acceptable."[4] Such a scenario has in fact already been played out.

In this country, one publicized case of altruistic surrogacy occurred in 1985 when Sherry King offered to become pregnant for her sister, Carole, who had undergone a hysterectomy eighteen years before. Sherry King provided both egg and womb. "I know I couldn't be a surrogate mother for money. . . . I'm doing this for love and for my sister."[5]

Such agreements have not been, confined only to sisters. In 1987, a forty-eight-year-old woman, Pat Anthony, acted as a surrogate mother for her daughter and gave birth to triplets in South Africa. The attending obstetrician, Dr. Bernstein, commented: "We feel that what Pat Anthony has done for Karen is the acceptable face of surrogacy. . . . There was no payment, no commercialism. It was an act of pure love."[6] Thus altruism becomes the ethical standard for an affirmative assessment of noncommercial surrogacy.

Altruism also is invoked to soften the pecuniary image of commercial surrogacy. Noel Keane, the well-known surrogate broker, has made an educational video called "A Special Lady," which is often shown to teenage girls in high schools and other contexts, encouraging them to consider "careers" as surrogates. The video promoted the idea that it takes a special kind of woman to bear babies for others, and that women who engage in surrogacy do so not mainly for the money but for the special joy it brings to the lives of those who can't have children themselves. A 1986 article in *The Australian* used exactly the same "special" appeal to argue "Why rent-a-uterus is a noble calling," Sonia Humphrey, the author stated:

> It does take a special kind of woman to conceive, carry under her heart and bear a child which she knows she won't see grow and develop. It also takes a special kind of woman to take a baby which is not hers by blood and rear is with all the commitment of a biological mother without the hormonal hit which nature so kindly provides. . . . But those special women do exist, both kinds. Why shouldn't both be honored?[7]

Altruism holds sway. Part of its dominance as an ethical norm derives from its accepted opposition to commercialism. Particularly in the current debate about legalizing surrogate contracts, opponents contend that these contracts make children into commodities to be bought and sold. They allege that this is tantamount to baby selling, and some have renamed the practice commercialized childbearing. Many have focused on the economic exploitation of the women who enter surrogate contracts, women who are in need of money or are financially dead-ended. In these perspectives, the ethical objection is restricted to the fact that a price tag is attached to that which should have no price. The corollary is often that surrogacy "for free" is morally and legally appropriate.

More significant for the dominance of altruism in the reproductive context, however, is the moral celebration of women's altruism. As Caroline Whitbeck has stated in a different context, "the moral expectation upon women is that they be nurturant, that is, that they ought to go beyond respecting rights and meet the needs of others."[8]

The Moral Celebration of Woman's Altruism

The cultural norm of the altruistic woman who is infinitely giving and eternally accessible derives from a social context in which women give and are given away, and from a moral tradition that celebrates women's duty to meet and satisfy the needs of others. The cultural expectation of altruism has fallen most heavily on pregnant women, so that one could say they are imaged as the archetypal altruists. As Beverly Harrison notes:

> Many philosophers and theologians, although decrying gender inequality, still unconsciously assume that women's lives should express a different moral norm than men's, that women should exemplify moral purity and self-sacrifice, whereas men may live by the more minimal rational standards of moral obligation . . . perfection and self-sacrifice are never taken to be a day-to-day moral requirement for any moral agent except, it would seem, a pregnant woman.[9]

Harrison calls this a "supererogatory morality," acts that are expected to go beyond the accepted standards of obligation. Although traditionally women have been exhorted to be passive, simultaneously they are expected to be more responsible than men for meeting the needs of others. "We live in a world where many, perhaps most, of the voluntary sacrifices on behalf of human well-being are made by women, but the assumption of a special obligation to self-giving or sacrifice . . . is male-generated ideology" (62). The other side of this altruistic coin is male self-interest. A man is allowed to be more self-seeking, to go to great lengths to fulfill his self-interests, and this has been rationalized, in the case of surrogacy, as genetic continuity and "biological fulfillment."[10]

This is not merely an ideological pronouncement about female self-giving and male self-seeking. It raises complex questions about moral double standards in a cultural context where men as a class set the standards and women live them out, where inequality is systemic, and where women have an investment in their own subordination. This does not mean that every women is altruistic. Were that the case, surely biological determinists would be right!

There is, moreover, a distinct moral language that is part of this tradition that celebrated women's altruism. It is the language of selflessness and responsibility toward others in which women's very possibilities are framed. It is the discourse of maternalism, which traditionally has been the discourse of devotion and dedication in which women turn away from their own needs. It is also the discourse of maternal destiny in which a real woman is a mother, or one who acts like a mother, or more specifically, like the self-sacrificing, nurturant, and care-taking mothers women are supposed to be. If a woman chooses a different destiny and directs herself elsewhere, she risks placing herself outside female nature and culture. This language also encases women's activities in mothering metaphors, framing many of the creative endeavors that women undertake. Motherhood becomes an inspirational metaphor or symbol for the caring, the nurturing, and the sensitivity that women bring to a world ravaged by conflict.

A body of recent feminist literature, exemplified in the work of Carol Gilligan, has valorized women's altruistic development as the morality of responsibility, emphasizing that this is morality "in a different voice" from men. Formerly a mainstay of separate but equal ideology—as in "vive la différence"—this same discourse is now being transformed by some feminists into an endorsement of women's difference in human and moral development. Yet as Catharine MacKinnon notes,

> For women to affirm difference, when difference means to dominance, as it does with gender, means to affirm the qualities and characteristics of powerlessness . . . So I am critical of affirming what we have been, which necessarily is what we have been permitted. . . .Women value care because men have valued us according to the care we give them.[11]

Altruism has been one of the most effective blocks to women's self-awareness and demand for self-determination. It has been an instrument structuring social organization and patterns of relationship in women's lives. The social relations set up by altruism and the giving of self have been among the most powerful forces that bind women to cultural roles and expectations.

The issue is not whether altruism can have any positive content in the lives of women, but rather that we cannot abstract this question from the gender-specific and gender-unequal situation of cultural values and structures in which new reproductive practices are arranged. This is not to claim that voluntary and genuine magnanimity does not exist among women. It is to say that more is at stake than the womb, the egg, or the child as gift—and the woman as gift giver.

Creating Women in the Image of Victim

Altruism is not crudely obligatory. The more complex issue is what kind of choices women make within the context of a culture and tradition that orients them to give and give of themselves. To paraphrase Marx, women make their own choices, but they often do not make them just as they please. They often do not make them under conditions they create but under constraints they are powerless to change. The social construction of women's altruism should not reduce to creating women in the victim image.

Yet when feminists stress how women's choices are influenced by the social system and how women are channeled into giving, for example, they are reproached for portraying women as passive victims. Lori Andrews in her essay "Alternative Modes of Reproduction" for the Rutgers *Reproductive Laws for the 1990s* project faults feminist critics of the new reproductive technologies for embracing arguments based on "a presumed incapacity of women to make decision."[12] For such detractors, pressure seems to exist only at the barrel of a gun.[13]

For women gifts play many roles. They generate identity, they protect status, and they often regulate guilt. Women who don't give—time, energy, care, sex—are often exposed to disapproval or penalty. But the more important element here is that on a cultural level women *are expected* to donate themselves in the form of time, energy, and body.

Emile Durkheim, in his classic work *Suicide*, maintained that suicide, seemingly the most individual of acts, must be viewed as the result of certain facts of the social milieu, what he called *courants suicidogénes*. One of these social currents was altruism. Durkheim discussed altruistic suicide as the manifestation of a *conscience collective*—the capacity of group values and forces to supersede the claims of individuality and, in the case of soldiers and widows, for example, to influence a tendency to suicide. Durkheim observed that altruistic suicide involved a group attachment of great strength, such that individual assertion and fulfillment and even life itself became secondary. The ego was given over to and eventually absorbed in another, having been stripped of its individuality. Altruism resulted when social integration was strong, so binding that the individual became not only absorbed in the group but in the group's expectations.[14]

Durkheim's analysis of social integration is especially applicable to the social construction of women's altruism of which I speak. For women, family expectations often generate this kind of social integration, with family values and inducements overriding a woman's individuality. This is especially evident in the context of family surrogacy arrangements.

Family Ties, Gifts, and the Inducement of Altruism

The potential for women's exploitation is not necessarily less because no money is involved and reproductive arrangements may take place within a family setting. The family has not always been a safe place for women. And there are unique affective "inducements" in familial contexts that do not exist elsewhere. Although there is no "coercion of contract" or "inducement " of money, there could be the coercion of family ties in which having a baby for a sister or another family member may be rationalized as the "greatest gift" one woman can give to another.

Thus we must also examine the power and role of gifts in shaping social life. In *The Gift: Forms and Functions of Exchange in Archaic Society*, Marcel Mauss contends that gifts fulfill certain obligations. These obligations vary, but in all these instances—whether gifts are used to maintain social affection or to promote unity or loyalty within the group—they are experiences as prescriptive and exacting.[15] This is true on a cultural level, as Mauss has pointed out, but it is even more true on a family level, the context most often cited as the desirable site of altruistic reproductive exchanges.

Family opinion may not force a woman, in the sense of being out-rightly coercive, to become pregnant for another family member. However, where family integration is strong, the nature of family opinion may be so engulfing that, for all practical purposes, it exacts a reproductive donation from a female source. And representing the surrogate arrangement as a gift holds the woman in tutelage to the norms of family duty, represented as giving to a family member in need.

Within family situations, it may also be considered selfish, uncaring, even dishonorable for a woman to deprive a relative of eggs of her gestating abilities. The category of altruism itself is *broadened* in family contexts to include all sorts of nontraditional reproductive "duties" that would be frowned on if women undertook them for money. Within families, it may be considered selfish for a woman to deprive her husband of children by not allowing the reproductive use of another female family member, especially *because* the arrangements will be kept within the family.

It is also highly likely that those with less power in the family will be expected to be more altruistic. Indeed they may be coerced to be so, as happened to Alejandra Munoz. Munoz, a poor, illiterate Mexican woman, was brought across the U.S. border illegally to bear a child for relatives at the urging of many family members. Munoz was deceived about her role, having been told by family members that when she became pregnant, the embryo would be flushed out and transferred to the womb of her infertile cousin, Nattie. When this did not happen, she vowed to end the pregnancy but was beleaguered and thwarted by family members. Her relatives kept her under house confinement until the delivery. When she fought to keep her child, she was threatened with exposure as a illegal alien.[16]

In 1989, a New Jersey State Task Force on New Reproductive Practices recommended that unpaid surrogate arrangements between friends, relatives, or others be made legally unenforceable. One task force member specifically directed her criticism of noncommercial surrogacy to the family context. Arguing that surrogate arrangements between family members portend the same "disastrous implications" as Baby M contract, Emily Arnow Alman said that she could foresee the "not-so-bright cousin" being exploited to bear a child for a relative.[17]

We might ask further what is suitable matter for exchange. When we speak of reproductive gifts and donations, but more especially in the case of surrogacy, where the gift and donation is the woman's body and ultimately the child who may be born of such a practice, we put the donation of persons side by side with the exchange of objects and things. The director of the New Jersey task force stated: "The task force feels that the state shouldn't confer any imprimatur of legitimacy on the practice of surrogacy in any form," and that "treating women and children and limiting their liberty by contracts enforceable by the state makes them less than human beings."[18]

Gender-Specific Ethics, Public Policy, and Legislation

While the altruistic woman may be at the center of noncommercial reproductive exchanges, so too is a portrait of science and technology as altruistic. A feature story on the mapping of the human genome in *The Economist* in May 1986 emphasized that "science's reputation—after *Challenger* and Chernobyl—could do with an altruistic megaplan."[19] The new reproductive technologies provide science with one part of this image: *in vitro* fertilization is represented as offering "new hope for the infertile"; surrogacy gives infertile couples the gift of a child; egg donation is helping others to have children. But it is not the technologies that are the sources of these reproductive gifts. It is women, and the historical medicalization of women's bodies in the reproductive context. Women are taken for granted in the name of reproductive research, the advancement of reproductive science, and of course, the giving of life.

Altruism cannot be separated from the history, the values, and the political structures reinforcing women's reproductive inequality in our society. Questions such as, Who is my stranger? which Titmuss designates as the altruistic question with respect to blood donation, cannot be asked within the context of reproductive donations without asking the prior question of Who is my Samaritan?

Reproductive gift relationships must be seen in their totality, not just as helping someone to have a child. Noncommercial surrogacy cannot be treated as a mere act of altruism, for more is at issue than the ethics of altruism. Any valorizing of altruistic surrogacy and reproductive gift giving for women must be assessed within a context of political inequality, lest it help dignify inequality. Moral meaning and public policy should not be governed by the mere absence of market values. Moral meaning and public policy should be guided by the presence of gender specificity.

What does this mean? For one thing, it means that any assessment of reproductive exchanges, whether they involve commerce or not, takes as its ethical starting point the question of women's status and how the exchange enhances or diminishes gender inequality. Gender-specific ethics devotes primary attention to the consequences to women. It recognizes not only the harm but the devaluation that happens to all women when some are used for reproductive exchanges.

In *Feminism Unmodified: Discourses on Life and Law*, Catharine MacKinnon develops this notion of gender specificity as a foundation for legislation. Gender specificity recognizes "the most sex-differential abuses of women as a gender" and the reality that this is not a mere sex "difference" but "a socially situated subjection of women."[20] It also recognizes that treating women and men as the same in law, as if all things are equal at the starting point, is gender neutrality.

A gender-specific ethics and public policy confronts the degradation of women in the "private" sphere of reproduction and recognizes the gender inequality that exists as a result, for example, of women's expected altruism. Validating altruistic surrogacy on the level of public policy leaves intact the image and reality of a woman as a *reproductive conduit*—someone through whom someone passes. The woman used as a conduit for someone else's procreative purposes, most evident in the case of surrogacy, becomes a mere instrument in reproductive exchanges, an incidental incubator detached from the total fabric of social, affective, and moral meanings associated with procreation. Thus the terminology of "donor" is inaccurate; women are more appropriately "sources" of eggs, wombs, and babies in the context of reproductive exchanges. Further, we are not really talking about "donations" here but about "procurement."

Surrogacy, situated within the larger context of gender inequality, is not simply the commercialization of women and children. On a political level, it reinforces the perception and use of women as a breeder class and reinforces the gender inequality of women as a group. This is not symbolic or intangible but strikes at the core of what a society allows women to be and become. Taking the commerce out of surrogacy but leaving the practice intact on a noncommercial and contractual basis glosses over that essential violation.

Proposals that the law keep clear of reproductive exchanges where no money changes hands are based on gender-neutral assumptions. If the harm of surrogacy, for example, is based only on the commercialization and commodification of reproduction, then the reality that *women* are always used in systems of surrogacy gets no fundamental legal notice. We must note that babies are not always born of surrogate contracts but women are always encumbered.

As a matter of public policy, the violation of a woman's person, dignity, and integrity have received no legal standing in most legislation opposed to surrogacy other than as mere allusion (the New Jersey Task Force recommendations are a notable exception). By not giving the violation of women primary standing in legislation opposing commercial surrogacy, women's systematic inequality is made invisible and kept in place. That inequality can then be romanticized as noble in so-called altruistic arrangements.

Gender-specific ethics and public policy raise serious doubt about the concept and reality of altruism and the ways it is used to dignify women's inequality. The focus on altruism sentimentalizes and thus obscures the ways women are medicalized and devalued by the new reproductive technologies and practices. An uncritical affirmation of reproductive gifts and gift givers— of egg donations, of "special ladies" who serve as so-called surrogate mothers for others who go to such lengths to have their own biological children, and of reproductive technology itself as a great gift to humanity—fails to examine the institutions of reproductive science, technology, and brokering that increasingly structure reproductive exchanges.

Women give their bodies over to painful and invasive IVF treatments when it is often their husbands who are infertile. Women are encouraged to offer their bodies in a myriad of ways so that others may have babies, health and life. These noble-calling and gift-giving arguments reinforce women as self-sacrificing and ontological donors of wombs and what issues from them.

Altruistic reproductive exchanges leave intact the status of women as a breeder class. Women's bodies are still the raw material for other's needs, desires, and purposes. The normalization of altruistic exchanges may have, in fact, the effect of promoting the view that women *should* engage in reproductive exchanges free of charge. In the surrogacy context, altruism reinforces the role of women as *mothers for others* and creates a new version of *relinquishing motherhood.*

The new reproductive altruism is very old in that it depends almost entirely upon women as the givers of these reproductive gifts. This is not to say that women cannot give freely. It is to say that things are not all that simple. It is also to say that this emphasis on giving has become an integral part of the technological propaganda performance. And finally it is to say that the altruistic pedestal on which women are placed by these reproductive practices is one more way of glorifying women's inequality.

QUESTIONS FOR CONSIDERATION

1. Why does Raymond contend that legislative committees and the courts find commercial surrogacy objectionable but not altruistic surrogacy? What is the special appeal of altruistic surrogacy?

2. How does Raymond characterize the altruistic woman in the "social context in which women give and are given away. . ."? How does this context represent a "supererogatory morality"?

3. What is the moral language of selflessness that contributes to the image of women as altruistic? Do you agree that altruism represents a major obstacle to women's self-awareness and self-determination? What risks do women take if they choose to live outside the role of a self-sacrificing caretaker, according to Raymond?

4. How does Raymond describe the family context as a coercive reproductive environment? Could surrogacy become coercive as a family obligation? Does the example of Alejandra Munoz illustrate this point?

5. What does Raymond mean by the expression "gender-specific ethics"? How does this expression relate to public policy involving altruistic surrogacy?

NOTES

1. Richard M. Titmuss, *The Gift Relationship: From Human Blood to Social Policy* (New York: Pantheon Books, 1971), 73.

2. Men donate sperm, of course, but sperm donation is simple and short-lived. As one commentator put it, comparing the donation of eggs and wombs to the donation of sperm is like comparing the giving of an eye to the shedding of a tear.

3. *Matter of Baby M,* 537 A2d 1265 (N.J. 1988).

4. George J. Annas, "Death Without Dignity for Commercial Surrogacy: The Case of Baby M," *Hastings Center Report* 18:2 (1988), 21–24, at 23.

5. "Florida Woman to Be Surrogate Mother for Sister," *Greenfield Recorder,* 12 November 1985.

6. Eric Levin, "Motherly Love Works a Miracle," *People,* 19 October 1987, 43.

7. Sonia Humphrey, "Why Rent-a-Uterus is a Noble Calling," *The Australian,* 19 December 1986.

8. Caroline Whitbeck. "The Moral Implications of Regarding Women as People: New Perspectives on Pregnancy and Personhood," in *Abortion and the Status of the Fetus,* William Bondeson *et al,* eds. (Dordrecht: D. Reidel Publishing Co., 1983), 249.

9. Beverly Wildung Harrison, *Our Right to Choose: Toward a New Ethic of Abortion* (Boston: Beacon Press, 1983), 39–40.

10. *Matter of Baby M,* 217 N.J. Super, 313.

11. Catharine A. MacKinnon, *Feminism Unmodified: Discourses on Life and Law* (Cambridge: Harvard University Press, 1987), 39.

12. Lori B. Andrews, "Alternative Modes of Reproduction," in *Reproductive Laws for the 1990's: A Briefing Handbook,* Nadine Taub and Sherrill Cohen eds. (Newark, N.J.: The State University, Rutgers, 1989), 269.

13. This reductionistic view has been challenged by many, including the New Jersey Supreme Court, which reversed the trial court's decision in the Whitehead-Stern surrogacy case. To its credit, the court recognized the complexity of consent in its assessment that for the so-called surrogate, money is an "inducement," as is the "coercion of contract."

14. Emile Durkheim, *Suicide: A Study in Sociology,* trans. John A. Spaulding and George Simpson (New York: The Free Press, 1951), 217–40

15. Marcel Mauss, *The Gift: Forms and Functions of Exchange in Archaic Societies,* trans. Ian Gunnison (New York: W.W. Norton & Co., 1967), see especially ch.1.

16. Alejandra Munoz, press conference on the founding of the National Coalition against Surrogacy, Washington, D.C., August 31, 1987.

17. Robert Hanley, "Limits on Unpaid Surrogacy Backed," *New York Times,* 12 March 1989.

18. Hanley, "Limits."

19. "How to Build a Human Being," *The Economist,* 24 May 1986, 87.

20. MacKinnon, *Feminism Unmodified,* 40–41.

ANDREA BONNICKSEN

Genetic Diagnosis of Human Embryos

On the top floor of the Gold Museum in Bogota, Colombia, visitors are ushered into a dark, windowless room; heavy doors are closed behind them. They stand in the darkness until gradually, like a ringed and rising sun, lights come on around them and they see they are surrounded by gold—glimmering, lustrous gold. Face masks, nose clips, amulets, and jewelry present a dazzling display of wealth and beauty.

We are at an analogous stage in medical genetics, when the lights come up and we marvel at the wealth of discoveries and what have been called "breathtaking" advances in DNA diagnosis. Experiments are underway to treat seriously ill patients with their own genetically corrected cells. More problematically, *in vitro* fertilization (IVF) clinics are either already analyzing egg cells for genetic defects or are poised shortly to begin DNA analysis of human embryos.

For all the worried talk about genetic engineering over the last two decades, it is surprising how quietly plans for the genetic diagnosis of human embryos have developed. The issues raised warrant careful examination: what needs are met through embryo diagnosis? Who bears responsibility for monitoring this technique? Under what overarching ethic should embryo diagnosis and, eventually, embryo therapy, be applied? What are the broader societal implications raised by the genetic diagnosis of human embryos?

The Rationale for Diagnosis

Preimplantation biopsies of human embryos are aimed at couples at high risk for having a child with a serious genetic disorder such as cystic fibrosis or Tay-Sachs disease but who will not terminate a pregnancy. A typical candidate is a couple who has one child with a serious disorder but who, for personal or religious reasons, will not undergo chorionic villus sampling (CVS) or amniocentesis and possible pregnancy termination. Traditionally, their options have been either to risk the birth of an affected child or not to conceive. Embryo biopsy gives the couple the third option of signing on with an IVF program and transferring to the wife's uterus only embryos deemed free from the genetic flaw.[1] Embryos can also be sexed in order to transfer only female embryos to couples at risk for passing a sex-linked genetic disease such as Duchenne muscular dystrophy.[2] Several IVF clinics here and abroad are offering preimplantation diagnosis or have set in motion institutional review of planned programs.[3]

Other motivations also underlie the effort to introduce embryo screening. Preimplantation diagnosis is part of a broader plan to reduce the prevalence of certain genetic diseases. Practitioners look at children with genetic disorders and, as one pediatrician said, "It is driving them crazy." He likened embryo diagnosis to the "ultimate measles vaccine": if we vaccinate children to prevent the spread of disease within a generation, should we not also discard embryos to avoid passing disease between generations? States the director of one IVF clinic, "The possibility of eliminating a fair number of genetic diseases by the end of the decade is exciting."

As IVF becomes more streamlined with extraction of eggs in the clinician's office, freezing of spare embryos, and improved implantation rates, screening of embryos presents an advantageous alternative to carrier or prenatal screening if the goal is eliminating lethal diseases. Arguably it is morally more acceptable to discard embryos than to abort pregnancies. Moreover, it allows a deleterious recessive gene to be eliminated from a family's genetic line. A second option is to use a donated embryo, but if IVF and embryo diagnosis are available, couples would probably prefer their own biological embryo.

Clinicians' more ambitious goal is to prevent disease by correcting genetic defects in embryos. Preimplantation diagnosis will prevent disease passively by discarding embryos with deleterious genes. Embryo therapy will prevent disease in a different way by treating genetic anomalies in embryos and then saving and transferring the embryos. Just as neonatologists use fetal therapy to fix defects detected through prenatal screening, so may specialists try embryo therapy in the future. For example, research aimed at correcting the CF gene in eggs is a not-too-distant possibility.[4] One clinic's draft consent form states that the embryo biopsy will "prevent genetic disease and . . . lay the foundation for site-specific gene therapy."

Nor should economic benefits be overlooked as a motivating factor behind the expected spread of preimplantation diagnosis. Although the targeted clientele is now couples at known risk who are so determined to avoid pregnancy termination that they will try repeated IVF attempts, we can predict that other groups will be targeted as well—some suggest preimplantation diagnosis could one day be a standard of care for women of advanced maternal age.[5]

The justification for routine embryo diagnosis in IVF is not difficult to imagine. If couples in IVF clinics plan to have CVS or amniocentesis anyway, it seems reasonable to examine embryos before transfer to avoid the potential trauma of a pregnancy termination, especially for couples with a history of loss due to infertility or for women over thirty-five who have special worries about chromosomal abnormalities. Couples need not wait weeks or months for the results of prenatal tests but can know at the outset that their embryos are free from major chromosomal or genetic disorders. The actual cost of embryo testing will be about the same as for fetal testing—$1,000 to $2,000. Even couples not planning on prenatal testing could see this as an attractive option. Deliberately discarding faulty embryos is arguably no worse than the constant threat in IVF of embryo loss due to biological fluke.

Thus, practitioners can present embryo diagnosis as a logical step for IVF couples planning on prenatal screening. The embryos are here, it can be said, why not test them now? Control over genetic screening remains in the IVF clinic, in contrast to present procedures, in which couples who conceive through IVF often go elsewhere for prenatal testing and care. Adding diagnosis to its IVF services can provide economic benefits for a clinic.

Although many practitioners are conservative in their predictions about the frequency and desirability of embryo testing, dreams can be ambitious. One practitioner, for example, visualizes a twenty-first century in which "sex will be for pleasure only" and conception will take place in the medical setting. To this practitioner, routine testing to secure healthy infants is a desirable future.

Embryo diagnosis will also receive an unwitting boost if access to abortion is curtailed by legislatures and courts. If it becomes difficult to terminate a pregnancy, embryo diagnosis will offer an alternative to prenatal screening. Moreover, laws defining life as beginning at the moment of conception provide a justification for embryo therapy. Whether intentionally or not, pro-life positions add to the pulse behind assisted conception, embryo diagnosis, and even therapy.

Questions for Policy Making

As with IVF, embryo freezing, and micromanipulation, a primary concern lies with the safety of the procedure. Embryo diagnosis has been studied systematically with mouse and other animal embryos. Ethical concerns about nontherapeutic research on human embryos, federal resistance to funding, and uncertainty about the legality of embryo experimentation mean that clinical application precedes systematic investigations on human embryos, although researchers study abnormal and donated normal embryos on an ad hoc basis in the U.S. and on a more systematic basis abroad.[6]

Another question relates to the accuracy of the procedure. Genetic diagnosis is complex, and the vast amount of new information from genomic studies will undoubtedly lead to premature conclusions. To suggest that disorders can be diagnosed in the human embryo when knowledge is still unfolding and the array of unknowns is great invites hubris, with weighty consequences for couples trying to have healthy children. The danger of both false positive and false negative results is real. A couple told their embryo has a genetic defect when in fact it does not will experience financial loss and emotional strain from IVF, although no one may ever know that a false positive result occurred. A couple told their embryo does not have the feared defect when in fact it does will be in a worse situation. If prenatal screening (generally a part of the embryo diagnosis research protocol) detects an affected fetus, the couple will either terminate the pregnancy after having been so motivated to avoid this that they tried a highly experimental procedure, or bear a child with the disease. That this might mean a couple will have two or more children with the same disorder magnifies the serious consequences of premature application of embryo diagnosis.

There are also concerns about the impact of embryo genetics on future generations. If embryo diagnosis becomes reasonably common for fatal disorders in which the child would not have grown up to procreate in the first place, the short-term impact will be minimal. If the range of tested disorders expands to include diseases that would not have precluded procreation, genetic diversity may be affected, though what effect this might ultimately have is not yet known. The same issue can be raised for prenatal screening (and pregnancy termination), but with an important difference: treatment of fetuses fixes the symptoms; treatment of embryos eliminates the gene.

Moreover, embryo diagnosis opens IVF to fertile couples. *In vitro* fertilization is expensive and rarely fully covered by insurance. Pregnancy rates remain low, the stress on couples is high, and hormonal hyperstimulation and egg extraction burden women physically. Embryo diagnosis is a window to new technological tinkering with reproduction that, while holding promise, opens the door to stress, discomfort, and expense for women in the short run and pressures for assisted conception as a standard procedure in the long run.

This new field opens virtually limitless possibilities for refining biopsy methods, expanding the range of disorders screened for, and correcting faulty genes. It also promises what Daniel Callahan calls the "ragged edge" of medical treatment and progress—a smooth edge is impossible when every advance creates first one and then another need to be addressed and fixed.[7] In this respect, embryo diagnosis is not so different from other areas of medicine. But trying to smooth the ragged embryo edge is different in at least one important respect: embryo manipulations are not, medically speaking, essential, and are not the simplest way of reducing illness. In a day of shrinking medical resources, their place in the hierarchy of medical priorities is open to debate.

Diagnosing and treating the embryo has few political limits. At present the federal government cannot fund research involving human embryos, and efforts to set up a structure to discuss the implications of genetic manipulations have been unsuccessful. State laws mentioning the embryo or conception were generally passed with the abortion controversy in mind and fail to provide a framework for reasoned discussion about the means and ends of embryo manipulation. One cannot realistically expect anticipatory policy to be developed in the public sector. Still, the implications of embryo genetics are too novel, far-reaching, and intimately connected with the human condition to be permitted to rise silently and by habitual degrees.

In the absence of public policy, then, a three-pronged approach to the questions raised by embryo diagnosis is in order that will (1) incorporate societal introspection about the goals of embryo diagnosis, (2) build an identity for embryo diagnosis that will place responsibility for overseeing it, and (3) develop ethically sound clinic policies.

What Needs? How Met?

Ideally, embryo genetics will be ushered into society by a cautious citizenry willing to question the goals of this new field and resist the lure of options raising troublesome implications. Embryo diagnosis is not patient-driven in the same way as IVF, nor does it have the sense of urgency of techniques designed to improve the medical status of individuals with AIDS or other terminal diseases. Introspection, then, can take place before embryo diagnosis becomes widespread in clinical practice and without the frenetic quality that comes when an immediate physical need is at issue. A critical mind, in place at the outset of embryo genetics, will ask these questions: What needs are served by embarking on embryo genetics? What priorities do these needs have in our society? Is this the best way of meeting those needs?

Embryo diagnosis is presented as a service to couples, yet a careful look should be given to how well it will actually serve couples' interests. There's no evidence to indicate a groundswell of support for the procedure among at-risk couples. In contrast to IVF, where tens of thousands of women were ready for a technique to circumvent blocked fallopian tubes, the clientele for embryo diagnosis is likely, initially at any rate, to be more narrowly defined. The technique will, in a word, need to be marketed and sold to people who may not realize they can benefit from it.

To get an idea of need, one practitioner sent a questionnaire to 123 women who had had prenatal testing because of previously abnormal conceptions. Of the 47 percent who responded, the initial impression of half, upon reading a summary of preimplantation diagnosis, was that the technique was a moderate or excellent improvement over prenatal testing. Women whose previous prenatal tests revealed abnormalities were twice as likely as other women to believe this. When asked how many IVF/embryo diagnosis procedures they themselves would undergo, 45 percent said none. They were wary about low pregnancy and birth success rates in IVF, risk to embryo, and cost.[8]

Pending further study, one may conclude that embryo diagnosis will be some time in the making inasmuch as IVF, biopsy techniques, and genetic tests on single cells all need improvement. One may expect a prolonged experimental phase during which couples will try diagnosis under varying conditions. This happened with IVF, where the patients were highly motivated and had little choice but to try this "last hope" for biological parenthood. With genetic risk, an alternative exists in the form of prenatal screening (itself being refined to detect abnormalities earlier in the pregnancy). Thus, one must consider the needs both of couples trying embryo diagnosis in the experimental stages and those trying it after the procedure becomes standard medical protocol. The former will predictably occupy much of this decade and are of more immediate concern.

For couples recruited to IVF to take part in experimental protocols, embryo diagnosis will minimize uncertainty if they cannot face the stress of waiting for prenatal screening and its results. The benefit of a shortened period of uncertainty may be outweighed, however, by new uncertainties introduced by the procedure, not least those of IVF itself. As an experimental procedure, embryo diagnosis also introduces worries about the accuracy of the results. Couples trying it will consent to CVS or amniocentesis as a routine backup, which makes embryo diagnosis a somewhat illusory relief from prenatal screening.

Couples already in IVF programs may be recruited to embryo diagnosis through monetary enticements (such as no charge for the diagnosis). However, embryo diagnosis will bring new dilemmas for people whose central mission is to have a baby. It is thought that much of the embryo loss that occurs in IVF is related to chromosomal or genetic abnormalities, so that unbeknownst to anyone, unseen flaws doom the embryo to be sloughed from the body. This natural selection occurs without choice or knowledge. Very few couples confront the dilemma of whether to continue or terminate a pregnancy when an embryo with abnormalities has implanted because most such pregnancies abort spontaneously.

With embryo diagnosis, the number and nature of people facing choices changes. More people will be given news of embryo abnormalities than fetal abnormalities. Again, this will become progressively more problematic as the number of diagnosable abnormalities grows to include not just major maladies such as Down syndrome but also moderate disorders and predispositions to disease. In short, with embryo diagnosis couples who did not necessarily place a priority on screening are drawn into the net and face problematic decisions.

In vitro fertilization and its variations have opened conception to people with a range of infertility problems. Embryo diagnosis opens conception to people with genetic problems. Yet embryo genetics will make a dent, at most, on single-locus disorders affecting select groups of people in advanced industrial countries who can afford to pay for IVF and embryo diagnosis. As an exciting and innovative field, will it be pursued at the expense of other means of protecting children's health?

Moreover, if embryo diagnosis is marketed for more than at-risk couples, it will take on a momentum of its own, leading to spiraling created needs, among other things, to have a supposedly risk-free pregnancy and birth (even though genetic mutations and teratogenic influences during pregnancy preclude the certainty of a healthful birth). Ultimately, genetically at-risk couples, such as carriers of the Tay-Sachs gene, may be only a small segment of the prospective clientele.

A type of affirmative action is in the works in which steps can be taken to help diverse groups of people have a child. This pushes procreation into the public arena and thus fosters an intense interest in fixing the numerous stages in reproduction where something can go wrong. Recent reports of high rates of chromosomal defects in eggs, sperm, and embryos inspire a problem-solving mode, a drive to fix conditions once thought natural, if unfortunate, or not even recognized as problems. With knowledge comes a widening of those deemed "at risk," which in turn leads to more needs to diagnose and fix. Far from recruiting more people to get help in conception, however, the opposite result might happen, inasmuch as couples faced with an expensive and complicated act of conception may simply remove themselves from the process and decide not to have children at all. The net gain of numbers of children born to high risk couples may not be as great as expected after all.

The lead time between theory and practice has narrowed to the point where discussion of ends and means is needed now. Beneath the excitement of embryo genetics lie fears that are shunted aside rather than confronted— the fear of having a child with an anomaly, the fear of being responsible for letting a child be born with a disorder, the fear of having disabled children in the society, and practitioners' fear of being left behind if they do not add embryo genetics to their list of services. Various needs are being cloaked by the addition of a new set of reproductive technologies. The impetus for the new genetics does not seem to be coming from groups of at-risk couples, but instead from intrigue over the promise of genetic inquiry. The genome project is the central symbol of an expected revolution in genetic medicine, yet the benefit to health and well-being may come mostly from somatic cell therapy and advances in carrier and prenatal screening. The rationale for inviting new couples into the IVF arena for preimplantation diagnosis is not compelling.

New Field or Refined Technique?

Beyond the general questioning of goals is the need to fix responsibility for integrating embryo diagnosis into society. If, indeed, embryo diagnosis is the first step toward embryo therapy, something new is afoot—an emerging body of applied knowledge with an uncertain identity. Embryo genetics may be one of three things: an extension of IVF, a distinct field of medicine, or an extension of prenatal screening. The professional and institutional identity of preimplantation diagnosis is important to study because it will color the ethic under which the technique is applied in the clinical setting.

Is embryo diagnosis an extension of IVF? If so, primary oversight lies with obstetricians, infertility specialists, and reproductive endocrinologists. Medical doctors head the clinics, and couples work with nurse coordinators. The "patient" is the couple experiencing infertility or genetic risk. Diagnosis is aimed at helping the couple have a healthy baby. The doctor and patient are partners and the couple's autonomy is valued, but the physician's professional competence determines which embryos are transferred right away, which are frozen, which are not transferred. Judging an embryo's transferability is a technical decision related to the embryo's morphology and other physical traits. The goal is to maximize, under safe conditions, the odds for a successful pregnancy and to minimize risks and false hopes for the couples.

An advantage of seeing embryo diagnosis as an extension of IVF is that a voluntary apparatus is already in place to oversee it. The American Fertility Society (AFS) and its Society for Assisted Reproduction, for example, yearly gather and publish data from member IVF clinics.[9] The AFS makes available to couples a list of questions to ask upon entering an IVF program, its ethics committee has published minimum standards governing IVF and ethics reports, and IVF clinicians are now meeting occasionally to discuss methods and procedures for starting embryo diagnosis.[10]

A disadvantage is that if marketed as just another facet of IVF, the heralding of embryo diagnosis as something new is missing and with it the opportunity to question the reasons behind its introduction and its contributions to individual and societal well-being. Moreover, it opens embryo diagnosis to IVF couples as a matter of course, which contravenes the original intention of embryo diagnosis as being for at-risk couples.

Is embryo diagnosis a new field of medicine? Although still early for speculation, it appears the stage is being set for the image of the embryo as "patient." Micromanipulations already create the context for correcting deficiencies in embryos. One day the twinning of embryos may be offered as medical insurance for the embryo. If an embryo is twinned before biopsy, one part can be biopsied and discarded while the intact part is transferred. Or the biopsied half can be transferred and the intact half frozen in the event the embryo does not cleave or implant. In either case, the technique protects the embryo proper, thereby enhancing its status as a "patient."

Seeing the embryo as patient complements evolving notions of the fetus as patient. Both advance the idea that entities are subject to protection and care before birth. Efforts to save a potential child or "rescu[e] an ailing embryo"[11] direct attention to the embryo or fetus as the object of attention rather than to the couple. Regarding the embryo as patient has analytic benefits. It presents a context for studying new techniques and gives embryo diagnosis a separate identity as a distinct field with identifiable dilemmas and rich possibilities for ethical analysis based on graduated definitions of "patient."

On the other hand, regarding the embryo as patient runs the danger of personalizing the embryo and further confusing the question of the beginnings of life. It also sets the stage for elevating the embryo to the status of an entity with rights. This restricts experimental protocols and defines the embryo as ill or needy, which in turn creates a new set of medical "needs" for embryo therapy. Moreover, if the embryo is the patient, this arguably enhances the clinician's authority in making decisions. When the embryo is something to which things (tests, manipulations) are done, the practitioner's judgment becomes more important than ever, which further mutes the couple's nonexpert voice.

Is embryo diagnosis an extension of prenatal screening and genetic counseling? If so, the context is less distinctly medical and the personnel more likely to be scientists and social workers or psychologists. Clinicians' goals are to help couples make choices about whether to conceive, provide information so couples understand the nature of their genetic risk, and set the stage for reproductive decisions. Genetic counselors use a model of nondirectionality and, at least in theory, maintain their impartiality. There is no real "patient," but instead a partnership between counselor and couple to allow a couple to make informed reproductive decisions based, among other things, on diagnostic tests. Genetic counseling allows couples to make choices, even though they may seem irrational.

If embryo diagnosis is an extension of prenatal screening, decisions will be made in a context where the couple's autonomy is valued. Genetic counselors, in general, guard individual choice. Thus, if a couple learns the fetus has an abnormality and asks the genetic counselor, "What would you do?" the counselor is inclined to defer the question and shift the conversation to the couple's needs and values.

One would expect a similar model to prevail if methods developed in relation to fetuses are used for embryos. Decisions regarding embryos will be presumed to be reproductive decisions, with autonomy paramount, rather than medical decisions, where expertise is a primary criterion. This protects the human interests in embryo diagnosis and acts as a brake to overeager expansion of embryo technologies. Each time a decision is to be made about what to do with embryos (whether and what to test, how to interpret results), the interests of the couple are built into the structure and the outcome is not predetermined. Critics have long claimed that new technologies depersonalize reproduction. The autonomy model of prenatal screening arguably helps protect against this.

On the other hand, maximizing individual choice is not an unrelieved blessing either. How far should individualism go? Should a couple in the future be able to select an embryo of the desired gender, say, and then twin it, freezing one twin for a later year to see the first child's personality and physical traits and then, if the child passes muster, have a genetically identical but younger twin?

A pure model of nondirectionality, with the presumption in favor of family choice, may not be desirable or even desired by couples in an era of increasing reproductive choices. What choices will people make if their array of options is not bounded? Will they find satisfaction from making these choices or might they instead be faced with unnecessary confusion and anxiety? Reproductive satisfaction is not necessarily achieved through more medical technology.

Ethics and Clinic Policies

Embryo diagnosis should take place in IVF clinics adhering to rigorous quality control in laboratories. The couples' autonomy should be respected, although the clinic teams bear the responsibility for setting borders on the range of decisions offered. Embryo diagnosis potentially creates a need for IVF among new groups of women, sets the stage for the spiraling development of new technologies (which is an elevator up or slippery slope down, depending on one's perspective), and creates new felt obligations for couples who might be happier conceiving through sexual intercourse and taking their chances on the usual outcome of having a healthy baby. Beneficence, then, expanding them. In placing limits, clinics are gatekeepers regulating the pace and substance of embryo manipulations. To be decided are matters of whom to invite into programs, what options to allow, what information to give, and to what extent team members should take societal interests into account in their informal policies.

Whom to admit? Assume a couple, at risk for having a child with the fatal condition of thalassemia, have experienced two terminations of affected fetuses and have two healthy children. Assume further that the husband wants a third child. The wife, who has medical problems and wants nothing more to do with prenatal screening, contacts the clinic about the possibility of embryo diagnosis. In asking whether the procedure is in the couple's best interest, one can understand their wariness over more prenatal screening. On the other hand, they have two healthy children, and the wife has been through prolonged emotional trauma. It may be that the couple is better off not knowing that the option of embryo diagnosis exists. Conservatism is warranted regarding whom to admit. One answer is to develop a criterion of "worthiness," measured in personal suffering and a legacy of loss, with the assumption that the "neediest" will be given the first opportunity to try this experimental protocol. The converse is to admit those with low emotional investment, inasmuch as the procedure is experimental and embryo loss is to be expected. This is a judgment call, but it should be articulated as part of the clinic's ethics.

What to offer? One clinic starts embryo diagnosis by testing embryos for sickle cell anemia. Another offers polar body biopsies for cystic fibrosis. A third offers sex-preselection for Duchenne muscular dystrophy. Two directions are possible. One is specialization, with individual centers specializing in a particular form of biopsy or a particular genetic disorder. Another is to focus on regional centers that offer several options. Strategy about expanding services ought to be developed deliberately as part of the clinic's policy. For example, a conservative course is to agree that new procedures will not be added until several healthy babies have been born from application of the core procedures. The expansion to different practices—different diseases, biopsy procedures, sex preselection—should be done gradually and with specified criteria in mind.

What should couples be told under conditions of uncertainty? The consent form at one clinic, for example, includes two general statements about the unforeseeability of risks to the patient, fetus, and child. The warning seems vague, but on the other hand, as Robert Veatch has noted, too much information can be "terribly tedious."[12] At some point in the development of IVF, practitioners blew the whistle on exploitive practices and inadequate or inaccurate information about success rates. These same warnings can be repeated with embryo diagnosis, and the same standards of full disclosure need to be developed. The content of information packets and consent forms will stand the greatest chance of being readable and informative if clinics share their forms and if practitioners talk with one another to present information that can be modified according to a clinic's own success rates and new technical developments.

Under what overarching ethics should decisions about clinic policies be made? Some IVF practitioners are reluctant to take embryo diagnosis seriously, thinking variously that (1) with no federal funding for embryo research, diagnosis will not develop, (2) crises should not be anticipated and cannot be predicted, (3) IVF has worked smoothly with no significant safety problems so embryo diagnosis will follow suit, and (4) genetic diagnosis is "pie in the sky." This sets the stage for trial and error muddling as happened in the early days of IVF and embryo freezing, where consent forms were spare, success rates misleading, and clinic policies ad hoc. A clinic policy should be constrained by the ethics of individual practitioners on the one hand and societal views about what is and is not appropriate on the other. Embryo diagnosis is a rapidly changing technology being introduced quietly in the clinical setting. This technology will ultimately affect the genetic composition of future humans, and it creates a new specially at a time when discrepancies in medical treatment between rich and poor are entrenched and growing. It brings the yearning to control the life course to a point so early in development that it negates the value of chance in everyday life.

Yet despite the importance of this field, there is a constitutional zone of protection around the technologies, the government is stymied about research involving embryos, and application is driven in no small measure by the promise of economic gain. Although patient advocacy groups can draw attention to the need for reforms, realistically the primary responsibility for framing coherent policies falls on the clinics that offer embryo diagnosis. These policies should be deliberate, crafted before the techniques of preimplantation diagnosis are applied in practice, and narrowly drawn regarding the options offered and patients accepted.

The ethics of individual clinicians should be articulated as a starting point for discussion within clinics with due humility about what is not known in genetics. Clinicians must bear the burden of showing the absence of harm to couples and potential children and the presence of clear benefit to specific groups of people. The ethics should protect the autonomy of couples who are not ill supplicants but healthy people making choices about reproduction. Efforts must be made to develop policies across clinics, communication should be open and free, and negative as well as positive results must be conveyed to clinicians and the public. Moreover, clear lines of responsibility should be developed within and across centers so that models of patient choice are clear, open to discussion, and consistent among team members.

Open, Critical Debate

The attitude of mind must come into play such that people rigorously ask and weigh questions about reasons for diagnosing human embryos, criteria for adding new genetic technologies in the future, distinctions between deeply felt needs and newly created ones, and the willingness to draw limits in the absence of legislation. Moreover, careful attention must be given to what, if anything, in embryo diagnosis and therapy is qualitatively different. One perspective holds that embryo diagnosis is not, in fact, distinctive: it merely pushes prenatal screening to an earlier stage and is just another step in IVF. A second perspective holds that embryo diagnosis is problematic because it will be used in embryo therapy (the long-debated genetic engineering).

A third perspective holds that embryo diagnostics are significant not so much because embryos or genetics are involved as because this opens a new set of labor-intensive technologies to the few in an era of scarce medical resources and growing respect for community as well as individual health concerns. Embryo diagnosis is indeed the ultimate in disease prevention, but it must be reconciled with other preventive measures designed to improve the health of the many.

The speculative wonderings of a generation are now faced with empirical realities. Embryo diagnosis on the eve of clinical application presents a challenge to reframe long-stated worries about genetic manipulation in ways consistent with the present medical reality. Pragmatic decisions must be made about who will be recruited as research subjects, how the protocol will be packaged, and what boundaries will define the choices developed and offered. Reflections on ethics need to take into account principles under which embryo diagnosis will be offered; the varying ethical frameworks used among practitioners, clinics, and professional associations; the identity of embryo diagnosis within medicine; the extent to which diagnosis furthers the goals envisioned for it; and the nature and importance of those goals themselves.

To return to the analogy of the Gold Museum, much of the new genetics is surrounded by dazzle and publicity, but embryo diagnosis is proceeding amid darkness and quiet. Our task is both to dim the glare and shed light on new applications. Reasoned policy governing medical innovations depends on open examination and reasoned understanding.

Acknowledgments

Interviews for this paper were conducted while I was a 1990–91 Rockefeller Foundation Fellow at the Institute for the Medical Humanities, University of Texas Medical Branch, Galveston, Tex. For their helpful comments, I would like to thank the Institute faculty and the following practitioners: Alan H. DeChemey, MD; Beth A. Fine, MS; Mark R. Hughes, MD; G. Laird Jackson, MD; Robert Kaufmann, MD; Susan Lanzendorf, PhD; Joe Leigh Simpson, MD; Charles H. Strom, MD; Yury Verlinsky, PhD; and Melody Ann White, MS.

QUESTIONS FOR CONSIDERATION

1. What is the significance of the analogy of the gold museum as applied to the advances in DNA diagnosis?
2. According to Bonnicksen, what is the value of "preimplantation biopsies of human embryos" for couples who are at risk of having children with

serious genetic disorders? How could such diagnoses become the "ultimate measles vaccine" for genetic disorders?

3. Do you agree that the screening of embryos is more of an advantage than prenatal screening and that discarding embryos is less of a moral problem than aborting pregnancies?

4. What would be the significance of embryo therapy in correcting genetic defects and preventing genetic disease?

5. What are Bonnicksen's concerns regarding the accuracy of genetic diagnosis? What are the dangers of false positive and a false negative results?

6. How could embryo diagnosis affect the genetic diversity of future generations?

7. What threefold approach does Bonnicksen recommend toward developing policy regarding genetic diagnosis, especially in the absence of public policy?

8. In examining the ethics of clinical policy, Bonnicksen focuses upon three questions: whom to admit, what to offer and what information should couples be given under conditions of uncertainty? How does she address these three questions?

NOTES

1. A variety of techniques may be employed in preimplantation diagnosis, including embryo analysis, trophectoderm biopsy, and polar body biopsy. For discussion, see Yury Verlinsky, Eugene Pergament, and Charles H. Strom, "The Preimplantation Genetic Diagnosis of Genetic Diseases," *Journal of In Vitro Fertilization and Embryo Transfer* 7, no. 1 (1990):1–5; A. Dokras et al., "Trophectoderm Biopsy in Human Blastocysts," *Human Reproduction* 5, no. 7 (1990): 821–25; Charles M. Strom et al., "DNA Analysis of Single Cells for Single Gene Diseases," Abstracts of the First International Symposium on Preimplantation Genetics, Chicago, 14–19 September 1990.

2. D. K. Griffin et al., "Fluorescent In-Situ Hybridization to Interphase Nuclei of Human Preimplantation Embryos with X and Y Chromosome Specific Probes," *Human Reproduction* 6, no. 1 (1991):101–5; A. H. Handyside et al., "Biopsy of Human Preimplantation Embryos and Sexing by DNA Amplification," *Lancet 1* (8 February 1989): 347–49; Svetlana Milayeva et al., "Successful Preimplantation Diagnosis for Gender Determination," Abstracts of the First International Symposium on Preimplantation Genetics, Chicago, 14–19 September 1990.

3. Illinois Masonic Medical Center in Chicago is offering polar body analysis for cystic fibrosis. Its team has attempted sex-preselection for X-linked genetic diseases. Several other clinics are planning to offer polar body or embryo biopsy in the near future. A healthy infant has been born in England following biopsy at the embryonic stage for cystic fibrosis (personal communication, Mark R. Hughes, MD).

4. "Germ Cell Gene Panel," *Science* 253 (23 August 1991): 841.

5. Verlinsky, Pergament, and Strom, "Preimplantation Genetic Diagnosis," p. 4.

6. See A. L. Muggleton-Harris and I. Findlay, "*In-Vitro* Studies on 'Spare' Human Preimplantation Embryos in Culture," *Human Reproduction* 6, no. 1 (1991): 85–92; Kate Hardy et al., "Human Implantation Development *In Vitro* Is Not Adversely Affected by Biopsy at the 8-Cell Stage," *Human Reproduction* 5, no.6(1990): 708–14. In polar body biopsy and trophectoderm biopsies, the embryo is left intact, but with embryo biopsy one or two cells are removed, with an uncertain long-term effect on the developing embryo. For discussion, see D. A. Melton, "Pattern Formation During Animal Development, " *Science* 252 (12 April 1991): 23441; Joel M. Schindler, "Basic Developmental Genetics and Early Embryonic Development: What's All the Excitement About?" *Journal of NIH Research* 2, no. 9 (1990): 49–55.

7. Daniel Callahan, What Kind *of Life? The Limits of Medical Progress* (New York: Touchstone, 1990), pp. 63–65.

8. E. Pergament, "Preimplantation Diagnosis: A Patient Perspective." Paper presented at the 5th International Congress on Early Fetal Diagnosis, July 1990, Prague, Czechoslovakia.

9. See, for example, Medical Research International, "In Vitro Fertilization-Embryo Transfer (IVF-ET) in the United States: 1989 Results from the IVF-ET Registry," *Fertility and Sterility* 55, no. 1 (1991): 14–23.

10. "Questions to Ask about an IVF/GIFT Program," American Fertility Society, Birmingham, Ala.; American Fertility Society, "Revised Minimum Standards for In Vitro Fertilization, Gamete Intrafallopian Transfer, and Related Procedures," *Fertility and Sterility* 53, no. 2 (1990): 225–26; Ethics Committee, American Fertility Society, "Ethical Considerations of the New Reproductive Technologies, " Supp. 2, *Fertility and Sterility* 53, no. 6 (1990).

11. E. Joshua Rosenkranz, "Custom Kids and the Moral Duty to Genetically Engineer Our Children," *High Technology Law Journal* 2, no. 1 (1987): 1–53.

12. Robert M. Veatch, *The Patient as Partner: A Theory of Human Experimentation* (Bloomington: Indiana University Press, 1987).

BARBARA KATZ ROTHMAN

Not All That Glitters Is Gold

I too want to begin with the example of the gold museum. Gold did not land in that museum from the sky. It came at great cost in human life and liberty. That is what is still left hidden in the dark, and in that sense the analogy works perhaps far better than was intended.

Embryo diagnosis also has costs in life and in liberty—that of the women on whose bodies these experiments are done. While the proven deaths to date from IVF-related treatments are quite small, the long-term risks are not yet in. And the costs of pain, illness, and physical and emotional suffering from these procedures go largely unremarked in Andrea Bonnicksen's discussion, collapsed into "financial loss and emotional strain" for the "couple." IVF and embryo retrieval procedures do not take place on a couple's body—it is a woman on the table, a woman who bears the costs of this treatment.

The new procreative technologies began with enormous fanfare, welcoming Louise Brown into the world, the first "test tube baby." What the technology has come to accomplish in just the fourteen years since her birth is indeed extraordinary. Originally, all they were doing (all!) was bypassing blocked fallopian tubes, letting sperm and egg join in a petri dish before continuing growth, *in utero* that is, in a woman, a mother. And now? The fastest growing use of this technology is for male infertility: most recently, with microinjection of a few living sperm, an otherwise infertile man can fertilize an egg. Fertilized eggs can now be frozen and stored indefinitely, and technologies are being developed to allow the freezing of unfertilized eggs. Ovaries can be stimulated to produce not the one or maybe two eggs of a normal cycle, but a dozen or even more. The plethora of eggs the drugs have created has spawned its own technology: pregnancy reduction, selectively aborting some embryos in a multiple pregnancy, turning potential quintuplets into more manageable twins.

The embryos themselves, while outside of the body, can now be examined, with the largest potential growth area for the technology being, as Bonnicksen points out, preimplantation diagnosis. Sex, chromosomal anomalies, and genetic disorders can be learned from embryo biopsy before the embryo is put back into the woman. Embryo diagnosis and embryo splitting can mean ordering specific embryos for growth, including the genetic twins of already born people, introducing a new level of quality control into procreation, and—combined with commercial surrogacy—making baby farms come to seem a real possibility. In a new twist that seems to fascinate the reproductive technologists themselves, with the use of hormones postmenopausal women can carry donated embryos.

Is all this science at its best?—NEW HOPE FOR THE CHILDLESS— or science at its worst?—SCIENTIST MAKES OLD WOMAN PREGNANT WITH ALIENS. Somewhere between the vision of *Scientific American* and that of the *National Enquirer*, women are groping their way through. If Louise Brown is the Eve of this story, there is also a Lillith—a first creation, a false start discarded by her creators. The first pregnancy from IVF produced an embryo with three sets of chromosomes, an anomaly incompatible with life. Leslie Brown, Louise's mother, had no idea that hers was the first baby that Steptoe and Edward's technology had produced. Nor did she know of the miscarriage that preceded this success. Another woman's false hopes, the deception by inference of Leslie Brown—this is a technology built on the blood, losses, and hopes of women.

The Costs of IVF

By now the costs of IVF and related technologies to infertile women themselves have started to show up. The first risks to consider are the immediate physical ones of the treatment. While the focus is on the petri dish or test tube and its contents, it is the woman's body that lies on the table. These are invasive treatments, involving powerful drugs and surgery, and deaths do occur.

Yet it is the longer term, as yet unknown risks—the "theoretical but unproven" risks—that worry me. These include the cancer risks of the drug use. In a technology so new, it is too soon to know much about long-term cancer risks. But more significantly no research has been done on these risks: as with immediate deaths or injuries from the treatment, no central records are kept.

How much should we worry about these cancer risks? Ann Pappert, a journalist who has been traveling around the world interviewing reproductive technologists, says that some of the doctors are themselves very concerned. One world-renowned specialist told her, "We're going to see an epidemic. Certainly we expect a cancer epidemic." It is not an unreasonable or unfounded worry: the drugs stimulate rapid cell growth, the hallmark of cancer. When research isn't being done, we are left only with easily dismissable anecdotal information. And with the connections not being made within the research community, it is easy for individuals also to overlook potential connections. Consider for example the much-publicized death of the actress Gilda Radner. She had gone through an unsuccessful IVF attempt just a few years before she was diagnosed with the ovarian cancer that killed her. She had a family history of cancer, including breast and ovarian cancer. But IVF programs do not always screen for cancer risks. Rita Arditti, reviewing IVF program applications, found that not all even ask on the history forms. Gilda Radner had previously had surgery for an ovarian cyst, but that did not rule her out.

What can one make of a story like this—a single anecdote or one of many? Without systematic research, one can draw no conclusions. But most striking is that questions are being systematically avoided. Radner, like so many other women, did not allow herself to consider the possible links. In her autobiography, she obsessed about cause:

> It runs through my mind constantly: why did I get this? I go from being realistic to being absurd. . . . I know I used a lot of saccharine and cyclamates in my life. . . . I have always loved red candies. . . . I ate an apple a day—even the ones that were thick-skinned with shiny wax. . . . These are the things that run through my mind, from the sensible to the ridiculous. I ate red meat. I used hairspray.

In all this searching for cause, she never wondered about the hormones that stimulated her ovaries to rapid, unnatural growth. And in the enormous publicity campaigns about ovarian cancer focusing on her case and offering dubious techniques for earlier diagnosis, the possible connection to her IVF treatment is never considered or discussed. Other women have experienced cancers after inferfility treatments; maybe they are and maybe they are not connected. The self-protective blocking of the thought is what fascinates me.

If there were careful follow-up research on the long-term consequences for women undergoing infertility treatments, we might have some answers instead of these anecdotes and suspicions, and might have more hesitation about expanding the use of the technologies yet further.

Long-term follow-up on the babies that are created is simply nonexistent. All we know about them is their pregnancy and birth status. According to Robert Lee Hotz (author *of Designs on Life*) and figures from IVF clinics around the world, IVF produced twice as many spontaneous miscarriages, five times as many babies with spina bifida, six times as many with transposition of the heart, and a rate of stillbirths and deaths in the first month of life that is three times higher than normal. And these are the babies of relatively wealthy parents, with access to pre- and postnatal care.

This is one of the contexts in which I believe we must place the push to develop new uses for these technologies. The "gold" may be impressive, but it is mined, not without cost, from the bodies of women.

Contexts and Consequences

Let us turn now from the physical to some of the social costs of expanding these technologies. Nolan and Bonnicksen are confident—far more confident than I could ever be at any rate—that there will be controls to regulate the spread of this technology to women without infertility problems, women who will be exposed to the risks of the technology solely for the purpose of embryo diagnosis. They feel that the voluntary apparatus put into place by the American Fertility Society works well enough to protect people who enter infertility programs and IVF clinics. Such is not my interpretation.

On the other hand, if embryo diagnosis is placed not in the context of infertility treatments, but of prenatal diagnosis, Bonnicksen feels that genetic counselors have done a fine job of preserving "couple" autonomy in decision-making. That too has not been my observation. Genetic counselors in general are, Bonnicksen says, guardians of individual choice. In observations of genetic counselors I found that not to be entirely true. Genetic counselors are the people hired by institutions to get the appropriate paperwork done and forms signed. That does not make them what one referred to as "amnio salesladies," but it does place constraints on their actions, if only dramatic time constraints. I saw more counselors choose not to speak of difficult issues than to open up talk of the ramifications of the counseling. I observed session after session in which the informed consent document was signed without the potential for abortion following a "bad diagnosis" ever having been discussed. And judging from the few clients who asked specifically, "So what could be done if a problem is found?" not all understood the agenda. Counselors virtually never discussed the possibility of the so-called ambiguous diagnoses—things like mosaics, sex chromosome anomalies, and other diagnoses considered "less severe" than Down syndrome—even though such diagnoses are at least as likely as the conditions ostensibly being tested for. Overworked counselors processed clients through. When a woman did have a problem diagnosed, physicians took over and counselors had little input into decisionmaking.

There is another particular bind here for women in the ways that both infertility treatments and prenatal diagnosis have operated. It is a bind that the language Bonnicksen uses should alert us to: "Couples" are not "individuals."

In the world of procreation, too often the terms are used interchangeably. But one of the greatest sources of pressure individual women face in procreative decisionmaking comes from their partners. Couple autonomy is in a sense an oxymoron. This is true in infertility diagnosis and is equally true in prenatal diagnosis. There is no reason to think it will be any less true under the combined pressures brought by embryo diagnosis.

In the world of infertility, Judith Lorber has written of the "patriarchal bargain" some women are forced to make: using the higher risk treatments of IVF for male infertility, rather than the safer and far more effective option of donor insemination (or adoption, for a nonmedical approach to infertility) in order to maintain the man's paternity. And unlike situations of, for example, kidney or other organ donation between family members, the "couple" is treated as a unit. In kidney donation, in contrast, family members are counseled separately and privately, and a "medical excuse" is offered for a family member who requests one after refusing to offer a donation. In IVF the couple is treated as one, and, as they say, he's the one.

In prenatal diagnosis, similar collapsing of the individuals into a unit occurs: for example, it is common to read in the medical and social science literature that "families break up" when a disabled child is born. That fact is sometimes used in support of prenatal diagnosis and selective abortion—as it will undoubtedly be used in support of embryo diagnosis and selective implantation—as evidence of the enormous stress imposed by the birth of a child with severe disabilities. But what exactly does it mean to say a family "breaks up"? Do all the family members go their separate ways? Do siblings pack up and move out? Do mothers leave home? Most usually what it means is that fathers leave. Pregnant women are being offered, sometimes subtly but sometimes quite openly, a choice by their husbands: the problem baby, or the husband. It is very, very much rarer for a husband to face the situation that if he wants to keep the baby, he will have to raise it without his wife's support and help.

I am not claiming that this is because women are finer people than men, but because women's experience of parenthood is very different. Women begin parenthood with nurturance and with attachment. The child begins as part of our bodies, with our feelings about the child deeply entangled in our feelings about ourselves. We are nurturing and caring for the baby before it is a baby. For women attempting conception, the nurturance begins before and without the presence of any product of conception.

But it is not women's language, not women's reality that is dominant, and men's view of procreation prevails. And so we speak of babies as if they arrived from Mars, or out of a black box. We speak of babies "arriving" when women experience babies *leaving*. We talk about "greeting" babies at birth, about "bonding" to them at the moment of separation.

Prenatal diagnosis was built on the idea that the baby does not exist until it is born or until it exists for other people. The unique relationship women experience is discounted. We ask women to adopt the traditional male model for parenting: holding back until the child earns approval and love, moving from separation to attachment.

My own research with women having amniocentesis for prenatal diagnosis showed the enormous costs this imposes on women as mothers. The mother grieves over an abortion following prenatal diagnosis as she does the death of a child. For the mother, it *is* the death of a child, a child she has held and cared for and nurtured and loved. It is not the same as an abortion to end an unwanted pregnancy, an abortion when the woman never identified herself as a mother, the pregnancy as bringing a baby. These "selective" abortions mean the loss of a baby, a true death. What women told me made this a particularly hard death to bear was that it was profoundly isolating. No one, the mothers reported, shared their sense of loss. For everyone else, including fathers, however much the baby was wanted it was not yet here. What others had lost was a baby who was expected. What mothers lost was a baby they had.

Now that we have earlier diagnosis, suddenly the tune has changed: late abortions are indeed traumatic, the old amnio was a problem. And, to take the next logical step forward, those who are writing about preimplantation diagnosis have begun to talk about the inherent trauma of all prenatal diagnosis after conception/implantation, and the grief of all abortions for genetic disorders. As is so often the case, having a solution enabled people to recognize or at least to acknowledge a problem. And preimplantation diagnosis does indeed solve some of the problems of later diagnosis. But that does not mean it has no problems of its own.

Preimplantation diagnosis comes from two fields that have not, I have argued, served the interests of women: work on IVF and work on prenatal diagnosis. Both have come in the guise of offering choice, but neither has had liberating consequences.

IVF has made the ability to accept infertility a sign of a weakness: infertility is no longer an ascribed characteristic but now more of a chosen status, if only one chosen by default whenever a woman decides to give up. This is of course only true for the women with financial access to these services; for other women, infertility is experienced as caused by the poverty that bars access to IVF services. It is one thing to say that one really would have loved to have given birth, but one cannot, and move on to adoption or to childless living. It is quite another thing to say one would have loved to have given birth but it was too expensive or too difficult or too painful or too dangerous to keep trying. The latter makes much greater demands on a woman's sense of self and of self-worth in this (and most) societies. Infertility becomes a test of character, of worth, and of commitment to maternalist ideals.

Prenatal diagnosis, as the other antecedent, is also supposed to offer "choice." Yet it too moves a sadness, grief, and loss from the realm of ascription, of things that just happen, to the realm of personal responsibility. A woman who chooses not to use the testing has in some sense come to be seen as having "chosen" to have a child with a disability. In choosing the risk, she is understood to have chosen the condition. This is part and parcel of a culture that separates, for example, "innocent victims" of AIDS from those who have acquired AIDS after having engaged in high-risk behavior. Taking the risk ensures culpability. For all the "nondirectionality" a given counselor may strive to achieve, the technology changes cultural meanings. Add to this the economic crisis in health care services, and the potential for increasing control in the form of economic coercion (can you afford a disabled child?) looms large.

These are just some of the costs—physical, psychological, and social—of preimplantation diagnosis. It would be a lovely world if Bonnicksen were right, and embryo diagnosis could be introduced *after* much thought and *after* some of these problems were addressed, even if not solved. But that is not going to happen. It has not happened before in the history of American medical services, and I cannot imagine it is going to happen here. The far more likely scenario is the technology beginning, as it has, with the few dramatic cases. A couple has a child with a serious disease, faces a one-in-four possibility of another such child, and cannot bear yet another selective abortion. Embryo diagnosis seems like the perfect solution. From there, as with all of these technologies, it is just a hop, skip, and a jump to broader application. The research questions are fascinating, careers are waiting to be made, and patient need—defined as loosely as "anxiety"—is highly malleable.

But let's say we could make preimplantation diagnosis and IVF safe, and we could make it accessible. Does this make sense as a goal?

Looking in the Right Places

There is an old story about a man looking for a quarter under a street lamp late at night. A second man comes along, sees the first searching the ground on hands and knees, and offers to help. After quite a few minutes of fruitless searching, the second man asks: "Are you sure this is where you dropped it?" "No," the first replies, "I dropped it on that other corner, but the light's better here."

Our current focus on finding the genetic causes of disease, illness, disability, maybe even general unhappiness, seems much the same—we are looking where the light is best. The light in this case is cast by the general social concern about and interest in genetic determinism, and the very specific shape that concern takes in the form of research. We are mapping the human genome, developing earlier and earlier prenatal testing for genetic disease, hunting down oncogenes, and generally trying to make more and more predictions about the course of a human life from reading the tea leaves of chromosomal patterns.

My concerns are twofold: first that we are looking in the wrong corner, and second that we might find what we seem to be hunting for.

First, by leaving important areas in relative darkness, we are less likely to find real solutions to our problems. For example, some of the concern that should go into cleaning up the workplace of hazardous chemicals has shifted to screening our workers with vulnerable genes. In a strikingly different approach to public health, the health of a population is maintained not by preventing the members of that population from becoming sick, but by keeping potentially sick people out of the population—in the case of occupational health, screening out the most vulnerable workers.

When we turn to the problem of prenatal and preimplantation diagnosis, there are similar issues involved. This too is quite a new approach to improving the health of the population (in this case the population of newborns). Rather than preventing or treating illness in existing newborns, the health of newborn babies is being improved by creating a situation in which potentially unhealthy babies are never born—they are identified as embryos and not implanted, or identified as fetuses and aborted. But genetic diseases are, in fundamental ways, the least of our problems. The high infant mortality rates in the United States are not due to genetic diseases. Our problems lie in darker corners, in poverty and the poor nutrition and inadequate health care and increasing homelessness that accompany poverty in America.

So my first concern with setting up safe and available embryo diagnosis as a goal is that the focus on genetic determinism shifts our attention away from what might be far more fruitful areas of research and action. We are simply not looking where the problems lie. My second concern is that not only will we not solve our problems, but we are indeed creating very serious new problems. I have addressed in this paper the costs to women as individuals facing the consequences of the technology we are developing for embryo diagnosis. But what about the costs to our understanding of ourselves as people, the costs of information and control?

We are a culture that values information. Knowledge is power, we say. That can certainly be true. But knowledge can also be disempowering, as I learned from interviews with women who got bad news from amniocentesis. Faced not with a baby with specific, albeit serious problems and needs, but with the potential of such a baby, some felt powerless to cope. Although the abortion was experienced, and expressed, not in the terms of abortion, of ending a pregnancy, but in terms of infanticide, of killing a baby, it was most often experienced as an "only choice," coming out of a sense not of empowerment, but of being trapped.

If we do earlier and earlier, more and more complete diagnosis would anyone dare give birth to anyone? There is of course no perfect child. Just suppose we could find the flaw(s) in each embryo: this one will be very fat, this one will have a tendency toward bladder cancer, this one will have this disability, this one another, this one is more likely to have this grief, that one that grief. In some crazy way the burden of responsibility shifts from fate, nature, the gods that be, to the person who chose to give birth to the child knowing what it might face. With earlier diagnosis, we ask not, "How can I bear to kill this baby?" but, "How can I bear to start a pregnancy with this baby?"

And even if we eliminate all the issues of abortion, is it empowering for parents to have this kind of information? If you know your child is twice as likely as most (or ten times, or a hundred times—it is in the nature of this information that it will always be expressed in probabilities) to develop a particular cancer, or to have depressions, or to be mildly retarded, what exactly are you supposed to do about it? You can eliminate all the additional risk factors under your control—and then you can wait. For some conditions, the specter of the self-fulfilling prophecy looms. Such was the case with the relatively simple "xyy" syndrome and its supposed link to aggressiveness. Tell a parent a child might become pathologically aggressive and you can virtually be assured that the child will not have a normal approach to aggression.

Life is very, very difficult. We are all born in a markedly similar way and in a markedly similar condition. And then some of us die quickly, and some live for a hundred years. We die of an extraordinary range of ills, having suffered an amazing amount of grief and pain, along with joy, over the years. Do parents *want* to know what grief awaits their children? Do we want to know how they are most likely to suffer or to die, or when?

I don't think most of what happens to us is just a simple matter of genes playing themselves out. I fall far on the side of nurture in the longstanding debate with nature. We can do more to control human destiny with economic, environmental, political, and social change than with all the embryo diagnosis in the world. So I do think we are looking on the wrong corner if we want to find our solutions. But I am not even sure that I want to find what the geneticists seem to be looking for: not a lost quarter, but the fortune-teller's crystal ball. And where some gaze in and see rooms of gold, others gaze in and see very dark mines and corners indeed.

QUESTIONS FOR CONSIDERATION

1. How does Rothman take the analogy of the gold museum (Bonnicksen) and offer a different interpretation? What does she mean by the statement "—it is a woman on the table. . ."?

2. What are some of the costs of IVF to infertile women identified by Rothman? What are the effects of IVF upon babies?

3. What are the social costs identified by Rothman? What did she mean by the expression "patriarchal bargain"?

4. Why does Rothman believe that IVF has made accepting infertility a sign of weakness? By contrast, how does she account for the existence of prenatal diagnosis as resulting in a woman appearing to have chosen to have a disabled child?

5. Describe Rothman's twofold concern regarding the genetic approach to solving our health problems.

John A. Robertson

Resolving Disputes over Frozen Embryos

Embryo—the term "embryo" rather than the technically more accurate term "preembryo" is used to refer to the postfertilization, preimplantation entities discussed in this paper—freezing as an adjunct to in vitro fertilization (IVF) is an important step forward in the treatment of infertility and control of human reproduction. Yet many questions concerning frozen embryos must be answered if the promise of this novel technology is to be realized.[1]

An immediate practical concern is decisional authority over frozen embryos. A recent dispute between a divorcing couple over custody of stored embryos highlights many of the issues that couples and IVF programs face when they cryopreserve human embryos.

The Tennessee Dispute

Mary Sue Davis, a twenty-eight-year-old secretary, and Junior Lewis Davis, a thirty-year-old housing authority employee, married in 1980. Their efforts to have a family over the last six years have been unsuccessful. Because of damage to Ms. Davis's fallopian tubes from ectopic pregnancies, six unsuccessful attempts at IVF have occurred. The last attempt resulted in seven extra embryos that were cryopreserved for possible use during later cycles. No document or consent form specifying disposition of these embryos was executed.[2]

The dispute over the fate of the embryos arose when the couple filed for divorce. The husband has sought to enjoin the fertility clinic from releasing the embryos to Ms. Davis or others for purposes of thawing and implantation. With divorce imminent, his concern is that neither his wife nor anyone else bear a child with these embryos, so that he will not end up a parent. Ms. Davis, on the other hand, wants very much to have a child with these embryos even if she is divorced. She insists that the embryos are living and that as the mother she has the right to initiate a pregnancy with them. If unable to use them herself, she wants to donate them to an infertile couple who could bring them to term.

Alternative Resolutions

Since few laws deal explicitly with the status and disposition of preimplantation embryos, direct precedents for deciding this case do not exist. The resulting decision, however, should clarify rules for IVF and embryo freezing generally or show the need for legislation or other policy solutions.

Several possible bases for resolving this dispute will not work. For example, there is no explicit prior agreement between the couple for disposition of embryos to which either could be bound. Nor can one imply an agreement to implant all embryos from the fact one has provided gametes for IVF, since so many contingencies could intervene to change original plans (death, divorce, illness, disability, financial reversal, etc.). Creation of embryos alone should not be taken as an irrevocable commitment to reproduction.

A presumption in favor of embryo transfer, to "protect" embryos by giving them the chance to implant and come to term, also is not persuasive in the absence of state law giving embryos such rights. Legally, extracorporeal embryos have no right to be implanted in Tennessee or most other states. Respected ethical advisory bodies in several countries have also concluded that embryos are not persons with rights.[3]

A policy of always discard in the case of dispute is also unsatisfactory. While postmortem anatomic gift laws and federal fetal research regulations require the consent of both parents, there is no inherent reason why one parent should have veto power in such matters.[4] Nor does the desirable goal of assuring every child two rearing parents justify such a rule, since the alternative for the child in question is never being born at all. Being raised by one parent does not amount to wrongful life, and other rearing parents may enter the picture later.

Equally unacceptable is a "sweat equity" position that always favors the woman's decision because she has put more effort into production of the embryo, having undergone ovarian stimulation and surgical retrieval of eggs. Great differences in physical burdens do not require that divorcing mothers always receive custody of children. Moreover, the difference in bodily burdens between the man and woman in IVF is not so great (especially with transvaginal aspiration of eggs) that it should automatically determine decisional authority over resulting embryos.

Finally, equal division of embryos, like division of other marital assets, will not do because embryos are a unique kind of marital "property." Equal division avoids the core conflict between producing or avoiding offspring, while implicitly resolving that conflict in favor of the party desiring to reproduce by assuring him or her some embryos to use in that effort. At the same time, it may so reduce the chance of a successful pregnancy that it is ultimately unsatisfactory to the party seeking to reproduce.

With these alternatives not applicable to the Tennessee case, its resolution requires a close look at the competing interests of each party: the one in avoiding the financial and psychosocial burdens of parenthood, and the other in using the embryos in question to become a parent. This analysis shows that the party wishing to avoid reproduction should prevail whenever the other party has a reasonable possibility of having offspring through other means.

Burdens of Unwanted Reproduction

A person who objects to transfer to a uterus of embryos formed from his or her gametes may experience significant financial and psychosocial burdens if the embryos lead to offspring.

Risks of Financial Liability

If the embryo implants and a child is born, the unwilling genetic father or mother may have legal obligations of support until the offspring reaches majority. Unless a statute provides an exemption, the traditional rule is that a man providing sperm for insemination or conception is the legal father, with rearing rights and duties, including support requirements.[5]

Since this rule is clearly established where conception occurs coitally, even when the woman has deceived the man about her ability to conceive, the rule is likely to be applied to noncoital conception as well.[6] The policy interest of holding men responsible for the consequences of their behavior and assuring offspring a male rearing parent also arises with noncoital insemination when no consenting male partner of the egg provider exists. Although the male is not engaging in sex, he is engaging in a transaction that makes offspring possible, and thus on policy grounds could be held responsible for resulting offspring.

Relieving the sperm source of financial responsibility is least likely to happen when there is no rearing male involved, as might happen when the sperm is provided to an unmarried woman, when a frozen embryo is used by a divorced wife, or when the embryo is donated to an unmarried woman. Under current law the sperm source for an embryo donation would be at substantial risk for financial liability in such situations.

The possibility of imposing support obligations on a woman who objects to transfer of embryos produced by her eggs is much less clear but cannot be ruled out in all situations. Precedents making the egg provider legally liable do not exist, because the egg source and the gestational mother have, until IVF made egg and embryo donation possible, always been identical.[7] Moreover, since the gestational mother will most likely have full rearing rights and duties the need to assure a responsible female parent for the child will not exist as it does with males.

Still, situations can be imagined in which the egg source would be financially liable if the unconsented transfer of embryos occurred. Suppose the father employs a gestational surrogate to bring the embryo to term, making him a single parent. Reversal of fortune could so diminish his resources that the child and the courts look to the genetic mother for support. Or suppose that the embryo were donated to an infertile couple, and that couple became incapable of supporting the child. Until it is clearly established that embryo donation severs all rearing rights and duties in the providers of the embryo, equal application of the rules applied to male gamete sources could lead to the female gamete source also being held liable for child support in these situations.

Psychosocial Impact

Whether or not the gamete source who opposes embryo transfer incurs child support obligations, he or she will still face the potentially significant psychosocial impact of unwanted biologic offspring. A marriage that had failed would have produced biologic offspring, for which the unconsenting partner may have strong feelings of attachment, responsibility, guilt, etc. Even if no rearing duties or even contact result, as might occur if the embryos are donated to another couple, the unconsenting partner may learn that biologic offspring exist, with the powerful attendant reverberations which that can ignite. The psychosocial burdens of unwanted parenthood are significant and should be given appropriate weight in deciding individual disputes.

The Burdens of Non-Transfer

Arrayed against the interest in avoiding the financial and psychosocial burdens of unwanted reproduction is the interest of the partner who wishes to use the embryos to reproduce. At stake for the woman wishing to use the embryos is gestation and rearing of her biologic offspring, while for the man there is the interest in rearing his biologic offspring. Let us assume that the interest of either the man or woman in reproducing is significant and ordinarily should be honored. The question, however, is whether it is of greater or lesser importance than the interest of the partner who wishes to avoid the financial and psychosocial burdens of reproduction. Since one person's loss is the other person's gain, it may appear that there is no objective way to arbitrate the dispute.

A way out of the dilemma exists if we consider the irreversibility of the respective losses at issue and the essential fungibility of the embryos. The party who wishes to avoid offspring is irreversibly harmed if embryo transfer and birth occur, for the burdens of unwanted parenthood cannot then be avoided. On the other hand, frustrating the ability of the willing partner to reproduce with these embryos will—in most instances—not prevent that partner from reproducing at a later time with other embryos. As long as the party wishing to reproduce could without undue burden create other embryos, the desire to avoid biologic offspring should take priority over the desire to reproduce with the embryos in question. If other embryos are reasonably available, there is no inherent reason to prefer already existing embryos over new ones that can be produced (given that the embryos themselves have no rights to be transferred).

In most instances the partner wishing to save the embryos to reproduce will be able to create new embryos to achieve his or her reproductive goals. For example, the male partner would be able to reproduce with another woman by remarrying, by obtaining an egg donation and surrogate gestator, or by serving as a sperm donor if no rearing is sought.

The woman, in most instances, should also be able to reproduce either with a new partner or a sperm donor. As long as her ovaries still function and hyperstimulation and egg retrieval are not medically contraindicated, she will be able to produce new embryos. Of course, she will have to undergo the moderate physical burdens of IVF stimulation and egg retrieval, but it does not appear unreasonable to ask her to bear moderate additional physical burdens to prevent the irreparable loss to the party seeking to avoid genetic offspring.

This solution is not available, however, if later reproductive opportunities do not exist for medical, financial, or social reasons. At that point the conflict between the right to reproduce and the right to avoid reproduction must be directly faced, with the argument for using the embryos against the wishes of the objecting partner then being strongest. One might then reasonably argue that the equities favor the party who has no alternative opportunity to reproduce, because the pleasures of parenthood will be deeper and more intense than the discomfort of unwanted genetic offspring.

Opting for reproduction when there is no other alternative assumes that the party wishing to reproduce will, if female, gestate and rear, or rear if male. The claim to reproduce against the wishes of the other is much less compelling if the party merely wishes the embryos donated to an infertile couple in order to have but not rear biologic offspring. The strongest argument in their favor, when they have no other reasonable reproductive opportunities, exists when they will assume all financial and childrearing burdens so that the unwilling party will have only the burden of genetic offspring *tout court*.

On this analysis the Tennessee case should be resolved in favor of the husband, who wishes the embryos not transferred, and against the wife, who wishes that they be transferred to her uterus or the uterus of a willing recipient. Her interest in reproduction can be satisfied by having her undergo yet another IVF cycle with a new partner or donor. She appears healthy and responds well to ovarian stimulation. The fact that she has already submitted to six attempt's at IVF is not determinative, since the burdens of any one additional retrieval cycle are moderate and acceptable, at least relative to the irreversible burdens of imposing fatherhood on the husband. Even if she ultimately prevails because of the many stimulation and retrieval cycles that she has undergone, cases in which the woman has undergone only one or two cycles should be decided in favor of the husband who now objects to reproduction with previously frozen embryos.

Whatever the balance struck by the Tennessee court, the Davis case is important for calling attention to the need for clear legal rules concerning disposition of frozen embryos. An essential starting point for such rules is recognition that the couple who provide the gametes jointly "own"—have dispositional authority over—the resulting embryos. Two legislative solutions to avoid future disputes should then be considered: embryo protection laws and prior directives.

The Couple's Ownership

Few persons would disagree that the gamete providers are the primary decisionmakers or "owners" of the resulting embryos, rather than the doctors or scientists who provide the technical skill to create the embryos, or the operators of the embryo bank where they are stored. They have provided the gametes, and the resulting embryos have great reproductive significance for them. In this context the terms "ownership" or "property" refer to the locus and not the scope of decisional authority over embryos.

The more interesting question is whether their decisional authority can be limited, so that their "property" or "ownership" in embryos is less than their ownership of other kinds of property. For example, limitations on buying or selling or use in research may be more appropriate with embryos than with other property. However, the couple might still retain the right to decide whether transfer of embryos to a uterus will occur, and to make advance binding commitments concerning future disposition of embryos. At a minimum, legislation and public policy should recognize the couple's authority to make those choices concerning embryos that are legally available.

It follows then that the couple retains dispositional authority or ownership over embryos until they relinquish it to others, or until the state has restricted their options. If so, IVF programs and embryo banks have no right to retain embryos against the couple's joint wishes or to make other dispositions unless the couple has specifically ceded that right to them.

An embryo bank thus has no right to refuse to release a stored embryo to a couple for thawing without transfer, or for transport to another location, unless the couple had specifically agreed to this limitation. Even then, one may question the reasonableness of the program or bank insisting on enforcing that condition, though there will be some situations in which legitimate interests of the IVF program would be harmed if the condition were not enforced.[8]

The *Jones v. York* case in Virginia should clarify the couple's dispositional authority over stored embryos when an IVF program or embryo bank refuses to follow their instructions.[9] An infertile couple had one frozen embryo remaining after three unsuccessful attempts at IVF pregnancy at a leading program in Norfolk. After the couple moved to California, they sought to transport their frozen embryo to a Los Angeles IVF program for thawing and placement in the wife's uterus. The Norfolk program refused, citing the signed consent form, lack of IRB approval, legal liability risks, and the demeaning effect of shipping human embryos by air "a la cattle embryos."

The court denied the Norfolk clinic's attempts to dismiss the couple's suit seeking release of their embryo. The judge found that the cryopreservation agreement between the couple and the program had created a bailor-bailee relationship, which imposed on the bailee an absolute obligation to return the subject matter of the bailment to the bailor when the purpose of the bailment had been terminated. Neither the state's human subject research law nor the terms of the agreement undercut the couple's property interest in the frozen embryo. Therefore, they had a *prima facie* claim to have their embryo released to them.

Jones v. York is significant because it assumes without question that embryos are the "property" of the gamete providers, and finds that any limitation of their dispositional authority in favor of an IVF program or embryo bank will be strictly construed against the IVF program. While a program could still insist that the embryos it creates not be transferred to other locations, such a restriction will be binding only if the program explicitly informs the couple that they are ceding their light to transport their embryos to other locations.

Prohibiting Embryo Discard?

The *Davis* case would have been easily resolved if Tennessee had enacted a law requiring that embryos be placed in a uterus whenever possible, either that of the woman providing the egg or a willing recipient. Louisiana currently bans the "intentional destruction" of IVF embryos, and mandates their donation in certain cases.[10] Other states may follow suit. But would such laws be constitutional? If so, is the limitation they place on a couple's dispositional authority justified?

The constitutional argument against such a statute rests on a right claimed by the couple or gamete providers individually to avoid the financial and psychosocial burdens of unwanted generic parenthood. Supreme Court cases recognizing the right to use contraceptives and have abortions may reasonably be taken as establishing a right to avoid reproduction because of the financial, social, and physical burdens that reproduction entails.[11] Even if parenthood entails only psychological burdens, as would occur with mandatory donation of unwanted embryos, the interest at stake is still of paramount importance to individual identity and therefore warrants protection as a fundamental right. If so, the state's desire to protect embryos and signify the importance of human life would not constitute the compelling interest necessary to justify infringement of the fundamental right to avoid reproduction.[12]

The counterargument appears stronger, even if *Roe v. Wade* remains intact. Since the right claimed is to be free of a purely psychological burden (no financial or other rearing burdens attach), it is unlikely that a Supreme Court disinclined to expand the menu of unwritten fundamental rights would give the interest in avoiding generic offspring *tout court* fundamental right status. If not a fundamental right, the state's interest in protecting embryos by requiring donation of unwanted extras would easily meet the rational basis test by which such a statute would be judged.[13] *Roe v. Wade* presents no obstacle to such a law as long as the woman is not herself forced to accept the embryos.

A variant on embryo protection laws might be to limit the number of embryos produced to avoid the problem of discard raised by extra embryos, for example, a law that prohibited insemination of more than five eggs during any one retrieval cycle. Such laws might have greater constitutional problems than mandatory embryo donation statutes, because they directly impair the couple's ability to become pregnant through IVF.[14] They might also effectively ban embryo freezing, since few extra embryos might result.

But are embryo protection laws desirable, even if they may be within the constitutional authority of the state? They would be a significant limitation on the couple's "ownership" or dispositional authority over their embryos, and could lead to imposition of unwanted parenting burdens. While a minority believes that a new person exists at fertilization, most people would disagree that the earliest stages of postfertilized human life, which consist of four to eight undifferentiated cells that are not yet biologically individual, are themselves persons or entities with rights. The consensus emerging from the Ethics Advisory Board, the Warnock Committee, the American Fertility Society, and most other ethics commissions throughout the world that have studied the matter is that special respect for embryos does not require treating them as actual persons or prohibiting couples from opposing transfer.[15]

If preimplantation embryos are too rudimentary in development to have interests, much less rights, protecting them can be justified only on symbolic or religious grounds that are not uniformly shared in a highly pluralistic society. In my view the argument for preferring early embryos over the competing concerns of couples or individuals who wish to prevent their placement in a uterus is not persuasive. Persons wishing to avoid reproduction have more to lose than society has to gain from laws that limit their dispositional authority over the embryos formed from their egg or sperm.

Advance Agreements on Disposition

A better policy solution would be to require couples to declare at the time that embryos are created or stored their instructions concerning disposition if they are unavailable or unable to agree when death, divorce, passage of time, or other contingencies occur. As part of the consent procedure, the gamete providers will be informed of the dispositional alternatives available at that program or bank, and asked to designate which alternatives they choose if certain stated contingencies occur. In some cases it may be possible for the couple to reserve the right jointly to change their designated disposition at later times, but until they do, the options selected would be binding when the specified events occur.

The argument for recognizing the binding effect of joint advance instructions rests on several grounds. The right to use embryos to reproduce or to avoid reproduction should include the right to give binding advance instructions because certainty about future outcomes is necessary to exercise reproductive options. In addition, all parties gain from the ability to plan for certain outcomes when future contingencies occur. Finally, it minimizes the frequency and cost of resolving disputes that arise over disposition of embryos.

But arguments against binding oneself in advance also exist. Advance instructions may be issued at a time relatively early in the IVF process, when a person's needs and interests may not be as fully realized as they would be when later events occur. One's interests and preferences might change as future events unfold, in ways that cannot be foreseen when the instructions are given. Since preconception agreements to abort, not abort, or give up for adoption are not enforceable, neither should preconception or preimplantation agreements for the disposition of embryos.[16] Also, there may be no easy way to assure that the parties are fully informed and aware of the legally binding choices they would be making.[17] Finally, IVF programs and embryo banks may have such monopoly power that the conditions they offer give couples little real choice.

To assess the desirability of having couples bind themselves in advance, consider two situations in which one party wishes to revise the original instruction and the other party is unavailable or disagrees.

Advance Agreements to Have Embryos Transferred

Suppose the couple has agreed that all embryos will be transferred to the uterus of the egg source, or to another woman if the former is unwilling or unable to have the embryos placed in her. Before transfer, however, divorce occurs, and the husband now objects to thawing of the embryos for implantation in the former wife or a willing recipient. May the embryo bank transfer stored embryos on the basis of the previously executed instructions?

Since agreeing to this disposition may be viewed as a material condition on which the other party and program relied in creating and storing embryos, the agreement should be binding. Indeed, enforcement is essential to provide the certainty about outcomes necessary for couples and IVF programs to proceed with embryo freezing. It is true that the husband may not have realized when the embryos were created that he would have had such strong feelings against post-divorce parenthood. But it is also true that neither partner may have been willing to create and freeze embryos unless they could rely on the certainty that all resulting embryos would be given a chance to implant.

The general unenforceability of preconception agreements not to abort by spouses or surrogate mothers should not apply to the very different situation of external embryos.[18] Enforcing a woman's agreement not to abort forces her to continue an unwanted pregnancy, but no bodily or gestational burdens are involved in enforcing the gamete sources' preimplantation agreement to have all stored embryos thawed and transferred to the uterus of a willing recipient.

Providing gametes to create embryos in this situation should thus be taken as a binding commitment to reproduce. The parties were informed of that consequence at the time of election, relied on the commitment to transfer, and knew that the spouse was relying on that commitment as well.

Advance Agreements Not to Transfer Embryos

Consider a second case in which the couple (and IVF program) have specifically agreed that in case of divorce, separation, death, inability to agree, or passage of time any stored embryos will be removed from storage and not transferred, that is, they will be allowed to die or be discarded. Avoiding the financial and psychosocial burdens of unwanted offspring is something that the parties may reasonably choose at the time of creation and storage. Since they may not undertake IVF and cryopreservation if they cannot be protected against unwanted offspring in those future situations, the agreement should be enforced, despite one party's change of mind and desire now to have the embryos transferred to a uterus. A suit by that party to enjoin thawing and nontransfer or for damages against the embryo bank that has thawed the embryos should fail.

Again an appeal to the unenforceability of agreements to abort fails because of the dissimilarity in the situation. A wife's agreement to abort if she becomes pregnant, or a surrogate mother's to abort if amniocentesis reveals a generic defect would not be specifically enforced because of the bodily intrusion that enforcement entails. Nor would the woman be legally liable for damages for continuing the pregnancy in violation of her agreement (though the opposite result could be justified).

But here the embryos are extracorporeal and not yet implanted. A woman's right to continue a pregnancy unwanted by the male partner is not implicated. Only her wish to become pregnant with extracorporeal embryos or have them donated to a willing recipient is at issue—an entirely different situation. The need for certainty in entering into embryo freezing and preventing the burdens of parenthood that one partner insisted on avoiding outweigh the interest of the party who has changed his or her mind and now wishes reproduction to occur. The need for certainty and efficient resolution of disputes over embryos demands that the prior commitment for embryo discard be honored. In this situation providing gametes to create embryos should not be viewed as a commitment to reproduce, because both parties explicitly agreed that it was not such a commitment.

Note that advance instructions should be binding by one party against another, or by the embryo bank or IVF program against the couple. The latter situation is important because IVF programs may have institutional or physician constraints on disposition of embryos, and thus need some certainty that couples will be held to limits on transfer, time of storage, donation, and the like. However, program-imposed restrictions should be binding only if they have been clearly disclosed to the couple at the start and are not inherently unreasonable.

The Best Guidelines

Because early embryos represent their potential offspring yet are too rudimentary in development to have interests in themselves, the couple's dispositional authority or ownership over extracorporeal embryos should be respected. They should have wide leeway in their decisions to form families through creation, storage, thawing, and transfer of embryos, yet should also be free to avoid reproduction with IVF embryos when their needs or circumstances have changed. Any limitation on their "ownership" must give due regard to their procreative freedom to have or to avoid having offspring.

Until the law prescribes otherwise, disputes over frozen embryos should be resolved first by looking to the joint wishes of the couple, and if they are not available or are unable to agree, to prior instructions which they gave for disposition of those embryos. If no instructions exist, we must then compare the relative burdens on each party of using or not using the embryos in question to see which party should prevail. These principles are the best guide for assimilating IVF technology into social practice while respecting family and reproductive choice.

QUESTIONS FOR CONSIDERATION

1. In what sense do couples have "ownership" (property rights) of frozen embryos produced by *in vitro* fertilization? Is the language of "custody of pre-born children" (used in the Davis case) more helpful?

2. Do the "burdens of an unwanted pregnancy" outweigh the "burdens of non-transfer" when settling disputes over frozen embryos? What com-

mitments are couples making to potential embryos when choosing *in vitro* fertilization?

3. What rights do clinics which preserve frozen embryos have in their disposition in times of dispute? Is an "always discard" policy morally defensible?

4. Are the types of advanced agreements proposed by Robertson practical? Will states recognize a binding legal authority in such agreements?

NOTES

1. John A. Robertson, "Ethical and Legal Issues in Cryopreservation of Human Embryos," *Fertility and Sterility* 47:3 (1987), 371–81.

2. R. Smothers, "Embryos in a Divorce Case: Joint Property or Offspring?," *New York Times*, 21 April 1989, 1.

3. Robertson, "Ethical and Legal Issues."

4. Uniform Anatomical Gift Act #3, 8A U.L.A. 8–9 (West Supp. 1987); 45 C.F.R. 46.209 (d).

5. John A. Robertson, *In the Beginning: The Legal Status of Early Embryos* (forthcoming).

6. *Hughes v. Hutt*, 500 Pa. 209, 455 A.2d 623 (1982); *In re Pamela P.*, 443 N.Y.S. 2d 343 (1981).

7. John A. Robertson, "Technology and Motherhood: Legal and Ethical Issues in Human Egg Donation," *Case Western Reserve Law Review* 39:1 (1988), 1–38.

8. Robertson, *In the Beginning*.

9. *Jones v. York*, No. 33455 (E.D. Va. 1989).

10. R.S. La. 9:125 (La. Supp. 1987).

11. John A. Robertson, "Procreative Liberty and the Control of Conception, Pregnancy and Childbirth," *Virginia Law Review* 69:3 (1983), 405–414.

12. John A. Robertson, "Embryos, Families and Procreative Liberty: The Legal Structure of the New Reproduction," *Southern California Law Review* 59:5 (1986), 939–1041.

13. Robertson, "Embryos, Families and Procreative Liberty."

14. Robertson, *In the Beginning*.

15. *Report of the Committee of Inquiry Into Human Fertilisation and Embryology*, (London: Her Majesty's Stationary Office, 1984), 53; Victoria Committee to Consider the Social, Ethical and Legal Issues Arising from In Vitro Fertilization, *Report on the Disposition of Embryos Produced by IVF*, 1984; Ontario Law Reform Commission, 1985; The Ethics Committee of The American Fertility Society, "Ethical Considerations of the New Reproductive Technology," *Fertility and Sterility* 46 Suppl. 1 (1986), IS–94S; U.S. Department of Health, Education, and Welfare (HEW), Ethics Advisory Board, "HEW Support of Research Involving Human In Vitro Fertilization and Embryo Transfer," 44 *Federal Register* 35, 033, 1979.

16. *In re Baby M*, 537 A.2d 1227 (N.J. 1988).

17. John A. Robertson, "Taking Consent Seriously: IRB Interventions in the Consent Process," *IRB: A Journal of Human Subjects Research* 4:5 (1982), 1–5.

18. Robertson, "Embryos, Families and Procreative Liberty."

David T. Ozar

The Case Against Thawing
Unused Frozen Embryos

The Rios case made headlines last year. A millionaire couple from the United States, Mario and Elsa Rios wanted to have children. Though each had had children by former marriages, they were unable to conceive together. In 1981 they sought the help of researchers at Queen Victoria Medical Center in Melbourne, Australia. Three of Mrs. Rios's egg cells were removed and successfully fertilized in the laboratory with sperm from an anonymous donor. One of the resulting live embryos was then implanted in Mrs. Rios's womb; the two remaining embryos were frozen to preserve them for future implantation if the first implanted embryo should abort.

The implanted embryo did spontaneously abort after about ten days but Mrs. Rios said she was not emotionally ready then to have a second embryo implanted. Some time later the Rioses went to South America to adopt a child. In the spring of 1983, Mr. and Mrs. Rios and their adopted child were killed in a crash of their private airplane (*New York Times*, October 24, 1984).

The legal question was: Who should inherit the considerable assets of their estate? The common law tradition, including both United States and Australian law, has long permitted those who have been conceived but have not yet been born to inherit. But their inheriting is contingent on their being born alive. "There is nothing in law," says William Salmond, "to prevent a man from owning property before he is born. His ownership is contingent, for he may never be born at all; but it is nonetheless a real and present ownership. . . . A posthumous child, for example, may inherit; but if he died in the womb, or is stillborn, his inheritance fails to take effect, and *no one can claim through him*, though it would be otherwise if he lived for an hour after his birth."[1]

A will, of course, identifies the heirs, regardless of their parentage. But when there is no will, as in the Rios case, is the embryo to be considered the child of the woman who bears it (and must she be bearing it when the deceased dies) or of the woman from whose ovum it has grown? And is the embryo the child of the man whose sperm fertilized that ovum or of some other? These are fascinating legal questions; but I shall not discuss them further here.[2]

Another question was: Who should decide the fate of the remaining frozen embryos? If the Rioses were still alive, it would be natural to conclude, both in law and from an ethical perspective, that they, together with the doctors and researchers involved, are the responsible parties.[3] With the Rioses now dead, should the executors appointed for the Rioses' estate or the Rioses' heirs or possibly the state take over the Rioses' role in these decisions?

A committee convened for the purpose later recommended that the embryos be destroyed. The legislators of the state of Victoria then rejected the committee's advice and passed an amendment to another bill, calling for an attempt to have the embryos implanted in surrogate mothers and then, if they came to term, placed for adoption. There has been no further word on whether they were actually implanted. Regardless of how this aspect of the matter is resolved, the doctors and researchers, who brought the sperm and ova together and who have preserved the embryos in their frozen state, will still have a role to play. I shall assume that, for our purposes, they bear the chief ethical responsibility for unused frozen embryos.

Is the fact that the Rioses are deceased of importance in determining what is the right thing to do with the remaining embryos? The answer is clearly, no. If it were determined that the embryos ought to be dealt with as pieces of property, organic goods duly owned by someone, then the fact that the Rioses are deceased means only that someone else owns them. By the same token, if it were determined that the embryos ought to be treated differently from pieces of property, then they ought to be so treated regardless of who has or has not died.

Suppose that the Rioses had lived, that the first implanted embryo had prospered and had been born a healthy baby, and that the Rioses had chosen to have only one child. The future of the two remaining embryos would still need to be decided. On this scenario the matter would probably have been decided privately between the Rioses and the hospital-laboratory team. A number of such decisions have undoubtedly been made in just this way, between the team and other couples. But the question is the same whether we as a community reflect on it or it is asked privately by doctors and researchers and the couples who are their patients; and its answer does not depend on the fate of Mr. and Mrs. Rios. How ought people to act, what ought people to do, in regard to unused frozen embryos?

Some might argue that this question misses the point, that the real issue concerns the morality of artificial reproductive techniques themselves, of which freezing live embryos is simply one example. From this perspective all forms of fertilization other than intercourse are profoundly unnatural and immoral.[4] The real point would be that these embryos should not have been fertilized and frozen in the first place. We are uncertain about how to proceed rightly from this point because the parties acted immorally at the outset.

This approach raises important questions about the reproductive technology that was offered to the Rioses. But this response is of little help to those who must now determine what to do about existing frozen embryos. Even if the acts that brought us to this pass were profoundly immoral, what we do next is still not a morally indifferent matter.

Obligation Toward Fetuses

In trying to answer this question, it is natural to examine the lines of thought that have been developed regarding our obligations toward fetuses. Unfortunately, many of these lines tell us little about a frozen eight- or sixteen-celled embryo. For example, any obligations that we might have toward a fetus by reason of its possession of neurological functions, and hence its possession of the beginnings of the most distinctive functions of the human species,[5] would not apply to an embryo whose cells have not yet begun to differentiate in terms of function. Even less could an embryo pass the test of actually engaging in acts of thinking, planning, choosing, or of being conscious and experiencing emotion, which some authors have made the key to a being's having rights and the rest of us having corresponding obligations.[6]

One approach that might seem helpful here focuses on viability outside the womb. The frozen embryo is obviously outside the womb and it is not dead or dying. Indeed it is being preserved in its frozen state precisely because of its potential for continued life.

Viability is one of the criteria employed by the United States Supreme Court in the ethical justification of the legal rulings in its landmark abortion decisions.[7] In *Roe v. Wade*, the Court held that the fetus is not a legal person, a bearer of legal rights, including the legal right not to be killed, at any point from conception until the moment of live birth. But the Court held that the state does have an "interest" in "protecting the potentiality of human life," and that this interest grows "in substantiality as the woman approaches term." Moreover, at some point in the pregnancy, the Court held, this interest may be considered "compelling," that is, sufficiently important that it may outweigh other fundamental values, in this case the mother's constitutional right to control her own body and thus to seek an abortion if she chooses.

The point at which the state's interest in protecting the potentiality of human life becomes "compelling," said the *Roe* Court, is "viability." Viability is in turn described as "the capability of meaningful life outside the womb"; but the term "meaningful" is not further defined by the *Roe* Court, so the Court's understanding of viability was still unclear. In *Danforth,* however, the Court upheld a Missouri statute containing this definition of viability: "that stage of fetal development when the life of the unborn child may be continued indefinitely outside of the womb by natural or artificial life-support systems."

But as Justice Sandra Day O'Connor has argued, there is still ambiguity here. In a dissent to the Court's 1983 *Akron* decision,[8] Justice O'Connor argues that "neither sound constitutional theory nor our need to decide cases based on the application of neutral principles can accommodate an analytic framework that varies according to the 'stages' of pregnancy, where those stages, and their concomitant standards of review, differ according to the level of medical technology at a particular time . . . . The *Roe* framework is clearly on a collision course with itself. As the medical risks of various abortion procedures decrease, the point at which the state may regulate for reasons of maternal health is moved further forward to actual childbirth. As medical science becomes better able to provide for the separate existence of the fetus, the point of viability is moved further back toward conception. . . ." Thus if medical science had developed an artificial womb, in which embryos could develop until they could live independently, the Rioses' frozen embryos would be viable under the *Danforth* definition.

But lacking an artificial womb, what are we to say? The most likely interpretation is that "life" in these definitions means not only that the organism under consideration is not dying, but also that it is able to continue to perform life functions (with or without mechanical assistance) outside of a womb. On this interpretation, the frozen embryo is not viable. For, while capable in their frozen state of not dying, these embryos cannot continue to perform life functions, even simple cell divisions, independent of the nutritive and protective environment of a woman's womb.

Consequently, to return to *Roe v. Wade*, the state would not have a "compelling" interest in protecting the potential life of frozen embryos. That is, the state's interest in protecting their potential life could not outweigh the fundamental constitutional right of a woman to control her own body. But in the case of frozen embryos, no woman is involved, and thus no woman's right to control her body. Might the state's interest then be strong enough to protect frozen embryos' lives? Here the competing rights would have to be the property rights of those who own the equipment that preserves the embryos' lives. Is the state's interest in protecting the potential life of the embryo great enough to outweigh the equipment owners' rights to control their property? Or are the frozen embryos to be considered property themselves, so that their owners may dispose of them more or less as they wish, and their lives would not have any special weight in relation to the property rights of the owners of the equipment? Obviously we are now asking questions that cannot be resolved in terms of the criterion of viability. So it turns out that this criterion, like the others mentioned above, cannot resolve our question about how to act rightly toward unused frozen embryos.

The "Instant of Conception" View

But there are two approaches to our obligations toward fetuses that are informative regarding frozen embryos as well. First is the most inclusive moral position regarding obligations toward the unborn—the position that holds that the conceptus has a moral right not to be killed, and the rest of us have a moral obligation not to kill the conceptus or to intend to kill it, from the first instant of its conception.[9] (This right, stated more completely, is a right not to be *directly* killed, and the obligation is an obligation not to *directly* kill or to intend to *directly* kill the conceptus. The added term, "directly," is very important in other contexts; but it is not important in the present discussion, and therefore I shall use the more simplified statement.)

This position is commonly called the "right to life" position; but I shall call it the "instant of conception" position. Many other positions on these matters affirm life-related rights, including rights not to be killed under various sets of circumstances. In calling it the "instant of conception" position, I am focusing on what is truly distinctive about it and on its substantive claims in the present discussion.

According to this position, a frozen embryo, as the fruit of human conception, has a moral right not to be killed. Therefore the doctors and researchers responsible for the care of such an embryo could not morally place it in an environment known to be lethal to it. This would preclude deliberately permitting a frozen embryo to be thawed without placing it in the only environment in which it could survive thawing, namely, a woman's womb. Nor could the parents (by any definition) or anyone else morally choose that a frozen embryo be dealt with in this way.

At the same time, the "instant of conception" position provides no basis for saying that an embryo has a moral right to be implanted in a womb. The moral right not to be killed does not automatically imply a right to the use of a womb. For an embryo may be implanted in a womb only by the free choice of the woman whose womb it is. Thus the obligation not to kill an embryo does not necessarily imply an obligation on anyone's part to offer her womb for its survival.

One possible exception is the genetic mother, the donor of the ovum whence the embryo has grown. It may be that, in bringing the embryo into being, she has undertaken an obligation to assist it in realizing its full potential for human life. But this obligation, if it exists, does not derive from a moral right of the embryo as the kind of being that it is, but rather from the mother's freely undertaking to bring it into being. (The genetic father might have a similar obligation, but since he cannot provide the womb that the embryo needs, I shall not consider his obligations further.)

I shall not attempt to resolve here the complicated questions about the degree of responsibility of genetic parents for their offspring.[10] The point is that, if the genetic mother does have such an obligation to the embryo, then she maybe obligated to accept the unused embryo into her womb. If the genetic mother refuses to do so, however, or if she dies as Mrs. Rios did, so that responsibility for the frozen embryos now falls upon the hospital-laboratory team, no one would have an *obligation* to accept the embryo into her womb. If anyone did accept it, this would be an act of charity toward the embryo, not an act of obligation or an act to which the embryo had a right.

There are then two possibilities. If no one volunteers her womb for the implantation of the unused frozen embryo, those responsible for its care will fulfill their obligations simply by not killing it, that is, by keeping it frozen. If, on the other hand, someone does volunteer for its implantation, the responsible parties would need to determine whether implantation in the womb of this particular volunteer would give the embryo a reasonable chance of survival and further development, as compared with continued freezing and the possibility of implantation in a future volunteer with more likelihood of success. It would be appropriate, also, for the responsible parties to seek out women who might desire to volunteer for implantation of unused embryos.

Since frozen embryos may deteriorate over time, let us assume that there is a point at which the hospital-laboratory team can accurately say that a particular embryo is no longer able to survive implantation. Such an embryo no longer has any potential for continued life. Because it is still frozen, it is not yet dead; yet death is its only conceivable prospect. I believe that the "instant of conception" position would conclude that such an embryo no longer has any moral right that would require its continued maintenance in the frozen state. Its condition is now analogous to that of someone who is irreversibly in the process of dying. The embryo may morally be thawed at this point, and the irreversible process of its death permitted to proceed to its conclusion.

The View that the Embryo Has No Moral Rights

The obligations that I have just outlined, based as they are on the most inclusive position regarding our obligations to the unborn, constitute the most extensive set of obligations toward unused frozen embryos that can reasonably be defended. Next we must ask: Is any lesser set of obligations toward unused frozen embryos more reasonable? In order to respond, I shall look at a position that accords no moral rights at all to the unborn.

If a frozen embryo has no moral rights of its own, if it is more like a piece of property (or is just like a piece of property) rather than a bearer of rights, still those who are responsible for it will have obligations regarding its use and the consequences of its use. If certain ways of dealing with it would lead to significantly more good than other ways, at relatively little cost in human effort, in monetary resources, and so on, then the responsible parties would be obligated to choose those ways of acting. If certain ways of acting would involve risk of significant harm, which could be avoided at relatively little cost in human effort, in monetary resources, and so on, then the responsible parties would be obligated to avoid them.

These straightforward moral principles point to the same conclusion as is defended by the "instant of conception" position, even if the embryo has no moral rights at all. My argument follows a pattern developed by Mary Anne Warren in a famous postscript to "On the Moral and Legal Status of Abortion." In response to criticisms that her criteria for having moral rights were so strict as to deny moral rights to infants, Warren argued that even when no moral rights are relevant, morality may require that human life be preserved and protected because of the negative consequences of doing otherwise.

Once the original outlay of expense and effort for freezing embryos has been made, embryos can be maintained in their frozen state at very little cost, in dollars or in human effort. Therefore if there are women who desire to bear a child and who might be successfully implanted with embryos unused by others, the moral principles just articulated argue strongly for maintaining unused embryos in their frozen state until they can be implanted. The costs of doing this are very small and the benefits to the mothers concerned (as well as to their spouses and other affected parties) are very great. In fact, if the good of enabling women to bear children can justify the sizable expense of developing or purchasing this technology in the first place, then it surely can justify the far smaller expense of maintaining unused embryos until other women who desire to bear a child have volunteered. It would also be reasonable for the doctors and researchers to seek out such women, especially if the frozen embryo does deteriorate over time, in the interests of maximizing the benefits and minimizing the costs of the process.

This same conclusion—that unused frozen embryos ought to be maintained in their frozen state for as long as they are able to survive implantation—can be reached in another way, which takes account of other consequences of the process. For even if frozen embryos do not have moral rights, they are still members of the human species with a potential for a full human life. Indeed it is precisely because of that potential that they were frozen in the first place. Consequently if hospital-laboratory teams, parents, or other responsible parties routinely followed a policy of simply disposing of unused frozen embryos, such a policy, if widely known, could have a negative impact on the ways in which we as individuals and as a community value and deal with human life generally, especially in other members of our species whose lives are in some way compromised.

Two questions need to be addressed here. One is a subtle question of social psychology. It asks how various policies concerning human life that are accepted within a community have an impact on individuals' values and future actions and on future policies within the community. The second is a normative question: What values, actions, and future policies regarding human life should we support and reinforce in our present policy making?

We are woefully short on answers to the first question. Some have argued that a community that values many other things over the life of a fetus will experience a gradual but significant lessening in the value of human life generally, so that previously unacceptable trade-offs between human life and other values will come to be accepted. Others have claimed that there is no such linkage in human feelings or in other parts of the human psyche between our valuation of human life in the unborn and the born.

I have no expert opinion to offer on the first question, but I believe that we do have some sense of the proper answer to the second, for it is clear that a great deal is at stake here. The value that we, as individuals and as a community, attach to human life is the most fundamental element of the social morality that makes it possible for us to live together in some measure of security. Such valuing of human life is nurtured in many subtle ways in our habits and mores, and in our institutions. Such valuing is probably vulnerable as well, at least over the long run; it may even be subject to significant change as habits, mores, and institutions change.

Thus it is not beyond the realm of possibility that widespread public acceptance of a practice in which human embryos are made when it is efficient and economical to make them and disposed of when it is efficient and economical to dispose of them would have an impact on the community's valuing of human life in other contexts, an impact that would put the lives of those already born at risk when trade-offs of efficiency and economics did not favor them. We know far too little to predict that something like this will certainly occur. But we also know far too little to predict that it certainly will not. Certainly enough is at stake that we would be foolish not to acknowledge the risk.

Only reasons of economy and efficiency support a policy of disposal. But a policy of maintaining the lives of frozen embryos for as long as they could survive implantation and of actively seeking out women who might desire to bear them would be far less expensive than the setup costs of the technology that enabled us to freeze embryos in the first place. Thus, given the possible negative impact of disposing of human embryos for reasons of efficiency and economics, clearly the far better course of action is to maintain the frozen embryos until they can no longer survive implantation and to actively support their implantation when women desiring to bear them volunteer. This course of action avoids risk of significant harm at relatively little cost.

From this it is clear that those who would accord to frozen embryos no moral rights whatsoever, but who would still be guided in their obligations by consideration of the outcomes of their actions, would reach the same conclusion regarding unused frozen embryos as those who affirm the embryos' moral rights from the instant of conception. From both perspectives, as well as each of the intermediate moral positions, the responsible parties have an obligation to preserve the frozen embryos in their frozen state until such time as they can no longer survive implantation. In addition, they should support implantation of unused embryos in women who volunteer to bear them and should make reasonable efforts to locate such women when there are implantable embryos.

Freezing Multiple Embryos

The issues discussed so far presuppose the value of fertilizing multiple ova and freezing the resulting embryos on the chance that an implanted embryo will subsequently abort. Since the risk of spontaneous abortion of implanted embryos is considerable, the fertilization and freezing of multiple embryos seem a reasonable efficiency. But the previous arguments suggest that the production of embryos is not something to be undertaken lightly. So we need to reflect on the ethical appropriateness of the multiple frozen embryo procedure itself.

Some authors have argued that in vitro fertilization and the implantation of the resulting embryo are, without exception, profoundly unnatural and immoral. Obviously if this view is correct, nearly every aspect of the procedure of freezing multiple embryos is immoral; but I do not find the arguments offered in support of this view to be persuasive. Putting considerations of the just allocation of health care resources aside for the moment, I consider it a reasonable and therapeutic intervention to assist a woman who desires to bear a child by fertilizing her ovum in vitro and implanting the resulting embryo in her womb. If freezing the embryo at some point in its development will give it a better chance of surviving implantation, without harming its development in other ways, this too seems reasonable to me.

The ethical issue that has not been adequately addressed is precisely the procedure of fertilizing and freezing of *multiple* embryos. The most obvious reason for this procedure is that it is easier and cheaper to fertilize several ova at the same time and to have the resulting embryos available for a second or third implantation whenever they are needed, rather than go back to fertilizing an ovum from the beginning if the first (second, third) implantation fails.

The problem is, as before, that the organisms being used to make the procedure cheaper and easier are genetically complete human organisms. It is, again, their very potential for full human life that prompts the hospital-laboratory team to fertilize and preserve them in the first place. Therefore the same considerations that argue for thoughtful caution in our dealings with unused embryos argue for a similar caution in our making and freezing of embryos at all.

If it becomes common knowledge that human embryos are fertilized and frozen in quantity in order to make a particular medical procedure easier and less expensive, could this not have a significant negative impact on individuals' and communities' values and future actions, at least over the long run? Are the benefits of such a procedure valuable enough to run the risks that the procedure involves?

In response, it could be argued that it is precisely in the interests of human life that human life is being used in this way. Everyone involved in this technology is striving to enable children to be born who otherwise could not have been born. The chances of a particular child's being born are multiplied by two or three or whatever the number, it would be argued, if we are able to fertilize and freeze two or three or more embryos at the start. Does not this goal of extending human life to those who would otherwise not have it justify the multiple frozen embryo procedure?

When we are dealing with those already born, we do not permit anyone's life to be used to improve another person's chances unless the helper undertakes the task voluntarily. If we are dealing with children or others who cannot choose on their own, we would permit ones life to be used in the interests of another in only the rarest of circumstances, if ever. Still, "using a life" usually does not mean giving a new life, as it does when multiple embryos are fertilized and frozen. On the other hand, the frozen embryo procedure is not the only way to obtain a second, third, or fourth living embryo if the first implantation should fail. So we are left with a question: If it was certain that every embryo fertilized and frozen in this procedure would have a chance for implantation, as in the policy argued for in the preceding section, then would the way in which the embryos' lives are "used" in this technology be morally acceptable? Or would manipulating the lives of human embryos in this way still pose a risk of negatively affecting the ways in which individuals and communities value and deal with human life? Considerations of efficiency and laboratory economy alone would not seem worth this risk.

But what about the value to the mothers involved, the value of bearing a child? To be sure, the good of childbearing is a great good; and the future of our species, itself a considerable good, depends on it. But a particular woman's ability to bear a child is not an absolute good; it can be outweighed by a variety of other considerations, singly or in combination. Nor is childbearing the only possible basis of parenting, which is the good that at least some candidates for this procedure seek. We must at least inquire whether adoption would not fulfill the most important needs of many who seek the assistance of reproductive technologies without the risks and costs of such technologies.

A single-minded commitment on the part of the physicians and researchers involved in reproductive technologies to enable women to bear children who would otherwise be unable to do so is understandable and perhaps even commendable. But in making policy the larger community must take more into account than the ability of patients to bear children and the ability of doctors and researchers to develop efficient procedures to this end.

The issue can be posed in a different way. Ought every woman who has healthy ova but who cannot bear children without such a procedure receive the benefits of multiple frozen embryo technology? As soon as we ask the question in this way, recognizing that many thousands of women might be candidates for the procedure (by some current estimates, 15 percent of all married couples are infertile),[11] we realize that we must consider the costs. Making the procedure available to every woman who might benefit would almost certainly draw significant resources away from other pressing health care needs or from other uses of resources within the larger community.

Is this procedure so valuable that we would be willing to close immunization programs or blood banks or a significant number of medical schools, or reduce the resources devoted to arthritis research or the like, in order to make it available to all who might benefit? Is it more valuable than efforts to provide better education to our disadvantaged young or decent survival to our elderly poor or basic foodstuffs and fresh water to the millions in the world community who cannot obtain them without assistance? We recognize immediately that the good that this technology pursues is a relative good; it must be weighed against other goods before we can know if pursuing it is worth the cost in resources, in human effort, and, as I have argued, in the risk of future harm.

At present the benefits of the multiple frozen embryo procedure are available only to the wealthy and to those who have been selected as research subjects. The latter pattern of allocating this therapy may be justified as long as the therapy is still experimental. But there is a clear injustice in giving the wealthy privileged access to an accepted therapeutic procedure. Admittedly some instances of "pure" research justify themselves only long afterwards by leading to benefits for many that could not have been foreseen. But we must ask who will benefit and how much, and how these benefits compare not only with the cost in resources and human effort, but also with the risk of future harm within the larger community.

An Unusual Opportunity

In the case of freezing multiple embryos we have an unusual opportunity for agreement on a question of reproductive morality. Richard McCormick, David Thomasma, and many others, have stressed that we cannot resolve by law and public policy a set of issues on which there is not, within the community at large, a consensus on the underlying values.[12] On the issue of the legality of abortion, and of the constitutionality of laws prohibiting or regulating it, our community appears to be profoundly divided; and this division has been deepened and entrenched by strident rhetoric on both sides.

But if I am correct in claiming that the two most frequently opposed moral positions about reproductive morality must reach the same conclusion regarding our obligations toward unused frozen embryos, then here is a possible starting point from which respectful conversation and the search for a broader consensus can begin. To be sure, different patterns of reasoning are involved in the two positions. But on this issue at least, the two sides need not begin their conversation at odds, committed to showing first of all that the other's position is without substance. On this issue there is a basis for agreement, and therefore for respect and for further conversation.

QUESTIONS FOR CONSIDERATION

1. Using the logic of the *Roe v. Wade* decision, do states have any "compelling interest" in protecting and preserving frozen embryos? Are frozen embryos "non-persons" and therefore possess no legal rights, including the right not to be killed? Or does their "potentiality of human life" demand some sort of protection?

2. How do the opposing views—the "instant of conception view" and the "embryo has no moral rights" view—differ on the issues of fetal rights and interests?

3. Can the two differing views—as the author suggests—agree that the best course of action in dealing with frozen embryos is to maintain them "in their frozen state for as long as they are able to survive implantation?"

4. Can a policy of disposal be defended morally? Is it true that "only reasons of economy and efficiency support a policy of disposal?"

NOTES

1. William Salmond, *Jurisprudence*, twelfth edition, edited by P.J. Fitzgerald (London: Sweet and Maxwell, 1966), p.303, emphasis in the original.

2. See George Annas, "Redefining Parenthood and Protecting Embryos: Why We Need Laws," *Hastings Center Report*, October 1984, pp. 50–51. See also Steven R. Fersz, "The Contract in Surrogate Motherhood: A Review of the Issues," *Law, Medicine, and Health Care*, June 1984, pp. 107–14; Flannery et.al., "Test Tube Babies: Legal Issues Raised by In Vitro Fertilization," *Georgetown Law Journal*, August 1979, pp.129ff.; "Note: Surrogate Mothers: The Legal Issues," *American Journal of Law and Medicine*, Fall 1981, pp.323ff.

3. See Mark E. Cohen, "The 'Brave New Baby,' and the Law: Fashioning Remedies for the Victims of In Vitro Fertilization," *American Journal of Law and Medicine*, 4:3(1978), 319–36.

4. A classic statement of this position appears in Pope Pius XXI's 1956 address to the Second World Congress on Fertility and Sterility, *Proceedings of the Second World Congress on Fertility and Sterility*, 2 vols. (Naples, Italy: University of Naples, 1957–1958), vol. I, p. 40. See also Leon Kass, "Making Babies—The New Biology and the 'Old' Morality," *Public Interest*, Winter 1979, pp. 44–60. But also see Anthony Kosnik, et al., *Human Sexuality: New Directions* in *American Catholic Thought* (New York: Paulist Press, 1977), pp. 137–40, and Margot Joan Fromer, *Ethical Issues in Sexuality and Reproduction* (St. Louis: Mosby, 1983), pp. 271–77. For a broad survey of ethical literature on in vitro fertilization, see LeRoy Walters, "Human In Vitro Fertilization: A Review of the Ethical Literature," *Hastings Center Report*, August 1979, pp. 23–43, and *Bioethics Reporter*, "Rights of Fetuses: Issues, Commentary, Literature, Court Cases, Legislation, and Bibliography," 1984.

5. See, for example, Baruch Brody, *Abortion and the Sanctity of Human Life: A Philosophical View* (Cambridge: MIT Press, 1975).

6. See, for example, Mary Anne Warren, "On the Moral and Legal Status of Abortion," *The Monist*, vol. 57 (1973), 43–61.

7. *Roe v. Wade*, 410 U.S. 113 (1973); *Doe v. Bolton*, 410 U.S. 179 (1973); *Planned Parenthood v. Danforth*, 428 U.S. 52 (1979).

8. *City of Akron v. Akron Center for Reproductive Health*, 103 U.S. 2481 (1983).

9. For examples of this position, see John T. Noonan, Jr., "An Almost Absolute Value in History," in his *The Morality of Abortion: Legal and Historical Perspectives* (Cambridge: Harvard University Press, 1970) and Teresa Iglesias, "*In Vitro* Fertilization: The Major Issues," *Journal of Medical Ethics* vol. 10 (1984).

10. This topic has not been carefully discussed in the literature. For a thoughtful discussion of voluntariness and responsibility in regard to a fetus conceived through intercourse, see Joel Feinberg, "Abortion," in Tom Regan, ed., *Matters of Life and Death*, (New York: Random House, 1980), pp. 209–14.

11. Lori Andrews, *New Conceptions: A Consumer's Guide to the Newest Infertility Treatments, Including In Vitro Fertilization, Artificial Insemination, and Surrogate Motherhood* (New York: St. Martins Press, 1984).

12. See Richard A. McCormick, S.J., "The Abortion Dossier," "Rules for Abortion Debate," and "Public Policy on Abortion," in his *How Brave a New World?* (Garden City, N.Y.; Doubleday, 1981), and David Thomasma, An Apology for the Value of Human Life (St. Louis: Catholic Health Association, 1983).

PART VII: Organ and Tissue Donation and Procurement and Transplantation

PART VII:1: The Human Body and Property Rights

LORI B. ANDREWS
My Body, My Property

MARGARET S. SWAIN AND RANDY W. MARUSYK
An Alternative to Property Rights in Human Tissue

PART VII:2: Organ and Tissue Procurement and Donation

ARTHUR L. CAPLAN
Organ Procurement: It's Not in the Cards

EIKE-HENNER W. KLUGE
Designated Organ Donation: Private Choice in Social Context

In 1976, John Moore received treatment at the University of California, Los Angeles Medical Center for a rare form of leukemia. The medical staff removed Moore's spleen and drew several samples of blood. Without his knowledge, these tissues were used in research that resulted in a commercially profitable treatment for some forms of leukemia. When UCLA and the researchers applied for a patent for the research results, Moore sued, arguing that he deserved a portion of the profits for the contribution of his tissues. The Medical Center responded that, in fact, Moore had been fully informed and had agreed to such use of his tissues when he signed the general consent form which granted the center the right to dispose of removed organs.

The *Moore* case raises the issue of property rights pertaining to removed organs and tissue. Traditionally, the language of "gifts" and voluntary consent has been applied to such tissue. But with the growing commercial possibilities of biotechnological research, the older language and metaphors are being challenged. Can voluntary donation provide the number of organs needed for transplant? Should a policy of presumed consent replace the existing policy of required request? Should a market for tissue and organs emerge? What principles would guide such a market and best protect the interests of the individuals involved?

These issues—the role of consent in organ procurement, the application of property rights to body parts, and the use of removed tissues in potentially profit-making research—will provide the focus of this discussion? The readings in this section address such issues from a variety of perspectives:

- Lori B. Andrews's **My Body, My Property** proposes guidelines for the creation of a market for organs and tissues that would meet the needs for transplantation but also protect the interests of donors.
- Margaret S. Swain's and Randy W. Marusyk **An Alternative to Property Rights in Human Tissue** offers a distinction between three levels of ownership which should be considered in the application of the language of property rights to human body parts.
- Arthur L. Caplan's **Organ Procurement: It's Not in the Cards** evaluates the successes and failures of required and presumed consent policies in organ donation.
- Eike-Henner W. Kluge's **Designated Organ Donation: Private Choice in Social Context** investigates the roles of the media, physicians, prospective recipients, and the donor in the organ procurement process.

LORI B. ANDREWS

My Body, My Property

In 1984 John Moore, a leukemia patient had his spleen removed at the University of California at Los Angeles School of Medicine.[1] Moore claims that, without his knowledge or explicit consent his physicians used his blood to develop the patented and commercially valuable Mo cell line. He began to suspect that his blood was being used for purposes beyond his personal care when the UCLA cancer specialists offered to pay his airfare and hotel expenses to Los Angeles in order to take further blood samples.[2] The physicians claimed that Moore waived his interest in his body parts when he signed a general consent form giving the UCLA pathology department the right to dispose of removed organs. This dispute is currently in litigation.

Moore's case is not unique. At the University of California, San Diego, Hideaki Hagiwara a postdoctoral biology student, suggested to faculty member Ivor Royston that a human monoclonal antibody be made with cancer cells from Hagiwara's mother. Once the new cell line was created, Dr. Hagiwara felt his family had an economic interest in the new cell line since he had proposed the project and his mother had provided the original cells. Dr. Royston disagreed, since he and his colleagues had invented the procedure and created the parent cell line that made the production of the human monoclonal antibodies possible. A settlement was ultimately reached, giving the University of California the patent and the Hagiwaras an exclusive license for the cell line in Japan and Asia.

Should a patient have a right to control what will be done to his or her body parts and receive compensation when they are put to research, diagnostic, or therapeutic uses? The issue has been debated in recent professional symposia[3] and congressional hearings,[4] and inspired the formation of an Office of Technology Assessment working group.[5] According to a survey conducted by a House subcommittee,[6] about half of the eighty-one responding medical schools now use patients' fluids or tissues for research, accounting for one-fifth of the patent applications the schools had filed in the previous five years. Overall, the schools reported a 300 percent increase in patents with origins in patients' tissues or fluids from 1975–1979 to 1980–1984. One way to grapple with questions of control and compensation is to consider the body as a form of property.

Tangible items are generally considered to be property. As new potentials for body parts unfold in research, diagnostics, and therapy, the question arises—should they be considered property as well? Current policy allows people to donate solid organs, but not to sell them. A federal law forbids sales of organs for transplant in interstate commerce[7] and certain state laws ban payment for specified organs as well.[8] This perspective—that bodily parts and products are gifts, not compensable items of property—underlies researchers' use of a patient's tissue to produce potentially marketable products.

The Property Approach and Individual Control

Throughout the legal lore, judges have reacted with horror to the idea that body parts may be property. Nevertheless, many legal decisions treat the body as a type of property. The law allows me to make gifts of certain body parts and even to destroy my body entirely. Not only do I have a property-like interest in my own body, I may have rights that could be considered property rights in other people's bodies. Tort law allows me to recover for harm to my child, much as it allows me recovery for damage to my car. In most instances, I can collect damages if an autopsy is performed on my next of kin without my consent.

Since the legal treatment of bodies and body parts sounds suspiciously like property treatment, why is there such a reluctance to label it as such? One major fear is that bodily property could be transferred to others (the legal term is alienable) and we could become slaves, not in a market for our bodies, but in a market for body parts. However, characterizing body parts as property does not mean that they must be completely transferable. As Susan Rose-Ackerman points out, many forms of property have restrictions on alienability.[9] There may be restrictions on who holds them, what actions are required or forbidden, and what kinds of transfers are permitted. Some types of properties can be given as gifts, but not sold (items made of the fur or feathers of endangered species, for example). Other types of properties (such as the holdings of a person who is bankrupt) can be sold, but not given as gifts.

Even under current policy, the body can be considered property, the kind of property that can be transferred without payment, but not sold.

However, restraints on payment need strong moral and legal justification. The Ontario Law Reform Commission recently faced the issue of paying for body parts in the context of artificial reproduction. After deciding that donating sperm, eggs, or embryos was ethically, morally, and socially acceptable, the Commission noted that any restriction on available services (for example, by prohibiting commercial banks for gametes and embryos) "must be scrutinized very carefully; it would be futile and frustrating to give with one hand, only to take with the other."[10]

The property approach recognizes people's interest in controlling what happens to their body parts. It provides a legal basis for a remedy as theories of privacy, autonomy, or assault do not when inappropriate actions are taken with respect to extracorporeal bodily materials. The presumption that the authority belongs to the individual who provided the body parts would be a starting point which would at least assure that the regulatory and institutional policies developed be measured against some standard.

Without characterizing the body as some form of property, theft or other harm to dead bodies or extracorporeal body parts is difficult to prosecute. Early American cases dealing with the disinterment of bodies recognized this problem and created the category of quasi-property to deal with it. For example, the court in an 1872 Rhode Island case noted:

> That there is no right of property in a dead body, using the word in its ordinary sense, may well be admitted. Yet the burial of the dead is a subject which interests the feelings of mankind to a much greater degree than many matters of actual property. There is a duty imposed by the universal feelings of mankind to be discharged by someone towards the dead; a duty, and we may also say a right, to protect from violation; it may, therefore, be considered as a sort of *quasi* property, and it would be discreditable to any system of law not to provide a remedy in such a case. . . .[11]

The Supreme Court of Minnesota in 1891 went one step further by holding that, to the person who has the right to possess the cadaver for burial, it "is his property in the broadest and most general sense of the term. . . ."[12]

If the body is not treated as property or at least quasi-property, we may be without remedies in some instances. Paul Matthews, pointing out that dead bodies and body parts are not considered goods under English law for purposes of the torts act or commercial code asks, "If the ashes of X, a celebrity, are without consent 'removed' and (say) later auctioned at a London auction-house, can anything be done by X's next-of-kin, or personal representatives?"[13] Matthews argues that dead bodies and body parts should be characterized as property so that interference with them could be considered a tort.

People have an interest in what will happen to their extracorporeal body parts, while they are alive and even after they die. Yet protection of that interest now tenuously rests on precarious doctrines that protect people from emotional distress. In a 1973 case, physicians at Columbia Presbyterian Hospital in New York City attempted to fertilize a woman's egg with her husband's sperm. Without consultation with the physicians or the couple, the department chairman removed the culture from the incubator and destroyed it. The couple, Mr. and Mrs. Del Zio, sued the department chairman and the hospital's trustees, charging conversion of personal property and intentional infliction of emotional distress.[14] The jury rejected the property claim but awarded plaintiffs damages for the emotional distress. Mrs. Del Zio was awarded $50,000 for emotional distress and Mr. Del Zio was awarded $3.00. It is ironic that Mr. Del Zio was compensated so poorly and that the contents of the petri dish were not considered property since sperm is sold; thus Mr. Del Zio's contribution could have been viewed as having had a market value exceeding $3.00.

Advances in reproductive technology now frequently require people to entrust their gametes or embryos to the care of the physician, laboratory worker, or health care facility. Yet if body parts are not considered property, there may be little protection for people who entrust their bodily materials to others. Traditionally, courts have allowed people to receive damages for emotional harm only if it accompanied an actual physical injury or physical impact to the party. If negligence brings about the loss of an embryo or other extracorporeal body part there will be a cause of action only in nine states;[15] the rest allow recovery only if the negligence caused a physical impact on the plaintiffs. Even if the harmful action was intentional, at least twelve states do not award damages absent physical impact.[16] In addition, there may be a cap on the amounts recoverable for emotional distress; thus the individual or couple may not be adequately compensated.

In the absence of a property approach, attempts have been made to limit the control people have over their extracorporeal body parts. Thus proposals have been made for transferring organs from a cadaver when the person did not grant consent before death or expressly refused consent. This apparently is already done without specific authorization in many instances in which physicians remove cartilage, tendons, bones, or corneas from cadavers.[17] In Hawaii, consent to an autopsy allows the physician to use the removed tissue, including fetal material, "for necessary or advisable scientific investigation, including research, teaching and therapeutic purposes."[18] Such takings may assault religious convictions and personal beliefs. Their proponents fall into the trap of considering the body as the sum of its physical parts without considering the emotional, intellectual, and religious nature of people before their deaths.

As policies covering inheritance make clear, our society recognizes the important psychological benefit to people when they are alive of determining what will happen to their property after death. There is a similar psychological benefit to them, and often to their relatives, in knowing that society will honor their wishes about disposing of their bodies after death.[19] The inappropriate treatment of a cadaver can cause psychological harm to relatives. In one incident, Mrs. Lott, an Orthodox Jew, and Mrs. Tumminelli, a Roman Catholic, died within an hour at the same hospital. The bodies were mixed up and Mrs. Lott's corpse was embalmed, made up with cosmetics, and put in a coffin with a rosary and crucifix. Mrs. Tumminelli's body was prepared for an Orthodox Jewish burial. The relatives of each woman sued and recovered damages for mental suffering.[20]

Joel Feinberg dismisses the psychological harm to dying people and their relatives of taking organs from a loved one. He argues that "it is difficult to understand how the thought of bodies having their organs removed before burial can be more depressing than the thought of them festering in the cold ground or going up in flames."[21] He criticizes people who object to routine organ salvaging as overly sentimental or superstitious. But this overlooks the importance that beliefs, acculturation, and values have on people's choices. From childhood, people grow accustomed to a certain view of how the dead should be treated, a view shaped by their familial and religious upbringing. Someone who has lived with a view that might emphasize the wholeness of the body at interment for a proper afterlife could understandably object to being condemned to a radically different fate.[22]

In a Gallup poll, 20 percent of respondents said they would not donate organs because they did not like the idea of being cut up after they died.[23] Psychological concern for body parts may be even greater among people who have undergone surgery. In one case, a patient's left eyeball had been surgically removed and was about to be examined for cancer when it was lost down a sink drain. The Texas Court of Civil Appeals, in acknowledging that the patient had a cause of action for negligence, recognized that individuals can be emotionally traumatized to the point of physical injury by the way their extracorporeal body parts are treated.[24]

Some lawyers and researchers argue that there is no need to inform people that body parts removed in the course of treatment may be used for research or commercial purposes, so long as the patient is not exposed to any additional physical risk due to the research. Currently, under federal regulations covering federally funded research, consent is not required to do research on such pathological or diagnostic specimens, so long as the subjects cannot be identified.[25] In such cases, consent is given under the general hospital admission form, which states that the part may be used for teaching or research before it is destroyed. But the hospital consent form does not say that the patient may refuse to allow bodily materials to be used and still retain the patient/physician relationship and be treated. Only when the human material is taken primarily for research purposes is consent required. Even then, if the research poses "no more than minimal risk" and involves only collection of some body excretions, including blood, placenta or amniotic fluid, it may be given an expedited review by an Institutional Review Board; while consent is not specifically required, presumably the IRB can seek consent if the subjects are identifiable.[26] The failure to extend consent to all categories of research on human body parts and the failure even to raise the issue of compensation puts patients at a distinct psychological and economic disadvantage.

In *The Mother Machine*, Gena Corea raises serious questions about whether doctors have obtained eggs and embryos from women without their consent. She points out that in the published studies on research using women's eggs, "there is, in almost every case, no indication that the women consented to the extraction of their eggs or even knew that their eggs had been taken."[27] In order to give weight to the biological parents' wishes regarding gametes and embryos, the American Fertility Society in its Ethical Statement on *In Vitro* Fertilization specifically refers to sperm, eggs, and embryos as the property of the individuals who provide them.[28]

The lack of additional physical harm to the patient should not be determinative of the ethical or legal rights of the patient. No physical harm comes to a woman if I snap her photo and sell it commercially, yet the law considers that I have taken something of value from her. It is even considered improper and actionable if a physician publishes a photo in a medical journal without the patient's permission.[29]

With a tangible body part, it is even easier to see the harm that may result from commercialization without the person's consent Some researchers argue that the patient need not be told of the possibility of profit since the body part was not of commercial value to the patient However, there are numerous markets where something valueless to one person is coveted by someone else. (This is the principle behind garage sales.) Moreover, it does not matter that the patient does not have the resources or opportunity to make the same use of the material as the researcher. If a person discovered oil in his back yard, it would not matter that he did not possess a refinery to process it. He would still expect payment for transfer of the resource to an oil company, and would be harmed if he did not receive it.

Nor should it make a difference that people did not expect compensation for body parts in the past. Scientists revel in the example of people wantonly parting with body wastes such as urine and feces all the time. Since people treat these excretions as valueless, they ask, why should scientists have to pay for them? This overlooks the fact that people might indeed view body products differently if they knew there was a possibility of a commercial market. Once valueless does not imply always valueless. Many markets have developed for seemingly worthless byproducts such as sawdust.

Similarly, a patient's right to information before consenting to a treatment is not contingent upon physical harm. Even if a treatment is beneficial, the physician breaches an ethical and legal duty by not providing sufficient information in advance. In some instances, the doctrine of informed consent itself might mandate disclosure of the physician's or colleague's intent to engage in research on, or commercially exploit, the excised organs, tissues, or fluids. One important purpose of the informed consent doctrine is to protect people from unnecessary procedures that serve the physicians' pecuniary or personal motives.[30] If a patient learns that her physician is engaged in research, she may legitimately wish to get a second opinion from another physician whose diagnosis is not colored by the need for a large sample size or the promise of commercialization. Or she may wish to have the surgery done by an equally competent physician/researcher who offers to compensate her for her participation in the research. Throughout medical care, the relative costs of alternative treatments or the same treatments performed by competing practitioners are becoming increasingly important There is support for informing patients about the potential uses of the body parts, even among groups that now gain commercially from using those parts. The licensing Executive Society Biotechnology Committee recently surveyed its members, who generally represent organizations that use human tissues, fluids, or cells for research or development purposes. Of those responding, twenty-two believed that research or commercialization should occur only with the patient's prior consent; two felt consent was unnecessary. Thirteen felt that a person has a right to receive compensation for the use of his or her fluid, tissues, or cells, while eight did not.

The Market's Effect on Donors

The property approach requires the individual's consent before her body parts can be used by others. But in some instances body parts—such as kidneys or corneas—may be in such short supply or a particular patient may have such a rare tissue or fluid type that the issue of payment to donors will arise, as it did in the Moore and Hagiwara cases.

The criticisms of a market for body parts focus on potential harms to the donor, the recipient, and society. In organ transplantation, Congress and some state legislatures have already decided to prohibit payment out of fear that poor, minority, or otherwise vulnerable people will be coerced to exchange body parts for money. Is this prohibition justified? And should it apply to the sale of bodily materials in other circumstances?

In its harshest form, allowing payment to living persons who donate solid organs could lead society to view poor people as suddenly having capital and consequently being ineligible for welfare benefits.[31] (A man with a $50,000 kidney, like a man with $50,000 in the bank, would not qualify for welfare.[32]) Such a society would include among its citizens walking human carcasses whose need for money has led them to go under the knife. These individuals would be doubly cursed. Not only would they have to give up precious body parts but, to the extent that the operations left them physically disabled or different looking (sans eye or limb, for example), they might be shunned.[33] Given society's deplorable track record in caring for the disabled, creating more disabled individuals seems immoral.

Suppose a person's body parts were not taken into account in determining his or her net worth. Even then there is concern that allowing payment for body parts could unduly coerce the poor to donate. The strongest argument against paying donors is that people in dire straits will consent to debilitating surgeries out of a desperate need for money. But banning payment on ethical grounds to prevent such scenarios overlooks one important fact: to the person who needs money to feed his children or to purchase medical care for her parent, the option of not selling a body part is worse than the option of selling it. Society has not benefitted individuals by banning organ sales unless it also provides a means to escape desperate conditions.

Naturally, the need for money is not a justification for any action (we would not want the person to become a contract killer for a fee). But it is difficult to justify a prohibition on payment for what otherwise would be a legal and ethical act—giving up body parts for someone else's valid use. Similarly, the analogy to slavery is inapposite. We do not want people to sell themselves into slavery nor do we want them to "give" themselves into slavery without pay. In contrast, with respect to organ donation or the development of a diagnostic or therapeutic product from bodily materials, the underlying activity is one we want to encourage.

Where regenerative bodily products are concerned—blood, sweat, and semen or, arguably, embryos—the criticism is even less justified, assuming that the product can be removed safely. In any paid labor, we are giving our body. For example, in response to the idea that a poor woman may be coerced into serving as a surrogate mother despite the risks due to the fee, Laurence Karp and Roger Donahue point out that "it seems inconsistent to categorically deny such women this kind of livelihood while we permit and even encourage people to earn money by such dangerous means as coal mining, or racing little cars around a track at 200 miles per hour."[34] In some instances—professional boxing—the assaults to the body are obvious. In others they may be more subtle. The scholar chugging coffee in front of a glowering word processor is damaging her body as well.

It is not the payment that harms the body, but the physical risk to the person of removing the body part or the subsequent risk of living without it. Neither of these risks is present where the sale of a body part becomes effective on the person's death. And when a person donates a body part while alive, the physical risks vary considerably depending on what the part is and how it is removed.

How much risk should a paid donor be allowed to run? One way of deciding would be to compare the level of risk people face when they donate organs with the risk of selling another product of their body, their labor. Along those lines, sales of regenerative body parts seem to present less potential physical harm than do many jobs (such as firefighting).

Giving up a heart or other nonregenerative body part that invariably causes death goes beyond the types of sacrifices that paid labor may demand. Arguably, such sacrifices should be prevented, whether for fee or for free. But an intermediary case—giving up kidneys or other nonregenerative body parts, which does not cause death—does not on its face justify such a drastic prohibition. The risk to a healthy thirty-five-year-old in donating a kidney is the same as the risk in driving a car sixteen miles every working day.[35] Moreover, allowing a market in body parts could reduce the use of (and thus the physical harms to) living donors, since more people may decide to sell their body parts upon death than currently donate them.

Physicians have adopted an odd view of risks to organ donors. Transplant surgeons traditionally have maintained that removing a kidney from a live donor presents minimal health risks. "However," Arthur Caplan points out, "when the proposal was made to buy and sell kidneys what had historically been deemed minimal risks suddenly escalated into intolerable dangers when profit became an obvious motive!"[36] I have found a similar shift in perspective among infertility specialists, who describe as safe the ovarian stimulation, laparoscopy, and anesthesia used to harvest eggs from patients undergoing *in vitro* fertilization. Yet they say that same process is too dangerous to be undertaken by a woman who wishes to be a paid egg donor.

Guarding Against Coercion

Part of the concern with selling body parts or doing risky paid labor rests on the belief that people should enter into these transactions voluntarily. Courts do not order specific performance when an individual, such as an opera singer, reneges on a job. Voluntariness should have its counterpart in body part donation as well. In 1890 a man sold the Royal Caroline Institute in Sweden the rights to his body after death. Later, he tried to refund the money and cancel the contract. In the subsequent lawsuit, the court held that he must turn his body over to the Institute and also ordered him to pay damages for diminishing the worth of his body by having two teeth removed.[37] In contrast, in the U.S., under the Uniform Anatomical Gift Act, promises to donate body parts upon death are revocable. With living donors, revocation should be allowed up until the time the transfer is made.

Just as we would not condone a labor system that did not allow people to choose their own employers, we should insist that paid donations from living people be voluntary: that is, made by the person himself or herself. It is one thing for people to have the right to treat their own bodies as property, quite another to allow others to treat a person as property. A hospital should not be allowed to take, sell, and use blood or eggs from a comatose woman to help pay her costs of hospitalization. People should be prohibited from selling their relative's body parts when the relative dies (unless the deceased left orders to that effect). Nor should judges be allowed to sentence offenders to pay their fines in body product donations (once the property approach has established a market value for them). If this seems farfetched, consider that there already have been instances in which judges sentenced defendants to give blood transfusions. Similarly, an eighteenth-century British statute allowed judges to order anatomical dissection of hanged murderers.[38] It is possible to maintain that people are priceless by not allowing others to treat a person's body commercially either before or after death and by giving people the power to refuse to sell their body parts.

A decision to sell certain types of body parts-nonregenerative ones (such as a kidney) or parts that could give rise to offspring (sperm, eggs, and embryos)—has lifelong implications. With respect to other decisions of long-lasting consequences (such as marriage), society has sometimes adopted added protections to assure that the decision has been carefully made. A similar approach might be used with regard to body parts. In this area, only competent adults should be allowed to decide to sell. There should be a short waiting period (like the cooling-off period that protects consumers from door-to-door salesmen) between the agreement to sell an organ and its removal, and the donor should be required to observe certain formalities (such as signing a witnessed consent form).

Only the person who owns the body part should be allowed to sell it. This approach has two goals. The first is to assure that others do not treat one's body as property. For example, it will prevent the harm associated with holding the body as security until funeral costs are paid.[39] The second is to attempt to assure that the individual is adequately compensated for the body part by limiting the amount any middleman receives. If the middleman cannot "sell" the part but can only be compensated for bringing together the donor and recipient, the donor may more likely receive adequate compensation and the transaction will less likely be viewed as excessively commercial. There might even be limitations on what the middleman (physician or entrepreneur) receives, similar to the statutory limitation in some states of "reasonableness" in the amount of money an attorney receives in connection with arranging a private adoption.

One state already has adopted an approach similar to the one I am advocating here. A California statute prohibits a person from knowingly acquiring, receiving, selling, or promoting the transfer or otherwise transferring any organ for transplantation for valuable consideration. The law is directed against brokering organs rather than the direct selling from a donor to a recipient. There is an exception to the ban on selling and buying for "the person from whom the organ is removed, [or] . . . the person who receives the transplant, or those persons' next-of-kin who assisted in obtaining the organ for purposes of transplantation."[40]

This approach may also have the additional benefit in rare instances of preventing crimes. Much of the original horror with recognizing commercial value in the body or its parts resulted from cases in which people fell prey to murderers who sold their bodies to medical schools for research. Even in the past decade, there have been cases where mortuary technicians have illicitly sold tissues and organs of corpses.[41] Limiting some parties' ability to sell the body parts does not undermine the property approach. Zoning laws restrict the uses that can be made of land, yet it is still considered property. Similarly, restrictions in a closed corporation on who may buy shares of stock or in a cooperative apartment on who may buy a unit do not undermine their status as property.

Giving an individual sole rights over his or her body parts is in keeping with attitudes toward the body held in other areas of law. Attempted suicide and suicide are no longer considered crimes.[42] However, aiding and abetting a suicide is a crime. Competent individuals can refuse a readily available lifesaving treatment, but their physicians cannot withhold it. Thus, people are allowed to control what is done to their bodies (even to the point of physical damage) in ways that other individuals are not.

Ironically, our current policy is just the reverse. Other people seem to have property rights in our body parts, but we do not In a British case, an accused man who poured his urine sample down the sink was found guilty of stealing it from the police department.[43] And although an individual has no property interest in his or her cell lines, scientists are quick to claim a property interest in those cell lines. Such a claim was the basis of a six-year conflict between microbiologist Leonard Hayflick and the National Institutes of Health. The conflict was over which side owned a cell line that Hayflick had developed with embryonic living tissue under NIH funding and then sold to scientists around the world.[44].

The notion that other people may own our body parts while we may not has an historical basis. In England, even though courts said people had no property rights in their body, until 1804 creditors apparently had such rights since they could arrest dead bodies for a debt. For example, the poet Dryden's body was arrested as it was being transported for burial.[45] And in feudal times, it was a crime to maim oneself because this rendered one less able to fight for the king.[46] Thus, the common law basis for preventing people from voluntarily transferring their body parts (which was later interpreted to prohibit even gratuitous organ donation) may not have its roots in the view that the body is sacred and that people should not be objectified as property. Rather, it may arise from the notion that people were the property of the Crown.

The Market's Effect on Recipients

We can protect potential donors from the market's effect by attempting to assure that donations are voluntary and by limiting donations to body parts that do not unreasonably affect the person's ability to function. But how does a market affect potential recipients? The policy of prohibiting payment for body parts and products has been justified as protecting potential recipients by raising the quality of donations and preventing a situation in which body parts are affordable only by the rich.

The work of Richard Titmuss on policies governing blood donation raised serious questions of quality control, when blood is sold.[47] Among other things, he argued that paid donors have an incentive not to disclose illnesses or characteristics that might make their blood of dubious quality. Subsequent work by Harvey Sapolsky and Stan Finkelstein[48] challenged Titmuss's conclusions. They pointed to a Government Accounting Office study in which some voluntary groups in the United States reported hepatitis rates as high as the worst paid groups; and some commercially collected blood was nearly as good as the best of the volunteer blood.

Even if paid donors are more likely to misrepresent their condition than are volunteer donors, payment need not be banned on quality control grounds since tests are available to assess the fitness of the donor. In this country we allow payment for blood and sperm, although it is easy to lie about their quality; yet we do not allow payment for body organs such as kidneys, although organ transplantation offers more independent checks on quality. Nor is banning payment the only mechanism to enhance quality, since if known risks are not disclosed, liability may follow. While this may not offer sufficient protection to the recipients of blood (since donors may not be solvent), organ donors would be better paid and a portion of that money could be used to buy insurance. When a person sells organs contingent on death, payment to an estate could be withheld if it was clear that he failed to disclose a known harmful condition. Already, the Ontario Law Reform Commission has recommended enacting a criminal law prohibiting people selling their gametes from knowingly concealing infectious and genetic disorders.

A market in solid organs is also thought harmful to potential recipients because of the possibility that only the rich will be able to afford organs. On the issue of the poor selling and the rich buying body parts, Thomas Murray says, "Our consciences can tolerate considerable injustice, but such naked, undisguised profiteering in life would be too much for us."[49] Yet other equally troublesome but less visible inequities are already occurring in allocating other kinds of medical care. When a drug company prices a medication necessary for someone's life beyond a person's reach or a physician with unique skills refuses to accept patients who receive Medicare, that is also profiteering in life, but the injustice may be overlooked. Currently at least fifty different types of artificial body parts (such as artificial blood vessels and joints) have been designed to substitute for human ones.[50] It is as important ethically to address discrimination between rich and poor recipients with respect to those products as it is with respect to human body parts. A visible market in body parts may lull people out of complacency to address more general issues of allocation in health care.

If we were to ban payment for all body parts (including blood) in this country, we could not sit back, assured that we had eliminated coercion of the poor. Even today, American drug companies undertake plasma collection in Third World countries throughout Latin America and Asia to meet the needs for plasma products here. People in poor countries are giving of their bodies for people in rich countries. Perhaps we should struggle to assure noncommercialization of human body products in all countries. But if this reduced the blood supply, doctors might have to turn down some patients who needed surgery. Would proponents of total market bans support that outcome?

Quality and cost issues raised by the sale of body parts are similar to issues raised by other medical treatments. Thus they should be handled in the same way with attempts to enhance the quality of care, the informed consent process, access to medical services, and so forth. A market for solid organs may even diminish risks to the recipient. If more organs were available, it would become easier to avoid rejection and recipients who would have died for lack of an organ might gain a chance to live.

The Market's Effect on Society

Will a market in body parts harm society by creating an attitude that people are commodities? The body is a symbol of the whole person and degrading it can be viewed as an assault to the whole person. Our distaste with viewing the body as property is, in part a reaction to our belief that human beings should have no price.

Certainly people are more than the sum of their parts.[51] But treating the body as property does not mean it is a person's only property. Cognitive functions can be included within the property characterization. Indeed, they already are, for example, under the legal doctrine of copyright, patent and other so-called "intellectual property" rights. I view my uniqueness as a person as more related to my intellectual products than my bodily products. (Definitions of personhood, for example, rarely revolve around the possession of body parts, but rather focus on sentience or other cognitive traits.) Arguably it commercializes me less as a person to sell my bone marrow than to sell my intellectual products. Thus, I do not view payment of body parts as commercializing people. The danger I see in the sale of a physical (as opposed to a mental) bodily product comes from the potential for physical harm in removing the bodily material or living without it. This danger can be handled by limiting the types of body parts that can be sold and the circumstances under which they can be sold.

Selling body parts has also been criticized as harmful to society because it could diminish altruism. But in our society, the basics of life—food, shelter, health care—are already sold. Nevertheless, many people continue to act altruistically, devoting time, money, or goods to provide needy people with those basics. The possibility of selling tissue or organs seems only a modest further step toward a market, unlikely to change vastly the impulse toward altruism. Even people who take advantage of the market may engage in altruistic behavior. One patient, Ted Slavin, received up to $10.00 per milliliter from commercial enterprises for his blood, which was used in manufacturing diagnostic kits for hepatitis B virus. At the same time, he provided additional blood—at no charge—to a research project at the Fox Chase Cancer Center, which used it to develop a vaccine against hepatitis B.[52]

Where a family member or friend is concerned, donation is likely to remain purely voluntary even if payment is allowed; thus the ban on payment cannot be justified as promoting personal altruism based on family or friendship ties. In contrast, donation to strangers is, as Kenneth Arrow notes, a "diffuse expression of confidence by individuals in the workings of society as a whole." Arrow questions whether there is merit to advancing that form of giving since "such an expression of impersonal altruism is as far removed from the feelings of personal altruism as any market place."[53]

Moreover, an argument can be made that neither personal nor societal altruism is furthered by a ban on payment Are people really more virtuous when they perform a particular act once the temptation to perform a contrary act has been removed by law? As Milton wrote in *Areopagitica*, "I cannot praise a fugitive and cloistered virtue . . . that never sallies out and sees her adversary."

Allowing individuals to treat parts of their bodies as property is also said to be conducive to allowing others to treat them as property. According to this argument, if we view the primary object, the body part as marketable, this will lead us to treat the secondary object, the individual person, as a commodity. As Joel Feinberg points out, however, "The weakness of the argument consists in the difficulty of showing that the alleged coarsening effects really do transfer from primary to secondary objects."

The issue of commodification goes far beyond the question of payment for human organs, tissues, and waste products. A variety of components of our social and legal structure have been criticized as commodifying people. The idea that biological parents have a greater right to control over their children than do other members of the community has been criticized by some feminists as treating children as property. Richard Abel, in a far-ranging critique of the American tort system, has argued that damages should not be allowed for pain and suffering because that inappropriately commodifies our emotions.[54]

To guard against the appearance that people are commodities we must not let other people treat one's body parts as property. Body parts will thus not be salable in the sense of cars, farm animals, or baseball cards. There will be no means for a tax man or physician to put a lien against a person's body parts. Nor can relatives choose to sell a person's parts after his or her death. This might better be called a quasiproperty approach. However, it differs from previous notions of quasi-property by recognizing the light of an individual to compensation for certain types of body parts. Under this approach human beings have the right to treat certain physical parts of their bodies as objects for possession, gift, and trade, but they do not become objects so long as others cannot treat them as property.

The Market's Effect on the Doctor/Patient Relationship

The treatment of body parts as property will help curtail activities by physicians, researchers, and their attorneys that deny individuals information about or control over body parts that will be removed.

Implicit in many arguments made by physician/researchers is that the removed body part belongs to the doctor, not the patient. Why do physicians feel that way? I can only speculate that it is because society allows medical practitioners to do things to a patient's body (for example, cut it up) that no one else (other than the patient) is allowed to do. Perhaps this gives physicians the feeling that the patient's body belongs in some sense to them.

Physicians argue that getting patients' permission to use their body parts and products would change the relationship between patients and physicians or researchers. Some argue that discussing the research with the patient may imply that a patient has a right to direct the scope or direction of the study. But that is absurd. Just because IBM is required to make certain disclosures to me when I buy a share of stock does not mean that I can set policy for the operation of the company.

Related to this is an argument that paying for the patient's cells, tissue, fluids, or organs would tie up physicians in endless negotiation with their patients. But when payment for human biological material is required, it is no more disastrous to the research enterprise than payment for pipettes, microscopes, animals, or laboratory equipment. It may represent a modest increase in the cost of doing business (just as an increase in fuel prices would raise the costs of lighting the laboratory). But the money paid would go to a good cause, slightly enhancing the resources of medical patients at a time when they need money to pay for medical care. If the patient is unwilling to sell rights to the biological materials, the physician need not barter; she can simply avoid using that specimen and approach other patients. Moreover, we allow the patient to pay the physician for services without being concerned that it will lead to endless negotiations.

Just as physicians raise the price of their services to cover rising malpractice insurance rates, so they will charge slightly more for the right to use the specimens of some patients for research. If it strikes you as unfair (it does me) to force patients to pay for the research by increasing medical costs, consider that under the current system the "cost" of the human specimens is born entirely by the patients who own them and who do not even get in return a right to refuse to participate.

Another reason has been advanced against disclosure: it would decrease patient-physician trust if the patient were aware that the physician might develop a commercial product from the patient's body parts. Yet this begs the question of whether the information is relevant. It might diminish the patient's trust to know the success rate and unnecessary surgery rates of a practitioner or health care facility; yet this information is clearly relevant to patient decision making.

There is a similar concern that disclosing the commercial potential of human body parts may tarnish the image of the researchers by making it appear that profit rather than scientific knowledge is their goal. However, the media is already informing the public about the relationship between researchers and the corporate sector. "The public cannot help but see that the goals of some scientists—clinical or basic—are different than in the past." says Leon Rosenberg, dean of the Yale University School of Medicine. "The biotechnology revolution has moved us, literally or figuratively, from the class room to the board room and from the *New England Journal* to the *Wall Street Journal*."[55]

Finally, people point to the difficulty of assigning values to body parts as an implicit barrier to the property approach. But the value of many items that are currently bought and sold (such as paintings or jewels) is difficult to assess. This is no reason to prohibit the market from developing a particular price.

Arguments about the difficulty in assessing the value of a patient's contribution to research take a variety of forms. Some argue that the patient's contribution is too small to warrant compensation compared to the contribution of researchers and other participants. Yet if a person designs and makes a car, she expects to have to pay for even the smallest screw she uses—though her contribution and the contribution of the other materials vastly overwhelms the role of the screw. Others argue that so many people contribute to a particular advance (for example, 7,000 pituitary glands were used to research the molecular structure of ACTH[56]) that it would be difficult to compensate all of them. Yet large companies have little trouble devising a means to allocate payment among thousands of employees, suppliers, and stockholders. It is also argued that it may be unfair to compensate the patient whose bodily material is used to make a commercially exploitable product, since many other patients' materials were used in research leading up to this advance (and thus it is difficult to measure that particular patient's contribution). That criticism has no more merit than claiming that a scientist should not be paid since he or she is building upon work done by previous researchers.

In fact, determining worth is problematic only when the contribution is evaluated after the fact. There is no compelling reason why before-the-fact contracts should not be made in which the buyer and seller themselves agree on a price (as they do in many other market transactions). Unless the contract involves unconscionable coercion, there is no ethical reason to intervene in the bargain struck between them. Nor does it seem appropriate for policy makers to grapple around in advance for a formula by which to set the price (such as a formula based on how much the bodily material had been altered by the scientist).

In a variation on the value argument physician/researchers seem to imply that the patient has already been paid for the body part by receiving the benefits of the surgery. John Moore, for example, was allegedly helped by his treatment at UCLA. (This argument is harder to make when the patient dies or otherwise does not recover.) But patients may feel they have already paid for their health benefits in the price of the surgery. The patient has a right to know about the research so that she can choose the "price" she is willing to pay for the surgery. Perhaps she would rather choose a surgeon whose price is set solely in terms of dollars and insurance coverage rather than one who commercially exploits, say, her ovaries.

The Future of the Body as Property

Some of the finest advances in society have resulted from a refusal to characterize human beings (blacks, women, children) as property. Why, then, am I arguing for a property approach here? Let me emphasize that I am advocating not that people be treated by others as property, but only that they have the autonomy to treat their own parts as property, particularly their regenerative parts. Such an approach is helpful, rather than harmful, to people's well-being. It offers potential psychological, physical, and economic benefits to individuals and provides a framework for handling evolving issues regarding the control of extracorporeal biological materials.

It is time to start acknowledging that people's body parts are their personal property. This is distinguishable from the past characterizations of people as property, which were immoral because they failed to take into account the nonbodily aspects of the individual (blacks and women were deemed incapable of rational thought) and they created the rights of ownership by others (masters, husbands, parents). Allowing people to transfer and sell their own body parts, while protecting them from coercion, does not present those dangers.

QUESTIONS FOR CONSIDERATION

1. Andrews argues that the property approach to the treatment of one's own body will provide protection for the individual's interests in what happens to his or her body parts. Do you agree that this approach provides the best protection for one's interests especially in light of the use of regenerative parts (blood, cell lines, urine, semen) parts without the patient's consent?

2. Andrews draws a sharp distinction between people treating their own bodies as property and their bodies being treated as property by others. Do you believe this distinction would be sufficient in avoiding the potential harms associated with creating a market for body parts?

3. Do you believe physicians/researchers should be able to use regenerative parts without the consent or compensation of the patient? Do patients give up the rights to disposable fluids once consent for treatment or surgery is given?

4. Does Andrews adequately justify a market for body parts (organs) against the concern that poor, minority, or otherwise vulnerable people will be forced to sell their body parts for money?

5. Do you agree that only the owner of the body part (organ) should be able to sell it? Does this adequately protect the individual against coercion?

6. If a market is created for body parts, will only the rich be able to afford organ transplants? Would such a market lead to a reduction of distribution based upon equality and fairness?

7. Would a market in body parts tend to reduce certain human beings to commodities?

NOTES

1. Barbara J. Culliton, "Mo Cell Case Has Its First Court Hearing," *Science* 813 (1984), 236.

2. "Whose Body Is It Anyway?" *Chicago Tribune,* May 9, 1985, p. 1A.

3. "Public Policy Symposium—The Legal, Ethical and Economic Impact of Patient Material Used for Product Development in the Biomedical Industry," *Clinical Research* 33:4 (October 1985), 442–458.

4. Subcommittee on Investigation and Oversight, Committee on Science and Technology, U.S. House of Representatives, October 29, 1985.

5. The Office of Technology Assessment's Working Group on Patients' Rights in Human Biological Materials: Legal and Ethical Issues met on January 17, 1986.

6. See, e.g., Alan Otten, "Researchers' Use of Blood, Bodily Tissues Raises Questions About Sharing Profits," *Wall Street Journal,* January 29, 1986.

7. 42 U.S.C. 274(e) (1984).

8. Cal. Penal Code §367f (West 1986) (exception for sale by patient); D.C. Code Ann. §6–2601(Supp. 1985); Fla. Stat. Ann. §873.01 (West Supp. 1986); La. Rev. Stat. Ann. §17.2280 (West 1982); Md. Health General Code Ann. §5.408 (Supp. 1985); Mich. Comp. Laws Ann. §333.10204 (West Supp. 1986); N.Y. Pub. Health Law §4307 (McKinney 1985); Va. Code §32.1-289.1 (1985). Additionally, in Arkansas, there is a specific prohibition on the sale of eyes after death. Ark. Stat. Ann. §82-410.2; §82-410.13 (1976).

9. Susan Rose-Ackerman, "Inalienability and the Theory of Property Rights," *Columbia Law Review* 931 (1985), 85.

10. Ontario Law Reform Commission, *Report on Human Artificial Reproduction and Related Matters* (Ontario: Ministry of the Attorney General, 1985).

11. *Pierce v. Properties of Swan Point Cemetery,* 10 R.I. 227, 14 Am. Rep. 667, 676–77 (1972).

12. *Larson v. Chase,* 47 Minn. 307, 50 N.W. 238, 239 (1891).

13. Paul Matthews, "Whose Body? People as Property," in Lord Lloyd of Hamstead and Roger W. Rideout with Jacqueline Dyson, *Current Legal Problems* 1983 36 (London: Stevens & Sons, 1983), 207.

14. *Del Zio v. Manhattan's Columbia Presbyterian Medical Center,* No. 74–3558 (S.D.N.Y. November 14, 1978).

15. William L. Prosser and W. Page Keeton, *The Law of Torts,* Ch. 9 §54 at 364–5 (5th ed. 1984).

16. 38 *Am. Law, Reports,* §1003 *et seq* (1985).

17. Russell Scott, *The Body as Property* (New York: Viking Press, 1981), p.228.

18. Hawaii Rev. Stat. §453–15 (1976).

19. See William May, "Attitudes Toward the New Dead," *Hastings Center Studies* 1:1 (1973), 3.

20. *Lott v. State and Tumminelli v. State,* 32 Misc. 2d 296, 225 N.Y.S.2d 434 (1962).

21. Joel Feinberg, "The Mistreatment of Dead Bodies," *Hastings Center Report,* 15:1 (February 1985), 31,36.

22. See William May, "Religious Justifications for Donating Body Parts," *Hastings Center Report,* 15:1 (February 1985), 38.

23. See "John Q. Public On Organ Donations," *Hastings Center Report,* 13:6 (December 1983), 25.

24. *Mokry v. University of Texas Health Science Center at Dallas,* 529 S.W.2d 802 (1975).

25. 45 C.F.R. 46.101(b)(5) (1985).

26. 45 C.F.R. 46.110(b) (1985).

27. Gena Corea, *The Mother Machine* (New York: Harper & Row, 1985) p. 135 n. 2.

28. American Fertility Society, "Ethical Statement on In Vitro Fertilization," *Fertility and Sterility* 41 (1984), 12.

29. *Griffen v. Medical Society of State of New York,* 11 N.Y.S. 109 (1939).

30. Theodore J. Schneyer, "Informed Consent and the Danger of Bias in the Formation of Medical Disclosure," *Wisconsin Law Review* (1976), pp. 124, 137–138.

31. I am grateful to Tom Merrill for bringing my attention to this point.

32. One commentator has suggested that if the body has a market value, all decedents would have to include that value in their gross estate for tax purposes. See "Tax Consequences of Transfers of Bodily Parts," *Columbia Law Review* 73 (1973), 842, 862.

33. See Same Gorovitz, "Will We Still Be 'Human' If We Have Engineered Genes and Animal Organs?" *The Washington Post,* December 9, 1984, p. C1.

34. Laurence E. Karp and Roger P. Donahue, "Preimplantation Ectogenesis: Science and Speculation Concerning *In Vitro* Fertilization and Related Procedures," *Western Journal of Medicine* 12 (1976), 295.

35. Jean Hamburger and Jean Crosnier, "Moral and Ethical Problems in Transplantation," in Felix Rapaport and Jean Dausset, eds., *Human Transplantation* (New York: Grune and Stratton, 1968), p. 38.

36. Arthur L. Caplan, "Blood, Sweat, Tears, and Profits: The Ethics of the Sale and Use of Patient Derived Materials in Biomedicine," *Clinical Research* 33:4 (October 1985), 448–50.

37. Scott, pp. 185–86.

38. Matthews, p. 205.

39. Such practices are described in *Jefferson County Burial Soc. v. Scott,* 218 Ala. 354, 118 S. 644 (1928).

40. Cal. Penal Code §367f(e) (West 1986).

41. Scott, p. 181.

42. A 1975 law review article, "Criminal Aspects of Suicide in the United States," 7 *North Carolina Central Law Journal* 156, 158 n. 19–21 (1975) listed only three states (Oklahoma, Texas, and Washington) which still had laws against attempted suicide. Those statutes have since been repealed.

43. *R. v. Welsh,* (1974) R.T.R. 478, reported in Matthews, pp. 223–24.

44. Constance Holden, "Hayflick Case Settled," *Science* 215 (1982), 271.

45. See Note, "The Sale of Human Body Parts," *Michigan Law Review* 72 (1974), 1182, 1243, n. 409.

46. Bernard Dickens, "The Control of Living Body Materials," *University of Toronto Law Journal* 27 (1977), 142, 164.

47. Richard Titmuss, *The Gift Relationship: From Human Blood to Special Policy* (New York: Vintage, 1972).

48. Harvey M. Sapolsky and Stan N. Finkelstein, "Blood Policy Revisited—A New Look at 'The Gift Relationship,'" *Public Interest,* 46 (1977), 15.

49. Thomas H. Murray, "The Gift of Life Must Always Remain a Gift," *Discover* 7:3 (March 1986), 90.

50. See, e.g., L.L. Hench, "Biomaterials," *Science* 208 (1980), 826.

51. See Leon R. Kass, "Thinking About the Body," *Hastings Center Report,* 15:1 (February 1985), 20.

52. Baruch S. Blumberg, Irving Millman, W. Thomas London, et al., "Ted Salvin's Blood and the Development of HBV Vaccine," *New England Journal of Medicine* 312 (1985), 189 (letter).

53. Kenneth J. Arrow, "Gifts and Exchanges," *Philosophy & Public Affairs* 1 343, (1972), 360.

54. Richard L. Abel, "A Critique of American Tort Law," *British Journal of Law & Society* 8 (1981), 199, 200, 210.

55. Leon E. Rosenberg, "Using Patient Materials for Production Development: A Dean's Perspective," *Clinical Research* 33:4 (October 1985), 452–54.

56. Angela R. Holder and Robert J. Levine, "Informed Consent for Research on Specimens Obtained At Autopsy or Surgery: A Case Study in the Overprotection of Human Subjects," 24(2) *Clinical Research* (February 1976), 68, 75.

Margaret S. Swain and Randy W. Marusyk

An Alternative to Property Rights in Human Tissue

Recent developments in biotechnology involving human tissue are sweeping our interactions with this material well beyond the boundaries of existing law. Some of these developments allow profit-oriented companies to use human tissue to generate lucrative products such as drugs, diagnostic tests, and human proteins. The profits obtained elevate the monetary worth of certain types of human tissue, which until very recently has had little or no monetary value, to incalculable levels.[1] Such changes require a society to reassess the present and future status of human tissue within the legal system.

As a free market society, we believe in the general principle of economic justice and attempt to render all individuals their economic due. Based on this general principle, some have argued for recognizing a limited form of property rights in human tissue, such that the profits can be shared amongst all who contribute to the development of the product, including the donor of the tissue.[2] Still others have called for full recognition of property rights in human tissue such that organs and other tissues can be sold as a source of revenue for the donor.[3]

This article investigates whether current ethical standards prohibiting a commercial market in transplantable organs and tissues can be maintained in a legal structure within which human tissue can also be used as a source to generate enormous profit. It is generally considered that the only options available are to recognize or not recognize property rights in human tissue.[4] We propose instead a legal structure in which transplantable human tissue entails no property rights, but in which such rights can be created in new forms of tissue through the investment of labor. This structure will be applied to the facts of *Moore v. The Regents of the University of California* to illustrate how a claim based upon the recognition of property rights in human tissue would be decided.[5]

Property Rights and the Body

Modern legal systems have consistently held that no property rights attach to the human body.[6] This standard has been affirmed regardless of whether the human body was alive or not. However, the courts have recognized that a temporary right of possession may exist in a dead body in favor of an executor until proper disposal of the body has occurred. In *Pierce v. Proprietors of Swan Point*, the Rhode Island Supreme Court held:

> Although . . . the body is not property in the usually recognized sense of the word, yet we may consider it as a sort of *quasi* property, to which certain persons may have rights, as they have duties to perform towards it, arising out of our common humanity. But the person having charge of it cannot be considered as the owner of it in any sense whatever; he holds it only as a sacred trust for the benefit of all who may from family or friendship have an interest in it . . .[7]

This supposed "right" is not only a very limited possessory right (for purposes of a proper burial, etc.), exercisable only by the executor of an estate, but is recognized for a limited time; the "right" is extinguished upon burial or cremation.

Courts have also consistently refused to recognize any form of property rights in a living human body. This reflects society's moral abhorrence toward any form of slavery. When faced with a plaintiff seeking the recognition of property rights in his or her body, the courts have classified the action as a tort and analyzed the matter through this legal framework.[8] Specific legislation, such as Congress's *National Organ Transplant Act,* builds upon this policy by explicitly prohibiting the *inter vivos* sale of many human organs.[9]

Nevertheless, developments in biotechnology hold great promise for both the advancement of scientific knowledge and the improvement of human health, and this eventually requires the use of human tissue in research. Private industry will typically participate only in research from which it can generate profit to recoup its investment of time and money. However, to generate profit, it must be able to claim property rights in its research products. Thus, when private industry develops a commercial product—regardless if such products were generated through direct or indirect utilization of human tissue—it demands some form of proprietary protection (patents or trade secrets) for these products. Given society's ethical standard of forbidding the recognition of property rights in human tissue, the question is how these standards can be maintained while allowing private industry to secure property rights in their inventions that directly or indirectly involve human tissue.

We can identify three distinct levels to classify the substance that makes up the whole human being. The first level is that of the person and persona.[10] The second is that of a functional bodily unit, such as blood, an organ, or cell, which can be transplanted into another person and carry out its function in the same capacity it did in its originator. At a third level, something must be produced from the human material, such as a cell line or cloned genetic material for it to become useful. It is through the labor of cultivating the tissue that the laborer could claim property rights in the final product.

The Level of Person

According to Kantian philosophy, it is imperative that a legal system distinguish natural persons from things. The concept of free will differentiates human beings from mere objects, and dictates that human beings receive nothing less than full human dignity. If free will is recognized as the basis of moral rights, then it is this free will that allows humans to exercise control over objects.

The legal recognition of property rights in the pecuniary value of one's name, voice, appearance, and personal features may appear contrary to this basic philosophy. However, these "rights of publicity" are property rights that attach to *the concept of* a human entity and not directly to the human body itself.[11] Such rights disappear upon the death of the natural person though the corpse may continue to exist, as exemplified in *Lugosi v. Universal Pictures* where it was questioned whether the persona of a movie actor—a proprietary right—could be passed on to his heirs. The court held that there did exist a right in an actor's name and likeness but that this right did not survive the actor.[12]

In this first level, then, the legal structure should view the human body in its entirety, including the persona. This level represents the most complex sum of the parts (that is, organs, tissue, proteins, genetic material, etc.) and could not be attained by any one of the parts independently. Although each of the parts are very similar, if not identical, from person to person, the *sum total collection* of these parts creates a unique individual. As long as the parts remain within that person, they serve the function of that total and hence fall under the classification of property rights for that total, viz., the "rights of publicity." However, once a part is removed from the total in such a way that it no longer functionally serves its original possessor, it would fall within the second level of the legal structure.

Res Nullius

The second level is constituted by functional bodily units capable of being transplanted. Upon removal from a person, human bodily material would be statutorily or judicially deemed *res nullius;* it would become a corporeal moveable owned by no one. If tissue is removed for transplantation into another person, the tissue would lose its *res nullius* status once the transplant was complete. Additionally, by having extracted tissue pass through the *res nullius* categorization, a donor would be prohibited from legally reclaiming rights in his transplanted tissue at some later date.

Under the classical definition of *res nullius*, ownership would be acquired by the first person who took possession of the tissue. However, for the purpose of transplantation, the legal system could deem those in possession of the excised tissue—physicians, nurses, or tissue transporters—as being possessors "in trust" of the tissue until the transplant was complete. During this period, the tissue would be classified as *trust res nullius*; a thing owned by nobody but held in trust for a recipient.[13]

A categorical distinction must be made regarding tissue that is permanently removed from the body as opposed to tissue that is temporarily removed with the intention of having it subsequently become part of the same person. A temporary removal may come about by an unintentional event such as the accidental amputation of a limb or by an intentional act such as the storage of blood for use in future surgery. In these situations, the patient would be both the donor and the recipient; the person in possession during the interim would be the trustee.

Some companies, such as those that concentrate bone marrow or blood factors, may be concerned that their products would fall under the second level of classification, prohibiting them from being able to protect their products for lack of property rights. These products are types of human tissue that have been temporarily removed with the intention of transplantation into another body. Furthermore, such products are composed of tissue maintained in its original form. However, these products could be protected through other means, such as the doctrine of unjust enrichments arising for a service performed.

The benefit of declaring a functional unit of bodily material *res nullius* is that this material will continue to serve humankind (for example, organ transplant and blood transfusion) under a traditional altruistic spirit without becoming a marketable commodity, as could occur if property rights were to be recognized in it. Furthermore, isolating human transplantable tissue within its own classification would serve to protect its status in the future where the unknowns of technological development might threaten its status. Tissue that is permanently removed from a body, however, would fall under a third level of classification.

Res Communes Omnium

A third level would deem permanently removed human tissue as *res communes omnium*: things that by natural law are the common property of all humans.[14] This classification would allow human material to be used in conjunction with high technology to generate property rights in the product. However, only after something is produced from tissue deemed *res communes omnium* could property rights be created in that thing. A key distinction between matter deemed *res communes omnium* and *res nullius* is that the latter need not be transformed in any way to be useful to humankind: it functions in much its original form.

This view of property reflects the philosophical justification of property expounded by John Locke's labor theory. Locke's justification rested upon two basic assumptions: A person has the right to maintain his life; and, God has provided us with the means to carry out this maintenance. The entire world is a common resource given by God to all persons to maintain themselves. These resources are the raw materials from which useful things are made through a person's labor. Since the labor is part of the person himself, as soon as the person mixes his labor with these raw materials to create a new product, he creates something that belongs only to him and nobody else. Locke stated that:

> It being by him removed from the common state Nature placed it in, it hath by this labour something annexed to it that excludes the common right of other men. For this labour being the unquestionable property of the labourer, no man but he can have a right to what that is once joined to . . .[15]

Thus the creation of a new thing through merging that thing with one's labor results in property that that person alone has the right to own; this is the case regardless if the labor is performed directly by the person, a servant under that person's control, or an animal (or machine) under that person's ownership.

How would this Lockean justification for the creation of property rights through labor apply to tissue permanently removed from the human body? Perhaps the following analogy will help us answer this question.

No one can claim exclusive property rights in information that is found in a common state, as this information is free for all to discover and utilize. This concept is expounded in the U.S. Supreme Court's decision of *International News Service v. The Associated Press*:

> The general rule of law is, that the noblest of human productions—knowledge, truths ascertained, conceptions and ideas—become, after voluntary communication to others, free as the air to common use. Upon these incorporeal productions the attribute of property is continued after such communication only in certain classes of cases where public policy has seemed to demand it. These exceptions are confined to productions which, in some degree, involve creation, invention, or discovery. But by no means all such are endowed with this attribute of property.[16]

Such information can be used to create property through the cultivation of this information into a report. This occurs every day within the business of news reporting. News can be recognized as having a dual character: the substance and the actual report. The substance of the information contained in the production is not the creation of the reporter, rather, as the court states, if it is a thing of "common property, so that none can make use of it, it is said to be *publici juris*, as in the case of light, air and public water."[17] However, property rights are created when a person transforms this common information into a report; the particular collocation of words in which the reporter has communicated the information is where property rights are created by virtue of the *Copyright Act*.[18]

Many parallels can be drawn between the information contained within a news report, and the utility contained within human matter, such as a cell line or particular sequence of genetic material. First, *res communes omnium* has been defined as "things incapable of appropriation, such as light or air.[19] The judicial pronouncement that the substance of a news report is *publici juris* parallels the proposal that permanently excised human substance be deemed *res communes omnium*, as both these substances belong to a common state.

Secondly, scientists could justify a claim for ownership in a cell line, and products generated therefrom, much in the same way that a news gathering agency claims rights in the news that it has collected and collocated. As stated in *International News Service*:

Not only do the acquisition and transmission of news require elaborate organization and a large expenditure of money, skill, and effort; not only has it an exchange value to the gatherer, dependent chiefly upon its novelty and freshness, the regularity of the service, its reputed reliability and thoroughness, and its adaptability to the public needs; but also, as is evident, the news has an exchange value to one who can misappropriate it.[20]

Thus, the transformation of this information into a news report or the transformation of a cell's genetic material into a viable product (for example, via cloning) would, through labor, produce a new thing capable of being owned. The newspaper article is property under the *Copyright Act*, whereas the new genetic material would enjoy property rights under the Patent Act or trade secret law.

Additional support for *res communes omnium* can be found in case law. In *Funk Brothers Seed Co. v. Kalo Inoculant Co.*, the court held that unmodified cells found in nature are free for all to use:

. . . these bacteria, like the heat of the sun, electricity, or the qualities of metals, are part of the storehouse of knowledge of all men. They are manifestations of laws of nature, free to all men and reserved exclusively to none.[21]

Furthermore, a series of cases, commonly referred to as the *Sears-Compco* doctrine, state that if a thing cannot be the subject of a patent in its current form, then such a thing is free to use by all (that is, is within "the common state of Nature").[22] It follows then, as unmodified human tissue cannot be patented, once it has been permanently removed from the body it is free for anyone to use; this use, however, is always subject to our legal, moral, and ethical standards.

Thus, case law exists that supports the proposal to classify human tissue permanently removed from the body as *res communes omnium*. In addition, Locke's theory for the creation of property through labor supports the concept of allowing human material to be used in conjunction with skill and effort to create property rights in the product.

DNA in the Legal Structure

The advent of a DNA fingerprint technology has allowed for the exact identification of an individual from a very small sample of tissue.[23] Given that a DNA fingerprint is unique for a particular person, how can the three-tiered structure claim that the information contained in an individual's genetic code is common to all humankind and thus *res communes omnium*? This apparent paradox is resolved by acknowledging that a major distinction exists between the uniqueness created by the organization of the total genetic material versus the nonuniqueness of components of the genetic material. A DNA fingerprint is an expression of a particular pattern of genetic material; nonetheless, each gene is common to humankind. In other words, though the parts are all the same, the way in which they are collected together makes the sum total unique.

The actual original strand of genetic material obtained from a donor is also problematic. Who owns this material? The third level dictates that substances contained within human tissue permanently removed from the body be deemed *res communes omnium* and are thus themselves incapable of becoming property. The original strand of genetic material would act as the initial template from which the laborers property would be generated. Newly formed strands of genetic material would, in turn, act as the template for successive generations of the product. Thus, the laborer would own everything produced except the original genetic material, which would continue to belong to nobody. If a human gene is cloned into a million copies of that gene, the laborer would own only the million copies but not the original gene. The same scenario would apply to human cell cultures. The original cell that initiated the culture could never be owned, though all copies of the cell would be owned by the laborer.

The Moore Case

How might this structure be applied to the facts of Moore, a case involving nonconsensual use of the plaintiff s cancerous spleen cells to develop lucrative pharmaceutical products? The crux of this dispute concerned whether the plaintiff held personal property rights in the tissue and substances of his body and, if so, whether these rights were breached when the defendant converted this tissue for commercial profit.

The first level of the structure is not applicable to the facts of Moore. A persona attaches to the whole person; these proprietary rights would not apply to a mere part of a person such as a cell or a strand of DNA. The second level pertains to tissue destined for transplantation and is also not applicable to the facts of the *Moore case.*

As Moore's spleen and blood were removed "with the intention of being permanently removed, this tissue would be classified as *res communes omnium.* This classification would not recognize the existence of property rights in human tissue, yet it would allow laborers to generate property rights through work—justified by a Lockean analysis. This would deny Moore any form of remuneration based upon property rights in his tissue. However, it would not deny the plaintiff the right to seek recourse through causes of actions independent of the need to have property rights in the human body.

Legally classifying the substances that make up humans into three distinct levels as we have suggested would thus allow us to preserve society's present ethical standards with regard to the transplantation of human tissue as an altruistic donation while at the same time allowing laborers to secure property rights in their inventions. Such a classification would, moreover, allow the legal system expressly to address our intuitive sense that while we each partake of universals of physiology, as unique personas we are more than the mere aggregation of our interchangeable parts.

QUESTIONS FOR CONSIDERATION

1. Do you agree with Swain and Marusyk that once a body part is removed from a person it belongs to no one and is placed in trust to the physicians or medical staff that removed it?
2. Should the original donor lose all claims over the removed body part, such as being able to reclaim the part or profit from the use of the part?
3. Does John Locke's theory of labor adequately justify the claim that secondary products created from body parts become the property of those who create the products?
4. Do you agree with Swain and Marusyk that the three tiered legal structure they recommen? (the person, functional bodily units that may be transplanted, that which is produced from the bodily units through labor) adequately justifies the use of patients spleen and blood for commercial profit in the *Moore v. The Regents of the University of California* case?

NOTES

1. Thomas P. Dillon, "Source Compensation for Tissue and Cells Used in Biotechnical Research: Why a Source Shouldn't Share in the Profits," *Notre Dame Law Review* 64 (1989), 628–45, at 630.

2. Roy Hardiman, "Towards the Rights of Commerciality: Recognizing Property Rights in the Commercial Value of Human Tissue," *UCLA Law Review 34* (1986), 207–64; Mary T. Danforth, "Cells, Sales, and Royalties: The Patient's Right to a Portion of the Profits," *Yale Law and Policy Review 6* (1988), 179–202.

3. Lori B. Andrews, "My Body, My Property," *Hastings Center Report* 16:5 (1986), 28–38; Ellen F. Paul, "Natural Rights and Property Rights," *Harvard Journal of Law and Public Policy 13* (1990), 10–16.

4. For discussion addressing why property rights should not be recognized in human tissue, see Allen B. Wagner, "Human Tissue Research: Who Owns the Results," *Journal of the Patent and Trademark Office Society* 69 (1987), 329–52; and Dillon, "Source Compensation for Tissue and Cells."

5. 249 Cal. Rptr. 494 (1988) (Cal.C.A.); File "S006987" (July 9, 1990) (Cal.Sup.Ct.).

6. In fact, the Supreme Court of California verified this position in its recent ruling in *Moore*. However, some jurisdictions have created statutory exception for such regenerative tissue as hair, blood, and semen. The monetary consideration involved in such transactions, however, can be explained as service charges; see the *Uniform Commercial Code*, the American Law Institute and National Conference of Commissioners on Uniform State Laws (Official Text–1978).

7. 14. Am. Rep. 667 at 681 (R.I.Sup. Ct 1872).

8. *Morky v. University of Texas Health Center at Dallas* 529 S.W. 2d 802 (1975) (Texas Ct. of Civ. App.); *Browning v. Norton Children's Hospital* 504 S.W. 2d 713 (1974) (Ky. C.A.).

9. *National Organ Transplant Act*, Public Law 98–507; Additionally a state's version of the *Uniform Anatomical Gift Act* or the *Uniform Commercial Code* usually classify the paid transfer of nonvital regenerative tissue as a service rather than a sale.

10. This right is a recognized and accepted form of incorporal property; see *Brown Chemical Co. v. Meyer* 139 U.S. 540 (1891).

11. *Price v. Hal Roach Studies Inc.* 400 F.Supp. 836 (1975) (S.D.N.Y.).

12. *Lugosi v. Universal Pictures* 603 P.2d 425 (1979) (Cal.Sup.Ct.) However, in 1984, the California legislature enacted §.990 *California Civil Code* which permitted limited rights in the personality to be passed to the heirs of the deceased (50 years post-death); furthermore, some other states have held the right of publicity to be descendible; see *Estate of Presley v.Russen* 513 F.Supp. 1339 (1981).

13. A subclassification of *res nullius* may better serve this function such as *hereditas iacens*— a thing belonging to nobody but part of a deceased's estate prior to its acquisition by an heir, or perhaps *res divini iuris*—things under divine law, thus making them non-negotiable and excluded from any legal transactions; Adolf Berger, ed *Transactions of the American Philosophical Society: Encyclopedic Dictionary of Roman Law* 43:2 (Philadelphia: The American Philosophical Society, 1953), 486, 677.

14. Berger, *Transactions*, at 677.

15. John Locke, *The Second Treatise of Civil Government: A Letter Concerning Toleration*, ed. J.W. Gough (Oxford: Basil Blackwell, 1946), 15.

16. *International News Service v. The Associated Press* 248 U.S. 215 (1918), at 235.

17. *International News Service*, 221.

18. *International News Service*, 239.

19. J.Burke, *Jowett's Dictionary of English Law*, 2nd ed. (London: Sweet & Maxwell Ltd., 1977), at 1556.

20. *International News Service*, at 221.

21. 333 U.S. 127 (1948), at 130.

22. *Sears, Roebuck & Co. v. Stiffel Co.* 376 U.S. 225 (1964); *Compco Corp. v. Day-Brite Lighting Inc.* 376 U.S. 234 (1964); Also William D. Noonan, "Ownership of Biological Tissue," *Journal of the Patent and Trademark Office* Society 72 (1990), 109–13.

23. Andrew G. Uitterlinden *et al.*, "Two-dimensional DNA Fingerprinting of Human Individuals" *Proceedings of the National Academy of Science* 86 (1989), 2742–46; Paivi Helminen et al., "Application of DNA 'Fingerprints' to Paternity Determinations" *The Lancet*, 21 March 1988, 574–76.

ARTHUR L. CAPLAN

Organ Procurement:
It's Not in the Cards

Not so long ago the distinguished Senator from Vermont, George Aiken, proposed a novel solution to the problem of ending the Vietnam War. He wryly observed that the fastest way to stop that conflict was simply to declare ourselves the winners and go home.

Defenders of the philosophy of voluntarism in the procurement of cadaver organs for transplantation seem to have taken to heart Aiken's ironic proposal for resolving an apparently intractable problem. Alfred and Blair Sadler declare that they are unable to see "any significant developments in transplantation [that] would justify discarding the principles of informed consent and encouraged voluntarism embodied in the Uniform Anatomical Gift Act." They are not looking carefully enough. The facts about both the supply of and the demand for cadaver organs do not support their decision to solve the crisis in organ procurement by declaring the system a success. Our society's decision in the late 1960s to rely on a public policy of voluntarism as the primary means for assuring an adequate supply of organs for transplantation is no longer tenable. Perhaps such a system was appropriate when organ transplantation was in its infancy, but this is no longer the case.

The Centers for Disease Control estimates that about 20,000 persons die each year under circumstances that would make them suitable for cadaver organ donation. This number should provide a maximum possible pool of 40,000 kidneys for transplant. Yet in 1982 only 3,691 cadaver kidney transplants were performed. The best estimates are that less than 15 percent of potential donors are utilized under the present policy.

Recent studies estimate that between 6,000 and 10,000 persons on hemodialysis are waiting for kidney transplants.[1] Some believe the number of possible recipients in the United States would be as high as 22,500 per year if transplant surgeons were not forced by the severe inadequacy of the present supply of cadaver kidneys to be so conservative in formulating criteria for eligibility for renal transplantation. Similar statistics exist concerning the shortfall of tissues for corneal transplants, hearts, lungs and, as the media remind us every day, livers. And unless something is done to modify the present reliance on a voluntary system, the shortage in cadaver organs will continue to worsen. Rapid progress in the development of surgical techniques, tissue matching, and immunosuppressive drugs will lead to incessant demands for more cadaver organs in the years ahead.

Transplantation may be, as the Sadlers observe, a "halfway" solution to the problem of organ failure. But for those suffering from renal failure, kidney transplants afford a better quality of life than dialysis, and they are far cheaper. Medicare's End-Stage Renal Disease Program has passed the $2 billion mark in reimbursing the costs of more than 70,000 dialysis patients. How can anyone possibly conclude that the present approach to procurement is adequate, acceptable, or working well?

Nor is it at all evident that donor cards have played a significant role in helping to produce even the small degree of procurement success that has been attained in the United States. Less than 15 percent of the population carry donor cards.[2] Transplant coordinators estimate that less than 3 percent of donors have cards in their possession at the time of death. Where data are available on the number of drivers designated as donors in states where organ donation boxes are provided on licenses the compliance rate is not impressive.[3]

Three Possible Alternatives

What then are the possible policy alternatives to the present system of voluntarism and donor cards? And more important, which of these alternatives is most consistent with the values of individual choice, altruism, and freedom?

One possible public policy alternative is to allow the creation of a market in cadaver organs. There are two variants of this approach. The "strong market approach" would allow individuals or, after death, their next of kin to auction organs for sale to the highest bidder. The "weak market approach," on the other hand, would discourage direct compensation of donors by recipients but would allow for the creation of various tax incentives or in-kind reimbursements (those who donate could guarantee their loved ones or friends priority for future transplants) to encourage donation.

A second approach—that of "presumed consent"—would grant medical personnel the authority to remove organs from cadavers for transplantation whenever usable organs were available at the time of death. Again, there are two variants. In "strong presumed consent" the state would grant physicians complete authority to remove usable tissues regardless of the wishes of the deceased or family members. In "weak presumed consent" the law would presume that organ procurement can be undertaken in the absence of some form of objection from the deceased or family members. Weak consent places the burden of opting out of organ donation on those who have objections to this procedure rather than, as is the case under the present system of voluntarism, upon those who wish to opt for organ donation.

A third approach, which has not been widely discussed in the current debate about organ procurement policies, is what I have termed "required request."[4] In the strong version, every citizen would be asked to indicate his or her willingness to participate in organ donation, perhaps by means of a mandatory check-off on applications for a driver's license, a social security card, or on tax returns.

In the weak version, current legislation pertaining to the definition of death might be modified to state that at the time death is declared a person who has no connection to the process of determining death would be required to ask family members about the possibility of organ donation.

What the Public Thinks

There has been a good deal of public debate about the moral acceptability of the strong market approach to procuring cadaver organs. Near unanimity of public opinion has emerged about the unacceptability of an open market in cadaver organs. At least one state, Virginia, banned the sale of organs for transplantation. Other states are considering such bans, as is the United States Congress. Transplant surgeons have repeatedly stated their adamant opposition to market solutions. The moral revulsion that has characterized discussions in the popular press and in professional journals about the spectacle of the desperately ill furiously bidding against one another for a kidney or a liver has, at least for the present, rendered both versions of this policy academic.

Similarly, little public enthusiasm has emerged for a system of strong presumed consent. In a recent survey the Battelle National Heart Transplantation Study found that less than 8 percent of those interviewed felt that "doctors should have the power to remove organs from people who died recently but have not signed an organ donor card without consulting the next-of-kin."[5]

Public opinion aside, the Sadlers argue that any form of presumed consent would have a corrosive effect on the trust that exists between the medical community and the public. They also note that presumed consent would not necessarily lead to an increase in the supply of cadaver organs for transplant. But in those European nations that have adopted versions of presumed consent we lack evidence to determine whether these concerns are justified.

The European Experience

Various European nations, including Austria, Denmark, Poland, Switzerland, and France, have legislation mandating a policy of strong presumed consent. Other nations such as Finland, Greece, Italy, Norway, Spain, and Sweden have adopted versions of weak presumed consent.[6] However, as the Sadlers correctly observe, the available empirical data does not show that these countries have dramatically increased their supply of cadaver organs.

The Swedes, for example, transplant nearly as many patients suffering from kidney failure as they maintain on hemodialysis.[7] This compares quite favorably with the one-to-nine ratio that prevails in the United States. However, statistics on the rates of organ procurement in Sweden and other European countries are not readily available. Indeed, all these countries still have waiting lists for those needing kidney transplants.

In June 1984 I visited France to discuss organ procurement with a number of transplant surgeons and nurses.[8] Organ transplantation in France has been confined almost exclusively to corneas and kidneys. French physicians and government officials estimated that approximately 800 kidney transplants were performed in 1982. This suggests a rate that is only slightly higher than the rate of kidney transplantation in the United States. There are indeed waiting lists for those on hemodialysis who hope for a transplant.

Why should this be so, given that France has a policy of strong presumed consent? French physicians offer two explanations. First, though the law has resulted in an increase in the number of cadaver organs available for transplant, this increase is not reflected in the overall rates because the additional organs have been utilized to decrease the numbers of live donors. Whereas live donors had provided about a third of the kidneys available for transplant in France in the late 1970s, today live donors make up less than 10 percent of the donor pool. (Live donors constitute nearly a third of the donor pool in the United States, Britain, and other nations with public policies of voluntarism based upon donor cards.)

Second, French physicians note that, despite a public policy allowing strong presumed consent, doctors are not willing to remove organs from cadavers without the consent of family members. Strong presumed consent exists only on paper in France. In practice French physicians find it psychologically intolerable to remove tissues from a body without obtaining the permission of next-of-kin.

In the view of both physicians and nurses, however, the French public strongly supports organ transplantation. The physicians I spoke with reported consent rates of between 90 and 95 percent when permission was sought to remove solid organs. In practice French physicians believe strongly in allowing family members to retain the right to object to organ removal. But few family members actually do object, indicating that a public policy of weak presumed consent is compatible with the moral values of both health professionals and the public in France.

Even if French physicians are only willing to participate in a system whose governing philosophy is one of weak presumed consent, why, given the low rate of refusal, are a larger number of organs not available for transplant? The answer is illuminating for its policy implications for the United States.

France, unlike the United States, does not have a cadre of highly trained personnel to handle the process of organ procurement. Health professionals, usually nurses, must bear the burdens of inquiring about objections to organ removal, locating a suitable recipient, and arranging the removal of organs. French hospital administrators, physicians, and nurses all reported that this process was both timeconsuming and costly. Given the growing concern in France over the rising costs of health care there is a reluctance to devote scarce medical resources to organ procurement. French transplant surgeons also noted that, at present, there were severe limits both in terms of personnel and hospital space on the number of transplants of all types that can now be performed. One surgeon noted that "if we had your resources and facilities for transplantation we would be much more aggressive in pursuing organ donors." Limits on the availability of transplant services in France seem to dampen the ardor with which organ procurement is undertaken.

Moreover, the French, like their American counterparts, find it psychologically difficult to approach grieving family members about the prospect of organ procurement even if only to ascertain whether the family objects to what is usually described in the consent process as a routine, customary, and legally sanctioned practice. Busy emergency room personnel are loathe to take the time necessary to fully discuss the subject of transplantation with distraught family members. In sum, despite the existence on paper of a strong version of presumed consent, health care professionals in France are only willing to operate within the boundaries of weak presumed consent. And while this approach has helped to increase the supply of available cadaver kidneys to the point where few live donations are utilized, economic, organizational, and psychological factors limit the willingness of French medical personnel to ask about objections to removing kidneys and other solid organs for transplantation.

The French experience with strong presumed consent legislation holds important lessons for those, such as myself, who believe that our system of organ procurement must be changed. The French physicians' unwillingness to act upon the authority granted them by the state to remove organs regardless of the wishes of family members parallels the unwillingness of American physicians to remove organs solely on the basis of the legal authority granted by donor cards. As organ procurement specialists know all too well, donor cards are almost never viewed by hospital administrators and physicians as adequate authorization for allowing organ retrieval. The permission of family members is always sought prior to organ removal whether or not a donor card or other legal document can be found.

On the other hand, the practical experience obtained by the French with a version of weak presumed consent does not support the sorts of concerns raised by the Sadlers about presumed consent. French physicians are impressed with the fact that objections have been raised by less than 10 per cent of the families who have been given the opportunity to refuse consent. The French press has not reported any dissatisfaction on the part of the public with presumed consent. And French physicians were uniformly relieved to be able to decrease their earlier dependence on live donors. A policy of weak presumed consent appears to have produced a significant amount of social good while allowing for family choice and autonomy in an atmosphere of mutual respect.

The organizational, financial, and psychological factors at work in the French system of organ procurement are also present in the United States. Unlike the French, we have a large number of highly trained and proficient specialists available in the field of organ procurement, but constant pressures to reduce costs in combination with an increasingly litigious atmosphere in medicine make it unlikely that the modest reforms of the present voluntary system proposed by the Sadlers and others[9] will lead to significant improvement in the supply of cadaver organs.

The Primacy of the Family

One key factor emerges from both the French and the American experience: the major obstacle to organ procurement is the failure to ask family members about organ donation. French physicians are entitled by law to take tissues without asking anyone but are unwilling to do so. American physicians are entitled by the Uniform Anatomical Gift Act to take tissues from those who sign donor cards but they are unwilling to do so. Whether or not one believes that the wishes of the family should supersede either the wishes of the public, as in France, or the wishes of the individual, as in the United States, in fact both countries always treat the family as the final authority insofar as the disposition of the dead is concerned.

The respect accorded family members' wishes in these two large and medically sophisticated nations would seem to dictate the kind of public policy change that has the greatest chance of alleviating the shortage in cadaver donors. The French experience indicates that the only practical policy options are those that recognize and respect the role of family members in participating in decisions about cadaver donation. The weak version of required request acknowledges the role of family members, while at the same time ensuring that an optimal environment exists for eliciting organ donations.

Physicians, nurses, or other hospital personnel should be required to inquire whether available family members will give their consent to organ donation. This could be accomplished by modifying the current legal process for declaring death in all states to include a provision requiring that a request concerning organ donation be made to available family members by a party not connected with the determination of death. When family members are not available, organs would be removed only if a donor card or other legal document were present. Or, hospital accreditation requirements could be revised to include a provision mandating that at death the families of potential donors be approached about their willingness to consent.

Linking Request and Consent

A public policy of weak required request could be merged with a further change in our current procurement policy. We could modify the consent process from the present system of opting in to one of opting out along the lines of the weak presumed consent approach used in Scandinavia and, de facto, in France. But weak required request need not be linked to any version of presumed consent. If, as the Sadlers apparently believe, there is something coercive about family members being asked to opt out of donations rather than being asked to opt in, our society might wish to see what the effects are of merely modifying the present emphasis on voluntarism to include required request.

In considering the alternatives of presumed consent or required request, four combinations of request and consent are possible:

Request	Consent
Optional	Opt in
Required	Opt out

The current system of donor cards is, in practice, an optional-opt-in approach. While sound moral arguments can be mounted in favor of the strongest alternative approach—a required-opt-out system—I believe that public and professional consensus could be achieved for a required-opt-in policy.

The Sadlers note that many philosophers, theologians. and social theorists have emphasized the importance of encouraging altruism on the part of every individual within a society. But, as those involved in blood donation in this country learned through years of hard-won efforts to improve the frequency with which blood is given, altruism is not sufficient to assure adequate supplies of necessary medical resources. People must be asked to act if their altruistic motivations are to make a significant difference in helping those in need.

Cadaver organ donation is, whether we like it or not, a family matter. Families should be given every opportunity to act upon their desire to transform the tragedy of death into the gift of life. But they must be asked. If our society were to institute a policy of weak required request, those who are, according to the public opinion polls, willing to give would have a maximal opportunity to do so. We should not allow our concern for the rights and values of the individual to blind us to policy options that can accommodate both individual autonomy and community good.

QUESTIONS FOR CONSIDERATION

1. Caplan quotes numerous statistics to demonstrate that the Sadlers' insistence upon voluntarism and informed consent is insufficient to meet today's demands. Do you agree?

2. Caplan suggests three alternatives to voluntarism: a market in cadavers, presumed consent, and required request. Which, if any, would you favor and why?

3. Why does Caplan conclude that organ donation is a family matter? Do you agree?

4. Caplan recommends that society should attempt a modification of voluntarism so that a requirement of requests for organ donations should be made of families upon the death of a potential donor. Do you believe

such a "weak required request" would significantly increase organ donors? Is such a policy ethically justifiable?

NOTES

1. G. Kolata, "Organ Shortage Clouds New Transplant Era," *Science* 221 (July 1, 1983), 32–33.

2. R. W. Evans, "Organ Scarcity and Issues of Distribution: An Overview," paper presented at a conference; "The Future of Technology in a New Payment Environment," American Enterprise Institute, Washington, D.C., January 24, 1984.

3. T. D. Overcast, R. W. Evans et al., "Problems in the Identification of Potential Organ Donors," JAMA (March 23–30, 1984), 1559–62.

4. See A. L. Caplan, "Public Policy and Organ Transplantation," Testimony to New York State Assembly Health Committee, April 26, 1984, and, "Morality Dissected: A Plea for Reform of Current Policies With Respect to Autopsy," *Human Pathology* 15, no. 12 (December 1984): 1105–06.

5. Evans, op.cit.

6. A. J. Matas and F. J. Veith, "Presumed Consent for Organ Retrieval," *Theoretical Medicine* 5 (1984), 155–66.

7. P. Safar, Hearings on Organ Transplants before the Subcommittee on Investigations and Oversight, Committee on Science and Technology, U. S. House of Representatives, April 23, 1983, Washington, D.C., pp. 653–59.

8. I would like to thank Claire Ambroselli at INSERM and the personnel at Hopital Necker and Hotel Dieu for providing information.

9. J. M. Prottas, "Obtaining Replacements: The Organizational Framework of Organ Procurement," Hearings on Organ Transplants before the Subcommittee on Investigations and Oversight of the Committee on Science and Technology, U. S. House of Representatives, April 1983, pp. 714–51.

EIKE-HENNER W. KLUGE

Designated Organ Donation: Private Choice in Social Context

A continuing feature of organ transplantation is the scarcity of available organs. Policies have attempted to manage the supply more efficiently as well as increase the supply itself. Thus, consciousness drives have been launched by various agencies to increase public awareness of the need for more organs and to increase the number of precommitted voluntary donors carrying donor cards; health care personnel, especially in the acute, intensive, and emergency care settings, have begun to be trained on how to approach the next-of-kin of moribund and of braindead patents about the possibility of donation; special units have been set up as flying recovery teams; and so on.

While all these efforts have ameliorated the shortage somewhat, they have certainly not solved the problem. The situation therefore raises the classic question of how to allocate scarce but vital resources in an ethically acceptable fashion.

In addressing this issue, the transplant community has set up waiting lists and developed criteria for ranking prospective recipients as to priority of access. These criteria usually focus on factors such as the urgency of the patient's medical status and the likelihood of a successful outcome of a transplantation. All other things being equal, those patients with the most acute need will receive the first available organ consistent with compatibility and likelihood of rejection, physiological fit, etc. But other factors are often considered, such as the psychological attitude of the prospective recipient toward transplantation, the existence and nature of a support group, and the ability to defray the costs that will arise in the post-transplantation period. In some countries, such as Great Britain, age is also considered—usually as an absolute and limiting criterion. Physiological suitability and likelihood of successful outcome are not, therefore, always decisive.

Evasive Maneuvers

The first thing a prospective recipient must do, therefore, is to get on a waiting list. But this provides no guarantee of receiving an organ. It has happened (and will continue to happen) that persons on waiting lists—even individuals high up in the ranking—have died before a transplantation.[1] Consequently it is not surprising that someone on a waiting list, and especially someone lower down, should attempt to shorten or even circumvent the allocation process entirely by initiating a public appeal for an organ to be donated specifically to him or her.[2] Or, particularly for pediatric patients, some individual or group of individuals—parents, next-of-kin, service groups—may launch an appeal on behalf of the affected person. These public appeals highlight the plight of the individual in the most graphic terms imaginable and utilize the whole gamut of available media services, particularly television, which cannot be surpassed in its ability to generate an emotional and direct response.

Such a campaign is eminently understandable. It both expresses the fundamental desire of the prospective recipient to live, and indicates concern and solidarity on the part of others.[3] Public appeals can be successful in producing an organ for the affected individual, and incidentally may result in an overall increase in the number of organs that are generally available, thereby improving the chances for other prospective recipients.

Nevertheless, serious ethical problems are raised not only with respect to such a campaign itself but for everyone involved in the process: the media, the physician, the prospective recipient—and even the donor. Nor are institutions in which the transplantation occurs immune from ethical challenge.

The Ethical Nature of Organ Donation

These concerns can be clarified if we first examine the nature of organ donation itself. Thomas H. Murray in particular has focused on organ donation as a gift relation, and suggested that it may be seen as serving a variety of social functions. It may "signal that self-interest is not the only significant human emotion" and that "it is good to minister to fundamental human needs"; "remind us that not all valuable things like love, a feeling of fellowship, trust, etc. can be purchased"; "affirm the solidarity of the community over and above the depersonalizing, alternating forces of mass society and market relationships"; or "create and sustain intimate personal relationships."[4]

Yet this correctly tells only part of the story; there is another aspect of organ donation that is crucial to understanding the ethical nature of organ donation itself. It concerns the meaningfulness of such donations.

Unlike most other gift transactions, organ donations are not complete within themselves. They are not like transactions where the value and significance—indeed the very nature of what is given—is a function solely of the interaction between the donor and the recipient and the gift transaction consists essentially in the transfer of these items from one person to another. For instance, gifts of clothing, food, and shelter are gifts of items that are significant in and by themselves. Although these gifts may also have various socially important purposes and functions, none impose an obligation on others to do something so that the gift may become meaningful and significant *as that kind of gift:* as a gift of the sort of thing the donor had in mind. To put this more concretely, the gift of a liver, a kidney, or a heart as such, to someone who requires an organ, is useless. Without active social involvement and intervention, it is merely the giving of a piece of human flesh. To become a gift in the sense that both we as members of society as well as the donor and the recipient understand, the donation must take place in a heavily institutionalized context consisting not only of the medical transplant team but of a whole array of support services without which transplantation itself would not be possible. These include recovery and delivery services. Then there is the planning, funding, and actual integration of the biotechnical support services that are necessary for the actual operation itself—a task that spans various departmental and administrative levels. Social and medical postoperative services are also implicated, as is counseling for next-of-kin and recipients—and sometimes even the health care professionals themselves. Furthermore, as a medical modality, transplantation is functionally dependent on historical developments that span millennia of social effort to advance the art and science of medicine. A myriad of other social developments and involvements stand behind transplantation and make organ donation possible and meaningful as an act. They are what give it significance as the gift of an organ rather than merely the discarding of human tissue.

Therefore organ donation is not only a personal action but also a social act. It is a social act not solely because it is embedded in a social context—most gift transactions have that nature—but because it requires society's direct and immediate participation. Society itself becomes a participant giver, and the organ, which as issue was merely a private good, becomes a social good when it is an organ-as-donated.

Access and Ranking

This fact of social involvement has important consequences. Procedurally, it entails that if there are formal constraints that govern social acts per se, then these will also apply to organ donation. Legal, social, and political parameters will here be implicated. But it also entails ethical constraints; constraints that derive from the principles of equality, justice, and respect for persons and which govern all social interactions in a fundamental way.

If we focus on the latter, the suspicion may arise that selective allocation in general and ranking in particular violate these ethical constraints. After all—so it might be argued—the principle of equality formally states that all persons are equal. Does this not entail that they must all be treated the same? Does this not in turn mean that there cannot be, even in principle, any way of distinguishing between prospective recipients, let alone of ranking them? For ranking, by its very nature, requires that individuals will be treated differently—namely, with respect to opportunity of access. Consequently, it might be concluded, we have only two ways of guaranteeing equality of treatment: to provide no one with an organ and abandon transplantation entirely until the problem of resource insufficiency has been solved, or to adopt a randomized lottery system of distribution in which there is no ranking at all.

The mistake in such reasoning lies in the interpretation of the principle of equality of persons. While the principle does prevent us from discriminating between persons as persons, it does not prevent us from discriminating between their competing claims. The strength of their claims may differ depending on such factors as degree of need, nature of the need, its origin,[5] and the probability of a successful outcome upon intervention.[6] Thus, the general rule is: so long as the characteristics on which the discrimination/ranking is based are not preselective in a way that violates equality and justice, they may be used as distinguishing parameters. To put it differently, all and only those characteristics may be used as ranking criteria that are condition-specific; person-specific characteristics, that is, those that by their very nature guarantee that only preselected persons will benefit, may not. Furthermore, it must be essentially a matter of chance, beyond the control of the individual or interested third parties, whether he or she has these characteristics.

These considerations allow us to allocate subjectively in the way that we have indicated: both by controlling entry into the pool of prospective recipients; and then by letting us construct a two-tier ranking system within the pool itself. Here, prospective recipients can first be ranked on the basis of criteria justified by the equality-and-justice rule. Then, if there are still candidates whose claims are indistinguishable, we can turn to an egalitarian lottery system: Since *ex hypothesi* the candidates that are left will have equal claims, any lottery approach that gives each the same chance will not subvert equality and yet at the same time will allow for selective allocation.[7]

Designated Donation

It is in this very regard, however, that designated organ donation differs. It is person-specific, and thereby abandons the general ethical framework. Rather than focusing on conditions that ultimately are defensible in terms of equality and justice, it ties access to an organ to the emotional appeal (or lack thereof) of the prospective recipient, the public relations skills of the physician(s) involved, of the next-of-kin and of those who orchestrate the media campaign, and the financial abilities of everyone concerned to mount such a campaign in the first place. Designated organ donation in effect singles out a specific individual and characterizes him or her as someone to whom an organ may be given independently of the established means of access. The assumption is that this person is ethically special; that he or she has some particular quality or characteristic that permits an exemption from the criteria that otherwise apply to all.

Of course, it is possible that such a person does have some special characteristic that makes him or her ethically unique—at least in this particular context. We cannot rule out *a priori* that there isn't some ethically relevant characteristic that was overlooked when the standard ranking criteria were formulated. However, to be compatible with equality and justice, such a characteristic must not be person-specific, but must be one that in principle anyone can have. This means the characteristic should be included in the criteria that determine the ranking in the first place. But if a new condition is added to the established set, there is then no need to go outside the proper ranking criteria to benefit this particular individual: Although in principle the characteristic could be had by anyone, it just so happens that at this time it is possessed only by this particular person.

In principle, then, there is nothing wrong with introducing a new criterion. However, such a move enjoins us to ask what the criterion is, and why it should apply to just this particular person. Photogenic appeal, having private funds available for a media campaign, or having a highly motivated personal physician certainly could not be considered appropriate criteria. Nor could frustration in waiting for an organ, the fear of not getting one in time, or extreme dissatisfaction with the current quality of life while waiting. These criteria either involve a violation of equality and justice, or are common to all prospective recipients, and therefore are not ethically distinguishing.

Family Ties

There is one characteristic that is ethically distinguishing and that does amount to a uniquely qualifying property in the case of a particular person: having an immediate family tie to a specific donor. Parents, in virtue of assuming the role of parents, have accepted an obligation of support and nurture for their child. This obligation may reasonably be understood as a requirement to do the best for the child so long as that does not involve undue, inordinate, or unreasonable risk for the parent. Since organ donation (in a medically acceptable fashion) does satisfy these conditions—all other things being equal, it will not involve the donation of the one remaining kidney, or of a heart by an as yet still living parent—and since donation itself can reasonably be interpreted as providing "the necessaries of life," it may be argued that it is merely the extension of an otherwise existing duty that does not hold for others or in other contexts.[8]

Following the suggestions of Murray and others, if the giving of a gift may raise reasonable expectations of return—especially in a social context where such an expectation is not only considered acceptable but is well-entrenched—then this also provides a unique and differentiating condition. While the parents may not expect support and the necessaries of life as a matter of payment, they do have a socially sanctioned expectation that does not exist in other cases. That expectation will be a variable that may legitimately count as an exception to the rule of otherwise impartial distribution. It honors the value that society places on the existence of the family unit itself.

This last consideration is important in the case of sibling donation. To be sure, there are practical considerations that play a role. The likelihood of a match is greater here than in other cases, and whatever the psychological factors might be that positively contribute to a better success rate, they are likely to be present to a greater degree in these contexts than in most others. Considered by themselves, these do not amount to ethical justifications for designated sibling donation in contravention of the equality-and-justice rule. However, the peculiar strength and nature of the interpersonal relationship within the immediate family context, coupled with the special role that society accords to the family unit itself, is such a justification. The fact of inter-sibling identification, which manifests itself in the supportive stance that siblings may take with respect to each other, and the mutually reciprocal relationship that has developed between them over the time of their growing together must also be considered.[9]

Interspousal designated donation is, of course, different. Whatever the exact formalization of their association as spouses may be—and here the various sociocultural and ethnic groups do differ—the spouses have agreed to provide mutual support and succor for each other to a degree that is not recognized outside of this sort of setting. And society, by recognizing the special nature of this association, acknowledges its uniqueness and strength. It would therefore be contradictory of society to recognize the special nature of this association, give it formal expression, place specific expectations upon it—and then deny the individual members of that association the right to act on it in actual practice. If one of the primary functions of gift-giving is to "create and sustain intimate personal relationships," and if society recognizes the spousal relationship as being of a uniquely intimate and exceptionally desirable sort, then the very act of so recognizing it creates just the special kind of relationship that ethically allows for an exception to the rule of impartial allocation.

Family ties, then, are uniquely privileging and identifying, and designated organ donation occurring within the immediate family context does not violate the equality-and-justice condition. However, when there is such a tie, and when there is a willing donor who falls under this rubric, there is no need of a *public* appeal for a designated donation. As an exceptive condition to the rule, therefore, family ties are acceptable—but practically speaking make no difference. No *public* appeal will be necessary or forthcoming.

The Media

When we examine the ethical positions of various parties outside of the family context for designated organ donation we immediately encounter a whole host of problems. Let us begin with the media. It can be argued that media involvement serves to heighten public awareness of the organ scarcity as well as of the particular need that exists. Thus, whether or not it is successful in producing an organ suitable for the designated individual, it often can effect an overall increase in the number of organs donated.

These possibilities should not be allowed to obscure several important ethical considerations. First, the need of the particular recipient is not isolated or unique. There exists a whole array of compelling needs of the same kind— namely the need of every other prospective recipient. By focusing on the need of one person, and participating in a campaign to satisfy specifically it, the media remove that need from the comparative context that allows the public to assess its ethical significance properly. By virtue of presenting the person's need in this fashion—isolated and divorced from its comparative context—the media would be characterizing it as something special: as something that not only invites a supererogatory act of donation in general, but an act focused on this particular need of a particular person. In this manner, therefore, the media would effectively falsify the true state of affairs.

As a result of this falsification, it may happen that someone who otherwise would have made an undesignated donation donates to this specific individual— thereby diminishing the overall organ pool. This however, means that someone who ethically would have been a more appropriate candidate—that is, someone who is higher on the waiting list—would lose what rightfully is his or hers. The person might even die as a result of this loss. A considerable part of the blame for this outcome would lie at the door-step of the media.

An additional problem with media participation in a designated organ donation campaign concerns the general ethical attitude that such involvement would foster: In championing the cause of the particular individual outside of the otherwise established allocation system, the media would be advancing the position that one may legitimately circumvent whatever ethically appropriate orders, limits, or procedures there are to achieve one's own private ends. The very fact of their participation would foster an attitude that private ends outweigh ethical rights. Not only is this false per se, it is also at least arguable that the media, by virtue of their social role, have an obligation not only to present information to the public but also to present it in an appropriate and truthful manner![10] There are situations in which this is difficult to do, especially when the data are themselves unclear. Here, however, that is not the case. Therefore while the media may present a specific individual to the public, they should do so only in such a way as to allow the public to appreciate his or her true ethical position. This means that the person may be presented only as one among many others who need organs, only as someone whose plight typifies the situation of those on waiting lists. Anything else would not only constitute participation in a subversion of the rights of those on waiting lists, but also involve misleading the public. By that very token, it would be a violation of a professional trust.

The Donor

At first glance, the donor's position seems unaffected by these considerations. After all, whatever the social functions and implications of his or her act may be, the person is performing a supererogatory act, for which he or she deserves praise, not blame. Moreover, the principle of autonomy affirms the right of self-determination, which may be extended to the right of disposing of what is one's own. Shouldn't this mean that the donor has a right of disposition with respect to his or her organs even in a donation to the recipient of his or her choice?[11]

This train of reasoning may initially strike us as extremely reasonable. Closer consideration, however, shows that it is based on the premise that the act of donation lies entirely within the power of the donor as to its nature and direction. That premise is mistaken. The fact that a donation *qua* act lies within the power and discretion of a donor does not entail that the donor may exercise that power as he or she may see fit. For the principle of autonomy does not mean that everyone has an unqualified right of self determination— of complete freedom of action, no matter what—but rather that this right of self-determination holds *subject to the compiling and legitimate rights of others*. In Rawlsian terms, "acting autonomously is acting from those principles that we would consent to as free and equal rational beings."[12] The principle of autonomy therefore carries a logic of limitation within itself. It requires a balancing between the rights of the individual who claims autonomy and the competing legitimate rights of all others, where that balancing must occur in terms of equality and justice. Hence, if the otherwise free and unconstrained choice of an individual infringes on equality and justice, it will not be a legitimate exercise of autonomy and must be rejected.

If we apply this logic to designated organ donation, we can see immediately why the donor cannot appeal to the principle of autonomy to ground his or her right to designate the nonfamilial recipient. Organ donation is not an act that is complete in itself. It is a social act. Directly or indirectly it involves all of society. Consequently it is subject to general ethical constraints, including equality and justice. The fact that the act originates voluntarily from the donor does not alter this.

If the donor wants to be ethical, he or she must act within these moral constraints. If the organ is donated outside of these constraints, then what was intended as an ethically praiseworthy act becomes a deplorable act of discrimination. While materially it will undoubtedly have importance, ethically it loses its value.

The Health Care Institution

The social nature of organ transplantation also is of relevance for health care institutions that are publicly funded or are part of a socialized health care system. In these cases, trivially, the institutions depend on society and operate under an express mandate to provide health care in an equitable fashion. By their very nature, such institutions will be barred from participating in nonfamilial designated organ donation schemes, whether in a procuring or a utilizing capacity. While on occasion it might be politically expedient to depart from this approach—for example, when a high-profile recipient or a financially powerful individual is involved—that very departure would signal the breakdown of the ethical mission of the institution.

Private health care institutions are equally not immune from these considerations, for they sill operate in a social context. This makes their actions subject to the limiting principles of equality and justice. Moreover, the organs that are to be transplanted derive their significance and meaningfulness as organs from the scientific, medical, and pharmacological developments that make donation possible. They are, in a very real sense, social goods. And, like any social agent, private health care institutions are subject to the principle of shared responsibility: If a first party engages in an unethical act which, as act, becomes materially possible only through the aid of a second party, then the second party shares in the guilt of the first to the degree that its participation is instrumental in allowing the act to take place.[13] Since any designated organ donation is dependent on the health care institution in which it occurs, it follows that if such an institution, whether public or private, participates in such an act, it will be subject to the principle of shared responsibility.

Under ordinary circumstances, with equitable and just allocation criteria in operation, the distribution of organs will still be selective—not everyone will get an organ—and because of that, some prospective recipient on the waiting lists will quite probably die. This death would in principle have been preventable in the sense that had the distribution been different, the patient would have received an organ and someone else who did not would have died. The distribution policy that follows from even just allocation criteria is therefore responsible for the death, in that it shifts the death from one person to another. But the fact that someone will die lies beyond the parameters of the situation itself. There will be a death, and whoever dies, the death will be tragic but not unethical. It will be the inevitable outcome of a tragic state of affairs with which society is dealing in the best way it can.

Designated organ donation, however (with the exception of the family context), alters all of this. It does not change the number of people who will die, but rather who particularly will die. Saving (or attempting to save) a specific individual who is not in the group of ranked prospective recipients creates a state of affairs that prevents relieving the need of someone in that group who but for the designation would have received the organ. And that is tragic as well as unethical: tragic because of the death; unethical because someone who according to equity and justice was entitled to the organ is deprived of it. And it is the institution that here is morally culpable. For had it acted ethically and refused to participate, the suggestion of designated organ donation would not have arisen in the first place. What is important and objectionable, therefore, is not *that* the pool of organs is being depleted but *how*.

Nothing we have argued entails that a health care institution may not become involved in media campaigns that highlight the plight of particular persons. The identified victim syndrome is too powerful to be ignored as a public relations tool. However, the institution must make clear that any organ resulting from such an appeal will be distributed according to appropriate ranking and distribution criteria that involve all transplant institutions. Institutional ethics demands no less.

The Physician

While the ethical implications of the social context apply also to physicians, there are in addition several considerations that apply uniquely to the physician. Indeed, these considerations are relevant irrespective of whether the physician works in a private fee-for-service setting or in a socialized health care system. They focus on the fact that medicine is a monopoly. Minimally, this implies that only those who fulfill certain criteria set by the profession itself and who have been licensed as practitioners by the profession are legally entitled to practice.[14] While it is arguable that some monopolies are granted by society for the benefit of the monopoly holders, this is not the case with public service monopolies. They are granted on the assumption that by allowing the profession to control entry into as well as the standards of the profession, society is assured of the best possible level of service. In addition, by accepting the monopoly, the holder binds him or herself to ensure not only quality of service but also ubiquity and universality.[15] That is, while quality of service may be society's primary consideration in granting a monopoly, society does not envision that the monopoly holder will offer the relevant service only in select locations, or only to select people who can afford to meet the (privately set) fees. The ethical basis on which society purports to operate requires that equality and justice be preserved in socially mandated actions.

Medicine as a social service monopoly is bound by these ethical constraints in a much tighter fashion than most other undertakings. Of course it is not the individual physician who is the actual monopoly holder. It is the profession as a whole, represented by the relevant professional organizations. What is important, however, and what should concern us, is that the actions of the individual physician must be in keeping with the obligations that bind the profession as a whole. Among other things, this means that individual physicians must not select patients entirely with an eye to profit but must at least attempt equity; and that actions on behalf of a particular patient must not only be professionally competent but also just and fair.

Therefore, while the individual physician has an obligation to do the best he or she can for the patient, whatever acts the physician undertakes must not be engaged in as though the patient existed in isolation, divorced as it were from the rest of society. The monopolistic nature of the profession requires that the possibility of meeting the needs of others in a just and equitable fashion be taken into account when it comes to resource allocation. At least, this must be the case with respect to those aspects of medical practice that involve drawing on nonrenewable social goods.

The ethically sensitive transplant physician, therefore—and indeed the ethically sensitive physician per se—cannot participate in a nonfamilial designated organ procurement and/or utilization process. It would jeopardize the ubiquity and universality of the health care services entailed by the fact of the monopoly. Furthermore, equality and justice would be denied through preferential access. Instead, the physician must actively reject any such undertaking and must *publicly* condemn any such attempt lest through professional silence on the matter a situation be allowed to develop that the profession itself could not ethically accept.

The Recipient

Given what we have already argued, the position of the designated recipient can be sketched rather quickly. Under normal circumstances of gift-giving, where the gift or *donum* is not a social good and does not depend for its significance as a gift on social involvement, the giver's intention to donate to a specific individual would be sufficient justification for the intended recipient to accept the gift should he or she feel so inclined. The situation here, however, is different The organ that is given as a gift is a social good, which means that the limiting parameters that affect the position of all other participants affect the prospective recipient as well. More specifically, it means that the individual cannot request a designated donation, and when designated as recipient with or without such a request, he or she cannot accept. He or she must gently reject the offer, that is, without denigrating the laudable spirit that underlies the donation as a donation, and without offending the sensibilities of the donating person. But reject it he or she must.

Two additional considerations may merit special attention. The first centers around the act of acceptance and what it suggests. To follow a point made by William Wollaston, "whoever acts as if things were so, or not, doth by his acts declare, that they are so, or not so; as plainly as he would by words, and with more reality. And if things are otherwise, his acts contradict those propositions, which assert them to be as they are."[16] That is to say, by accepting the designated donation, the intended recipient in effect holds him or herself as ethically so special that he or she is not subject to the general constraints that govern social interactions. In that sense, and to that degree, the act of acceptance has an inherent and ineluctable fraudulent parameter. It is, so to speak, a lie.

A second point is analogous to a consideration that we adduced on the position of health care institutions. Since the pool of available organs is limited, any interference with its ethical distribution will result in a shift in the distribution pattern, so that someone who ethically is entitled to an organ will not in fact receive it. To accept a designated donation is to interfere in the distribution pattern and to take something that, all other things being equal, someone else should have. Unless there are extenuating circumstances, to take something to which one is not entitled and away from someone who is, is to commit theft. Since there is here no question of entitlement on the part of the intended recipient—*ex hypothesi* the criteria that would confer entitlement are here not being met—the latter, by accepting the designated donation, will be committing theft.

It could, of course, be argued that since the organ is freely given by the donor but only to the designated recipient, the situation is altered: The donation is either for this individual or not at all. Thus, talk about theft is entirely out of place. This reasoning, however, fails. The donor is free to give or not, as he or she pleases; and in that sense, the size of the available organ pool is not a predetermined matter. However, once he or she has decided to give, the donation is subject to the constraints of equality and justice. This means that if it really is given—if it really is to be used as an organ—it does become part of the pool whose distribution must adhere to these ethical principles. It also means that if the designated recipient accepts the organ in violation of these, he or she will be committing theft. The claim that it is better that the designated recipient accept the organ and be saved than that the designated recipient refuse, the donation be withdrawn (because it was intended only for this person) and therefore a person who could have been saved now die without any compensating saving relative to the ranked prospective recipients, has little to recommend it ethically. Not even a utilitarian would accept this view, because it would mean abandoning equality and justice as operational principles.

Whatever its sociological and psychological functions, organ donation is an ethically praiseworthy act whose purpose is to benefit others. It sets into motion a train of events that is designed to ensure that the donated organ will not be wasted, precisely because the gift is so precious and the need so great. However, neither the fact that the gift is precious nor that in itself the act is praiseworthy should be allowed to obscure the further fact that organ donation does not occur in a social vacuum. Its meaningfulness as an act, to say nothing of its possibility, presupposes a health care delivery system that has ineluctable social parameters. These parameters entail considerations of equality and justice and therefore imply an ethical ban against procedures that do not abide by them. Organ donation is an ethically praiseworthy act, to be sure; but only when it remains within the ethical framework that governs all social interactions.

QUESTIONS FOR CONSIDERATION

1. Kluge stresses that organ donation is not merely a private act but very much a social good. What bearing would organ donation as a social good have on legal, social, political, and especially ethical concerns?
2. Kluge contrasts ranking and discrimination based upon condition, specific criteria, and a persons specific characteristics. What is the ethical difference between the two forms of ranking.
3. Why does Kluge consider designated organ donation to be unjust? Do you agree?
4. Kluge considers certain family ties to be exceptions to the ethical objections to designated organ donation. Do you agree?
5. What responsibilities would Kluge place upon the media, the donor, the health care institution, the physician, and the recipient in in maintaining the principles of equality and justice in organ donation?

NOTES

1. See Jeffrey M. Prottas, "Organ Procurement in Europe and the United States." *The Milbank Memorial Fund Quarterly* 63:1 (1985), 95–126.

2. A celebrated Canadian case involved a man from Edmonton who, in the spring of 1987, advertised nationally for a kidney and indicated his willingness to pay.

3. For a discussion of various factors involved here, see Thomas H. Murray, "Gifts of the Body and the Needs of Strangers," *Hastings Center Report* 17:2 (1987), 30–38.

4. Murray, "Gifts," 35–37.

5. But see Dan E. Beauchamp, "Public Health and Social Justice," *Inquiry* 13:1 (1976), 3–14.

6. See Nicholas P. Rescher, "The Allocation of Exotic Lifesaving Therapy," *Ethics* 79:3 (1969), 173–86.

7. See Frank A. Sloan and Judith D. Benthkover, *Access to Care and the U.S. Economy* (Lexington, MA: Lexington Books, 1979).

8. The situation of foster homes and/or institutions is different because both of these are acting as representatives of the state in its *parens patriae* role. The obligation, therefore, is not their's but the state's; and the state is fulfilling its role by providing appropriate medical/transplantation care.

9. Mary A. Lewis, "Comments on Some Ethical Legal, and Clinical Issues Affecting Consent in Treatment, Organ Transplants, and Research in Children," *Journal of the American Academy of Child Psychologists* 20 (1981), 581–96.

10. Stephen H. Daniel, "Ethical Theory and Journalistic Ethics," *Applied Philosophy* 1 (1982), 19–25; see also Michael Bayles, *Professional Ethics* (Belmont Calif.: Wadsworth, 1981).

11. See Section 4(c) of the U.A.G.A. which states in part that "The gift may be made to a specific donee or without specifying a donee." However, since the very tenability is here at issue, this can hardly be adduced without begging the question.

12. John Rawls, *A Theory of Justice* (Cambridge, MA: Harvard University Press, 1976), 516.

13. This is what apparently underlies the so-called Good-Samaritan statutes proposed by the Law Reform Commission of Canada in Working Paper 46 *Omission, Negligence, and Endangering* (Ottawa, 1985).

14. For some other considerations, see E.H.W. Kluge, "The Profession of Nursing and the Right to Strike," *Westminster Institute Review* 2:1 (1982), 3–6.

15. For a different approach, see the Report of the President's Commission for the Study of Ethical Problems in Medicine and Biomedical and Behavioral Research, *Access to Medical Care* (Washington, DC: U.S. Government Printing Office, 1983).

16. William Wollaston, *The Religion of Nature Delineated* [1028], reprinted in *British Moralists*, L.A. Selby-Bigge, ed., 2 vols. (Oxford: Oxford University Press, 1897), 364.

PART VIII: Genetics, Human Nature, Human Destiny

PART VIII:1: Genetic Diagnosis and Screening

KATHLEEN NOLAN
First Fruits: Genetic Screening

ELAINE DRAPER
Genetic Secrets: Social Issues of Medical Screening in a Genetic Age

PART VIII:2: Genetic Engineering and the Human Future

C. KEITH BOONE
Bad Axioms in Genetic Engineering

W. FRENCH ANDERSON
Genetics and Human Malleability

ERIK PARENS
Taking Behavioral Genetics Seriously

In the early 1990s, the United States government committed 3 billion dollars to fund the 15-year Human Genome Project. This program, which is part of a larger international effort, seeks to map out the hereditary information on the 23 pairs of human chromosomes and eventually to determine the DNA sequences that create this information. The technical challenges of the project are enormous. But the ethical questions raised by the deluge of genetic information promised by the project have proven even more challenging. How will this new knowledge be managed? What purposes will this knowledge serve? Will it be used for good—as in new gene therapies for diseases? Does this knowledge have the potential for harm—as in the notification of individuals with genetic disorders where no therapy is available, or in discrimination by employers or insurance companies based on genetic screening? What guidelines will control the use of this information?

Genetic Diagnosis and Screening

Prenatal testing for the detection of certain genetic diseases such as Down's syndrome, spina bifida, and anencephaly provide prospective parents with information that may lead to selective abortions. The genetic information that will be made available through the Human Genome Project has the potential to significantly increase the burden of choice on the part of parents and to dramatically alter the practice of prenatal care.

This new genetic information derived from the Genome Project will identify not only current conditions but will also detect contingency conditions: potential problems, such as cancer or heart disease, that may develop later in life. Such information poses serious concerns that individuals will be identified as "high risk" and thus excluded from insurance and employment benefits.

Genetic Engineering and the Human Future

Ashanthi De Silva was born with ADA deficiency, which prevents the T-cells—white blood cells that fight disease—from functioning as an effective immune system. By extracting samples of her blood, Drs. Michael Blaese, French Anderson and Kenneth Culver were able to splice a healthy ADA gene into her DNA. This recombined healthy gene was inserted into Ashanthi's T-cells by means of a virus that spread the gene into each cell. The success of this treatment promises hope for the treatment of many diseases including some forms of cancer, AIDS and sickle cell anemia.

Should gene therapy be limited to serious diseases? Are there moral problems with genetic enhancement—the improvement of mental and physical traits? Should gene therapy be limited to somatic cell alterations—changes that affect only the cells of the individual and are not passed on to future generations? Or should gene therapy also be used for germline alterations—changes that can be passed on to future generations—to improve the genetic pool of the human race? Are there dangers in altering the genetic make-up of the human race?

The readings for this section include the following:

Genetic Diagnosis and Screening

- Kathleen Nolan's **First Fruits: Genetic Screening** identifies the problems that new diagnostic tests will bring to normal prenatal care.
- Elaine Draper's **Genetic Secrets: Social Issues of Medical Screening in a Genetic Age** examines problems of discrimination in the workplace as genetic information becomes widespread.

Genetic Engineering and the Human Future

- C. Keith Boone's **Bad Axioms in Genetic Engineering** acknowledges the new moral challenges of genetic engineering while objecting to the reductionist and partial truths of what he calls "bad axioms" that create an unrealistic fear of genetic engineering.
- W. French Anderson's **Genetics and Human Malleability** examines the potential for human genetic engineering and differentiates between somatic cell gene therapy for serious diseases and enhancement genetic engineering.
- Erik Parens' **Taking Behavioral Genetics Seriously** responds to two errors committed in discussions of genetic research: that genetic technology can only affect our bodies and not our minds (soul) and that genetic reseach will undermine political ideas of freedom and equality. He argues that genes are one component in a complex system that accounts for human behavior.

KATHLEEN NOLAN

First Fruits: Genetic Screening

One of the first fruits of the Human Genome Project will be many new markers for traits and diseases believed to have a genetic base but so far lacking an identified gene (or genes). Most of these markers can be developed into diagnostic tests quite easily, greatly expanding the range of genetic diagnostic options potentially available to individuals for themselves, or as parents and prospective parents.

However, the sheer mass of genetic information that may become available, along with the complex patterns of information offered by many of the new markers, has generated concern about the extent and rapidity with which these new markers should move from the laboratory bench into various clinical uses. In particular, critics of modern obstetric practices have taken note of the ways in which increased diagnostic surveillance can change the character and mood of pregnancy, and they have urged special caution about increased prenatal genetic testing. This paper explores these issues and suggests the need for national standards articulating criteria for introducing and funding new genetic tests as a part of normal prenatal care.

Genetic Testing in Prenatal Care

Having a baby is an exciting and emotionally demanding process for parents. Here is a new life, forged from complex physical and emotional bonds between its parents, and manifesting the powerful and mysterious intertwining of their previously distinct genetic heritages. Whether planned or unanticipated, pregnancy emerges replete with potential: a potential child with an almost infinite range of needs, desires, and attributes.

From a parent's perspective, pregnancy is thus filled with both curiosity and concern. What kind of baby will this be? Who will it look like? Will it be a girl or a boy? Will it be healthy?

This last question—Will my baby be healthy?"—helps propel parents into the obstetrician's or midwife's office, as they seek to fulfill their responsibility to protect and promote the well-being of their developing offspring. Joining with the health professional, they construct a history of the developing fetus via a series of physical examinations and selected diagnostic tests.

Although few parents realize it, none of these tests, singly or in combination, can prove that the pregnancy is proceeding normally. In fact, even directly examining the baby after birth is not fool-proof against unsuspected conditions. Nonetheless, prenatal and even preconceptual screening of various sorts can identify many problems, sometimes at very early stages. Parents and health care professionals have therefore increasingly turned to amniocentesis, ultrasound, alpha-fetoprotein assays, and other tests in an attempt to gain information and to detect and treat conditions for which prenatal interventions are available.

Genetic screening has until recently played a relatively minor role in this process. Because genetic testing was expensive and time-consuming, and because most detectable conditions were quite rare, specialized testing for inherited disorders (other than chromosomal analysis and the diagnosis of disorders of hemoglobin formation, such as sickle cell disease) has not generally been recommended as a part of normal prenatal care, except in those situations where a family history or a previously affected child indicates an increased risk.

However, this aspect of prenatal care may undergo enormous change over the next two decades. The prospect of dozens or even hundreds of relatively inexpensive new genetic diagnostic tests emerging rapidly from the genome project has been held out as likely by both the project's advocates and its opponents. Many of these markers will identify genes related to common illnesses and other traits and conditions that were previously well outside prenatal health professionals' routine range of concern.

Various professional, political, and policy stances can influence the degree to which the introduction of more genetic markers into normal prenatal care is accepted, or indeed, encouraged. The question is, then, Will such markers actually improve the quality of prenatal care, and at what cost? The need for an answer to this question will only become more pressing if, as some hope, it soon becomes possible to screen maternal blood for fetal lymphocytes, which can be safely and easily subjected to testing with genetic markers.

Diagnostic Options

What prenatal diagnostic tests to pursue has always been something of a judgment question. Risks for Down syndrome and other chromosomal abnormalities increase precipitously at a maternal age of approximately thirty-five years, leading health care professionals to recommend amniocentesis at that point; nonetheless, the majority of infants with Down syndrome in the United States are actually born to younger mothers, where the frequency of chromosomal abnormalities is lower but the number of births is much higher. Alpha-fetoprotein screening is also becoming more common despite concerns about its low predictive value (requiring expensive follow-up testing for many women whose pregnancies will ultimately prove uneventful) and despite the absence of treatment (other than abortion) for many of the problems the screening identifies.

In addition, serious debate has attended consideration of both routine prenatal screening for HIV infection, which some health professionals advocate, and elective screening for identification of fetal sex, which some parents request for personal reasons (including the desire to abort a fetus of an unacceptable sex).

The fruits of the genome project hold the potential to multiply these options exponentially. We can reasonably expect the development of genetic probes for most major, early onset genetic diseases caused by a single gene, but researchers will also likely discover markers that provide some degree of information about the genetics of a wide range of other conditions, of varying severity and of complex etiology. In fact, genome project and other federally sponsored research has already led to the development of markers for late onset diseases such as Huntington chorea and adult onset polycystic kidney disease, as well as for susceptibility or vulnerability to various abnormal blood lipid patterns and certain forms of cancer.

Markers for these "contingent conditions"—conditions that are related to the presence of certain genes but not fully or immediately predicted by them—may turn out to be very plentiful. Moreover, markers will likely be available for behavioral conditions, such as schizophrenia and manic depressive disorder, and conditions of relatively minor severity, such as obesity, freckling, myopia, and some learning disorders. It will also be possible to identify carriers of recessive and sex-linked disorders; they will not themselves manifest the condition, but they will be capable of transmitting its gene(s) to future generations.

Which of these markers to develop into diagnostic tests for widespread use has already proved to be a difficult question for postnatal populations. For example, widespread screening for adult carriers of cystic fibrosis was recently discouraged by two national scientific organizations after substantial study, despite great media excitement about the new developments and the readiness of several biotechnology firms to begin marketing their new diagnostic probes.

Moving the question to prenatal populations introduces several additional layers of complication. First, it is much less clear who is being served by diagnostic testing: is it the parents, who acquire information about their pregnancy and subsequent offspring, or is it the offspring, considered as a second (fetal, embryonic, or preembryonic) patient?

Similarly, how are the benefits and burdens of testing to be estimated? Can we say anything intelligent about the importance of diagnosing late onset and other contingent conditions, or conditions of limited severity? What about conditions for which successful postnatal treatment is available? And, again, whose perspective on benefits and burdens should we consider: the parents'? the offspring's? geneticists'? other health professionals'? society's?

We can also responsibly ask, Should any limits be placed on the availability of such probes or the use of such information? Will parents understand what the markers do and do not offer in terms of diagnosis and prognosis? Do we want to have large panels of markers available for prenatal use? Are we willing to have pregnancy decisions, including abortion, turn on the presence or absence of genes for late onset conditions, contingent conditions, or conditions of limited or questionable severity? And, finally, who will pay for whatever testing is available?

Planning for the Introduction of New Markers

One of the main grounds offered in support of efforts to obtain funding for the genome project has been the potential for genetic information to improve medical care. Thus, the very existence of the project serves as an impetus to move newly discovered markers rapidly into the clinical arena. In the absence of prospective planning, new diagnostic tests will likely be introduced rapidly, in response to both market and professional forces.

The market forces are obvious: if biotechnology firms own patents on either the new markers or on techniques for bringing them into the clinical arena, there are clear financial incentives to make testing a more routine part of prenatal care.

The professional forces are also straightforward. First, there is a general tendency in medicine to view new developments, especially those perceived to be of low risk, as beneficial. Despite theoretical support for pilot studies and even randomized clinical trials of new diagnostic or dierapeutic interventions, many clinicians assume that care will be improved by offering the new "services," and they are frequently reluctant to wait for formal evaluations of them. Of course, the Food and Drug Administration includes formal testing in the process for licensing new drugs, but its jurisdiction over and willingness to review diagnostic tests arising from the genome project are uncertain.

Perhaps more importantly, health care professionals providing prenatal care may feel compelled to use new tests as soon as they become available so they can obtain increased security against possible malpractice suits for failure to diagnose a given condition. The fear of possible wrongful birth suits (and "wrongful life" suits in the few states that allow children as well as parents a cause of action) has been cited as a major factor in the dissemination of alpha-fetoprotein screening, and harried clinicians may attempt to reduce their perceived threat of liability by offering the broadest possible panel of diagnostic tests. This problem is exacerbated by the current absence of any professional or societal guidance about which tests should be considered essential, and which optional, unnecessary, or relatively contraindicated. Even if patients are offered the option of refusing testing, in the absence of mechanisms to provide education about the value of obtaining various types of genetic information, the tendency will likely be for patients to accept everything available, since that is what appears to be recommended." Moreover, when ignorance is the only alternative, patients may actually prefer a full range of "information," no matter what its relevance and quality.

Providing Guidance

Traditionally, the ethics of prenatal genetic counseling has required that prospective parents be given full information and then be allowed to choose which, if any, genetic diagnostic tests to pursue. Out of respect for reproductive decisionmaking and genetic privacy, and to prevent abuses such as attempts at eugenic control, virtually all genetic counselors espouse the ideals of value-neutral counseling and autonomous decisionmaking. This model is theoretically extremely appealing, and it works well in settings where well-trained counselors are available and affordable, and where counselors and clients share a common cultural background.

Yet the demands of routine prenatal care make it difficult simply to transpose this ethical framework into the obstetric or primary care clinic. The volume of patients is large, there is little enough time as it is to attend to patients' physical and psychological needs, and there are frequently quite prominent gaps between the social and cultural backgrounds of prenatal health care professionals and their patients. Moreover, genetic counselors have in the past generally been able, based on specific clinical indications, to focus their attention on one disease or syndrome at a time, while in the future, decisionmaking will likely encompass a broad spectrum of conditions for which prospective parents may be at no particularly increased risk. In the language of public health specialists, the issue will thus be one of *screening* rather than *testing.*

There are also matters of substance that argue in favor of a new model for providing guidance to prospective parents. Most importantly, the benefits of widespread screening have yet to be documented, and there are potential burdens that also need investigation, including increased anxiety about the pregnancy or about the parent's own health, risks associated with follow-up testing, possible changes in insurance coverage, overall increased costs, and the general effect on families and society of having parents prospectively evaluate their offspring in this fashion. Thus, while *access* to a broad range of genetic screening should remain available to those who specifically request it, new markers should not be offered as part of normal prenatal care.

Who, then, should decide which markers to incorporate into routine practice? Individual health professionals are poorly suited, both because of financial and liability pressures and because most lack sufficient information to guide such decisionmaking. Geneticists have a useful role to play, but are likely to be reluctant to issue sweeping recommendations without public input lest they rekindle fears of eugenics. Regulatory agencies are too insulated and also too bureaucratic, lacking the flexibility that will be necessary if recommendations are to be based on information somewhat less rigorous than formal pilot studies and controlled trials.

The default solution would be to let financial matters take precedence, considering as routine only those markers that are covered through state or federal funding or through private insurance. Yet this alternative too is unresponsive to the desire to have public input into decisionmaking, and it is unclear that it would totally alleviate clinicians' concerns about liability.

No doubt a perfect solution is unattainable. A reasonable pragmatic approach, however, might be to seek out the guidance of professional genetics and genetic counseling organizations, asking them to help develop procedures for gathering information, generating interdisciplinary and public comment, and making nonbinding recommendations about which tests *need* to be offered routinely in order to meet standards of normal prenatal care. Examples of such a process can be seen in the American Academy of Pediatrics' "Red Book Committee," which publishes recommendations for routine pediatric immunization practices, and the American Fertility Society's Committee on Ethics, which has formulated voluntary but highly influential guidelines for those involved in infertility services and research. For genetic screening issues, substantial collaboration with consumer groups, such as the Alliance of Genetic Support Groups, would be essential to insure a balanced representation of values. Such efforts could proceed at both the state and federal level, perhaps with funding from the genome project itself.

Leaving the Garden

When Adam and Eve ate of the fruit of the tree of knowledge of good and evil, they were expelled from the Garden of Paradise and entered a world of suffering and toil. So too may we be leaving behind what some would consider blissful days of ignorance about our future genetic legacies. We will soon have the power to evaluate ourselves and our prospective offspring, to peer into previously opaque genetic mysteries, to gain an understanding that seems clear. Whether we will reap benefits from seeking this knowledge, collectively and as individuals, is still quite uncertain. Thus, if we truly seek wisdom, we must consider most carefully in what manner and how deeply we will taste the genome project's tempting fruits.

QUESTIONS FOR CONSIDERATION

1. Nolan identifies one of the first fruits of the Human Genome Project to be new markers for genetic traits and diseases. Why does she believe a national standard for introducing and funding new genetic tests in prenatal care should be developed?

2. Characterize the "enormous change" she believes genetic diagnostic tests will have on prenatal care over the next two decades.

3. Nolan believes the Human Genome Project will multiply the diagnostic options currently available exponentially. What did she mean by markers for "contingent conditions"? Why would such markers differ in significance from traditional genetic tests? How do you respond to her question regarding "who is being served by diagnostic testing"?

4. What does Nolan see as the role of market and professional forces upon the new developments in biotechnology? How could the failure to administer the new tests result in "wrongful birth suits"?

5. What are the complications of prenatal genetic counseling Nolan identifies with widespread genetic screening? What is the "reasonable pragmatic approach" she recommends?

Elaine Draper

Genetic Secrets: Social Issues of Medical Screening in a Genetic Age

In the 1990s, as the multi-billion-dollar Human Genome Project has made more and more genetic information available, we would do well to look closely at the social context of power dynamics, control, and economic interests within which that information will be used.

Let us consider four specific questions. How does social stratification by race, ethnicity, gender, and social class affect the use of genetic information in the workplace? In what ways are perspectives on genetic testing socially located? What can fetal exclusion policies teach us about how genetic information might be used to identify high-risk individuals? What social and political challenges are posed by new information about genetic abnormalities, and how might that information be distributed fairly?

The Genetic Scarlet Letter

Genetic information can be used to screen workers who might be predisposed to disease. In pre-employment genetic testing, job applicants who have genetic traits such as G–6–PD deficiency or sickle cell trait can be screened out of jobs for two main reasons: to prevent on-the-job health damage to especially vulnerable individuals, and to protect employers from the medical costs and possible lawsuits that stem from worker disease.

Employers have a strong interest in requiring employees to report any genetic traits that may make them more vulnerable to work hazards, in part because such information may absolve management of responsibility for contributing to workers' disease. Even when employers are reluctant to use genetic information to exclude workers, insurers may pressure companies to collect genetic information and to differentiate between high-risk and low-risk individuals. Within an employment context, management typically has access to much of the information from medical tests that employees undergo. When physicians are employed by private corporations, their legal responsibility to keep test results confidential has been quite limited: in the workplace, genetic information is unlikely to be kept secret.

As genetic information accumulates, spurred on by the Human Genome Project's resources, many more people will find themselves stigmatized as a bad risk for employment, sometimes with grave economic consequences for themselves and their families. They may find it virtually impossible to obtain health insurance. They may also be stigmatized within their families and friendship circles. Thus employment and the broader social context of medical testing will have a strong effect on how people perceive the possible benefits and dangers of genetic information.

Employers and insurance companies treat individuals they identify as high risk in ways that depend not simply on biology, but on race, ethnicity, and gender. For example, G–6-PD deficiency and sickle cell trait are found in higher proportions among blacks, so that screening out people with those traits will mean screening out a disproportionate number of blacks. They claim to be screening out only individuals who may be genetically susceptible to damage from working conditions. But in using genetic information they are more likely to exclude people from relatively high-paying jobs, and the individuals screened out are most likely to be blacks or women, who have entered those jobs in large numbers only in recent years.[1] Thus in airline, chemical, and steel companies, blacks or women have been identified as genetically at high risk in relatively high-paying production jobs, which they have entered only recently. But in those same companies and in many others, genetic information has seldom been used to screen people out of low-paying, hazardous jobs.

Lessons from Johnson Controls

The *Johnson Controls* case that the Supreme Court decided in 1991 is instructive for understanding how genetic information is used to identify high-risk groups. The Johnson Controls Company, which manufactures batteries, had a policy of excluding fertile women from relatively high-paying jobs that involve exposure to lead, in the belief that exposing women to lead might damage fetuses. The company was also concerned that they could be sued for damage to the fetus. The employer excluded all women except those who showed proof of surgical sterilization. The Supreme Court ruled in a unanimous decision that it is unlawful discrimination to ban all fertile women from specific jobs because of possible fetal damage.[2] Two points about this case relate to our discussion of health risk and genetic information.

First, even if it can be shown that a particular group is at high risk because of their biology, there may be many others at risk and we should not lose sight of that important fact in conducting research, in setting priorities for fighting disease, and in putting forth alternative social policies. At Johnson Controls, only women were being excluded from lead exposure on preliminary indications of hazards to fetuses, even though there is strong evidence of the damage that lead causes to all adults, and some evidence of damage to children whose *fathers* have been exposed. In the case of genetic screening, it may be true that some workers are somewhat more likely than others to develop disease. But typically the exposures in question are carcinogenic or otherwise toxic to all workers. In *Johnson Controls,* the Supreme Court ruled that employers should not discriminate against only one possible high-risk group. In the case of genetic screening for susceptibility, rather than put considerable time, research, and money into gathering information on genetically high-risk groups, more effort could be focused on reducing the hazard to the work force and general public.

The second insight we might derive from fetal exclusion policies concerns individual choice. The justices were unwilling to give fetuses priority over women's right to equal employment opportunity. The Court held that women's employment choices had been unfairly curtailed by a policy that systematically excluded them from jobs which are clearly hazardous to both men and women as well as to fetuses. But the rhetoric of choice raises complicated questions. To what extent should people be allowed to endanger themselves or their children for wages? Given the fact of limited job opportunity and the economic necessity of working, is it sufficient to inform individuals that they may be at special risk genetically, and that they have a "choice" to keep or quit a hazardous job?

The skewed framing of genetic risk—which in practice excludes racial minorities and women from relatively high-paying jobs—penalizes economically disadvantaged groups and deepens divisions in society based on race, ethnicity, and gender. Further, when new genetic information makes a person appear to be at high risk, he or she is likely to experience as a personal medical problem what is in fact a social problem—a social dynamic that reflects stratification in the broader society by race, gender, and social class. Workers also have little access to the aggregate genetic data which may show that specific racial or ethnic groups are disproportionately screened out. This makes it even more difficult to recognize the social dimensions of genetic screening that go beyond issues of medical risks to individuals.

Social Place and Point of View

The belief that gaining information regarding individual risks should be given a high priority is not universally shared, and beliefs in this area are shaped by economic and other social interests. Four examples will help make this point.

1. As part of a study on genetic testing in the workplace, I found that corporate managers tend to support genetic screening technologies that labor opposes.[3] Employers and scientists working for corporations maintain that workers and labor officials oppose genetic screening out of technophobia, an ideological distrust based on fear and ignorance. But workers do not condemn all genetic testing in principle. Organized labor does generally oppose genetic screening for inherited traits, where the unspoken agenda is to exclude people from jobs and to blame workers' diseases on genetic susceptibility, but it tends to favor genetic monitoring, which seeks to uncover genetic damage from pollutants. The charge of technophobia is largely false and obscures the real reasons some types of people oppose and others favor screening workers' genes. An individual's economic interests and position in the labor force tell us a great deal more. They tell us whether he or she is likely to support screening for genetic defects or, in contrast, to support a focus on conditions that affect workers in general, not just those with specific genetic traits.

2. Employers and many scientists in corporations tend to subscribe to what I call a new genetic orthodoxy, which acknowledges that both genetics and the environment contribute to disease, but in fact represents a model of genetic causation. Scientists and employers who favor genetic screening no longer say that genes alone cause disease, for that would make them appear to be extremists. Instead, they mention occasionally that disease may have an environmental component, but then focus on the genetics and routinely ignore the environmental contributions. For example, sickle cell disease is called "genetic" despite the fact that it protects people against the environmental threat of malaria; PKU is called "genetic" even though it can be effectively prevented through diet; and spina bifida is called "genetic" despite the fact that it is found in very high concentrations in areas of high industrial pollution, such as South Wales.[4] Despite considerable evidence of the importance of environmental factors, employers and many scientists genetic screening, of course, are far less likely to share this faith.

3. The views of scientists on important social questions about health risk and information tend to differ dramatically depending on where they work. With regard to health hazards in the workplace, for example, Frances Lynn's 1986 survey indicates that scientists who work in corporations are very likely

to share opinions held by corporate executives—for example, that chemicals are overregulated and that current work exposure causes little disease. In contrast, scientists employed by universities seldom hold these views. Government scientists fall midway between these two groups in their views regarding health risks.[5] It is true that corporations, government, and universities each attract different kinds of people, but these differences are likely to become much greater once employers, coworkers, the political environment, and economic interests come into play on the job.

4. A fourth example concerns estimates of cancer causation. Estimates of the proportion of cancer cases attributable to work and the environment range from 40 percent to less than 1 percent; estimates of the percentage attributable to genetic factors also range widely. In our current climate of scientific uncertainty, which estimates are to be believed? It turns out that employers are much more likely than workers to believe that job applicants should be excluded from jobs because of genetic information obtained through screening.[6] One's employment, social networks, and economic interests affect whether one believes that inborn genetic defects cause a large proportion of cancer, that we must seek much more genetic information to help us determine who are individuals at high risk, or that high-risk individuals should be excluded from jobs.

The Burden of Genetic Information

Our system of stratification by social class as well as by race and ethnicity helps to determine the way genetic information is generated and applied. Social dynamics pertaining to power and wealth—as expressed in rules limiting access to information, in the practices of insurance companies, and in the hiring and medical testing practices of employers—contribute to genetic information's being used in ways that deepen economic and racial inequality. Currently, workers bear not only the health burden of occupational disease but also its costs. In 1990 OSHA counted almost 300,000 new cases of occupational disease. Most of the expense of this disease and disability is not borne by employers, but by individuals, their families, and the public in the form of Social Security and disability. Since there is little evidence that genetic screening can make a significant contribution to reducing this burden, how can we, as a society, begin to deal with it more equitably? There are, I believe, four directions in which we can make progress.

First, priorities in health policy could be redirected toward reducing disease without needlessly penalizing individuals and groups perceived to be genetically at high risk. For example, reducing exposure hazards through engineering controls on chemical emissions can make the workplace safer for everyone. This approach reduces risk without falsely making it appear that individuals' genetic inheritance is the problem, when in fact broad health hazards continue to arise from environmental conditions. Beyond the workplace too the search for genetic predisposition should not limit the use of effective and widely recognized but underfunded strategies for reducing disease. Second, the scientific merits of screening for genetic abnormalities could be investigated more carefully. Genetic traits should be linked to disease risks only when there is a sound scientific reason for doing so. Excitement over scientific breakthroughs and the potential uses of new genetic information produces a halo effect for proposed genetic screening tests, but employers and scientists need solid evidence to support their claim that an individual or a group is in danger and must be removed from the workplace. Companies should be accountable for their claims that there are special risks to which only certain individuals are subject. Further, genetic tests should be truly predictive and should be related to relatively common exposures and ailments. This is true whether genetic information pertains to the workplace or to more general health risks.

Third, individuals have the right to know the results of medical tests and the disease risks they face. Expanding patients' and workers' access to information about their own health is important but by no means sufficient. Most employees now have the right to obtain medical records if they request them, so they can find out what genetic tests have been conducted. But workers also need independent evidence of health hazards, for otherwise they cannot evaluate employers' warnings of hazards or assurances of safety. Moreover, individuals should have the right to keep their test results confidential much more frequently than current laws provide.

Fourth, and finally, even individuals with access to new genetic test results need more protection than information alone can give them. As genetic information expands with the Human Genome Project, individuals increasingly will be identified as at low risk or high risk for a widening array of diseases. Measures could be instituted to limit the discriminatory effects of exclusionary policies based on genetic information. The impact of the power dynamics and economic interests I have discussed should be acknowledged. If we recognize that most jobs are fundamentally insecure and that current evidence regarding links between genetic abnormalities and occupational health hazards is uncertain, we can see the value of protecting workers who are removed for reasons related to their health. In some cases certain individuals *may be* at special risk.

These workers could be given other jobs if any are available, but in no case should they lose their pay, benefits, or seniority. Meanwhile, the company could be setting up engineering controls to reduce exposure and collecting scientific information on ways to prevent harmful effects. A good model is the OSHA lead standard, which has medical removal and rate retention provisions that offer this protection. Without such provisions, any worker or group who is removed is heavily penalized.

Genetic information and environmental health hazards do not simply present questions of policy. They also present questions of power: for example, who can enforce the distribution of costs associated with a policy change? New policies for controlling health hazards and for preventing genetic secrets from being divulged inappropriately will emerge only from a complex process of legal challenges, government regulation, education, and collective bargaining. Government and employer decisions as to which policies are chosen, and how they are carried out, will depend only in part on the scientific evidence of genetic risks. They will also be shaped in significant ways by the social and political terrain on which employment and medical decisions are made. We must make this recognition a part of our public discourse.

QUESTIONS FOR CONSIDERATION

1. What does Draper mean by the expression, "the genetic scarlet letter"? What concerns does she identify with genetic screening in the workplace?
2. How does Draper reason that genetic screening will likely exclude women and blacks? Does the *Johnson Controls* case illustrate her point? How does this case also exemplify limits on individual choice?
3. What does Draper mean by "a new genetic orthodoxy"? How does she contrast the views of management and labor with regard to genetic screening?
4. Draper calls for a more equitable distribution of the burden of disease and disability, especially in light of the additional burden of genetic information. What are the ways she suggests would make the burden more equitable?

NOTES

1. Elaine Draper, *Risky Business: Genetic Testing and Exclusionary Practices in the Hazardous Workplace* (New York: Cambridge University Press, 1991). The study draws on interviews with 120 U.S. scientists and managers, government and union officials, and production workers.

2. *United Automobile Workers v. Johnson Controls, Inc.* 111 S. Ct. 1 196 (1991).

3. Draper, *Risky Business.*

4. See Troy Duster, *Back Door to Eugenics* (New York: Routledge, Chapman, and Hall, 1990); and Edward J. Calabrese, *Ecogenetics: Genetic Variation in Susceptibility to Environmental Agents* (New York: John Wiley and Sons, 1984).

5. Frances M. Lynn, "The Interplay of Science and Values in Assessing and Regulating Environmental Risks," *Science, Technology, and Human Values 11*, no. 2 (Spring 1986): 40–50.

6. See Richard Peto and Marvin Schneiderman, eds., *Quantification of Occupational Cancer Banbury* 9 (Cold Spring Harbor, N.Y: Cold Spring Harbor Laboratory, 1981); and Draper, *Risky Business.*

C. Keith Boone

Bad Axioms in Genetic Engineering

The parade of wonders mounted by biological science marches by at an increasingly rapid pace. In a kind of mimicry of Genesis, we have synthesized a living, functioning gene from shelf chemicals in the laboratory. Through improved cloning techniques we are able to produce exact copies of lower life forms—genetic replicas down to the very shape and location of spots on the backs of leopard frogs. Even more significantly, recent techniques for gene mapping and recombination ("gene splicing") are throwing open doors to the treatment of diseases, ecological control, and the technological production of a wide range of goods from pharmaceuticals to peanuts.

In short, we are now able to control the destinies of ourselves, our offspring, and our environment in ways that are much more direct and trait-specific than previously imagined.

Profound and fascinating moral dilemmas accompany the new biotechnical achievements, particularly those that involve manipulating the human genome, going to the very heart of who we are and how we think about ourselves. Many have argued that our technical advances have outpaced our ability to deal ethically with them. But they have not said why this is so, or what we ought to do about it. In fact, no ethical tradition seems sufficient to comprehend either the peculiarity of the genetic dilemma or the multiplicity of moral conundrums it presents.

New Moral Challenges

The new methods of genetic engineering pose difficult ethical problems in part because they offer technological options that never before existed. Still, it is not the *fact* of options that is problematic, but rather their nature. What revisionist social philosophers and theologians of hope have described as the category of the novum, the generation of the qualitatively new, independent of any organic evolution from what already exists, has seen its first genuine demonstration in the realm of the biological sciences. Inasmuch as many of the new genetic techniques allow scientists to bypass *development* in creating novel life forms, some scientific achievements can be appreciated only in these nonorganic, nonontologic terms. In the new biology, we confront in its most irreducible form the direct, minute, and purposeful design of life. That fact presents us with moral problems that are not just new in history, but new in kind.

As it applies specifically to human genetic manipulations, genetic engineering presents an unprecedented technological leap from merely designing the environment to "designing the designer."[1] These prospects threaten wholly to subvert traditional philosophical paradigms and undermine the standard ethical touchstones of "human nature," "humanity," and "rationality." These would become synthetic products rather than points of common reference. Of course, this scenario would result from proposed eugenic manipulations to alter human capacities in "positive" ways. It may be precisely such scenarios that give us a distinct basis for deciding where we would balk at further interventions.

An additional complicating feature is that genetic engineering is not a single problem at all, but rather a complex set of problems occurring in quite different domains of inquiry—epidemiological, ecological, evolutionary, human-genetic, and political. Many of the original concerns about recombinant DNA arose on the epidemiological level, involving fears about the accidental dissemination of altered, pathogenic bacteria for which there is no known antidote. And fear of the consequences of human germline alteration led fifty-six clergy and several scientists in 1983 to adopt a "Resolution," delivered to Congress, requesting a ban on all such interventions.

Finally, what Willard Gaylin has called the "Frankenstein factor" has influenced the tone of the genetic debate in negative ways. The specter of new life forms somehow "threatens our sense of identity, our sense of uniqueness, and our sense of primacy among the creatures of the earth."[2] Perhaps this is as it should be, that some nonrational element in our respect for extant genomes be maintained alongside our rational affirmations of them. But to the extent that these premonitions become exaggerated beyond what the facts can support, they tend to generate peremptory condemnations. The recombinant DNA controversy in this country was instantly polarized by disputants who charged that scientists were conspiring to create the master race and take control of our genetic futures. In response, many scientists joined battle and categorized their critics as anti-science ideologues.

Bad Axioms

The combination of these characteristics of genetic engineering—its newness, its potential for manipulation of the "human," its complexity, and its capacity for arousing fear and recrimination—has proven fertile soil for the growth of an assortment of bad axioms whose distinguishing feature is that they are reductionistic. They substitute invocation of formula for careful analysis and in the process cut off precisely the kind of balanced scrutiny called for by this complex set of problems.

It is not the case that bad axioms contain no truth, however. Quite the contrary, it is their tendency to encapsulate a partial truth that makes them alluring. The problem with bad axioms is precisely their power to convince the hearer that a partial insight comprises the whole truth, that looking through a single porthole provides panoramic vision. Thus the initial step in an appropriate ethical assessment of genetic prospects is to identify the axioms that have most obscured the issues. The second step is to consign them, as *axioms,* to history. The final step is to discern what element of truth they may contain in their nonaxiomatic forms.

Playing God

In the Jewish and Christian traditions "playing God" is characteristically associated with pride and arrogance, the aping of divine power, or the attempt to gain salvation without the help of the divinity. It is not the *use* of power and creativity that offends, but rather attributing power to one's own resources, denying its origin in what Jews and Christians believe is God's continuing creation. Those who object to any genetic medicine on religious grounds need to be clear that "playing God" is not, in this usage, an act against morality, but rather one against faith. Its verbal counterpart is blasphemy. However, it would not seem that individual genetic pursuits would be forbidden in any necessary sense, unless the motive were an attempt to stand in God's place. Therapeutic interventions are, in fact, consonant with the benevolent, other-regarding impulses of Judaism and Christianity.

Yet these traditions might well morally object to particular applications of genetic science, or point to problems with human conceits about our ability to predict or control the outcomes of our actions.

Such legitimate concerns are similar to those expressed in the secular usage of "playing God," in which the phrase is often used to remind us that it is only with caution that we should tamper with the most elemental organic forces in the universe. It intends to point to the great uncertainties we face as we consider how genetic science may eventually shape our physical being, our social structure, and our moral culture.

If these sorts of concerns lie beneath "playing God," then the concept has valid standing. Used in this sense, it ceases to be a bad axiom insofar as it rightly recommends a cautionary posture. The appropriate response, however, is not that we should not "play God," but that we must do so intelligently. That is the essence of making choices, and it undeniably is our destiny, whether we choose to accept genetic options or reject them.

Interfering with Nature

There is nothing problematic in this axiom in its descriptive sense. *Homo faber* is, by definition, one who interacts with and reshapes the environment. But in the genetic context the phrase is often used as an indictment.

Behind such use of "interfering with nature" usually lies the notion that nature has a prescribed telos and a single program for reaching that telos. But it is not clear that the uncontrolled reign of nature produces the most humane world we can imagine. As molecular geneticist Stanley Cohen has noted, it is nature that gave us the genetic combinations for such afflictions as yellow fever, typhoid, and diabetes.[3] Humans have always danced a delicate ecological minuet with various other potent life forms, including bacteria and viruses. Deadly microorganisms have their own survivalistic ecology, and nowhere in nature's book is it written that human survival is the most preferred. The emergence of *Homo sapiens* in the evolutionary drama does not, according to biologists, represent a necessary, end-directed process. And we have always interfered with nature to protect the species and its likelihood, from the medical use of antibiotics to the draining of swamps that festered with malaria-bearing mosquitos.

The issue is not whether we interfere, but whether or not our incursions enhance or diminish the human prospect. Erwin Chargaff has put it eloquently: "This world is given to us on loan. We come and we go; and after a time we leave earth and air and water to others who come after us."[4] We have the ability to make genetic choices in symbiotic rhythm with nature, or to assault our contingent relationship with nature. We also have the ability to make intergenerationally sensitive choices or to take the short-term perspective.

This is not to underestimate the difficulty of deciding what is or is not an assault upon nature, particularly with regard to human genetic engineering. For example, whose definition of what is "natural" shall we accept? And as the President's Commission to study the question of gene splicing noted, the widely accepted belief that there is a fixed human genome is faulty, given that the "genetic basis of what is distinctively human continually changes through the interplay of random mutation and natural selection."[5] Our choices, then, should be based on some human conception of what is natural, not on a naturalistic definition of what is human. It is in the latter sense that the charge of "interfering with nature" becomes a bad axiom.

The truth in the axiom lies in its implicit invocation of the basic rule, *primum non nocere,* and in its explicit dual challenges for critical examination prior to action. First, it suggests an honest self-examination of motives for "intrusions" into the natural. Such motives can be venal and short-sighted, as has been frequently alleged against eugenics programs, or they can give relief to those who are or will be genetically crippled. Second, it suggests a careful examination of the external world for impacts and outcomes, not only on the physical, but on the social and cultural environments as well.

Slippery Slopes

Those who use the "slippery slope" argument seem to imply two principles at work, one of momentum and one of logic. The principle of momentum states that, once you perform X, you will not be able to restrain yourself from doing Y, even though X does not necessarily imply Y. The principle of logic states that Y will inevitably follow from X, since doing X contains the *principle of permission* for doing Y. It is the latter that is more ethically relevant and seems to be operative in the following passage from the "Resolution":

> Once we decide to begin the process of human genetic engineering, there is really no logical place to stop. If diabetes, sickle cell anemia, and cancer are to be cured by altering the genetic make-up of an individual, why not proceed to other "disorders": myopia, color blindness, left handedness. Indeed, what is to preclude a society from deciding that a certain skin color is a disorder? . . . What is the price we pay for embarking on a course whose final goal is the "perfection" of the human species?[6]

This line of reasoning mistakenly assumes that beginning the process of human genetic engineering means carrying it through to any conceivable application. It claims that if the principle of permission allows *some* kinds of interventions it will hold for all kinds of interventions. But morally to endorse positive eugenic measures would require justification by a very different, and certainly more disputable, principle. There is a seismic moral difference between treating leukemia and enhancing IQ, and to recognize that difference is one of the preeminent purposes of moral reasoning. The moral gulf between these two classes of action suggests that there is, in fact, a "logical place to stop"; it is just prior to the leap from therapeutic to eugenic measures. Once this boundary has been crossed, then there really is no logical place to stop. To be sure, in practice there are gray areas in what constitutes "eugenics." The better part of wisdom may tell us that we should not enter even that territory.

When used to refer to genetic enhancement of characteristics, the slope argument is no longer a bad axiom. It functions correctly in alerting us to the fact that permission for one eugenic measure inevitably establishes the principle of permission for other eugenic measures. Once the new moral rationale is in place, license would be the order of the day. It is not clear what could prevent us at that point from engaging in genetic wanderlust.

To assert that our final goal is the "'perfection' of the human species" does not accurately report the motivation behind genetic research, except in the sense that all our endeavors aim at making the world a more hospitable place. Most of our genetic efforts are not even aimed at "final goals." They are more immediate attempts to find cures for diseases that disfigure, kill, or deny individuals the basic capacities to realize a minimally recognizable human existence. To deny afflicted individuals these therapies on the ground that we cannot make distinctions between remedial germline alterations and eugenic enhancements indicates a lack of trust in the human ability to act discriminately on the basis of distinctive ethical classifications.

The Ethical Neutrality of Science

Taken in its most literal sense, the claim that science is ethically neutral is accurate. We would be hard put to defend the proposition that knowledge alone has a moral value or disvalue. But the claim is not usually made in this pure sense. It almost always conveys the notion that scientists do not have responsibility for the production of knowledge. As Jacob Bronowski has noted, however, this belief confuses the *findings* of science, which are ethically neutral, with the *activity* of science, which is not.[7]

Even so, the argument continues, it is not the activity of science to which notions of responsibility attach, but rather to the applications of the products of that activity. Knowledge itself is value-neutral and "ambipotent"; for example, the same chemicals used to create nerve gases in the Great Wars turned out to be "elegant research weapons in the protein biochemistry revolution."[8] Therefore, the moral burden lies with those who choose to implement scientific information for ill purposes.

This argument combines a prima facie plausibility with some degree of disingenuity. The source of each is the attempt to form a cleavage between scientist *qua* scientist and scientist *qua* moral agent. But scientist *qua* scientist does not really exist except as a heuristic notion. The scientist in the laboratory is always moral agent at the same time that he or she is scientist. It is not possible for the scientist to hang the moral self on a coatrack on the way into the laboratory and then proceed indiscriminately with the scientific venture.

But in what precise sense is the scientist responsible for this production of knowledge? In his *Double Image of the Double Helix,* Clifford Grobstein distinguishes three kinds of research with recombinant DNA—basic, applied, and technological—and suggests that only the latter two be considered for any kind of external regulation, leaving the search for pure knowledge unfettered except for certain judicious forms of self-regulation.[9] Reasonable scientists may well agree with this recommendation, concurring that the connections between some kinds of applied or technological research and scientists' accountability can be readily established. For example, it is not hard to see the direct and predictable link between applied research on nerve gases and their use on human populations. But the same reasonable scientists may insist, along with Grobstein, that there is no such obvious connection between basic research and its unpredictable—perhaps even improbable—applications. Can the inventor of diesel engines be held responsible for Nazi submarines?

Still, the inability to predict the uses of pure knowledge does not relieve scientists of the responsibility for thinking in advance about how such knowledge might be used. The scientist, no less than other professionals, is required to exercise the "imagination principle" in projecting potential uses of scientific information."[10] I am speaking here of ordinary responsibility as a moral agent. In actual practice, scientists cannot be expected to think in terms of infinite causal chains into the future ("Only God can be a good utilitarian"). Since the eventual permutations of discovering pure knowledge are highly speculative, we would not expect to find frequent moral deterrence in the pursuit of basic knowledge. Nor is the moral responsibility to imagine uses the same as the moral responsibility to refrain from doing.

In its axiomatic form, then, the claim that scientific activity is ethically neutral is not accurate. Yet hidden within this bad axiom is often a more modest claim, that most knowledge may be used for good or ill, and that scientists should not shoulder the burden of responsibility for harmful applications. Corrupt persons, societies, and political regimes may misuse even the most innocent knowledge for deplorable ends, and therein lies considerable responsibility. If that is what is meant by the claim, then it ceases to be a bad axiom. Still, far from relieving scientists of all responsibility, it merely confirms that all share responsibility.

Genetics Is the Answer

For many, the biological revolution has signaled the dawn of a bold new era of omnipotence. The euphoria of the 1970s, generated by rapid developments in genetic science, was for many a result of prospective applications in medicine, reproduction, agriculture, industry, and pharmacology. For others, it was the result of imagining these heady genetic technologies as the long-awaited solutions to perennial human problems and aspirations. Theoretical biologist James Danielli contended that "from the point of view of genetics, man is a barbarian," and it is only such radical interventions as genetic alteration that will allow civilization to "advance to a modestly stable state."[11] In a recent letter to the *New York Times,* Robert Davis spotted divine intentionality behind the new genetic powers:

> God has put into our hands the possibility of what has so long been demanded by the great world religions, a change in man himself . . . . To succeed will be to begin a new and glorious stage in the history of what has been so defective a humanity.[12]

Among others, Joshua Lederberg and Joseph Fletcher have argued for the direct, asexual copying of superior human traits, or of entire individuals, in the place of the genetic dice roll of ordinary reproduction.

In both their milder and more extreme expressions, these views share hope for instant genetic remedies that are themselves problematic. There are no single, discrete genes that code the complex arrangements of proteins that produce given human traits; and to manipulate one is to change the original, fragile configuration in unforeseeable ways. But even if such Promethean methods were developed in the distant future, who would decide what traits should be preferred? Who would decide what makes a person a more fit specimen, and under what idealized plan for human harmony and well-being? What would be the criteria for choosing alternatives that seem to some a social boon, to others a form of dehumanization?

Use of genetic methods for positive, eugenic purposes should give us sudden pause for another reason. It would involve us in the historic and shameful confession that we have not been able to resolve problems of social intercourse in ways that rely on human intelligence and character. Whatever problems we may have defining what is "human," it would be clear that use of these technological shortcuts would signal the repudiation of our current human abilities—in both material and immaterial senses. The legitimate desire to improve the human lot need not evolve into this sort of collective humiliation. Long before teleological thirst deteriorates into technological lust, it will need tempering by the acknowledgment of human finitude and by the willful determination to resolve problems by means that realize human integrity, not ones that undermine it.

Every such argument for "technological fix" merits counterargument from the fact of technological tragedy. The latter occurs in at least three senses. First, all inventions are two-edged swords. The obvious example is nuclear energy; on balance, it is not clear that the capability to split the atom nets human good. A second sense of technological tragedy is summarized in Chargaff's complaint about the microorganisms produced through the inexact and serendipitous methods of gene splicing:

> You can stop splitting the atom; you can stop visiting the moon; you can stop using aerosols; you may even decide not to kill entire populations by the use of a few bombs. But you cannot recall a new form of life.[13]

It is not just new forms of life that are dubious in this respect, however. Once introduced, no unit of technological knowledge can be recalled, even if particular technologies can. In that sense, all technology is a new organism that insinuates itself into living cultures through altering them irrevocably.

Finally, the third meaning of technological tragedy is that technology's problem-solving innovations seem persistently to create new problems. What Reinhold Niebuhr articulated as a general social principle is equally true for genetic discovery: Every advance in the fulfillment of human aspirations creates problems at an entirely new level. An urgent example in the world of medical ethics is the host of moral dilemmas issuing from the new life-prolonging and resuscitative devices. We are still novices at resolving the legion of problems that accompany these otherwise beneficent technologies.

Of course, the fact that technology creates rich and challenging new problems is in no way determinative for the case against invention, either in genetics or in any other pursuit. But it does serve us notice to be perspicacious in the applications of science, and temperate in our expectations of it. Knowledge of tragic implications need not and should not paralyze action. To "know sin" is our ineluctable fate and fortune, and to lose nerve in the face of such knowledge would only enlarge the tragedy. On the other hand, that knowledge should take some of the color out of glib fantasies about what genetic science will do for us, as well as inform moral decisions about what we want to do with it.

QUESTIONS FOR CONSIDERATION

1. Explain Boone's expression "bad axioms" with regard to genetic engineering. Why do such axioms have the power to convince those who hear them?
2. Why does Boone consider the expression "playing God" to be a bad axiom? What would be an appropriate use of that expression relative to genetic engineering?
3. How does Boone criticize the axiom "interfering with nature"? What did he mean by the statement, ". . . nowhere in nature's book is it written that human survival is the most preferred"?
4. What are the two principles of the slippery slope argument related to genetic engineering? How does Boone respond to these two principles?
5. How does Boone characterize "the ethical neutrality of science"? What is the significance of Grobstein's three kinds of research? What is the moral burden that scientists share?
6. In responding to the axiom "genetics is the answer," Boone identifies three technological tragedies. How does he respond to each of these tragedies?

NOTES

1. Leon Kass notes that "engineering the engineer seems to differ in kind from engineering his engine," "The New Biology: What Price Relieving Man's Estate?," *Science* 174 (November 19,1971), 780.

2. Willard Gaylin, "The Frankenstein Factor," *New England Journal of Medicine* 97:12 (September 22, 1977), 665–66.

3. Stanley Cohen, "Recombinant DNA: Fact and Fiction," *Science* 195 (February 18,1977), 655.

4. Erwin Chargaff, "On the Dangers of Genetic Meddling." *Science* 192 June 14, 1976), 904.

5. President's Commission for the Study of Ethical Problems in Medicine and Biomedical and Behavioral Research, Splicing *Life: A Report on the Social and Ethical Issues of Genetic Engineering with Human* Beings (Washington, DC: U.S. Government Printing Office, 1982), 70.

6. Jeremy Rifkin, "Resolution" (June 8, 1983), Foundation on Economic Trends.

7. Jacob Bronowski, *The Identity of Man* (Garden City, NY.: Doubleday Press, 1965), ix. Quoted in William Lowrance, *Modern Science and Human Values* (New York: Oxford University Press, 1985), 5.

8. Lowrance, *Modern Science*, p. 5, uses this example to show the dual uses of scientific knowledge, not to argue that science is value-neutral, a position with which he does not identify.

9. Clifford Grobstein, *Double Image of the Double Helix* (San Francisco: W. H. Freeman and Company, 1979).

10. Daniel Callahan, "The Social Responsibility of Science in the Face of Uncertain Consequences," *Annals of the New York Academy of Science* 265 (January 23, 1976), 4.

11. James Danielli, "Industry, Society, and Genetic Engineering," *Hastings Center Report* 2:6 (December 1972), 5–7.

12. Robert Davis, "What New Adam Lurks Inside the Gene Splice?," *New York Times,* March 15, 1987.

13. Chargaff. "On the Dangers of Genetic Meddling," 938.

W. FRENCH ANDERSON

Genetics and Human Malleability

Just how much can, and should we change human nature . . . by genetic engineering? Our response to that hinges on the answers to three further questions: (1) What *can* we do now? Or more precisely, what *are* we doing now in the area of human genetic engineering? (2) What *will* we be able to do? In other words, what technical advances are we likely to achieve over the next five to ten years? (3) What *should* we do? I will argue that a line can be drawn and should be drawn to use gene transfer only for the treament of serious disease, and not for any other purpose. Gene transfer should never be undertaken in an attempt to enhance or "improve" human beings.

What Can We Do?

In 1980 John Fletcher and I published a paper in the *New England Journal of Medicine* in which we delineated what would be necessary before it would be ethical to carry out human gene therapy.[1] As with any other new therapeutic procedure, the fundamental principle is that it should be determined in advance that the probable benefits outweigh the probable risks. We analyzed the risk/benefit determination for somatic cell gene therapy and proposed three questions that need to have been answered from prior animal experimentation: Can the new gene be inserted stably into the correct target cells? Will the new gene be expressed (that is, function) in the cells at an appropriate level? Will the new gene harm the cell or the animal? These criteria are very similar to those required before use of any new therapeutic procedure, surgical operation, or drug. They simply require that the new treatment should get to the area of disease, correct it, and do more good than harm.

A great deal of scientific progress has occurred in the nine years since that paper was published. The technology does now exist for inserting genes into some types of target cells.[2] The procedure being used is called "retroviral-mediated gene transfer." In brief, a disabled murine retrovirus serves as a delivery vehicle for transporting a gene into a population of cells that have been removed from a patient. The gene-engineered cells are then returned to the patient.

The first clinical application of this procedure was approved by the National Institutes of Health and the Food and Drug Administration on January 19, 1989.[3] Our protocol received the most thorough prior review of any clinical protocol in history: It was approved only after being reviewed fifteen times by seven different regulatory bodies. In the end it received unanimous approval from every one of those committees. But the simple fact that the NIH and FDA, as well as the public, felt that the protocol needed such extensive review demonstrates that the concept of gene therapy raises serious concerns.

We can answer our initial question, "What can we do now in the area of human genetic engineering?," by examining this approved clinical protocol. Gene transfer is used to mark cancer-fighting cells in the body as a way of better understanding a new form of cancer therapy. The cancer-fighting cells are called TIL (tumor-infiltrating-lymphocytes), and are isolated from a patient's own tumor, grown up to a large number, and then given back to the patient along with one of the body's immune growth factors, a molecule called interleukin 2 (IL–2). The procedure, developed by Steven Rosenberg of the NIH, is known to help about half the patients treated.[4]

The difficulty is that there is at present no way to study theTIL once they are returned to the patient to determine why they work when they do work (that is, kill cancer cells), and why they do not work when they do not work. The goal of the gene transfer protocol was to put a label on the infused TIL that is, to mark these cells so that they could be studied in blood and tumor specimens from the patient over time.

The TIL were marked with a vector (called N2) containing a bacterial gene that could be easily identified through recombinant DNA techniques. Our protocol was called, therefore, the N2—TIL Human Gene Transfer Clinical Protocol. The first patient received gene-marked TIL on May 22, 1989. Five patients have now received marked cells. No side effects or problems have thus far arisen from the gene transfer portion of the therapy. Useful data on the fate of the gene-marked TIL are being obtained.

But what was done that was new? Simply, a single gene was inserted into a population of cells that had been obtained from a patient's body. There are an estimated 100,000 genes in every human cell. Therefore the actual addition of material was extremely minute, nothing to correspond to the fears expressed by some that human beings would be "reengineered." Nonetheless, a functioning piece of genetic material was successfully inserted into human cells and the gene-engineered cells did survive in human patients.

What Will We Be Able to Do?

Although only one clinical protocol is presently being conducted, it is clear that there are several applications for gene transfer that probably will be carried out over the next five to ten years. Many genetic diseases that are caused by a defect in a single gene should be treatable, such as ADA deficiency (a severe immune deficiency disease of children), sickle cell anemia, hemophilia, and Gaucher disease. Some types of cancer, viral diseases such as AIDS, and some forms of cardiovascular disease are targets for treatment by gene therapy. In addition, germline gene therapy, that is, the insertion of a gene into the reproductive cells of a patient, will probably be technically possible in the foreseeable future. My position on the ethics of germline gene therapy is published elsewhere.[5] But successful somatic cell gene therapy also opens the door for enhancement genetic engineering, that is, for supplying a specific characteristic that individuals might want for themselves (somatic cell engineering) or their children (germline engineering) which would not involve the treatment of a disease. The most obvious example at the moment would be the insertion of a growth hormone gene into a normal child in the hope that this would make the child grow larger. Should parents be allowed to choose (if the science should ever make it possible) whatever useful characteristics they wish for their children?

What Should We Do?

A line can and should be drawn between somatic cell gene therapy and enhancement genetic engineering.[6] Our society has repeatedly demonstrated that it can draw a line in biomedical research when necessary. The Belmont Report illustrates how guidelines were formulated to delineate ethical from unethical clinical research and to distinguish clinical research from clinical practice. Our responsibility is to determine how and where to draw lines with respect to genetic engineering.

Somatic cell gene therapy for the treatment of severe disease is considered ethical because it can be supported by the fundamental moral principle of beneficence: It would relieve human suffering. Gene therapy would be, therefore, a moral good. Under what circumstances would human genetic engineering not be a moral good? In the broadest sense, when it detracts from, rather than contributes to, the dignity of man. Whether viewed from a theological perspective or a secular humanist one, the justification for drawing a line is founded on the argument that, beyond the line, human values that our society considers important for the dignity of man would be significantly threatened.

Somatic cell enhancement engineering would threaten important human values in two ways: It could be medically hazardous, in that the risks could exceed the potential benefits and the procedure therefore cause harm. And it would be morally precarious, in that it would require moral decisions our society is not now prepared to make, and it could lead to an increase in inequality and discriminatory practices.

Medicine is a very inexact science. We understand roughly how a simple gene works and that there are many thousands of housekeeping genes, that is, genes that do the job of running a cell. We predict that there are genes which make regulatory messages that are involved in the overall control and regulation of the many housekeeping genes. Yet we have only limited understanding of how a body organ develops into the size and shape it does. We know many things about how the central nervous system works—for example, we are beginning to comprehend how molecules are involved in electric circuits, in memory storage, in transmission of signals. But we are a long way from understanding thought and consciousness. And we are even further from understanding the spiritual side of our existence.

Even though we do not understand how a thinking, loving, interacting organism can be derived from its molecules, we are approaching the time when we can change some of those molecules. Might there be genes that influence the brain's organization or structure or metabolism or circuitry in some way so as to allow abstract thinking, contemplation of good and evil, fear of death, awe of a 'God'? What if in our innocent attempts to improve our genetic make-up we alter one or more of those genes? Could we test for the alteration? Certainly not at present If we caused a problem that would affect the individual or his or her offspring, could we repair the damage? Certainly not at present. Every parent who has several children knows that some babies accept and give more affection than others, in the same environment. Do genes control this? What if these genes were accidentally altered? How would we even know if such a gene were altered?

My concern is that, at this point in the development of our culture's scientific expertise, we might be like the young boy who loves to take things apart. He is bright enough to disassemble a watch, and maybe even bright enough to get it back together again so that it works. But what if he tries to "improve" it? Maybe put on bigger hands so that the time can be read more easily. But if the hands are too heavy for the mechanism, the watch will run slowly, erratically, or not at all. The boy can understand what is visible, but he cannot comprehend the precise engineering calculations that determined exactly how strong each spring should be, why the gears interact in the ways that they do, etc. Attempts on his part to improve the watch will probably only harm it. We are now able to provide a new gene so that a property involved in a human life would be changed, for example, a growth hormone gene. If we were to do so simply because we could, I fear we would be like that young boy who changed the watch's hands. We, too, do not really understand what makes the object we are tinkering with tick.

In summary, it could be harmful to insert a gene into humans. In somatic cell gene therapy for an already existing disease the potential benefits could outweigh the risks. In enhancement engineering, however, the risks would be greater while the benefits would be considerably less clear.

Yet even aside from the medical risks, somatic cell enhancement engineering should not be performed because it would be morally precarious. Let us assume that there were no medical risks at all from somatic cell enhancement engineering. There would still be reasons for objecting to this procedure. To illustrate, let us consider some examples. What if a human gene were cloned that could produce a brain chemical resulting in markedly increased memory capacity in monkeys after gene transfer? Should a person be allowed to receive such a gene on request? Should a pubescent adolescent whose parents are both five feet tall be provided with a growth hormone gene on request? Should a worker who is continually exposed to an industrial toxin receive a gene to give him resistance on his, or his employer's request?

These scenarios suggest three problems that would be difficult to resolve: What genes should be provided; who should receive a gene; and, how to prevent discrimination against individuals who do or do not receive a gene.

We allow that it would be ethically appropriate to use somatic cell gene therapy for treatment of serious disease. But what distinguishes a serious disease from a "minor" disease from cultural "discomfort"? What is suffering? What is significant suffering? Does the absence of growth hormone that results in a growth limitation to two feet in height represent a genetic disease? What about a limitation to a height of four feet, to five feet? Each observer might draw the lines between serious disease, minor disease, and genetic variation differently. But all can agree that there are extreme cases that produce significant suffering and premature death. Here then is where an initial line should be drawn for determining what genes should be provided: treatment of serious disease.

If the position is established that only patients suffering from serious diseases are candidates for gene insertion, then the issues of patient selection are no different than in other medical situations: the determination is based on medical need within a supply and demand framework. But if the use of gene transfer extends to allow a normal individual to acquire, for example, a memory-enhancing gene, profound problems would result. On what basis is the decision made to allow one individual to receive the gene but not another: Should it go to those best able to benefit society (the smartest already?) To those most in need (those with low intelligence? But how low? Will enhancing memory help a mentally retarded child?)? To those chosen by a lottery, To those who can afford to pay? As long as our society lacks a significant consensus about these answers, the best way to make equitable decisions in this case should be to base them on the seriousness of the objective medical need, rather than on the personal wishes or resources of an individual.

Discrimination can occur in many forms. If individuals are carriers of a disease (for example, sickle-cell anemia), would they be pressured to be treated? Would they have difficulty in obtaining health insurance unless they agreed to be treated? These are ethical issues raised also by genetic screening and by the Human Genome Project. But the concerns would become even more troublesome if there were the possibility for "correction" by the use of human genetic engineering.

Finally, we must face the issue of eugenics, the attempt to make hereditary "improvements." The abuse of power that societies have histotically demonstrated in the pursuit of eugenic goals is well documented.[7] Might we slide into a new age of eugenic thinking by starting with small "improvements"? It would be difficult, if not impossible, to determine where to draw a line once enhancement engineering had begun. Therefore, gene transfer should be used only for the treatment of serious disease and not for putative improvements.

Our society is comfortable with the use of genetic engineering to treat individuals with serious disease. On medical and ethical grounds we should draw a line excluding any form of enhancement engineering. We should not step over the line that delineates treatment from enhancement.

QUESTIONS FOR CONSIDERATION

1. What is Anderson's answer to the question "what can we do now in the area of human genetic engineering"?
2. What does Anderson believe can be done in gene transfer in the next five to ten years? What diseases does he believe will be treatable? What will be possible in germline gene therapy?
3. Why does Anderson draw a line between somatic cell gene therapy and enhancement genetic engineering? Why does he argue that somatic cell

gene therapy for serious diseases could be morally justified but not enhancement engineering?

4. What implications would Anderson's objections to enhancement genetic engineering have on possible germline gene therapy?

NOTES

1. W. French Anderson and John C. Hatcher, "Gene Therapy in Human Beings: When Is It Ethical to Begin?," *New England Journal of Medicine* 303:22 (1980),1293–97.

2. See also W. French Anderson, "Prospects for Human Gene Therapy," *Science* (26 October 1984), 401–409; T. Friedman, "Progress Towards Human Gene Therapy," *Science* (16 June 1989), 1275–81.

3. J. Wyngaarden, "Human Gene Transfer Protocol," *Federal Register* (1989) vol. 54 no. 47, pp. 10508–10510.

4. Steven A. Rosenberg et al., "Use of Tumor Infiltrating Lymphocytes and Interleukin–2 in the Immunotherapy of Patients with Metastatic Melanoma," *New England Joumal of Medicine* 319:25 (1988), 1676–80.

5. W. French Anderson, "Human Gene Therapy: Scientific and Ethical Considerations." *Jounal of Medicine and Philosophy* 10 (1985), 275–91.

6. W. French Anderson, "Human Gene Therapy: Why Draw a Line?," *Journal of Medicine and Philosophy* 14 (1989), 681–93.

7. See, for example, Kenneth M. Ludmerer, *Genetics and American Society* (Baltimore, MD: The Johns Hopkins University Press, 1972), and Daniel J. Kevles, *In the Name of Eugenics* (New York: Alfred A. Knopf, 1985).

Erik Parens

Taking Behavioral Genetics Seriously

As information about the genetic component of human behavior increases, so, of course, does the number of opportunities for its abuse. It is troubling to imagine simple-minded criminologists who aspire to use genetic information about behavior to identify and control "antisocial" individuals. It is perhaps more troubling because far more practicable to imagine insurers and employers who use such information to deny insurance or employment to people deemed "predisposed to" costly behaviors. Given the sordid history of attempts to use pseudobiological explanations to justify the stratification of our society,[1] perhaps most troubling of all is to imagine that our society will use such information to reinforce the view that current forms of stratification are "natural." Peter Breggin, director of the Center for the Study of Psychiatry in Bethesda Maryland, suggests this last fear in vivid terms: "Behavioral genetics is the same old stuff in new clothes. . . It's another way for a violent, racist society to say people's problems are their own fault, because they carry 'bad' genes."[2]

Such pronouncements may tempt some to ignore research that explores the genetic component of human behavior. Merely taking such research seriously could be construed as legitimating an inherently evil enterprise. But ignoring such research won't make the abuses go away. Indeed, the crafting of careful critiques will be needed to effectively fight the abuses. In this essay I attempt to make a small contribution to that project by calling attention to two errors that are sometimes made in discussions of the implications of genetics research in general, and behavioral genetics research in particular. Actually, the first error is not usually made by critics of behavioral genetics, but by those who tend to be its friends. They make their error in the course of trying to fend off critics, who in their view exaggerate the power of genetics to alter important human behaviors. Their error is to conceive of the body and soul (or mind) as separable—and to assume. For example, that no matter how much altering of the body we might do with genetics, altering the soul (and the complex behaviors associated with it) is forever beyond our reach.

The second error tends to be made by those who are largely unfriendly toward genetics research, and who want to expose its dangers. That error is to think that facts and policies are related in an obvious and inevitable manner—to think, for example, that facts about the genetics of behavior will inevitably be used to undermine valuable political ideas or to undergird hateful social programs.

Before turning to those errors, I should say a word about the modest contribution that molecular genetics has already made, and is expected to make, toward understanding some complex behaviors.[3] It has already contributed toward understanding some behaviors associated with some forms of, for example, Alzheimer disease, Tourette syndrome, and Lesch-Nyhan syndrome. Further, much research suggests that genetics may help to explain a partial but significant component of some forms of, for example, schizophrenia, bipolar disorder, and depression.[4] Probably more disturbing to traditional ways of thinking about complex behaviors will be the discovery of genes or groups of genes that correlate, not with well-recognized disease states, but rather with "normal" personality traits, such as impulsivity or shyness[5]—or as recent research suggests, "novelty seeking."[6]

When speaking about the contribution that genetics can make toward understanding such complex behaviors, it is enormously important to remember that genes are but one component of fabulously complex biological, and ultimately biopsychosocial, systems. Even if there are strong correlations between single-gene defects and certain dispositions to some complex behaviors, such correlations will never provide anything approximating a full account of those behaviors. To begin with, a fuller account will require thinking in terms of nonlinear and dynamic interactions among many genes, hormones, nutrients, and other biological factors in the "internal" environment that is the body. And as genetics always will be only one important part of biology, biology always will be only one important part of any richer account of human behavior.

Such an account will have to consider not only interactions among social and biological factors in the "external" environment, but will have to consider the complex interactions between the internal and external environments. Indeed, insofar as research into gene expression reveals the extent to which such expression is affected by the internal and external environments, the study of genetics ought to expand, not constrict, our appreciation of the importance of our environments. In light of such complexity, it should be clear that even if there were a correlation between, say, a single-gene defect and a predisposition to impulsivity, no amount of behavioral genetics could

predict whether such a predisposition will gain expression in a bar room—
or a board room—fight.

To reiterate: we need not adopt simplistic or reductionistic conceptions
of the relationship between single genes and complex behaviors to take seriously
the information produced by behavioral genetics research. But we do need
to avoid two errors often advanced in discussions of this information.

Body and Soul

The first simple but fundamental error that threatens to keep us from
taking seriously the information produced by behavioral genetics is to conceive
of the human body and soul (or mind) as two distinct entities. The most
notorious perpetrator of this error, of course, is Rene Descartes. After
announcing that he had discovered that he was not deceived and that he did
indeed exist, Descartes wrote:

> From that I knew that I was a substance, the whole essence or nature of
> which is to think, *and that for its existence there is no need of any place, nor
> does it depend on any material thing so that this "me," that is to say, the soul
> by which I am what I am, is entirely distinct from body,* and is even more
> easy to know than is the latter; and even if body were not, the soul
> would not cease to be what it is. (my italics)[7]

According to Descartes, body and soul are entirely distinct. Soul needs
no place called body.

Kant, too, at least the Kant of the *Grundlegung*, understood human beings
in terms of two utterly distinct realms: the realms of nature (or body) and
freedom (or soul). "The science of the first," he said, "is called *physics*, that
of the second *ethics*."[8] Like Descartes, Kant thought that to understand the
realm of ethics or freedom or soul, one didn't have to concern oneself with
the realm of nature or body.

Now these would be no more than familiar philosophical anecdotes if it
weren't that the ideas encapsulated in them are often at work in our current
discussions of genetics and behavior. Usually those ideas are implicit. Sometimes, however, versions of them are fairly explicit. For instance, when the
Council of Europe recommended that persons have "a right to a genome that
has not been 'tampered' with," two critics argued:

> [T]he recommendation invokes the "rights to life and to human dignity
> protected by . . . the European Convention on Human Rights," and claims
> that these "imply" the right to a pristine genetic inheritance. We fail to

see the "implication." For philosophers like Kant, human dignity is equated with our dignity as rational beings, and not with the whole of our biological nature as homo sapiens. Thus as rational beings, we are ends in ourselves, and have a right not to be treated as mere means to the ends of others. This may entail that others ought not to interfere (unjustifiably) with our pursuit of our own legitimate ends. It does not entail that others ought not to have interfered with our chances to have been conceived, say, with genes for hazel eye color.[9]

The relevant argument thus goes something like this: because our dignity resides in our rationality, and because it is dignity, not mere body, that requires protection, it is unreasonable to criticize "genetic tampering" on the grounds that it contravenes the obligation to protect dignity. Worries about tampering with future bodies thus need not concern those who want to protect the dignity of future human beings. Critics of the Council of Europe's recommendation assume what I take to be an erroneous conception of human beings: the view that our dignity—or whatever else you want to call that about us which requires respect—resides in some part of us that is separable from our bodies.

That same mistaken conception is seen even more easily in a recent piece by W. French Anderson, "Genetic Engineering and Our Humanness."[10] In it he poses the question, "Is it possible that we could alter our humanness itself by genetic engineering?" Proceeding from the distinction between the body, which does *not* "make one human being unique from another," and the soul, which is that "spiritual part of us that makes us uniquely human," he makes the following argument: "If what is uniquely important about humanness . . . is not defined by the physical hardware of our body, and since we can only alter the physical hardware, it follows that we cannot alter that which is uniquely human by genetic engineering" (p. 758). In other words, Anderson claims: because genetic technology cannot alter what is "uniquely human," there is no good reason to worry that it will "alter our humanness." But what does he mean by the phrase "alter our humanness"? "Our humanness," he tells us, is that "spiritual" and "nonquantifiable" part of us that makes "one human being unique from another." According to this account, our "humanness" is a thing that, not only in words but in fact, can be extricated and distinguished from the mere physical hardware that is our body.

In an attempt to make patent why this idea is untenable, allow me a nongenetic example. It is reported that, by inhibiting the reuptake of serotonin, fluoxetine (Prozac) transforms the personalities of a significant minority of users. More specifically, it enables those users to feel "better than well";[11] it makes them less sensitive to rejection, more competitive, more aggressive, etc. These personality traits contribute significantly to our experience of ourselves and others; the ways in which we are aggressive or competitive or sensitive make us who we are. Thus Prozac can be understood to "alter our humanness," not by giving us new capacities (say, the capacity to fly), but by altering traits that, to use Anderson's language, make "one human being unique from another."

The significant minority of users whose experience is altered in these ways is a vivid example of the ability of such drugs to transform just that "part" of us Anderson thinks is unalterable. But even if one goes "only" from being profoundly depressed to feeling well, one's self has undergone a significant alteration. While that sort of alteration may be less vivid than the sort where individuals come to feel "better than well," both manifest the inextricable entwinement of "body and soul." If one accepts that using a drug to inhibit the reuptake of a neurotransmitter can alter some complex behaviors, then it is plausible to suppose that by manipulating genes that code for enzymes that regulate neurotransmitters, we will be able to do the same—even if there are terrible side effects and even if we do not thoroughly understand why what we are doing works.

The more general point is this: if the complex behaviors we traditionally associate with soul are in an important respect a function of the body, and if the new genetic technologies will be able—however bluntly—to alter the body in ways such as those just suggested, then there is reason to suppose that it will be possible to use genetic technologies to alter some complex human behaviors. In other words, it is an error to assume that altering the complex behaviors that we associate with the soul or mind is somehow forever beyond our reach.

Fact and Policy

The second error is more complex than the first. It is the error of assuming that the facts produced by research in behavioral genetics inevitably will be used to undermine cherished political ideas (in particular, freedom and equality) and to justify social policies that further disenfranchise the already disenfranchised.

Some of those who voice the greatest skepticism about the possibility that genetics could tell us anything interesting about complex human behaviors seem to be motivated in part by a concern that if we give up the idea that the soul (or mind) is a thing independent of "mere" body, then we necessarily will have to give up some other ideas as well. We will have to stop thinking that choice is free, in the sense of uninfluenced by body. And we will find it increasingly diffcult to think of people as moral equals as we increasingly understand that who they are and what they do is intimately related to their different bodies.

I want to suggest the respect in which these worries are and are not legitimate. I should emphasize that the theoretical moves I want to criticize are being made by people I think of as fellow travelers,[12] people who devote considerable energy to thinking about how scientific information has and can be used to hurt people who already hurt.

Freedom. Many people are concerned about the impact of "genetic determinism" on our traditional ideas about freedom of the will and about related ideas concerning responsibility and guilt, praise and blame. Dorothy Nelkin and Susan Lindee advance a version of this concern. They write:

> The notion of biological predisposition can relieve personal guilt by implying compulsion, an inborn inability to resist specific behaviors. Biological explanations deflect attention away from the social and economic circumstances that may drive people to violence, depression, overeating, or drink, but they also provide an excuse for those who, driven by their predispositions, their irresistible biological drives, need not blame themselves.[13]

According to Nelkin and Lindee, the notion of biological predisposition can be used to relieve society of its responsibility to the disempowered, and also can be used to relieve us all of responsibility for our actions. Neither concern is unreasonable. Notions of biological predisposition can indeed be used in these ways. It would be unreasonable (and as I will suggest later ironic), however, to assume that such notions *must* be used in these ways, or that attending to such information "dictates"[14] social policy.

It is by now, as Troy Duster suggests, "almost a truism that science both shapes and is shaped by social, economic, and political conditions."[15] What we call facts both shape and are shaped by those conditions. I think it is, however, a theoretical and tactical mistake to assume that facts about the genetics of behavior will necessarily be used to further disempower the already disempowered—to assume that, as Duster says elsewhere, "no matter how one slices it, just underneath the talk of a paradigmatic shift [from the old-style eugenics to the new-style genetics], society seems *inexorably pulled back* to the ancient concern for trying to explain what could be called 'trouble at the bottom, virtue at the top,' by reference to the properties of individuals" (my emphasis).[16] I appreciate that Duster and most of us who worry about the abuse of behavioral genetics are not in the end making a deductive claim about the nature of behavioral genetics, but instead are making an inductive claim based on the history of the abuses of such research. My concern is that if we overstate the extent to which such research "inexorably" will lead to abuse, then we risk undermining our concerns insofar as overstated claims are easily ignored.

In fact, many people from traditionally disempowered communities have themselves argued that genetic information can be used to show how the categories of praise and blame are irrelevant to the behaviors on account of which these communities have been discriminated against. As Nelkin and Lindee acknowledge, many gay activists welcome the attempt to identify a genetic contribution to homosexuality because they not unreasonably think that gays will be discriminated against less if it is understood that they have no more "freely chosen" their sexual preference than heterosexuals have theirs.[17]

Similarly, many activists for the mentally ill welcome the attempt to identify the genetic component of mental illness.[18] Indeed, the same genetic information about any given behavior can fuel arguments on both sides of any policy question. Those who want to further disempower schizophrenics, for example, can use information about the genetic component of schizophrenia to "demonstrate" that the current disempowerment of schizophrenics reflects their scientifically described "genetic deviance." And those who want to em-power people with schizophrenia can use that same information to argue that it is absurd to discriminate against people on the grounds that they have made a "deviant choice" since it makes little sense to say that they have "chosen" their patterns of behavior.

In a word, while it is true and important that genetic information can be used to further disempower the already disempowered, it does not follow that it must be so used. Moreover, to say that genetic information calls into question some traditional ideas about freedom, guilt, responsibility, and the like does not discredit that information. It may be that some of the dominant ways of thinking about those ideas have been simplistic and are no longer tenable. It may be that the tradition of linking up absolute freedom of the will and absolute separation of the soul and body—a tradition stretching at least from Augustine to Kant and into the present—is discredited and can no longer form a basis for morality. (It should go without saying that there is not just one tradition of thinking about such matters; for thinkers like Aristotle, for whom "pleasure and nobility between them supply the motives of all actions,"[19] there is no talk of absolute freedom of the will nor any absolute separation of the body and soul.)

To say that one dominant way of thinking about free will, guilt, responsibility, and the like is no longer tenable does not commit anyone to abandoning those ideas.[20] The idea of an absolutely free and disembodied will is not a necessary condition for having, for example, a concept of responsibility. Indeed, our society has for some time now accepted that some actions are not simply freely chosen insofar as economic and social forces constrain individual actions, while simultaneously insisting that citizens must be held responsible for their actions. Today we need to grapple with the respect in which, like economic and social factors, some genetic factors to some extent constrain how we act. With new vigor we will have to grapple with a question that is not at all new: How can we simultaneously accept the respect in which our behaviors are not freely chosen, and also insist that, as members of communities, we must act as if they were? To say that question is difficult does not discredit the genetic information that prompts it.

Equality. Another version of the argument about facts dictating policy emerges in discussions of equality. Many worry that if we take too seriously the claims about the genetic roots of various complex and prized traits (such as intelligence), we will undermine the idea of moral equality. At the root of this concern seems to be an assumption that with regard to important traits, human beings are pretty much equal, in the sense of the same. According to this view, apparent differences or inequalities in complex traits can be explained largely in terms of contingent social and historical forces. Further, according to this view, genetic information that suggests biological roots to such behaviors will be used only to defend the status quo or further blame the victims of the status quo. Such information will be used to give a "scientific" account of why the poor are poor, why those who suffer are destined to suffer.

Perhaps the most notorious example of genetic information posing a putative threat to equality arises in the context of the IQ debate. In the wake of Herrnstein and Murray's ugly book, *The Bell Curve*,[21] some thinkers on the left have floated the idea that not just Herrnstein and Murray's attempt, but any attempt to speak about the genetics of intelligence is inherently racist, or a threat to the political idea of equality.[22]

But it is simply not true that acknowledging that there is a correlation between a number like the intelligence quotient and certain abilities valued by our society necessarily entails or dictates racist policies. As Adrian Wooldridge has recently suggested, it is an unhappy but utterly contingent fact that the political right has stolen the tool of such tests from the left. In mid-nineteenth-century England, for example, as reformers tried to wrest control of the civil service from the aristocracy, they argued "that positions should be allocated on the basis of examination results and that the exams should be designed to test 'the candidate's powers of mind' rather than to 'ascertain the extent of his metaphysical reading.' "[23] In that context (and well into the twentieth century), intelligence tests were a tool used by progressives to battle an aristocratic system built on the idea that class (one sort of environment) was determinative of intelligence and its prerequisites.

It would be absurd to ignore the differences between mid-nineteenth century England and late-twentieth century America. But even today in this country, with its history of systematic oppression of people of African descent, it is possible to recognize that test scores to some extent reflect both genotype and ability—while simultaneously recognizing that, for example, blacks in this country on average score lower on such tests due to what the liberal social psychologist Claude Steele calls "stereotype vulnerability."[24] One can accept that the difference between the scores of *individuals* can partly be explained in terms of genes, and simultaneously accept that the difference between the average scores of white and black *populations* cannot be explained in terms of genes—but in terms of a culture that systematically depresses the scores of black students by telling those students they don't do as well on such tests as do their white counterparts.

Again, my first point is to urge us to remember that to believe such tests are one indicator of real abilities valued by this society—and to believe that those scores can partly be understood in genetic and other biological terms—does not necessarily entail or dictate any one social policy. My second point is to insist that genetics only threatens the idea of equality if one takes equality to mean something like "the same with respect to all significant capacities." This society might do well to adopt Howard Gardner's view that we need to stop thinking that intelligence is monolithic, and start thinking about many different kinds of intelligence,[25] one of which may to some extent be reflected in IQ tests and correlated to particular genotypes. It would be supremely ironic if those of us who profess to affirm difference were incapable of accepting that different people have different capacities, and that those capacities can to some extent be correlated with genetic differences.

While talking about the genetic component of individual differences may be politically risky in this society at this time, talking about the genetic component of population (that is, ethnic or racial) differences is no doubt even riskier. The history of the abuse of such talk is so horrible and long that it is not unreasonable to entertain the idea that any information pertinent to such talk ought to be suppressed. Yet we ought to remember that the suppression of scientific information is something most of us would resist most of the time and that some benign information about population differences is already emerging. For example, some research suggests that genetic differences among different ethnic groups can be correlated with the different rates at which those groups tend to metabolize drugs.[26] Thus, when prescribing medications, it may be appropriate for doctors to consider the "ethnicity" of patients in those cases where the category is useful. If our society decides to suppress genetic information about population differences on the grounds that in general such information is harmful, then it also will have to factor in the harm done by suppressing some information that may be helpful. Leaving aside the practicability of suppressing such information, I suspect that it would be exceedingly difficult to make the argument for suppressing helpful information in the name of protecting a simplistic understanding of equality—one that denies the fact of different capacities.

Criticizing bodiless conceptions of equality does not mean abandoning equal respect. To say that genes play a significant role in, for example, different people having different levels of the same sort of intelligence or having different sorts of intelligence (as Gardner would put it) need not diminish anyone's commitment to the moral equality of all humans. We can both be dismayed that only one sort of intelligence gets highly valued in this society and also accept the genetic component of those multiple intelligences. We can both be outraged at socially constructed and reinforced inequalities and accept the genetic component of difference.

Conversation on the Political High Wire

Such a balancing act will always be threatened by the hateful uses to which some people will try to put information about the genetic component of different traits and behaviors. There is no denying, for example, that in the imagination of many Americans there are powerful links among the categories of race, crime, and genes.[27] There is therefore good reason to worry that some Americans will intentionally or unintentionally use the conversation concerning behavioral genetics to prop up their fantasies about those links. When such information is discussed in a racist society such as this one, those who engage in it must be prepared to battle the hateful uses to which that conversation will be put—even when, as in the case of African Americans and criminal behavior, no research has been done, nor can one imagine any creditable research being done.

Yet justifiable worries about the public's imagination concerning research that is not being done ought not to be used as grounds for ignoring research that is being done. We cannot powerfully criticize what we inadequately understand or inaccurately describe. Research suggests, for example, that the drug Clonidine can be used to treat children whose hyperactivity and attention deficit can be linked to genetic defects affecting norepinephrine levels.[28] Attention deficit hyperactivity disorder (ADHD) makes it difficult if not impossible for some children to succeed in school. Clonidine (like Ritalin) could in principle be used not only to cure sick children, but to "calm down" children who are hyperactive and unfocused because their stomachs are empty, their classrooms full, and their teachers demoralized. Those who ignore research into the genetics of ADHD will be ill prepared to insist, for example, that whereas children who are sick and unable to thrive in school should be given treatment, children who are "hyperactive and inattentive" because their environments are cruel should be given better schools.

Summing up what is perhaps the fundamental worry shared by those of us committed to fighting the abuses of behavioral genetic information, Patricia King asserts: "the danger to racial and ethnic minorities and the poor from current gene mapping efforts is . . . that greater attention will be paid to genetic explanations than to more complex explanations for differences."[29] As long as our society seeks simple explanations for phenomena as complex as the differences between individuals and groups, danger surely looms. But those of us committed to combatting that variety of simplicity need to be careful to avoid introducing simplifications of our own. Our lives would be easier if, for example, it were true that complex human behaviors in principle could not be manipulated by genetic means. We would not need to worry about the extent to which we ought to engage in such manipulation because such manipulations would be impossible. Likewise, our lives would be easier if it were true that genetic information about complex behaviors were inherently dangerous. We could then be spared the difficult work of distinguishing between hurtful and helpful uses of it. Unfortunately, the evidence does not point in the direction of such simplicity.

Strangely enough, research into the genetics of behavior could actually help make our accounts of different ways of being in the world more complex. After all, as I suggested in the beginning, behavioral genetics is helping us to learn that any rich account of human behavior must, at a minimum, recognize the nonlinear and dynamic interactions *within and between* our "internal" and "external" environments. Such a science could be one among many useful tools for those of us who, like Patricia King, want to promote complex explanations for different ways of being in the world. Just as surely as our society is not fated to be stratified in the ways it is now, neither is it fated to use genetic information about human behavior in the simplistic and hateful ways it has in the past.

Acknowledgments

I gratefully thank the following people for reading and commenting on earlier versions of this essay: Erika Blacksher, Daniel Callahan, Maria Deknatel, Eric Juengst, Karen Lebacqz, Hilde Lindemann Nelson, Andrea Kott Parens, and the *Report's* anonymous readers.

QUESTIONS FOR CONSIDERATION

1. What are some of the "modest" contributions of molecular genetics that Parens identifies?
2. Parens states that ". . .genes are but one component of fabulously complex biological, and ultimately biopsychosocial systems." What are other components that account for human behavior?
3. How does Parens criticize the argument that genetic technology can only affect our bodies and not our minds (souls)? How does the example of Prozac illustrate his point?
4. How does Parens respond to the argument that research in genetic technology will undermine political ideas such as freedom and equality?
5. What are his arguments against suppressing genetic information?

NOTES

1. Stephen Jay Gould, *The Mismeasure of Man* (New York: W. VW. Norton, 1981); Daniel J. Kevles, *In the Name of Eugenics: Genetics and the Uses of Human Heredity* (New York: Alfred A. Knopf, 1985); Troy Duster, Backdoor to Eugenics (New York: Routledge, 1990); Diane B. Paul, *Controlling Human Heredity: 1865 to the Present* (Atlantic Highlands, NJ.: Humanities Press International, 1995).

2. Quoted in Charles C. Mann, "Behavioral Genetics in Transition," *Science* 264 (1994): 1686–89, at 1686.

3. For a succinct overview of the aspirations and limitations of the field, see all of volume 264 (17 June 1994) of *Science*.

4. U.S. Congress, Office of Technology Assessment, *Mental Disorders and Genetics: Bridging the Gap Between Research and Society*, OTA-BP-H-133 (Washington, D.C.: U.S. Government Printing Office, September 1994); Robert Plomin and Gerald E. McClearn, *Nature, Nurture and Psychology* (Washington, D.C.: American Psychological Association, 1993).

5. See, for example, Roger D. Masters and Michael T. McGuire, eds., *The Neurotransmitter Revolution: Serotonin, Social Behavior and the Law* (Carbondale and Edwardsville, Ill.: Southern Illinois University Press,1994) and Robert Plomin, Michael J. Owen, and Peter McGuffin, "The Genetic Basis of Complex Human Behaviors," *Science* 264 (1994): 1733–39.

6. C. Robert Cloniger, Rolf Adolfsson, and Nenad M. Svrakic, "Mapping Genes for Human Personality," *Nature Genetics* 12 (1996): 34.

7. Cited in Antonio R. Damasio, *Descartes' Error: Emotion, Reason, and the Human Brain* (New York: G. P. Putnam's Sons, 1994), p. 249 (see part four of *Discourse on the Method*).

8. Immanuel Kant, *Groundwork of the Metaphysics of Morals*, trans. H. J. Patton (New York: Harper and Row, 1964), p. 55.

9. Ronald Munson and Lawrence H. Davis, "Germ-Line Gene Therapy and the Medical Imperative," *Kennedy Institute of Ethics Journal* 2, no. 2 (1992): 137–58, at 142.

10. W. French Anderson, "Genetic Engineering and Our Humanness," *Human Gene Therapy* 5 (1994): 755–60, at 755.

11. Peter D. Kramer, *Listening to Prozac* (New York: Viking, 1993).

12. For example: R. C. Lewontin, Steven Rose, and Leon J. Kamin, *Not in Our Genes: Biology, Ideology, and Human Nature* (New York: Pantheon Books, 1984); Ruth Hubbard and Elijah Wald, *Exploding the Gene Myth* (Boston, Beacon Press, 1993); Dorothy Nelkin and M. Susan Lindee, *The DNA Mystique* (New York: W. H. Freeman, 1995).

13. Nelkin and Lindee, *The DNA Mystique*, p. 144.

14. R. C. Lewontin, "The Dream of the Human Genome," *New York Review of Books*, 28 May 1994.

15. Duster, *Backdoor to Eugenics*, p. 2.

16. Troy Duster, "Human Genetics, Evolutionary Theory, and Social Stratification," in *The Genetic Frontier: Ethics, Law, and Policy*, ed. Mark S. Frankel and Albert Teich (Washington: American Association for the Advancement of Science, 1994), pp. 131–53, at 132.

17. See, for example, David Gelman et al., "Born or Bred? *Newsweek*, 24 February 1992. According to J. Michael Bailey, one of the genetics of homosexuality researchers, some gay and lesbian bookstores sold a T-shirt proclaiming, "Xq28—Thanks for the genes, mom"; see J. Michael Bailey, "Sexual Orientation Revolution," *Nature Genetics* 11 (December 1995): 353–54, at 353.

18. U.S. Congress, Office of Technology Assessment, *Mental Disorders and Genetics*, p. la.

19. Aristotle, *Nichomachean Ethics* III.i.ll.

20. Patricia S. Greenspan, "Free Will and the Genome Project," *Philosophy and Public Affairs* 22, no. 1(1993): 31–43; Dan W. Brock, "The Human Genome Project and Human Identity," *Houston Law Review* 29, no.1 (1992): 7–22; Norval Morris, "Linking Genetics, Behavior, and Responsibility: Legal Implications," in *The Genetic Frontier*.

21. Richard J. Herrnstein and Charles Murray, The *Bell Curve: Intelligence and Class Structure in American Life* (New York: The Free Press, 1994).

22. For example, see Adolph Reed, Jr., "Looking Backward," *The Nation*, 28 November 1994.

23. Adrian Wooldridge, "Bell Curve Liberals: How the Left Betrayed I.Q.," *The New Republic*, 27 February 1995, p. 22.

24. Claude M. Steele and Joshua Aronson, "Stereotype Threat and the Intellectual Test Performance of African Americans," *Journal of Personality and Social Psychology* 69, no. 5 (1995): 797–811.

25. Howard Gardner, *Frames of Mind: The Theory of Multiple Intelligences* (New York: Basic Books, 1983).

26. For example, Keh-Ming Lin and Russell E. Poland, "Ethnicity, Culture and Psychopharmacology," *Psychiatric Times*, March 1995: 20–23; see also, however, Gregory Carey, "Genetics and Violence," *in Understanding and Preventing Violence*, vol. 2, ed. Albert J. Reiss, Jr., Klaus A. Miczek, and Jeffrey A. Roth (Washington D.C.: National Academy Press, 1994): "[T]here is no positive evidence to suggest that heritability plays an important role in group differences in violence within the United States" (p. 50).

27. This point was made by Professor Katheryn Russell (University of Maryland's Department of Criminal Justice and Criminology) at the University of Maryland's September 1995 conference on "Research on Genetics and Criminal Behavior: Scientific Issues, Social and Political Implications."

28. Personal communication with David E. Comings, M.D., Department of Medical Genetics, City of Hope Medical Center, Duarte, California, October 1995.

29. Patricia King, "The Past as Prologue: Race, Class and Gene Discrimination," *in Gene Mapping: Using Law and Ethics as Guides*, ed. George Annas and Sherman Elias (New York: Oxford University Press, 1992), pp. 94–111, at 102.

PART IX: Cloning Human Beings: Responding to the National Bioethics Advisory Commission's Report

Executive Summary

JAMES F. CHILDRESS

The Challenges of Public Ethics: Reflections on NABC's Report

SUSAN M. WOLF

Ban Cloning? Why NABC Is Wrong

The successful cloning of a sheep by Ian Wilmut and his colleagues raises significant ethical dilemmas regarding the possible use of somatic cell nuclear transfer cloning to create children. The NABC report is primarily concerned with the safety of children. However, other concerns were identified: individual identity, family integrity, the manipulation of children, and the effects upon moral, religious, and cultural values in society.

While in agreement that cloning requires regulation, Susan M. Wolf argues that a ban on somatic cell nuclear transfer will reduce cloning to a political issue, chill important research, and infringe upon important constitutional rights.

- **Executive Summary** is an overview of the NBAC's report. It summarizes the harm issues raised by somatic cell nuclear transfer cloning to create children. It also recommends federal legislation that would prohibit such cloning for a specific period of time. The commission also seeks to protect other important areas of scientific research.
- James F. Childress' **The Challenges of Public Ethics: Reflections on NABC's Report** is a response to the NABC's report by a member of the Commission. Childress raises several issues based upon the Commission report: safety as an ethical issue, the intrinsic wrongness or limited acceptance of human cloning, principled or casuistical analysis, public policy in a political context, and religious perspectives on human cloning.

- Susan M. Wolf's **Ban Cloning? Why NBAC Is Wrong** raises objections to the Commission's ban on human cloning. She recommends, instead, that regulation by an advisory body would be more acceptable. She insists that such regulations should be extended to protect human subjects in private research and to regulate the use of reproductive technologies in private clinics.

Executive Summary

In February of this year two figures were added to our daily life. Dolly, a cloned sheep, and her maker, Scottish scientist Ian Wilmut, could be found in our newspapers, on our televisions, across the Internet, and in our conversations. What Wilmut had done was indeed new, if not fantastic. By transferring the nucleus of a somatic cell from an adult animal into an egg from which the nucleus had been removed, Wilmut successfully cloned a mammal—a technique that had never before succeeded.

The drama of this scientific capability, and its potential reach toward human beings, prompted President Clinton to ask his newly formed National Bioethics Advisory Commission to spend ninety days examining the ethical and legal issues raised by the possibility of cloning human beings. This collection of essays responds to NBAC's report.

Though the science that made Dolly possible is unprecedented, two authors remind us that much of this debate is not new. By the late 1960s and 1970s, scholars Leon Kass, Paul Ramsey, and others had already started to speculate, and worry, about the possibility of cloning human beings. Though they did not have the details of Wilmut's technique, which NBAC called "somatic cell nuclear transfer" (SCNT), to guide their analyses, they nonetheless foresaw with clarity many of the issues.

And, according to some, the ethical issues are profound. Reiterating the report, one author clearly lays out those raised by SCNT. Parents hoping to clone using Wilmut's technique can "circumvent the chance events of meiosis and fertilization" and enter the baby making enterprise with a tremendous amount of control over and knowledge about their future child's characteristics. Both the prospect for increased control and knowledge are worrisome, particularly for those who believe, as one author says, that the practice of cloning children threatens the "moral significance of the family, the meaning of parenthood, and the ethics of unchosen obligations."

Both prospects are possible because the technique uses *adult* cells. Indeed, NBAC's analysis hangs on the subtle but crucial distinction between adult and embryonic or fetal cells. While one author lauds the commissioners' attempts to make clear the boundaries of their analysis and recommended temporary ban only to techniques using adult cells aimed at producing a child—another thinks the commissioners have been anything but clear. The ban is overly broad and overly vague, likely to chill important research both inside and outside these parameters, and for an unlimited time. And the ban's "sunset" provision fails to satisfy. Some worry that Congress will never muster the political will to lift the ban after the specified three to five years; others, to keep it in place. Much will depend on the "national dialogue" that NBAC has urged us to undertake.

Executive Summary

From Cloning Human Beings: The Report and Recommendations of the National Bioethics Advisory Commission (Rockville, Md., June 1997)

The idea that humans might someday be cloned—created from a single somatic cell without sexual reproduction—moved further away from science fiction and closer to a genuine scientific possibility on February 23, 1997. On that date, *The Observer* broke the news that Ian Wilmut, a Scottish scientist, and his colleagues at the Roslin Institute were about to announce the successful cloning of a sheep by a technique which had never before been fully successful in mammals. The technique involved transplanting the genetic material of an adult sheep, apparently obtained from a differentiated somatic cell, into an egg from which the nucleus had been removed. The resulting birth of the sheep, named Dolly, on July 5, 1996, was different from prior attempts to create identical offspring since Dolly contained the genetic material of only one parent, and was, therefore, a "delayed" genetic twin of a single adult sheep.

This cloning technique is an extension of research that had been ongoing for over 40 years using nuclei derived from non-human embryonic and fetal cells. The demonstration that nuclei from cells derived from an adult animal could be "reprogrammed," or that the full genetic complement of such a cell could be reactivated well into the chronological life of the cell, is what sets the results of this experiment apart from prior work. In this report we refer to the technique, first described by Wilmut, of nuclear transplantation using nuclei derived from somatic cells other than those of any embryo or fetus as "somatic cell nuclear transfer."

Within days of the published report of Dolly, President Clinton instituted a ban on federal funding related to attempts to clone human beings in this manner. In addition, the President asked the recently appointed National Bioethics Advisory Commission (NBAC) to address within ninety days the ethical and legal issues that surround the subject of cloning human beings. This provided a welcome opportunity for initiating a thoughtful analysis of the many dimensions of the issue, including a careful consideration of the potential risks and benefits. It also presented an occasion to review the current legal status of cloning and the potential constitutional challenges that might be raised if new legislation were enacted to restrict the creation of a child through somatic cell nuclear transfer cloning.

The Commission began its discussion fully recognizing that any effort in humans to transfer a somatic cell nucleus into an enucleated egg involves the creation of an embryo, with the apparent potential to be implanted in utero and developed to term. Ethical concerns surrounding issues of embryo research have recently received extensive analysis and deliberation in our country. Indeed, federal funding for human embryo research is severely restricted, although there are few restrictions on human embryo research carried out in the private sector. Thus, under current law, the use of somatic cell nuclear transfer to create an embryo solely for research purposes is already restricted in cases involving federal funds. There are, however, no current federal regulations on the use of private funds for this purpose.

The unique prospect, vividly raised by Dolly, is the creation of a new individual genetically identical to an existing (or previously existing) person—a "delayed" genetic twin. This prospect has been the source of the overwhelming public concern about such cloning. While the creation of embryos for research purposes alone always raises serious ethical questions, the use of somatic cell nuclear transfer to create embryos raises no new issues in this respect. The unique and distinctive ethical issues raised by the use of somatic cell nuclear transfer to create children relate to, for example, serious safety concerns, individuality, family integrity, and treating children as objects. Consequently, the Commission focused its attention on the use of such techniques for the purpose of creating an embryo which would then be implanted in a woman's uterus and brought to term. It also expanded its analysis of this particular issue to encompass activities in both the public and private sector.

In its deliberations, NBAC reviewed the scientific developments which preceded the Roslin announcement, as well as those likely to follow in its path. It also considered the many moral concerns raised by the possibility that this technique could be used to clone human beings. Much of the initial reaction to this possibility was negative. Careful assessment of that response revealed fears about harms to the children who may be created in this manner, particularly psychological harms associated with a possibly diminished sense of individuality and personal autonomy. Others expressed concern about a degradation in the quality of parenting and family life.

In addition to concern about specific harms to children, people have frequently expressed fears that the widespread practice of somatic cell nuclear transfer cloning would undermine important social values by opening the door to a form of eugenics or by tempting some to manipulate others as if they were objects instead of persons. Arrayed against these concerns are other important social values, such as protecting the widest possible sphere of personal choice, particularly in matters pertaining to procreation and child rearing, maintaining privacy and the freedom of scientific inquiry, and encouraging the possible development of new biomedical breakthroughs.

To arrive at its recommendations concerning the use of somatic cell nuclear transfer techniques to create children, NBAC also examined longstanding religious traditions that guide many citizens' responses to new technologies and found that religious positions on human cloning are pluralistic in their premises, modes of argument, and conclusions. Some religious thinkers argue that the use of somatic cell nuclear transfer cloning to create a child would be intrinsically immoral and thus could never be morally justified. Other religious thinkers contend that human cloning to create a child could be morally justified under some circumstances, but hold that it should be strictly regulated in order to prevent abuses.

The public policies recommended with respect to the creation of a child using somatic cell nuclear transfer reflect the Commission's best judgments about both the ethics of attempting such an experiment and our view of traditions regarding limitations on individual actions in the name of the common good. At present, the use of this technique to create a child would be a premature experiment that would expose the fetus and the developing child to unacceptable risks. This in itself might be sufficient to justify a prohibition on cloning human beings at this time, even if such efforts were to be characterized as the exercise of a fundamental right to attempt to procreate.

Beyond the issue of the safety of the procedure, however, NBAC found that concerns relating to the potential psychological harms to children and effects on the moral, religious, and cultural values of society merited further reflection and deliberation. Whether upon such further deliberation our nation will conclude that the use of cloning techniques to create children should be allowed or permanently banned is, for the moment, an open question. Time is an ally in this regard, allowing for the accrual of further data from animal experimentation, enabling an assessment of the prospective safety and efficacy of the procedure in humans, as well as granting a period of fuller national debate on ethical and social concerns. The Commission therefore concluded that there should be imposed a period of time in which no attempt is made to create a child using somatic cell nuclear transfer.[1]

Within this overall framework the Commission came to the following conclusions and recommendations:

I. The Commission concludes that at this time it is morally unacceptable for anyone in the public or private sector, whether in a research or clinical setting, to attempt to create a child using somatic cell nuclear transfer cloning. We have reached a consensus on this point because current scientific information indicates that this technique is not safe to use in humans at this time.

Indeed, we believe it would violate important ethical obligations were clinicians or researchers to attempt to create a child using these particular technologies, which are likely to involve unacceptable risks to the fetus and/ or potential child. Moreover, in addition to safety concerns, many other serious ethical concerns have been identified, which require much more widespread and careful public deliberation before this technology may be used.

The Commission, therefore, recommends the following for immediate action:

*A continuation of the current moratorium on the use of federal funding in support of any attempt to create a child by somatic cell nuclear transfer.

*An immediate request to all firms, clinicians, investigators, and professional societies in the private and non-federally funded sectors to comply voluntarily with the intent of the federal moratorium. Professional and scientific societies should make clear that any attempt to create a child by somatic nuclear transfer and implantation into a woman's body would at this time be an irresponsible, unethical, and unprofessional act.

II. The Commission further recommends that:

*Federal legislation should be enacted to prohibit anyone from attempting, whether in a research or clinical setting, to create a child through somatic cell nuclear cloning. It is critical, however, that such legislation include a sunset clause to ensure that Congress will review the issue after a specified time period (three to five years) in order to decide whether the prohibition continues to be needed. If state legislation is enacted, it should also contain such a sunset provision. Any such legislation or associated regulation also ought to require that at some point prior to the expiration of the sunset period, an appropriate oversight body will evaluate and report on the current status of somatic cell nuclear transfer technology and on the ethical and social issues that its potential use to create human beings would raise in light of public understandings at that time.

III. The Commission also concludes that:

*Any regulatory or legislative actions undertaken to effect the foregoing prohibition on creating a child by somatic cell nuclear transfer should be carefully written so as not to interfere with other important areas of scientific research. In particular, no new regulations are required regarding the cloning of human DNA sequences and cell lines, since neither activity raises the scientific and ethical issues that arise from the attempt to create children through somatic cell nuclear transfer, and these fields of research have already provided important scientific and biomedical advances. Likewise, research on cloning animals by somatic cell nuclear transfer does not raise the issues implicated in attempting to use this technique for human cloning, and its continuation should only be subject to existing regulations regarding the humane use of animals and review by institution-based animal protection committees.

*If a legislative ban is not enacted, or if a legislative ban is ever lifted, clinical use of somatic cell nuclear transfer techniques to create a child should be preceded by research trials that are governed by twin protections of independent review and informed consent, consistent with existing norms of human subjects protection.

*The United States Government should cooperate with other nations and international organizations to enforce any common aspects of their respective policies on the cloning of human beings.

IV. The Commission also concludes that different ethical and religious perspectives and traditions are divided on many of the important moral issues that surround any attempt to create a child using somatic cell nuclear transfer techniques. Therefore, we recommend that:

*The federal government, and all interested and concerned parties, encourage widespread and continuing deliberation on these issues in order to further our understanding of the ethical and social implications of this technology and to enable society to produce appropriate long-term policies regarding this technology should the time come when present concerns about safety have been addressed.

V. Finally, because scientific knowledge is essential for all citizens to participate in a full and informed fashion in the governance of our complex society, the Commission recommends that:

*Federal departments and agencies concerned with science should cooperate in seeking out and supporting opportunities to provide information and education to the public in the areas of genetics, and on other developments in the biomedical sciences, especially where these affect important cultural practices, values, and beliefs.

QUESTIONS FOR CONSIDERATION

1. What are some of the unique ethical issues raised by the Commission regarding the use of somatic cell nuclear transfer to create children?
2. What kind of harms to children did the Commission identify related to human cloning?
3. What were the major recommendations of the Commission?
4. How did the Commission seek to protect other important scientific research?

NOTE

1. The Commission also observes that the use of any other technique to create a child genetically identical to an existing (or previously existing) individual would raise many, if not all, of the same non-safety-related ethical concerns raised by the creation of a child by somatic cell nuclear transfer.

JAMES F. CHILDRESS

The Challenges of Public Ethics: Reflections on NBAC's Report

These reflections build on my participation in the commission, but I do not profess to speak for the commission in my attempt to illuminate its discourse, deliberations, and conclusions about cloning humans. Others inside and outside the commission may have quite different interpretations.

NBAC's report, *Cloning Human Beings*, recommended continuing the moratorium on the use of federal funds for human cloning to create children, continuing the call for a voluntary private moratorium, and passing federal legislation to prohibit somatic cell nuclear transfer to create children. (When I use the phrases "human cloning" or "cloning humans" I am referring to somatic cell nuclear transfer cloning to create children, unless otherwise indicated.) NBAC concluded that "at this time it is morally unacceptable for anyone . . . to attempt to create a child using somatic cell nuclear transfer cloning . . . because current scientific information indicates that this technique is not safe to use in humans at this time."

In light of the available scientific evidence, NBAC reached a *moral* conclusion, based on the ethical obligation not to harm, or impose serious risks of harm on, fetuses and/or potential children. *Safety is a fundamental ethical consideration.* It is not merely a scientific consideration, even though it obviously requires scientific evidence. Any procedure that creates a substantial risk of harm to children is morally problematic.

To be sure, other important ethical issues also arise from the prospect of human cloning, and these require careful, thoughtful, and imaginative reflection over time so that society will be ready to respond appropriately to human cloning if the technique appears to be safe. Hence, NBAC recommended a sunset clause in federal legislation, review by "an appropriate oversight body" prior to the expiration of the sunset period, and "widespread and continuing [public] deliberation"—in short, a national dialogue—on the whole range of ethical and social issues so that society can formulate appropriate long-term policies regarding human cloning if the safety concerns are adequately addressed. And it attempted to identify, at least in a preliminary way, some of these issues and to start to build a framework in which to address them. However, it did not attempt to resolve—nor is it likely that it could have resolved—these other ethical and social issues that emerge once the safety threshold is crossed.

Is Human Cloning Intrinsically Wrong or Does It Depend on the Circumstances?

There is disagreement in this society and possibly also in NBAC about whether any conceivable acts of human cloning could ever be justified if the technique were safe for the children so created. On the one hand, some thinkers, especially but not only in the Roman Catholic tradition, hold that cloning humans is wrong in and of itself (intrinsically wrong), and that it would thus be wrong under any conceivable circumstances. Any use would violate human dignity, the natural law, the natural order, or some other fundamental principle or value, perception of this violation often being expressed, as Leon Kass suggests, in the language of repugnance and revulsion.

On the other hand, many hold that human cloning would be wrong in some, perhaps most, circumstances but not in others that could be imagined. Although there are numerous variations, a number of Protestant and Jewish thinkers, along with many secular thinkers, take this second position and worry about inappropriate uses or abuses of human cloning rather than about every single use. Some who take this second position view human cloning as a morally "neutral" technology, as Rabbi Elliot Dorff does, while others, such as Protestant ethicist Nancy Duff, view it as morally problematic but not intrinsically wrong (both in testimony to NBAC, 13 and 14 March 1997).

Several scenarios are considered: cloning because of problems of infertility; cloning to provide a compatible source of biological material, such as bone marrow, for treatment; cloning a dying child; cloning to prevent genetic diseases. Many who hold that human cloning could be justified under some circumstances would not view all these scenarios as ethically acceptable. In any event, most religious and secular positions that accept some possible cases of human cloning presuppose that the procedure is sufficiently safe for the child created by cloning and that the child's rights and interests will be adequately protected. Otherwise human cloning even for legitimate purposes would be morally unjustifiable.

Those who reject all human cloning as immoral tend to favor a permanent legislative ban. By contrast, those who believe that human cloning could sometimes be ethically justified may argue for a ban (usually temporary), or regulation, or permission, depending on the circumstances. At this time, in view of the great uncertainty about the safety of human cloning, a temporary ban or strict regulation seems plausible to many. Nevertheless, concerns quite properly arise about the range and scope of any ban or regulation as well as about its potential effectiveness.

Practical Reasoning: Principled or Casuistical or Both?

After NBAC's deliberations, one commissioner suggested to me that we had not appealed to principles at all in our reasoning and wondered whether I wanted to reconsider my defense of a principle-based approach. I responded that NBAC's concern for safety reflects the principle of nonmaleficence and that NBAC at this time could not identify benefits of human cloning that outweigh the risks to children (a consideration of beneficence) or claims of autonomy in reproduction or in scientific inquiry strong enough to outweigh the risks to children. In addition, concerns about respect for persons, including their dignity as well as their autonomy, surfaced in discussions about objectifying and commodifying children.

I would argue that these principles, and others, were transparent in NBAC's deliberations. To suppose that they are irrelevant when they are not explicitly and directly invoked in jargonistic formulations misses the richness of our ordinary moral language and discourse. At the very least, the commission's consensus reflects its views about the respective weights of three prominent moral principles—nonmaleficence, beneficence, and respect for autonomy—in the context of recommending public policies regarding human cloning. Furthermore, the commission focused not only on the weights of these and other principles but also on how they might be specified—for example, in debates about whether reproductive or procreative rights are expressions of autonomy rights and whether they might include a right to self-replication.

Much of our discourse also moved casuistically, as we looked for settled cases that could provide helpful analogies. For instance, we referred to what was more or less settled in the 1994 federal policy regarding embryo splitting, and to what is currently accepted in various reproductive and genetic technologies. These two approaches—principled and casuistical—are, in my judgment, quite compatible with and even essential to each other in deliberations about public policy.

Moral Reasoning About Public Policy in a Particular Political Context

It was not always easy to determine and keep in clear view our primary target, which I would identify as recommending and justifying a prohibitive, a restrictive, or a permissive public policy with regard to somatic cell nuclear transfer cloning to create a child. In doing public ethics, it is also necessary to explicate the premises and presumptions of moral discourse in a particular society. Commissioners need to ask which acts and policies are justifiable within the society's moral framework, not merely which they themselves view as morally justifiable. For several commissioners, the premises and presumptions of a liberal democratic society placed the burden of proof on those who argued for restrictive or prohibitive legislation directed against human cloning. For them, that burden of proof was met by the safety argument.

Consensus on the safety argument meant, however, that NBAC did not have to try to resolve the larger debate about the probable impact of acts and especially of widespread practices of human cloning on social values that are not reducible to harms or wrongs to individuals. One major concern is the potential impact of human cloning on the family, especially if it were to become a widespread practice rather than an occasional act. Among the risks, which some commissioners considered speculative, are threats to fundamental responsibilities within the family, including intergenerational relationships.

Religious Perspectives on Human Cloning

When President Clinton asked NBAC to consider the cloning of human beings, he commented that "any discovery that touches upon human creation is not simply a matter of scientific inquiry, it is a matter of morality and spirituality as well." Shortly thereafter, the commission set up two days of hearings, with particular attention to scientific, ethical, and religious perspectives.

Some were surprised that NBAC solicited religious perspectives along with the expected philosophical perspectives. However, attention to religious perspectives is not unprecedented in debates about public policies for new technologies—for instance, the President's Commission for the Study of Ethical Problems in Biomedical and Behavioral Research included religious perspectives when it examined genetic engineering. While recognizing that public policy in the United States cannot be based on considerations that are purely religious in nature, NBAC believed that it was important to examine religious as well as philosophical perspectives on human cloning for several reasons.

First, religious communities, several with ancient roots and long traditions of moral reflection, significantly shape the moral positions taken by many U.S. citizens on new technological developments. Hence, it is important to understand how these communities view human cloning, including how they argue for their positions as well as the conclusions they reach. NBAC wanted to hear and read various religious and philosophical arguments in their own integrity. Though some questions pressed for translation into a more secular idiom, NBAC was interested in the arguments that religious communities actually use to guide their own adherents as well as to guide public policy.

Second, religious traditions often present moral arguments that rest on premises that are not merely or exclusively religious in nature. For instance, they may invoke categories such as "nature" or "basic human values" or "family values" that are not reducible to particular faith commitments and that are accessible to citizens of different or no faith commitments.

Third, NBAC sought to determine the extent to which religious traditions—and secular traditions—overlap on moral positions on human cloning to create children. It wanted to learn whether these diverse traditions have reached a moral consensus on human cloning—and, if so, the nature of that consensus.

Fourth, NBAC sought to engender and sustain in its own meetings and in its report serious national moral discourse about human cloning and about public policies regarding human cloning. Hence, it listened to and attempted to understand as fully as possible various religious and philosophical positions.

Fifth, many different factors determine whether particular public policies are feasible and effective and whether their social benefits outweigh their social costs. One such factor is the nature, extent, and depth of opposition to those policies by various religious and secular communities. It was thus important to NBAC to identify the basic concerns both religious and secular communities have about human cloning.

For all these reasons NBAC invited testimony from several religious thinkers, with particular attention to Jewish, Protestant, Roman Catholic, and Islamic perspectives; it contracted with Professor Courtney Campbell of Oregon State University for a paper on these and other religious perspectives, including, for example, Eastern Orthodox, Buddhist, Hindu, and Native American perspectives; and public testimony often reflected religious perspectives. As a follow-up to NBAC's report, Senator Bill Frist (Rep., Tenn.) organized a hearing before the U.S. Senate Labor and Human Resources Subcommittee on Public Health and Safety titled "Ethics and Theology: A Continuation of the National Discussion on Human Cloning."

Sociologist James Hunter has observed that conservatives in a particular religious tradition may share more with conservatives in other religious traditions than with liberals in their own tradition; the same point covers liberals too. However, it is striking that this pattern does not uniformly hold for human cloning. Conservative Rabbi Byron Sherwin has observed that, in general, on the basis of their legal tradition, orthodox and conservative Jewish thinkers find it difficult to condemn human cloning per se, and that much opposition to human cloning, particularly in Reform Judaism, reflects categories outside Jewish law, such as human dignity.

On one point a strong consensus, perhaps even unanimity, exists among Jewish, Roman Catholic, and Protestant thinkers: A child created through somatic cell nuclear transfer cloning would still be created in the image of God. It is important to make this point because so many commentators on religious perspectives miss or neglect it. Even when religious thinkers maintain that cloning would always or at least sometimes violate the dignity of the child created this way, they also contend that it would not diminish that child's dignity (Pope John Center testimony to NBAC, 13 March 1997). In different language, Rabbi Elliot Dorff (also in testimony to NBAC, 14 March 1997) stressed that cloning would create "a new person, an integrated body and mind, with unique experiences," however difficult it may be for such persons to "establish their own identity and for their creators to acknowledge and respect it."

Religious and secular thinkers alike insist that it is morally obligatory not to inflict serious harm on children created through human cloning. One such harm is physical. Cloning would be wrong at least for now because cloners could not be sure that they would not be doing unacceptable harm to children. This is also the position NBAC took, based on broad societal moral norms, in holding that safety is a fundamental ethical issue, and that, at least for the time being, human cloning to create a child should not be undertaken and should even be prohibited through legislation. Such prohibitive legislation would provide a window of opportunity for society to determine whether safe human cloning would have unacceptable moral costs and should be severely restricted or even banned.

QUESTIONS FOR CONSIDERATION

1. What is the ethical issue of safety that Childress raises?

2. What is the contrast that Childress draws between cloning as intrinsically wrong and wrong under certain circumstances?

3. Childress indicated that the Commission deliberated on three important moral principles and also deliberated casuistically regarding human cloning. What are the three moral principles and what is the difference between an appeal to principle and casuistry?

4. What did Childress identify as the primary target of the Commission? Why was it difficult to keep a clear view of this target in a liberal democratic society?

5. Why did Childress believe it was important for the Commission to hear religious as well as philosophical perspectives on human cloning?

Susan M. Wolf

Ban Cloning? Why NBAC Is Wrong

In its report on cloning, NBAC recommended a ban of unprecedented scope.[1] Based on commission consensus that human cloning would currently be unsafe, NBAC called for congressional prohibition throughout the public and private sectors of all somatic cell nuclear transfer with the intent of creating a child. President Clinton promptly responded by proposing legislation to enact such a ban for five years.

NBAC was wrong to urge a ban. Cloning undoubtedly warrants regulation. But the ban proposed will not yield the sort of regulation required. Instead, it will reduce cloning to a political football in Congress, raise serious constitutional problems, and chill important research. NBAC defends its ban as a limited one, prohibiting somatic cell nuclear transfer (not all forms of cloning), when used to create a child (not in research), and for three to five years (not indefinitely). A congressional ban, however, is likely to be far broader.

NBAC erred by taking cloning out of context. Like any technology, cloning needs to be safe before used. But that counsels regulation, not a ban, which merely slows development of safe procedures. And cloning demands we deal with issues beyond safety on which NBAC achieved no consensus, issues bound up in the ethics of human experimentation and reproductive technologies.

A better approach would extend human subjects protection into the private sphere and regulate reproductive technologies effectively, with a central advisory body for novel issues such as cloning. By failing to tackle private research and reproductive technologies, NBAC avoided the real job and instead proposed an isolated and misguided response to cloning.

The Regulatory Challenge

Human cloning clearly requires regulation. Indeed, some regulation already applies. President Clinton has barred all federal funds for cloning, covering both research and clinical application.[2] Earlier prohibitions on the use of federal money to create human embryos for research purposes would also impede cloning research with federal funds.[3] And federal regulations protecting human subjects would seem to block cloning in research covered by those regulations because cloning remains unsafe, at least for now.[4] This leaves two regulatory gaps that properly troubled NBAC: private sector research outside federal oversight and private clinical activity, especially infertility programs using reproductive technologies.

But by responding to these worries with a congressional ban, NBAC missed the target. Protecting human subjects in private research and regulating reproductive technologies are both long overdue. A ban on cloning just suppresses one technology, while these two systemic problems guarantee the development of other technologies in need of regulation. Some would argue that somatic cell cloning deserves to be singled out as the most threatening possibility. But that assumes a conclusion we have not had time to reach, that Dolly-style cloning raises radically more difficult problems than, for example, cloning by embryo splitting (which can also lead to a delayed twin, with cryopreservation).[5]

NBAC admits that protecting human subjects in private research offers advantages over a ban on cloning (pp. 99-100). Yet the commission balks. It first complains that extending human subjects protections requires legislation and thus delay. But Senator John Glenn (Dem., Ohio) has already proposed legislation,[6] and enacting a congressional ban involves delay as well. The commission further complains that human subjects legislation would rely on decentralized institutional review boards (IRBs). But others have suggested creating a national IRB for novel questions,[7] and NBAC ought to be considering this among other improvements in human subjects protection anyway. Moreover, IRBs are actually part of a larger mechanism providing centralized federal agency review when needed. The commission's final objection is that human subjects legislation would not reach beyond research activity to clinical use, as in infertility clinics. But this merely counsels supplemental regulation of those clinics.

NBAC's report, in fact, suffers from minimal consideration of infertility programs and reproductive technologies.[8] The commission acknowledges that the federal statute requiring fertility clinic reporting would seem to require reporting of cloning (p. 88).[9] But it ignores the broader issues plaguing reproductive technologies: the inadequacy of federal and state regulation, state-to-state inconsistencies, and conflicts of interest inherent in industry self-regulation. The report overlooks the burgeoning literature on those problems and, indeed, reflects little input from infertility programs.[10]

Instead of developing a legal response to cloning that addresses the core problems of private research and underregulated reproductive technologies,

NBAC simply called for a ban of cloning itself. That skirts the central problems, while adding new ones.

The Error in a Ban

No other bioethics controversy has been addressed by a ban as broad as the one NBAC advocates and the president now proposes. Its prohibition reaches all public and private institutions, whether or not federal money is involved or FDA approval is required. Limits on the use of federal money are common, but federal prohibitions on medical and scientific work in the private sector are not.

Moreover, the ban threatens substantial damage. The president's bill prohibits "somatic cell nuclear transfer with the intent of introducing the product of that transfer into a woman's womb or in any other way creating a human being," and would impose significant fines. Though NBAC insists it does not want to tamper with research in the private sphere, merely baby-making, this ban cannot avoid the former. The policing necessary to enforce the ban will require intruding into labs and monitoring the "intent" of scientists. Research will thus be chilled. It will be chilled further by the vagueness of a prohibition that is meant to ban baby-making, but seems to reach intent to "transfer," even if a researcher knows no child will result, plus the intent to create a human being in any unspecified "other way."

Beyond the ban's breadth and potential damage, NBAC and the president have placed this weapon in the wrong hands. The ban is to be imposed by Congress itself, not a regulatory body poised to respond to developments in the technology. That turns cloning into a political football. Past congressional brawls over the related areas of embryo research and abortion predict the same for cloning. This means that although the president and NBAC would ban private-sector application not research, Congress is likely to ban research too, as one of the pending federal bills seems to propose.[11] And though the president and commission would ban only somatic cell nuclear transfer, Congress may well include other technologies such as embryo splitting (which, after all, is another form of cloning and may also produce a delayed twin). Two of the three federal bills pending appear to do exactly that.[12] But embryo splitting may allow a woman undergoing in vitro fertilization to avoid repeated exposure to drugs inducing superovulation, which may reduce her risk of ovarian cancer later in life. Finally, though NBAC and the president would limit the ban to five years, there is little reason to expect Congress to develop the political bravery to lift the ban at that point.

The ban proposed thus raises serious constitutional questions. The ban's prohibition of somatic cell nuclear transfer with the wrong intent and its unavoidable chilling effect on research may infringe freedom of scientific inquiry in violation of the First Amendment.[13] And the ban as proposed by the president may well be unconstitutionally vague in its statement of the prohibited intent.[14] The ban may also represent an unconstitutional infringement on the procreative liberty of infertile couples.[15] In any case, it may exceed the limits of federal power, especially since the regulation of health and clinical practice has traditionally fallen to the states.[16]

Beyond the constitutional questions, a ban at this point is bad policy. NBAC's advocacy of this ban contradicts its call for careful study and debate in our pluralistic society. With only ninety days to report on cloning, NBAC admits more analysis is needed. Yet by calling now for a ban that is likely to sweep more broadly and last much longer than NBAC wants, the commission has in effect already yielded to those who claim cloning is wrong in all cases and for the indefinite future. This ends the important deliberation, embraces one absolutist moral perspective, and writes it into law.[17]

NBAC defends the ban as a safety measure preventing harm to potential children. But that reasoning does not justify this result. Indeed, the ban may well cause harm. A ban that inevitably chills research will prevent the development of a cloning technology that is physically safe for the children it produces. Some may protest that even physically safe cloning may threaten psychological harms. But that claim is purely speculative and can ground regulation and research, but not a ban; cloning may in fact save children from psychological difficulties involved in having an anonymous genetic parent through donor egg or sperm.

Moreover, a ban may cause harm to infertile couples, especially if it hardens into an indefinite prohibition. After all, cloning offers potential benefit in infertility cases. NBAC points to a couple each carrying a recessive gene for a serious disorder. Cloning would allow them to avoid conceiving an embryo with the disorder and facing selective abortion. In another case, a woman might carry a dominant gene for a disorder. Cloning would permit her to avoid genetic contribution from an egg donor and thus would keep the genetic parenting between the woman and her partner, something of value to many couples. Other cases would include a couple entirely lacking gametes.

All of these potential uses for cloning are controversial and might ultimately be rejected. But for NBAC to ban cloning because it currently is unsafe, with no agreement on the future benefits and harms if it becomes safe, is ill-advised. Stalling development of reproductive technologies may trap us in halfway measures, such as donors' genetic involvement, that may cause more harm than cloning.

A federal ban on cloning thus misses the big picture. Cloning is only one of many reproductive technologies that should be safe before application, be it intracytoplasmic sperm injection, cytoplasm transfer, or beyond. The task is to devise a regulatory approach that addresses safety while permitting research and progress in a sphere of immense importance to couples. Cloning should spur us to that delicate balancing act. Simply lowering the boom on cloning does the opposite.

A Better Model

There is a better way. Certainly we need improved regulation of assisted reproduction and human subjects experimentation in the private sphere.[18] But we have to combine that regulation with an advisory body providing oversight for cloning and other novel reproductive and genetic technologies.

The commission, president, and Congress should consider a model we have used before: agency regulation guided by an advisory body able to respond to improvements in the technology over time and more removed than Congress from partisan politics. Though NBAC's report compared policy options, strangely this was not among them.[19]

The Recombinant DNA Advisory Committee (RAC) is one example of such a body. RAC was formed over twenty years ago as an NIH advisory panel. When concern later erupted over human gene therapy, RAC (with its Working Group on Human Gene Therapy) showed how an advisory committee can hold the line, by refusing to consider germ-line gene therapy protocols for approval. It used not a legislative ban, but the committee's declared moratorium, continually subject to debate and reconsideration.

RAC's very accomplishments have fed criticism. As some forms of gene therapy became better understood (in part thanks to RAC), the committee's review began to seem an obstacle to scientific progress. The director of NIH restructured RAC earlier this year.[20] Now a smaller RAC will advise on ethical issues, surrendering authority to approve protocols to the FDA. Though RAC's authority has been reduced, this is a success story. A mechanism appropriate at the introduction of a controversial technology may require revamping later. What we use now to govern cloning must have the flexibility to evolve.

RAC is merely one example. And it is narrower than what we need for cloning: RAC's jurisdiction has been confined to protocols requiring NIH approval. On cloning, as I have argued, we need to extend human subjects protections to private research and regulate reproductive technologies, with an advisory body for novel issues such as cloning.[21]

Certainly the details of the model can be debated. Indeed, rather than create a new advisory body, using a reinvigorated RAC, another preexisting entity, or NBAC itself (if its mission were restructured) might be considered. And some may argue we need two bodies, one for human subjects and the other for reproductive technologies. But surrendering cloning to a congressional ban, as NBAC suggests, attempts a delicate operation with far too blunt an instrument. It is slim consolation that under the president's proposal, NBAC will be continuing discussion on the sidelines.

NBAC might respond that it favored a limited ban to head off worse proposals in Congress. But a national bioethics commission should call for what is right, not merely what is expedient. Congressional bills in the panicked days after the announcement of Dolly should not drive the national bioethics agenda.

A congressional ban may seem simple and safe. Yet the issues posed by cloning are not simple. We have to balance the promise of research and the potential benefits against the need for regulation and caution. We have to do better than NBAC's ban.

Acknowledgments

My thanks to George Annas, Arthur Caplan, Jim Childress, Alan Fleischman, Jeffrey Kahn, and John Robertson for advice at various stages, including on my related op-ed, "Why the Bioethics Commission is Wrong to Seek a Ban on Cloning," [Minneapolis] *Star Tribune*, 19 June 1997. They bear no responsibility for these views. Ryan Johnson of the University of Minnesota Law School provided able research assistance. Portions of this article are based on the earlier op-ed.

QUESTIONS FOR CONSIDERATION

1. What are two regulatory gaps that Wolf identifies that should be regulated along with cloning?
2. Why does Wolf argue that a ban on human cloning will result in a chill on important scientific research?
3. How would the ban turn cloning into a political football?

4. What are the serious constitutional questions that Wolf raises regarding the ban on human cloning?

5. How does Wolf respond to the charge that the ban prevents harm to children?

6. How does Wolf consider the Recombinant DNA Advisory Committee as model for regulating human cloning?

NOTES

1. National Bioethics Advisory Commission, *Cloning Human Beings: Report and Recommendations of the National Bioethics Advisory Commission* (Rockville, Md., June 1997).

2. The White House, Office of Communications, Directive on Cloning, 4 March 1997, 1997 *Westlaw* 91957 (White House).

3. See "Statement by the President on NIH Recommendation Regarding Human Embryo Research," *U.S. Newswire* (2 December 1994); Omnibus Consolidated Appropriations Act, 1997, Pub. L. No. 104-208, 512, 110 Stat. 3009, 831.

4. 45 C.ER. Part 46 (1996). These regulations cover only research that is federally funded, at institutions offering assurances that all research will be subject to the regulations, or on drugs and devices needing FDA approval.

5. NBAC's report leaves unclear the proper policy approach to embryo splitting. Chairman Shapiro's transmittal letter states, "We do not revisit . . . cloning . . . by embryo splitting." However, a report footnote ambiguously "observes that . . . any other technique to create a child genetically identical to an existing . . . individual would raise many, if not all, of the same non-safety-related ethical concerns raised by . . . somatic cell nuclear transfer" (p. iii, n. 1). One would think that "any other technique" could include embryo splitting with cryopreservation to produce a delayed genetic twin. However, the report claims that the capacity to produce a delayed genetic twin is a prospect "unique" to Dolly-style cloning, i.e., somatic cell nuclear transfer (pp. 3, 64). This leaves NBAC's approach to embryo splitting in confusion.

6. S. 193, 105th Cong. (1997).

7. See Carol Levine and Arthur L. Caplan, "Beyond Localism: A Proposal for a National Research Review Board," *IRB* 8, no. 2 (1986): 7–9; Alexander Morgan Capron, "An Egg Takes Flight: The Once and Future Life of the National Bioethics Advisory Commission," *Kennedy Institute of Ethics Journal* 7 (1997): 63–80, at 69.

8. NBAC might respond that its mandated areas of study are human subjects research and genetic information, not reproductive technologies. But one cannot do justice to cloning without considering its most likely use in treating infertility. And a national commission should bring to cloning the necessary bioethics analysis, not just bureaucratically designated topic areas.

9. See 42 U.S.C.A. 263a-1 et seq.

10. NBAC asserts, for example, that most reproductive technologies aside from in vitro techniques for fertilization involve no micromanipulation as substantial as somatic cell nuclear transfer (p. 32), without even analyzing techniques such as assisted hatching and cytoplasm transfer. The report also makes the startling suggestion that childlessness condemns one to immaturity: "Without reproduction one remains a child . . . With reproduction . . . one becomes a parent, taking on responsibilities for another that necessarily require abandoning some of the personal freedoms enjoyed before" (p. 77). An infertile adult does not automatically remain a "child" and may take on numerous responsibilities requiring self-sacrifice. Surely, these remarks would not have survived serious engagement with clinicians in infertility programs. NBAC's witness list includes none. Cf. Gina Kolata, "Ethics Panel Recommends a Ban on Human Cloning," *New York Times*, 8 June 1997, at 22 (quoting an NBAC member remarking that no IVF physicians addressed the commission).

11. See H.B. 923: "It shall be unlawful. to use a human somatic cell for the process of producing a human clone." This seems to prohibit making even an embryo clone for research.

12. See H.B. 922, S. 368.

13. See generally Ira H. Carmen, *Cloning and the Constitution: An Inquiry into Governmental Policymaking and Genetic Experimentation* (Madison: University of Wisconsin Press, 1985); Richard Delgado and David R. Millen, "God, Galileo, and Government: Toward Constitutional Protection for Scientific Inquiry," *Washington Law Review* 53 (1978): 349–404.

14. Cf Lifchez v. Harrigan, 735 E Supp. 1381 (N.D. 111*.), aff'd without opinion*, 914 F.2d 260 (7th Cir. 1990), *cert. denied sub nom.* Scholberg v. Lifchez, 498 U.S. 1069 (1991) (striking down a statute on fetal experimentation as unconstitutionally vague).

15. The shape of this argument is suggested by John A. Robertson in *Children of Choice: Freedom and the New Reproductive Technologies* (Princeton: Princeton University Press, 1994), though he questions whether cloning is so different from other forms of reproduction as to fall outside of constitutional protection for procreative liberty (pp. 169–70). On constitutional protection for reproductive technologies, see also *Lifchez*, above.

16. For the limits of federal power based on the Constitution's commerce clause, see, for example, U.S. v. Lopez, 514 U.S. 549 (1995).

17. See also Alexander Morgan Capron, "Inside the Beltway Again: A Sheep of a Different Feather," *Kennedy Institute of Ethics Journal* 7 (1997): 171–79, at 176 ("[I]t would be a mistake to say everything we believe would be wrong to do should be a wrong to do. This is particularly true of cloning.").

18. See also George J. Annas, "Regulatory Models for Human Embryo Cloning: The Free Market, Professional Guidelines, and Government Restrictions," *Kennedy Institute of Ethics Journal* 4 (1994): 235–49, 245–46

19. NBAC did mention RAC (p. 97), but in its discussion of voluntary moratoria (and even though RAC's moratorium on germ-line gene therapy proposals has been binding on researchers seeking federal funds, not voluntary).

20. National Institutes of Health, "Notice of Action under the NIH Guidelines for Research Involving DNA Molecules," 62 Fed. Reg. 4782 (31 January 1997).

21. Unlike a ban on cloning, my suggested approach is likely to survive constitutional scrutiny. Research is routinely disseminated interstate with substantial commercial effects. And the terrible history of research scandals would seem to justify extending protection to subjects in private research as a matter of civil and human rights. Moreover, there is little reason to suspect infringement on researchers' freedom of inquiry from application of our current protective framework. Augmenting regulation of reproductive technologies, if carefully done to respect the constitutional need for a compelling justification to restrict access to procreative technologies, would seem defensible given extensive interstate commerce in reproductive services.

Contributors

Anderson, W. French is director of Gene Therapy Laboratories and is professor of biochemistry and pediatrics at the University of California School of Medicine in Los Angles, California.

Andrews, Lori B. is professor of law at Chicago-Kent College of Law and is senior scholar at the Center for Clinical Medical Ethics at the University of Chicago in Chicago. Illinois.

Blustein, Jeffrey is associate professor of philosophy at Mercy College in Dobbs Ferry, New York, and is a bioethics consultant at the Weiler Division of Montefiore Medical Center in Bronx, New York.

Bonnicksen, Andrea is professor of political science at Northern Illinois University in DeKalb, Illinois.

Boone, C. Keith is associate dean of the College of Arts and Sciences at Denison University in Granville, Ohio.

Brock, Dan W. is director of the Center for Biomedical Ethics and professor of philosophy at Brown University in Providence, Rhode Island.

Brody, Baruch is Leon Jaworski professor of Biomedical Ethics and director of the Center for Ethics, Medicine, and Public Issues at Baylor College of Medicine.

Callahan, Daniel is co-founder and former president of the Hastings Center. He is currently the director of International Programs at the Hastings Center.

Callahan, Sidney is professor of psychology at Mercy College in Dobbs Ferry, New York.

Caplan, Arthur L. is director of the Center for Bioethics at the University of Pennsylvania in Philadelphia, Pennsylvania.

Capron, Alexander Morgan is Henry W. Bruce University Professor of Law and Medicine at the University of Southern California and director of the Pacific Center for Health Policy and Ethics in Los Angeles, California.

Childress, James F. is Kyle Professor of Religious Studies and professor medical education at the University of Virginia in Charlottesville, Virginia.

Cohen, Cynthia B. is a senior research fellow at the Kennedy Institute of Ethics at Georgetown University, Washington, D.C., and an adjunct associate at The Hastings Center.

Daniels, Norman teaches ethics and political philosophy at Tufts University in Medford, Massachusetts.

Doerflinger, Richard is associate director for policy development of the Office for Pro-Life Activities of the National Conference of Catholic Bishops in Washington, D.C.

Draper, Elaine is associate professor of sociology at the University of Southern California in Los Angeles, California.

Elliott, Carl is research fellow, faculty of medicine at the University of Natal, Durban, South Africa.

Hardwig, John is associate professor of medical ethics at the James H. Quillen College of Medicine at East Tennesee State University in Johnson City, Tennessee.

Kluge, Eike-Henner W. is director of the Division of Ethics and Legal Affairs for the Canadian Medical Association in Ottawa, Ontario, Canada.

Langerak, Edward A. is professor philosophy at Saint Olaf College in Northfield, Minnesota.

Lynn, Joanne is senior associate in the Center for Evaluative Clinical Sciences and professor of medicine at Dartmouth Medical School in Hanover, New Hampshire.

Macklin, Ruth is professor of bioethics at Albert Einstein College of Medicine in Bronx, New York, and an adjunct associate of The Hastings Center.

Mahowald, Mary B. is assistant director of the Center for Clinical Medical Ethics at the University of Chicago in Chicago, Illinois.

Mann, Jonathan M. directs the Francois-Xavier Bagnoud Center for Health and Human Rights, Harvard University in Boston, Massachusetts.

Marusyk, Randy W. is an attorney practicing biotechnology law in Ottawa, Ontario, Canada.

Menzel, Paul T. is professor of philosophy at Pacific Lutheran University in Tacoma, Washington.

Meilaender, Gilbert is professor of religion at Oberlin College in Oberlin, Ohio.

Nolan, Kathleen is an adjunct associate of The Hastings Center.

Ozar, David T. is associate professor of philosophy, director of the Center for Ethics Across the Curriculum, and codirector of the masters program in health care ethics at Loyola University of Chicago in Chicago, Illinois.

Parens, Erik is associate for philosophical studies at The Hastings Center.

Rachels, James is professor of philosophy at the University of Alabama in Birmingham, Alabama.

Raymond, Janice G. is professor of women's studies and medical ethics at the University of Massachusetts in Amherst, Massachusetts.

Robertson, John A. is professor of law at the University of Texas School of Law in Austin, Texas.

Rothman, Barbara Katz is professor of sociology at Baruch College and the Graduate Center of the City University of New York in New York, New York.

Sabin, James E. is codirector of the Center for Ethics in Managed Care at Harvard Pilgrim Health Care and Harvard Medical School and associate clinical professor of psychiatry at Harvard Medical School in Boston, Massachusetts.

Scofield, Giles R. is associate professor of law at the Pace University law School in White Plains, New York.

Swain, Margaret S. is an attorney practicing biotechnology law in Ottawa, Ontario, Canada.

Truog, Robert D. is associate professor of anaesthesia and pediatrics at Harvard Medical School and also directs the Multidisciplinary Intensive Care Unit at Children's Hospital in Boston, Massachusetts.

Wolf, Susan M. teaches bioethics and health law at the University of Minnesota, where she is associate professor of law and medicine in the law school and a faculty member at the Center for Bioethics.

Articles from the
Hastings Center Report

Can Ethics Provide Answers?

James Rachels, "Can Ethics Provide Answers?" June 1980, pp. 33–39.
Sidney Callahan, "The Role of Emotions in Ethical Decisionmaking," June–July 1988, pp. 9–14.
Carl Elliott, "Where Ethics Comes From," July 1992, pp. 28–35.

The Goals and Allocation of Medicine

A Hastings Center Project Report, "Setting New Priorities," November–December 1996, pp. S2–S3.
A Hastings Center Project Report, "Specifying the Goals of Medicine," November–December 1996, pp. S9–S14.
Jonathan M. Mann, "Medicine and Public Health, Ethics and Human Rights," May–June 1997, pp. 6–13.
Norman Daniels and James E. Sabin, "Last Chance Therapies and Managed Care," March–April 1998, pp. 27–41.
Paul T. Menzel, "Rescuing Lives: Can't We Count?" January 1994, pp. 22–23.
Baruch Brody, "Public Goods and Fair Prices: Balancing Technological Innovation with Social Well Being," March 1996, pp. 5–11.

Biomedicine, Rights, and Responsibilities

Alexander Morgan Capron, "The Burden of Decision," May–June 1990, pp. 36–41.
John Hardwig, "What About the Family?" March–April 1990, pp. 5–10.
Jeffrey Blustein, "The Family in Medical Decisionmaking," May–June 1993, pp. 6–13.

Reproductive Freedom and Responsibility

Gilbert Meilaender, "Abortion: The Right to an Argument," November–December 1989, pp. 13–16.

Mary B. Mahowald, "Is There Life After *Roe v. Wade?*" July–August 1989, pp. 22–29.
Edward Langerak, "Abortion: Listing to the Middle," October 1979, pp. 24–28.

Termination of Treatment

John Hardwig, "Is There a Duty to Die?" March–April 1997, pp. 34–42.
Daniel Callahan, "Terminating Treatment: Age as a Standard," October–November 1987, pp. 21–25.
Robert D. Truog, "Triage in the ICU," May–June 1992, pp. 13–17.
Giles R. Scofield, "Is Consent Useful When Resuscitation Isn't?" November–December 1991, pp. 28–36.
Kathleen Nolan, "In Death's Shadow: The Meanings of Withholding Resuscitation?" November 1987, pp. 9–14.
Joanne Lynn and James F. Childress, "Must Patients Always Be Given Food and Water?" October 1983, pp. 17–21.
Arthur L. Caplan and Cynthia B. Cohen, eds., Imperiled Newborns. 3. Standards of Judgement for Treatment," December 1987, pp. 13–16.
Arthur L. Caplan and Cynthia B. Cohen, eds. Imperiled Newborns. 5. Deciding Not to Employ Aggressive measures," December 1987, pp. 22–25.
Alexander Morgan Capron, "Anencephalic Donors: Separating the Dead from the Dying," February 1987, pp. 5–8.
Richard Doerflinger, "Assisted Suicide: Pro-Choice or Anti-Life?" January–February 1988, pp. 16–19.
Dan W. Brock, "Voluntary Active Euthanasia," March–April 1992, pp. 10–22.
Daniel Callahan, "When Self-Determination Runs Amok," March–April 1992, pp. 52–55.

Family, Parenthood, and New Reproductive Technologies

Ruth Macklin, "Artificial Means of Reproduction and Our Understanding of the Family," January–February 1991, pp. 5–11.
Janice G. Raymond, "Reproductive Gifts and Gift Giving: The Altruistic Woman," November–December 1990, pp. 7–11.
Andrea Bonnicksen,"Genetic Diagnosis of Human Embryos," July–August 1992, pp. S5–S11.
Barbara Katz Rothman, "Not All that Glitters Is Gold," July–August 1992, pp. S11–S15.
John A. Robertson, "Resolving Disputes Over Frozen Embryos," November–December 1989, pp. 7–12.
David T. Ozar, "The Case Against Thawing Unused Frozen Embryos," August 1985, pp. 2–7.

Organ Procurement and Transplantation

Lori B. Andrews, "My Body, My Property," October 1989, pp. 28–38.

Margaret S. Swain and Randy W. Marusyk, "An Alternative to Property Rights in Human Tissue," September–October 1990, pp. 12–15.

Arthur L. Caplan, "Organ Procurement: It's Not in the Cards," October 1984, pp. 9–12.

Eike-Henner W. Kluge, "Designated Organ Donation: Private Choice in a social Context," September–October 1989, pp. 10–16.

Genetics, Human Nature, Human Destiny

Kathleen Nolan, "First Fruits: Genetic Screening," July–August, 1992, pp. S2–S4.

Elaine Draper, "Genetic Secrets: Social Issues of Medical Screening in a Genetic Age," July–August, 1992, pp. S15–S18.

C. Keith Boone, "Bad Axioms in Genetic Engineering," August–September 1988, pp. 9–13.

W. French Anderson, "Genetics and Human Malleability," January–February 1990, pp. 21–24.

Erik Parens, "Taking Behavioral Genetics Seriously," July–August 1996, pp. 13–18.

Cloning Human Beings

"Executive Summary," September–October 1997, pp. 7–9.

James Childress, "The Challenges of Public Ethics: Reflections on NBAC's Report," September–October 1997, pp. 9–11.

Susan M. Wolf, "Ban Cloning? Why NBAC Is Wrong," September–October 1997, pp. 12–15.